Interventional and Therapeutic Gastrointestinal Endoscopy

Frontiers of Gastrointestinal Research

Vol. 27

Series Editor

Markus M. Lerch Greifswald

Interventional and Therapeutic Gastrointestinal Endoscopy

Volume Editors

Klaus Mönkemüller Bottrop, Germany
C. Mel Wilcox Birmingham, Ala., USA
Miguel Muñoz-Navas Pamplona, Spain

386 figures, 270 in color, and 88 tables, 2010

KARGER Basel · Freiburg · Paris · London · New York · Bangalore · Bangkok · Shanghai · Singapore · Tokyo · Sydney

Frontiers of Gastrointestinal Research
Founded 1975 by L. van der Reis, San Francisco, Calif.

Klaus Mönkemüller
Chief, Department of Internal
Medicine and Gastroenterology
Marienhospital, Bottrop
Josef-Albers-Str. 70
DE-46236 Bottrop

C. Mel Wilcox
Division of Gastroenterology and
Hepatology
University of Alabama at
Birmingham
703 19th Street, South ZRB 633
Birmingham, AL 35294–0007

Miguel Muñoz-Navas
Director del Servicio de Digestivo
Clínica Universitaria de Navarra
Avda. Pío XII, 36
ES-31008 Pamplona

Library of Congress Cataloging-in-Publication Data

Interventional and therapeutic gastrointestinal endoscopy / volume editors,
Klaus Mönkemüller, C. Mel Wilcox, Miguel Muñoz-Navas.
p. ; cm. -- (Frontiers of gastrointestinal research, ISSN 0302-0665
; vol. 27)
Includes bibliographical references and indexes.
ISBN 978-3-8055-9308-3 (hardcover : alk. paper)
1. Gastrointestinal system--Endoscopic surgery. 2. Gastroscopy. I.
Mönkemüller, Klaus. II. Wilcox, C. Mel. III. Muñoz-Navas, Miguel. IV.
Series: Frontiers of gastrointestinal research, vol. 27. 0302-0665 ;
[DNLM: 1. Gastrointestinal Diseases--surgery. 2. Endoscopy,
Gastrointestinal--methods. W1 FR946E v.27 2010 / WI 140 I615 2010]
RD540.I587 2010
617.4'30597--dc22
2009037556

Bibliographic Indices. This publication is listed in bibliographic services, including Current Contents®.

Drug Dosage. The authors and the publisher have exerted every effort to ensure that drug selection and dosage set forth in this text are in accord with current recommendations and practice at the time of publication. However, in view of ongoing research, changes in government regulations, and the constant flow of information relating to drug therapy and drug reactions, the reader is urged to check the package insert for each drug for any change in indications and dosage and for added warnings and precautions. This is particularly important when the recommended agent is a new and/or infrequently employed drug.

www.karger.com
Printed in Switzerland on acid-free and non-aging paper (ISO 9706) by Reinhardt Druck, Basel
ISSN 0302–0665
ISBN 978–3–8055–9308–3
e-ISBN 978–3–8055–9309–0

Contents

Introduction

The introduction of the fiberoptic gastroscope by our teacher, friend and chief Basil Hirschowitz 50 years ago dramatically changed the practice of gastroenterology and that of many other medical disciplines. Although it was previously possible to visualize the inner organs with rigid endoscopes, the flexibility of the fiberoptic endoscope greatly improved manipulation and hence the extent of organ examination. Fiberoptic technology has been replaced by video endoscopy, and today there is a myriad of advanced imaging techniques available. Approximately a decade after the introduction of the fiberoptic gastroscope, endoscopists around the world began to use this instrument to perform therapeutics in the gastrointestinal (GI) tract, such as injecting bleeding ulcers or resecting colon polyps. Thus, GI endoscopy rapidly progressed from a specialty focused on diagnosis to one dealing with intervention and therapeutics. The reader may ask her- or himself why this book is called 'interventional and therapeutic' GI endoscopy, as the title seems to be an oxymoron. However, there are three types of endoscopies being performed today. For example, diagnostic endoscopy refers to procedures such as esophagogastroduodenoscopy for dyspepsia and screening colonoscopy; interventional endoscopy refers to those endoscopies that imply more manipulation or require more technical skills such as endoscopic cholangiography, pancreatography, endosonography-guided fine-needle aspiration or balloon-assisted enteroscopy, and therapeutic GI endoscopy implies the performance of an active treatment through an endoscope such as transmural drainage of pancreatic fluid collections, dilation of esophageal strictures and polypectomy.

The type of endoscopic interventions in the GI tract has dramatically increased over the last decades. The aim of this book is to present a concise yet instructive overview of the most common interventional and therapeutic GI endoscopic procedures. Although there are many books dealing with therapeutic endoscopy, this one is different for several reasons. First, it is written by a highly selected group of prominent experts from around the world. The reader will notice that every tip and trick detailed by these experts has either been personally invented and developed or practiced with great expertise. Second, the description of the techniques follows a homogeneous approach, making it easy for the endoscopists to 'grab out' the important aspects for their own practice. The majority of the procedures described here are 'classic' and have stood the proof of time. Thus, the reader can be confident that this 'cookbook' will accompany her or him during many years to come. Third, despite being a 'cookbook', the data presented follow evidence-based medical guidelines, but do not inundate the reader with confusing facts and numbers. Fourth, the book is illustrated like an atlas, using real-life pictures and when necessary nice drawings and algorithms.

We are aware that it is impossible to cover the entire spectrum of therapeutic endoscopy in one concise book, but this was not our aim. We want this book to become part of the daily routine; that it is carried around and used at the bedside and in the endoscopic suite, and hopefully it contributes to fulfill the major aim of every endoscopist, which is to deliver the best possible care to patients who are in need of an interventional or therapeutic GI endoscopy.

Klaus Mönkemüller, MD, PhD, FASGE
Bottrop, Germany
C. Mel Wilcox, MD, MPH, FASGE
Birmingham, Ala., USA
Miguel Muñoz-Navas, MD, PhD
Pamplona, Spain

Mönkemüller K, Wilcox CM, Muñoz-Navas M (eds): Interventional and Therapeutic Gastrointestinal Endoscopy.
Front Gastrointest Res. Basel, Karger, 2010, vol 27, pp 1–8

Periendoscopic Use of Anticoagulants and Antiplatelet Agents

Andrew Veitch

New Cross Hospital, Wolverhampton, UK

Abstract

Anticoagulants and antiplatelet agents are very commonly prescribed. They have clear benefits in cardiovascular disease but confer a risk of haemorrhage, particularly in the context of therapeutic procedures. Therapeutic endoscopic procedures also have clear benefits but confer a risk of haemorrhage, which is increased by anticoagulants and antiplatelet therapy. Discontinuation of anticoagulants or antiplatelet agents may result in thrombosis. In the context of clopidogrel therapy for coronary artery stents, discontinuation of therapy could lead to acute myocardial infarction or death. There is therefore a risk:benefit scenario in the case of patients undergoing endoscopy while taking these medications. Here a practical evidenced-based approach is discussed to resolve these issues and offer clinical guidance

Anticoagulants and antiplatelet agents are very widely prescribed. It is estimated that there are more than 1 million individuals in the United Kingdom, and more than 2 million in the United States taking warfarin. Clopidogrel has been prescribed to millions of individuals worldwide. These drugs are of proven benefit in reducing risks associated with cardiovascular disease, but confer an increased risk of bleeding; spontaneously or after therapeutic interventional procedures. When planning endoscopic procedures in patients taking these drugs it is important to consider the potential increased risks of the procedure in relation to the risks of discontinuing drug therapy. However, evidence for the risks associated with continuing or discontinuing these drugs in the periendoscopic period is limited. Following published guidance from the American Society for Gastrointestinal Endoscopy (ASGE) [1, 2] there has been wide variation in practice noted in surveys in the United Kingdom and the Far East [3, 4]. Guidance produced by the ASGE and the British Society of Gastroenterology (BSG) [1, 2, 5] forms the basis of the advice in this chapter. Discussion will be limited to the most widely prescribed anticoagulants, warfarin and heparin, and to the most widely prescribed antiplatelet agents, aspirin and clopidogrel.

Benefits and Risks of Therapy

Anticoagulants

Warfarin is widely prescribed to patients at risk of cardiovascular and cerebrovascular disease. The risk of stroke associated with atrial fibrillation (AF) varies from 1.9 to

18.2%/annum depending on comorbidity. Hypertension, heart failure and diabetes mellitus increase this risk, which can be estimated using the CHADS2 score [6]. A retrospective study of anticoagulated AF patients, whose anticoagulation was adjusted pre-endoscopy, examined the subsequent risk of stroke [7]. This ranged from 0.13% in those with uncomplicated AF to 2.93% in complex patients of advanced age. Mitral stenosis increases the risk of stroke associated with AF by 3–7 times [8, 9]. In a meta-analysis involving greater than 9,000 patients, warfarin reduced the risk of stroke associated with AF by 62% [10]. Venous thromboembolism is a major source of morbidity and mortality, resulting in approximately 25,000 deaths/year in the UK and 200,000 in the US. Warfarin is the mainstay of treatment, initially co-prescribed with heparin until satisfactory anticoagulation levels are achieved with warfarin.

Metal prosthetic heart valves confer a risk of thromboembolism, and anticoagulation is indicated. Biological valve prostheses generally require only aspirin therapy in the absence of other indications for anticoagulation. Metal prostheses in the aortic position are at lower risk of thromboembolism than those in the mitral position [11]. The relative risk of thromboembolism associated with metal prosthetic heart valves is high, but the absolute risk low: a meta-analysis of studies covering more than 50,000 patient years estimated the risk of thromboembolism when not on warfarin to be only 4 events/100 patient years. This is reduced to 2.2 events/100 patient years on aspirin and 1 on warfarin [12]. Over a 7-day period of discontinuation of anticoagulation the risk of thromboembolism would be approximately 0.2%. This has not been tested prospectively in the context of endoscopy.

In the elderly, warfarin confers an annual risk of severe haemorrhage of 1.5%, including cerebral haemorrhage of 0.3% [13]. Response to warfarin therapy is measured by the international normalised ratio (INR). This is used to monitor treatment, and the level required depends on the indication. A high INR confers a higher risk of spontaneous haemorrhage but is a poor predictor of haemorrhage in response to interventional medical procedures [14].

Heparin is available in unfractionated (UFH) and low molecular weight (LMWH) forms. UFH has to be administered by continuous intravenous injection, compared to subcutaneously once daily for LMWH. In addition, UFH therapy has to be monitored by measurement of the activated partial thromboplastin time, and this is unnecessary for LMWH. LMWH has therefore superseded UFH for most indications. LMWH is widely used for the prevention and treatment of deep vein thrombosis and pulmonary embolism, and in the treatment of unstable coronary syndromes. Traditionally UFH has been used as bridging therapy for patients with metal prosthetic heart valves who need temporary discontinuation of warfarin for a therapeutic procedure. One study of greater than 1,000 patients in this situation found no thromboembolic events during short-term bridging with LMWH [15]. Substitution of LMWH rather than UFH in this context is widely practiced, but there have been no randomised controlled trials.

LMWH can be administered as a temporary substitute for warfarin in patients who require continued anticoagulation prior to an endoscopic procedure with a high risk of haemorrhage. It can be administered where necessary on an outpatient basis with appropriate nursing input, or by the patient themselves. The short half-life of LMWH (5 h) compared to warfarin (2.5 days) allows this to be administered safely until the day before the procedure, omitting the dose on the morning of the procedure. Warfarin can be recommenced that evening and LMWH recommenced the following day until the INR is within the therapeutic range.

Antiplatelet Agents

The most commonly prescribed antiplatelet agents are aspirin and clopidogrel. Aspirin is effective in the treatment and prevention of cardiovascular and cerebrovascular disease, and is very widely prescribed. Fortunately, aspirin therapy is safe in the context of both diagnostic and therapeutic endoscopic procedures. This has been demonstrated in large series involving endoscopic polypectomies or sphincterotomies [16–19].

Clopidogrel inhibits platelet aggregation. Its effects last for the life of the platelets, and platelet function has been demonstrated to return to normal 7 days after discontinuation of therapy. Clopidogrel is indicated in the treatment and prevention of acute coronary syndromes, and in the prevention of occlusion of coronary artery stents. Coronary stents are at risk of occlusion, but this is diminished in the case of drug-eluting stents, with a reduction in the need for repeat intervention from 20 to 5% in randomised controlled trials [20, 21]. The risk of stent thrombosis is present until the stent has undergone re-endothelialisation; this takes approximately 1 month for bare metal stents and at least 6 months for drug-eluting stents. Dual therapy with aspirin and clopidogrel must be prescribed until this process has occurred; discontinuation of therapy is associated with a 50% risk of myocardial infarction or death [22]. Case reports of late stent thrombosis have prompted the Food and Drug Administration in the United States and the British Cardiovascular Intervention Society to recommend continuation of aspirin and clopidogrel for 1 year. The risk of stent thrombosis on discontinuation of clopidogrel is greatest after 5 days. In the event of cessation of therapy for an emergency endoscopic procedure, the endoscopy should be carried out as soon as possible within that time period.

Antiplatelet agents confer an increased risk of bleeding, but the risk of spontaneous gastrointestinal haemorrhage is less for clopidogrel than with aspirin [23]. Clopidogrel is widely held to increase the risk of haemorrhage during operative procedures but there are limited data, and none for gastrointestinal endoscopy. Data from studies of cardiac surgery demonstrate an increase in perioperative haemorrhage in those patients who remained on clopidogrel [24, 25]. For any interventional procedure with a risk of haemorrhage, the benefit of the procedure must be balanced against the risk of discontinuing clopidogrel, and this will be dependent on the indication for clopidogrel therapy.

Endoscopic Procedures

The benefits of endoscopy in the diagnosis and therapy of diseases within the gastrointestinal tract are well recognised, and the boundaries are continually expanded by new and improved technologies. This also applies to non-endoscopic diagnostic techniques, particularly radiology, where effective alternatives to diagnostic endoscopy exist, and continue to be developed. Alternative diagnostic modalities are important to consider in patients at high risk of thrombosis if discontinuing anticoagulants or antiplatelet agents, although they may ultimately require a therapeutic intervention if pathology is found. Data on the risks of haemorrhage associated with endoscopic procedures are generally good for commonly performed interventions such as colonoscopic polypectomy or endoscopic sphincterotomy. For newer and less frequently performed procedures, however, data are limited and tend to be less universally applicable due to the influence of local expertise or case mix in the published series. Minor haemorrhage during endoscopic procedures is not uncommon, but for the purposes of this discussion, haemorrhage which requires an unplanned admission to hospital, or transfusion, will be considered. Haemorrhage may occur at the time of the procedure, or be delayed by up to 2 weeks or more.

Table 1. Risk of haemorrhage associated with therapeutic endoscopic procedures

Procedure	Risk of haemorrhage %	References
Colonoscopic polypectomy	0.07–1.7	26, 27
Endoscopic mucosal resection	5.3	32
Endoscopic submucosal dissection	0.15–6	29, 30, 31
ERCP + sphincterotomy	1.13–5.3	17, 33–36
Oesophageal dilatation	2.2	39
Oesophageal stent	7.3–8	40, 41
Pecutaneous endoscopic gastrostomy	≤2	42
Endoscopic ultrasound with FNA	6	37, 38

ERCP = Endoscopic retrograde cholangiopancreatography; FNA = fine needle aspiration.

Before considering the risks of endoscopy on anticoagulation or antiplatelet therapy it is helpful to consider the risks associated with therapeutic procedures undertaken in patients not taking these medications (table 1). Haemorrhage following colonscopic polypectomy has been reported in large prospective series. A British study of 9,223 colonoscopies reported an incidence of 1.7% [26], and an American series of 13,580 reported 0.07% [27]. A number of factors will influence the risk of haemorrhage, including endoscopic technique and the size of polyp. Experience suggests that diathermy using 'coagulation' current results in a lower risk of haemorrhage than 'blend' or 'cut' current, but there are no prospective data to support this. Injection of adrenaline into the base or stalks of large polyps has been demonstrated to reduce the incidence of haemorrhage in one small randomised study [28]. Endoscopic submucosal dissection (ESD) is a relatively new technique associated with a high incidence of intra-procedural haemorrhage, although this is usually controlled by coagulation diathermy during the procedure. Delayed haemorrhage can, however, be problematic. The greatest experience to date comes from Japan. In a series of gastric ESDs only 1/655 (0.15%) experienced haemorrhage requiring transfusion [29]. In a series of colonic ESDs 4/200 (2%) had delayed bleeding after 1–3 days which required endoscopic haemostasis; none required transfusion [30]. The incidence of delayed haemorrhage has been reported to be as high as 6% after ESD [31] and 5.3% after endoscopic mucosal resection [32].

Several large series have examined post-sphincterotomy haemorrhage at endoscopic retrograde cholangiopancreatography: range 1.13–5.3% [17, 33–36]. Biliary or pancreatic stenting has not been demonstrated to be associated with significant haemorrhage. Diagnostic endoscopic ultrasound is not associated with haemorrhage, but this has been reported in association with fine needle aspiration performed at the time of the procedure [37, 38]. Emergency banding of oesophageal varices occurs in the context of acute haemorrhage. Elective therapy of oesophageal varices can provoke immediate haemorrhage but there are no data available regarding the incidence of this, and it is usually resolved by the procedure. Oesophageal dilatation carries a small risk of haemorrhage but recent data on incidence are lacking. A study of balloon dilatation of oesophageal strictures published in 1986 demonstrated post-procedural haemorrhage in 2.2% [39]. Oesophageal stenting has been reported as being associated with a risk of fatal haemorrhage of 7.3–8% [40, 41], but in many of these cases haemorrhage occurred weeks after stent insertion. Haemorrhage due to percutaneous endoscopic gastroenterostomy insertion has been reported at 2% [42], but again many of these instances occurred at a delayed interval, and due to pathology such as local ulceration rather than the endoscopic intervention itself. Diagnostic procedures, including endoscopic pinch biopsies, are generally not associated with significant haemorrhage [43]. There have been isolated case reports of splenic haemorrhage due to trauma during colonoscopy [44–46], but this complication has not been reported in very large case series [26, 27].

Anticoagulants or antiplatelet agents are likely to increase the risks of haemorrhage described above. Diagnostic biopsies are considered safe while on anticoagulant or antiplatelet therapy [1, 47, 48] but there are no prospective data. There are very few studies on the risks of haemorrhage due to therapeutic endoscopic procedures while on warfarin as this is usually discontinued, or substituted with heparin. In a retrospective study of 1,657 patients undergoing colonoscopic polypectomy, the risk of post-polypectomy haemorrhage while on warfarin was increased by a factor of 13.37 [16]. One small study, however, demonstrated safe removal of small polyps while on warfarin after endoscopic clipping of the polypectomy site [48]. However, it should be considered generally that therapy with warfarin or clopidogrel will increase the risks of haemorrhage associated with the above procedures.

Risk:Benefit Analysis

Emergency Procedures

In the context of acute severe gastrointestinal haemorrhage in a patient on anticoagulants or antiplatelet therapy, the immediate risk to the patient is from bleeding rather than thrombosis. For those patients on therapy for conditions with a relatively low risk of thrombosis, then temporary discontinuation of anticoagulation or antiplatelet therapy is clearly indicated. Indeed for patients on warfarin it may be necessary to administer fresh frozen plasma if the haemorrhage is life-threatening. As discussed above, even in the instance of anticoagulation for metal prosthetic heart valves, temporary discontinuation confers a small absolute risk of thrombosis [12]. Adequate resuscitation of the patient is of course paramount, as is early endoscopic intervention to achieve haemostasis.

In the event of acute gastrointestinal haemorrhage in a patient on clopidogrel for coronary artery stents, then discontinuation of therapy might result in a life-threatening occlusion of a coronary stent. It is recommended that a senior cardiologist is involved in the patient's management at an early stage. If clopidogrel needs to be discontinued then endoscopy should be performed as soon as possible. Clopidogrel therapy should be discontinued for as short an interval as possible, and not beyond 5 days, as the risk of stent thrombosis increases markedly after this period. It may be that, with early effective endoscopic haemostasis, clopidogrel can be continued in many cases.

Elective Procedures

The decision whether to continue or discontinue anticoagulant or antiplatelet therapy in a patient due to undergo endoscopy depends on the relative risk of thrombosis on stopping therapy vs. the risk of haemorrhage due to the procedure. Figure 1 summarises these risk categories and advises on management in each instance. In applying this guidance the individual clinical situation should be taken into consideration, as should the limited data upon which this guidance is based. In the context of clopidogrel for coronary artery stents, it is advisable to liaise with the patient's cardiologist as there may be additional risk factors pertinent to that patient. In the American and British guidelines [1, 2, 5], AF without valvular disease is considered a low risk condition, but additional comorbidity such as heart failure and diabetes increase the risk of thrombosis. If

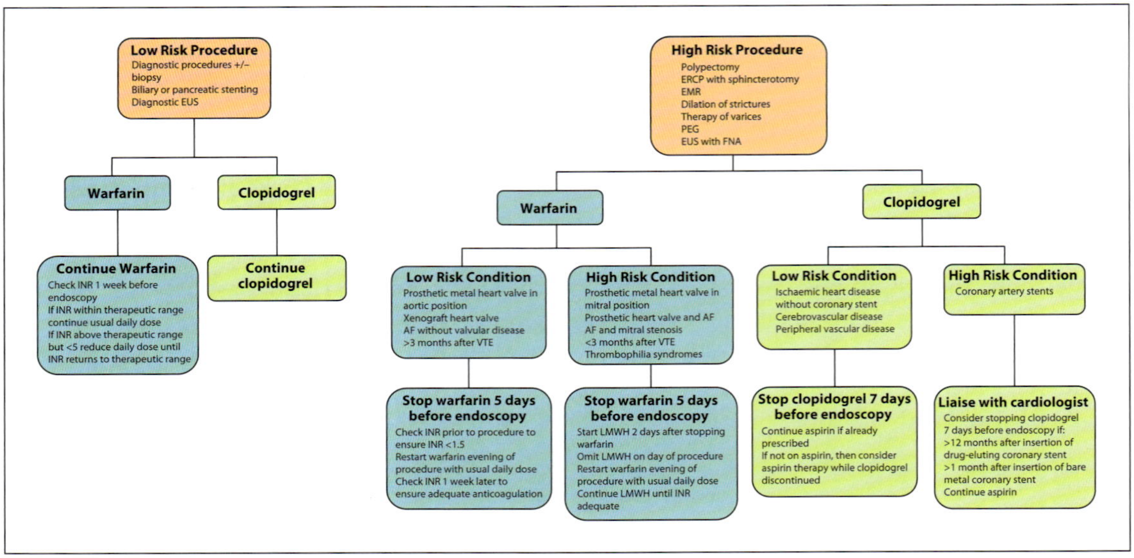

Fig. 1. Periendoscopic use of anticoagulants and antiplatelet agents. EUS = Endoscopic ultrasound; ERCP = endoscopic retrograde cholangiopancreatography; EMR = endoscopic mucosal resection; PEG = percutaneous endoscopic gastroenterostomy; FNA = fine needle aspiration; INR = international normalised ratio; AF = atrial fibrillation; VTE = venous thromboembolism; LMWH = low molecular weight heparin. Reproduced from Veitch et al. [5] with permission from BMJ publishing.

desired, further categorisation according to CHADS2 score could be undertaken to quantify this risk [6]. In patients with coronary artery stents receiving clopidogrel, an alternative radiological investigation could be considered in the first instance. Removal of a small colonic polyp may be delayed until clopidogrel is no longer required. If malignant disease is found then the risks of surgery will need to be considered. Diagnostic colonoscopy is considered low risk, but polyps are likely to be present in 22.5–34.2% [26, 27]. One could pragmatically categorise colonoscopy as high risk on this basis, but on an individual level, a young patient with undiagnosed diarrhoea or known inflammatory bowel disease is likely to just need diagnostic biopsies. For endoscopic retrograde cholangiopancreatography in a patient with a known malignant stricture, then stenting is required which is low risk. If stones are suspected, or the diagnosis uncertain, then a sphincterotomy may be required, which is high risk.

In patients in whom warfarin is temporarily discontinued, it is advised to restart anticoagulation on the night of the procedure. In one study 41/4,592 (0.9%) colonoscopic polypectomies developed severe post-polypectomy haemorrhage [49]. Case-control analysis identified that 34% of patients who bled had resumed anticoagulation within 1 week of the procedure compared to 9% of controls (OR 5.2). It would be prudent to advise all patients resuming anticoagulant therapy after endoscopic therapy that they have an increased risk of delayed haemorrhage.

The time intervals advised for discontinuation or substitution of drug therapy (fig. 1) are based on the pharmacology of the drugs involved. A safe level of INR of <1.5 for therapeutic procedures is arbitrary, and based on anecdotal experience. This has not been prospectively tested, but moderately elevated INR levels have been found to be a poor predictor of subsequent haemorrhage in a variety of non-endoscopic invasive procedures [14].

Conclusion

The periendoscopic management of patients on anticoagulant or antiplatelet agents depends on a balance of risk factors. There is a risk of thrombosis on discontinuation of these drugs, and a risk of haemorrhage associated with the endoscopic procedure. The clinical context, including comorbidity and the likelihood of detecting pathology in individual patients, should also be considered. The guidance in this chapter is based on that published by the ASGE [1, 2] and the BSG [5]. None of the guidance has been rigorously prospectively tested, but neither have there been case reports to refute it.

References

1 Eisen GM, Baron TH, Dominitz JA, et al: Guideline on the management of anticoagulation and antiplatelet therapy for endoscopic procedures. Gastrointest Endosc 2002;55:775–779.

2 Zuckerman MJ, Hirota WK, Adler DG, et al: ASGE guideline: the management of low-molecular-weight heparin and nonaspirin antiplatelet agents for endoscopic procedures. Gastrointest Endosc 2005;61:189–194.

3 Goel A, Barnes CJ, Osman H, et al: National survey of anticoagulation policy in endoscopy. Eur J Gastroenterol Hepatol 2007;19:51–56.

4 Lee SY, Tang SJ, Rockey DC, et al: Managing anticoagulation and antiplatelet medications in GI endoscopy: a survey comparing the East and the West. Gastrointest Endosc 2008;67:1076–1081.

5 Veitch AM, Baglin TP, Gershlick AH, et al: Guidelines for the management of anticoagulant and antiplatelet therapy in patients undergoing endoscopic procedures. Gut 2009;57:1322–1329.

6 Gage BF, Waterman AD, Shannon W, et al: Validation of clinical classification schemes for predicting stroke: results from the National Registry of Atrial Fibrillation. JAMA 2001;285:2864–2870.

7 Blacker DJ, Wijdicks EF, McClelland RL: Stroke risk in anticoagulated patients with atrial fibrillation undergoing endoscopy. Neurology 2003;61:964–968.

8 Szekely P: Systemic embolism and anticoagulant prophylaxis in rheumatic heart disease. Br Med J 1964;i: 1209–1212.

9 Salem DN, Stein PD, Al-Ahmad A, et al: Antithrombotic therapy in valvular heart disease–native and prosthetic: the Seventh ACCP Conference on Antithrombotic and Thrombolytic Therapy. Chest 2004;126(suppl):457S-482S.

10 Hart RG, Benavente O, McBride R, et al: Antithrombotic therapy to prevent stroke in patients with atrial fibrillation: a meta-analysis. Ann Intern Med 1999;131:492–501.

11 Bonow RO, Carabello BA, Kanu C, et al: ACC/AHA 2006 guidelines for the management of patients with valvular heart disease: a report of the American College of Cardiology/American Heart Association Task Force on Practice Guidelines. Circulation 2006;114:e84–e231.

12 Cannegieter SC, Rosendaal FR, Briet E: Thromboembolic and bleeding complications in patients with mechanical heart valve prostheses. Circulation 1994;89: 635–641.

13 Shireman TI, Howard PA, Kresowik TF, et al: Combined anticoagulant-antiplatelet use and major bleeding events in elderly atrial fibrillation patients. Stroke 2004;35:2362–2367.

14 Segal JB, Dzik WH: Paucity of studies to support that abnormal coagulation test results predict bleeding in the setting of invasive procedures: an evidence-based review. Transfusion 2005;45:1413–1425.

15 Seshadri N, Goldhaber SZ, Elkayam U, et al: The clinical challenge of bridging anticoagulation with low-molecular-weight heparin in patients with mechanical prosthetic heart valves: an evidence-based comparative review focusing on anticoagulation options in pregnant and nonpregnant patients. Am Heart J 2005;150:27–34.

16 Hui AJ, Wong RM, Ching JY, et al: Risk of colonoscopic polypectomy bleeding with anticoagulants and antiplatelet agents: analysis of 1657 cases. Gastrointest Endosc 2004;59:44–48.

17 Nelson DB, Freeman ML: Major hemorrhage from endoscopic sphincterotomy: risk factor analysis. J Clin Gastroenterol 1994;19:283–287.

18 Shiffman ML, Farrel MT, Yee YS: Risk of bleeding after endoscopic biopsy or polypectomy in patients taking aspirin or other NSAIDS. Gastrointest Endosc 1994;40: 458–462.

19 Yousfi M, Gostout CJ, Baron TH, et al: Postpolypectomy lower gastrointestinal bleeding: potential role of aspirin. Am J Gastroenterol 2004;99: 1785–1789.

20 Babapulle MN, Joseph L, Belisle P, et al: A hierarchical Bayesian meta-analysis of randomised clinical trials of drug-eluting stents. Lancet 2004;364:583–591.

21 Maeng M, Okkels JL, Rasmussen K, et al: Target lesion revascularisation in patients treated with a sirolimus-eluting or paclitaxel-eluting stent. Heart 2007;93:694–697.

22 Gershlick AH, Richardson G: Drug eluting stents. BMJ 2006;333(7581):1233–4.

23 A randomised, blinded, trial of clopidogrel versus aspirin in patients at risk of ischaemic events (CAPRIE). CAPRIE Steering Committee. Lancet 1996;348:1329–1339.
24 Yende S, Wunderink RG: Effect of clopidogrel on bleeding after coronary artery bypass surgery. Crit Care Med 2001;29:2271–2275.
25 Chu MW, Wilson SR, Novick RJ, et al: Does clopidogrel increase blood loss following coronary artery bypass surgery? Ann Thorac Surg 2004;78:1536–1541.
26 Bowles CJ, Leicester R, Romaya C, et al: A prospective study of colonoscopy practice in the UK today: are we adequately prepared for national colorectal cancer screening tomorrow? Gut 2004;53:277–283.
27 Wexner SD, Garbus JE, Singh JJ: A prospective analysis of 13,580 colonoscopies. Reevaluation of credentialing guidelines. Surg Endosc 2001;15:251–261.
28 Hsieh YH, Lin HJ, Tseng GY, et al: Is submucosal epinephrine injection necessary before polypectomy? A prospective, comparative study. Hepatogastroenterology 2001;48:1379–1382.
29 Oda I, Saito D, Tada M, et al: A multicenter retrospective study of endoscopic resection for early gastric cancer. Gastric Cancer 2006;9:262–270.
30 Saito Y, Uraoka T, Matsuda T, et al: Endoscopic treatment of large superficial colorectal tumors: a case series of 200 endoscopic submucosal dissections (with video). Gastrointest Endosc 2007;66:966–973.
31 Oda I, Gotoda T, Hamanaka H, et al: Endoscopic submucosal dissection for early gastric cancer: technical feasibility, operation time and complications from a large prospective series. Dig Endosc 2005; 17:54–58.
32 Okano A, Hajiro K, Takakuwa H, et al: Predictors of bleeding after endoscopic mucosal resection of gastric tumors. Gastrointest Endosc 2003;57:687–690.
33 Cotton PB, Lehman G, Vennes J, et al: Endoscopic sphincterotomy complications and their management: an attempt at consensus. Gastrointest Endosc 1991;37:383–393.
34 Freeman ML, Nelson DB, Sherman S, et al: Complications of endoscopic biliary sphincterotomy. N Engl J Med 1996;335:909–918.
35 Masci E, Toti G, Mariani A, et al: Complications of diagnostic and therapeutic ERCP: a prospective multicenter study. Am J Gastroenterol 2001;96:417–423.
36 Vaira D, D'Anna L, Ainley C, et al: Endoscopic sphincterotomy in 1000 consecutive patients. Lancet 1989;ii:431–434.
37 Affi A, Vazquez-Sequeiros E, Norton ID, et al: Acute extraluminal hemorrhage associated with EUS-guided fine needle aspiration: frequency and clinical significance. Gastrointest Endosc 2001;53:221–225.
38 Varadarajulu S, Eloubeidi MA: Frequency and significance of acute intracystic hemorrhage during EUS-FNA of cystic lesions of the pancreas. Gastrointest Endosc 2004;60:631–635.
39 Kozarek RA: Hydrostatic balloon dilation of gastrointestinal stenoses: a national survey. Gastrointest Endosc 1986;32:15–19.
40 Neale JC, Goulden JW, Allan SG, et al: Esophageal stents in malignant dysphagia: a two-edged sword? J Palliat Care 2004;20:28–31.
41 Wang MQ, Sze DY, Wang ZP, et al: Delayed complications after esophageal stent placement for treatment of malignant esophageal obstructions and esophagorespiratory fistulas. J Vasc Interv Radiol 2001;12:465–474.
42 Schapiro GD, Edmundowicz SA: Complications of percutaneous endoscopic gastrostomy. Gastrointest Endosc Clin N Am 1996;6:409–422.
43 Cappell MS, Abdullah M: Management of gastrointestinal bleeding induced by gastrointestinal endoscopy. Gastroenterol Clin North Am 2000;29:125–127, vi–vii.
44 Ellis WR, Harrison JM, Williams RS: Rupture of spleen at colonoscopy. Br Med J 1979;i:307–308.
45 Janes SE, Cowan IA, Dijkstra B: A life threatening complication after colonoscopy. BMJ 2005;330:889–890.
46 Tuso P, McElligott J, Marignani P: Splenic rupture at colonoscopy. J Clin Gastroenterol 1987;9:559–562.
47 Hittelet A, Deviere J: Management of anticoagulants before and after endoscopy. Can J Gastroenterol 2003;17:329–332.
48 Friedland S, Soetikno R: Colonoscopy with polypectomy in anticoagulated patients. Gastrointest Endosc 2006;64:98–100.
49 Sawhney MS, Salfiti N, Nelson DB, et al: Risk factors for severe delayed postpolypectomy bleeding. Endoscopy 2008;40:115–119.

Dr. Andrew Veitch, BSc, MD, FRCP, Consultant Gastroenterologist
Clinical Director of Endoscopy and Bowel Cancer Screening
New Cross Hospital,
Wolverhampton WV10 0QP (UK)
Tel. +44 1902 694121, Fax +44 1902 695738, E-Mail andrew.veitch@rwh-tr.nhs.uk

Mönkemüller K, Wilcox CM, Muñoz-Navas M (eds): Interventional and Therapeutic Gastrointestinal Endoscopy.
Front Gastrointest Res. Basel, Karger, 2010, vol 27, pp 9–17

Use of Antibiotics in Therapeutic Endoscopy

Klaus Mönkemüller[a,b] · Qasim Akbar[b] · Lucia C. Fry[a,b]

[a]Department of Internal Medicine, Gastroenterology, Hepatology and Infectious Diseases, Marienhospital, Bottrop, and [b]Department of Gastroenterology, Hepatology and Infectious Diseases, Otto-von-Guericke University, Magdeburg, Germany

Abstract

The gastrointestinal (GI) tract harbors about 10–100 trillion bacteria, which surpass the number of cells in a human being. The intestinal microflora is a complex ecosystem containing over 500 bacterial species. Most pathogenic bacteria are kept under control by the host immune system, the gut microenvironment and the help of non-pathogenic commensal microorganisms. In addition, entrance of pathogenic bacteria into the lymphatic and blood system is impeded by several types of mucosal and immunological barriers. Occasionally, the endoscopist partially or entirely destroys these barriers to perform a therapeutic intervention (e.g. skin incision for PEG tube placement, endoscopic resection of polyps or tumors, perforation). Under these circumstances, bacteria can cause infections such as cellulitis, abscess and peritonitis. Thus, antibiotics are helpful to decrease the risk of infection in such circumstances. However, the use of prophylaxis for bacterial endocarditis has been a matter of debate. Currently, the routine use of prophylactic antibiotics during GI procedures is no longer recommended by the American Heart Association. On other occasions the endoscopist needs to treat specific GI infections such as cholangitis and diverticulitis. The objective here is to provide the therapeutic endoscopist with a summary of conditions commonly encountered in therapeutic endoscopy which will require prophylactic or specific antibiotic use, describe the rationale and principles of antibiotic choice and provide a useful guide on appropriate antibiotic utilization.

Prophylactic Use of Antibiotics in Therapeutic Endoscopy

Currently there are very few situations in which prophylactic antibiotic use is indicated (table 1) [1–3]. As a rule antibiotic prophylaxis, or prompt antibiotic use, is indicated when the risk of infection as a result of an endoscopic intervention is very high.

Prevention of Bacterial Endocarditis

The use of antibiotics for the prevention of bacterial endocarditis has been a matter of debate for the last decades [4–6]. This resulted in complex and inconclusive guidelines over the years [2, 7]. However, recently the guidelines for endocarditis prophylaxis of the American Heart Association were updated and also endorsed by the Infectious Disease Society of America, Society of Cardiovascular Anesthesiologists, Society for Cardiovascular Angiography and Interventions, and Society of Thoracic Surgeons [1, 3]. These guidelines take a significant departure from

Table 1. Conditions for which antibiotic prophylaxis is indicated

Condition	Microorganism	Choice of antibiotic	Alternative antibiotic
Bacterial endocarditis	Enterococci	Penicillin, ampicillin, amoxicillin	Piperacillin, vancomycin
Bacterial endocarditis *Enterococcus faecalis*	Resistant to vancomycin and streptomycin/GM (>500 µg/ml)	Penicillin G or Ampicillin (systemic infection)	Ampicillin and ceftriaxone (adequate for SBE, even if high level AG resistance), Linezolid (effective in 70%)
Enterococcus faecium	Resistant to vancomycin and streptomycin/gentamycin (>500 µg/ml)	Penicillin G, ampicillin (systemic infection)	Penicillin/ampicillin resistance >8 <64 MIC: high dose ampicillin (300 mg/kg/day) Penicillin G or ampicillin + FQ or cloramfenicol or rifampycin or doxicyclin Synercid (70%)[1] Linezolid[2] (58%)[1]
PEG	Staphylococci	Cefazolin, cefoxitin, cefotetan, cefuroxime or ceftizoxime	
Necrotizing pancreatitis	Enterbacteriacea, streptococci, anaerobic bacteria	Imipenem, carbapenems	Treat based on culture results
Bleeding gastric or esophageal varices	Oral bacteria[3] (peptostreptoocci, anaerobic streptococci, enterobacteria)	Ceftriaxone fluorquinolones	
ERCP in the setting of obstructed biliary tree	Enterobacteriacea (68%) (e.g. *Escherichia coli, Klebsiella pneumoniae*) Enteroccocci, 14% Bacteroides spp, 10% Clostridium spp 7%	Ciprofloxacin, piperacillin-tazobactam, ceftizoxime	
Drainage of PFC	Same as above, also peptostreptocci	Ciprofloxacin, piperacillin-tazobactam	
EUS-guided FNA	Same as PFC and ERCP	Fluoroquinolones	Ceftriaxone

GM = Gentamycin; MIC = minimum inhibitory concentration; SBE = spontaneous bacterial endocarditis; ERCP = endoscopic retrograde cholangiopancreatography; PFC = pancreatic fluid collection. Data adapted from Gilbert et al. [3].

[1] Resistance can develop in monotherapy regimens.

[2] Useful for β-lactamase-positive vancomycin-resistant enterococci, faecalis strains.

[3] The oral bacteria of patients with cirrhosis, alcoholics, immunosuppressed and elderly patients may contain more gram negative bacteria.

previous ones as the indications for antibiotics have been significantly cut down, being recommended only for cardiac conditions with the greatest risks of complications and for dental procedures that involve perforation of oral mucosa, manipulation of gingival tissue or periapical region of the teeth [1, 3].

In patients undergoing endoscopic procedures, prophylaxis is no longer recommended, even in patients deemed at high risk, e.g. those with previous spontaneous bacterial peritonitis, prosthetic valve, valvulopathy following heart transplant, and congenital heart disease with one of the following: completely repaired cardiac defect using prosthetic material, partially corrected but with residual defect near prosthetic material, uncorrected cyanotic congenital heart disease, surgically constructed shunts and conduits [1, 3]. However, in patients who have an active infection with enterococci, it is important to treat before an elective procedure or, if the procedure is emergent, use an accepted enterococcal regimen [1, 3]. Also if a patient undergoes procedures involving infected skin or soft tissues, include coverage against staphylococci and β-hemolytic streptococci in the treatment regimen [1, 3].

Percutaneous Endoscopic Gastrostomy or Percutaneous Endoscopic Jejunostomy Placement

The rate of infection after percutaneous endoscopic gastrostomy or percutaneous endoscopic jejunostomy placement is significantly decreased with the use of prophylactic antibiotics [8, 9]. The recommended agents are those with activity against skin flora (staphylococci): first-generation cephalosporins (table 1). Most experts use only one dose of antibiotic 6 h before the procedure. However, others prefer to use 'prophylactic' antibiotics for 3 days [3, 6, 8].

Endoscopic Manipulation of the Biliary Tract

Conditions that increase of cholangitis in the setting of endoscopic retrograde cholangiopancreatography (ERCP) are: obstructed biliary tree due cholangiocellular carcinoma, pancreatic head cancer, and practically any common bile duct (CBD) or hilar lesion that impedes adequate bile flow (metastasis, lymph nodes, sclerosis, fibrosis). The incidence of cholangitis and sepsis after ERCP is as high as 3% [2, 10–12]. In addition, choledocolithiasis, acute cholecystitis, a non-functioning gallbladder, and increased age (>65 years) increase the risk of biliary sepsis [2, 3, 10–13]. However, if adequate bile flow is guaranteed after ERCP the risk of infection is minimal. Thus, most biliary tract interventions do not result in cholangitis. Nevertheless, one can never assume that all ERCPs performed in patients with obstructive cholestasis will result in adequate drainage, and thus antibiotic prophylaxis is recommended for the above-mentioned conditions [2, 3]. The antibiotics should have coverage against enterobacteriacea and enterococci. Ciprofloxacin has the advantage of excellent absorption, and therefore can be administered orally [3, 10–12]. Piperacillin has additional coverage against many enterococci [3].

Drainage of Pancreatic Fluid Collections

Antibiotic prophylaxis should be administered before endoscopic, endosonographic or percutaneous drainage of any pancreatic fluid condition [3]. Generally, these fluid collections are sterile, but puncture and drainage will automatically results in contamination of this contained fluid collection. Commonly employed antibiotic prophylactic agents are fluorquinolones [2, 3].

Endoscopic Ultrasound-Guided Fine Needle Aspiration

No clear guidelines exist regarding the use of antibiotic prophylaxis during endoscopic ultrasound-guided fine needle aspiration. However, experts routinely use prophylaxis [14, 15]. The most commonly used antibiotic in this situation is ciprofloxacin, 400 mg one dose before the procedure [14, 15].

Bleeding Gastric or Esophageal Varices
Bacteremia has been reported to occur in up to 50% of patients undergoing sclerotherapy and 25% of patients undergoing endoscopic variceal ligation [16–20]. Currently, endoscopic variceal ligation is the standard therapy to treat esophageal varices [18]. Whether antibiotics decrease the risk of spontaneous bacterial peritonitis is not known. However, the existing data clearly support the use of antibiotics to decrease infectious complications, rebleeding and mortality in cirrhotic patients presenting with gastrointestinal hemorrhage [2, 3]. Quinolones are the preferred prophylactic antibiotics in cirrhotic patients with gastrointestinal hemorrhage.

Endoscopic Dilation of Esophageal Strictures
Esophageal dilation is frequently associated with bacteremia [21–23]. However, no studies to date have demonstrated a clinically significant reduction in the incidence of infections by the use of prophylactic antibiotics in patients undergoing esophageal dilation. Nevertheless, the author prefers to use antibiotic prophylaxis in cirrhotic patients with ascites and those with primary or secondary immunosuppression (e.g. steroids, antineoplastic agents, azathioprine).

Pancreatitis
Antibiotics in acute pancreatitis are rarely indicated. Even in the presence of significant pancreatic necrosis or severe acute pancreatitis (SAP) there is controversy on the utility of prophylactic antibiotics [24–28]. Based on results of double-blind, randomized, placebo-controlled trials, antibiotic prophylaxis in SAP is ineffective for reducing the frequency of infected necrosis and to decrease hospital mortality [28]. In patients with SAP and multi-organ failure on admission and in those with hemodynamic shock, it is advisable to use antibiotic treatment with carbapenems and quinolones on demand [28]. In addition, patients with biliary sepsis (acute biliary pancreatitis and acute cholecystitis and/or cholangitis) also benefit from antibiotic treatment [2, 3, 28]. In addition, SAP patients with documented bacteremia, urinary tract positive or a positive bronchoalveolar lavage infection should also be treated with antibiotics [28]. In essence, the most important issue in patients with SAP is to follow them closely and start antibiotics once there are clinical and laboratory signs of infection. If there is suspicion of pancreatic infection, a CT-guided fine needle aspiration with gram stain and cultures are mandatory [29, 30]. The most commonly used antibiotics are listed in table 1.

Specific (Non-Prophylactic) Use of Antibiotics in Therapeutic Endoscopy

Biliary Tract Infections
The most common biliary tract infections encountered by the therapeutic endoscopist are cholecystitis and cholangitis. Cholecystitis usually results from the obstruction of a stone at the level of the cystic duct. However, up to one third of cholecystitis are acalculous. Acalculous cholecystitis is seen more frequently in the elderly, immunosuppressed and diabetic patients [31]. Thus, patients with typical clinical presentation may still have acute cholecystitis, even in the absence of radiographically documented gallstones.

Acute Suppurative Cholangitis
Acute suppurative cholangitis can develop when one or more types of organisms enter the CDB [3, 13]. Bile is usually sterile but it is a nice culture media for bacteria. In fact, most culture media are enriched with bile to promote the growth of bacteria. Thus, it is logical to infer that cholangitis can result when the biliary tract is manipulated either percutaneously or endoscopically or when stones remain trapped inside the CBD and get impacted in the ampulla of Vater. Occasionally, a stone gets impacted in Hartmann's pouch, which is small indentation at the junction of a cystic duct and CBD. This impaction results in obstruction of the proximal bile duct (i.e. common hepatic duct), while the distal bile duct (CBD) remains patent. This condition is known as Mirizzi's syndrome [32]. Albeit less common, cholangitis can also develop spontaneously in the setting of malignant CBD obstruction [3, 13].

Sclerosing Cholangitis
The most common types of sclerosing cholangitis are primary sclerosing cholangitis, secondary sclerosing cholangitis and Caroli's disease or syndrome [13, 33]. Patients with these conditions are at risk of developing recurrent bacterial cholangitis because of diminished bile flow resulting from one or multiple strictures and bacterial super-infection [3]. Whereas in Caroli's disease resection of the affected segment can result in improvement of the condition, in patients with diffuse sclerosing biliary changes, recurrent bacterial cholangitis is common. In this scenario it is important to relieve the stenosis through endoscopic biliary dilation. However, a significant number of patients will have multiple strictures. Thus, chronic, intermittent use of antibiotics is recommended to prevent acute, recurrent cholangitis [33]. The most commonly employed antibiotic is ciprofloxacin.

Cholangitis Resulting from Parasites
Parasites are probably one of the most common causes of cholangitis worldwide [3, 13, 34, 35]. The problem when parasites enter the biliary tract is threefold. First, the parasite itself can lead to an inflammatory reaction and fibrosis, resulting in acute and chronic cholangitis [34]. Second, the parasite transports organisms into the biliary tract, potentially resulting in acute suppurative cholangitis. And third, the parasite itself can result in acute mechanical obstruction, such as *Ascaris lumbricoides* [35]. The workup and therapy of this type of cholangitis depends on the infecting organism and the timing of diagnosis. In case of acute mechanical obstruction, endoscopic removal of the parasites is mandatory [35]. Specific antiparasitic therapy is also indicated, even in patients with chronic, sclerosing cholangitis [3, 34]. Infestation with *Clonorchis sinensis* organisms can cause such complications as intrahepatic stones, recurrent pyogenic cholangitis, cirrhosis, cholelithiasis, pancreatitis, and cholangiocarcinoma [34]. *Opisthorchis viverrini*, *Opisthorchis felineus*, and *Dicrocoelium dendriticum* are closely related to *C. sinensis* and can also lead to cholangitis. Fascioliasis, caused by *Fasciola hepatica* and *F. gigantica*, is a zoonotic helminthiasis that can result in significant liver fibrosis and lead to acute hepatic or chronic biliary tract infection [35].

Choice of Antibiotics for Biliary Infections
The choice of antibiotics depends on the etiologic microorganism. The most common microorganisms infecting the gallbladder and biliary tract are: Enterobacteriacea (such as *Escherichia coli* and *Klebsiella pneumoniae*), 68%; enteroccocci, 14%, Bacteroides spp, 10% and Clostridium spp 7% [3]. First-line antibiotics include: piperacillin-tazobactam, ticarcillin-clavulanic acid, ampicillin-sulbactam and ertapenem [3]. Life-threatening infections should be treated with antibiotics such as imipenen or meronem [3] (table 2).

Table 2. Antibiotics used for specific gastrointestinal infections

Condition	Microorganism	Choice of antibiotic	Alternative antibiotic
Cholecystitis[1] Cholangitis[1]	Enterobacteriacea (68%) (e.g. *Escherichia coli*, *Klebsiella pneumoniae*) Enteroccocci, 14% Bacteroides spp, 10% Clostridium spp 7%	Piperacillin-tazobactam, ticarcillin-clavulanic acid Ampicillin-sulbactam ertapenem	Third-generation cephalosporin and metro or aztreonam and metro, or cipro and metro or moxifloxacin
Pancreatic necrosis	Enterobacteriacea, enterococci, *Staphylococcus aureus*, *S. epidermidis*, anaerobes, candida	Base antibiotic coverage on gram stain and culture	
Diverticulitis and perirectal abscess; small bowel/colon perforation	Enterobacteriacea, Bacteroides, enterococci, occasionally *Pseudomonas aeruginosa*	Mild: (always drain perirectal abscess): TMP-SMX DS or cipro or levofloxacin + metro	Ampicillin clavulanate or moxifloxacin
		Moderate: pip-tazobactam, ampSB, tic-clavulanic acid, or moxifloxacin	Cipro or levofloxacin plus metro or moxifloxacin or tigecyline
		Severe: Imipenem or meronem	Amp + metro + cipro or levofloxacin oder amp + metron + aminogylcosides
Esophageal perforation	Oropharyngeal anaerobes, peptostreptococci, in elderly and immunosuppressed patients also gram-negative bacteria	pip-tazobactam, tic-clavulanic acid amp-sulbactam ERTA	
Liver abscess	Monobacterial and polybacterial (80%)	Depends on isolated microorganism(s) If culture results pending use coverage against enterobacteria, streptococci, enteococci and anaerobes (see cholangitis)	
Amebic liver abscess	*Entamoeba histolytica*	Metro or tinidazole, followed by paromomycin	
Parasites	*Ascaris lumbricoides* *Clonorchis sinensis* *Fasciola hepatica* *Opsitorchis viverrini* Schistomiasis Intestinal tapeworms Echinococcosis	Mebendazole, albendazole Praziquantel or albendazole Praziquantel Praziquantel Praziquantel Praziquantel Albenadazole	Ivermectin, nitazoxanide

amp = Ampicillin; metro = metronidazole; cipro = ciprofloxacin; pip = piperacillin; tic = ticarcillin; TMP-SMX DS = trimetoprim-sulfametoxazole double strength; ampSB = ampicillin sulbactam.
Data adapted from Gilbert et al. [3].
[1] Life-threatening infections should be treated with imipenen or meronem.

Diverticulitis and Perirectal Abscess

The most common bacteria in diverticulitis and perirectal abscess are enterobacteiacea and bacteroides. *Pseudomonas aeruginosa* and enterococci may also be present (table 2) [3, 36, 37]. Thus, the choice of antibiotics is dictated by these bacteria. Diverticulitis is categorized into mild, moderate and severe. Patients with mild diverticulitis can be treated on an ambulatory basis and receive trimetoprim sulfamethoxazole (double strength) twice a day for 7–10 days [3, 36, 37]. Patients with moderate to severe disease and patients with pelvic abscess should be treated initially in the hospital. Table 2 lists the antibiotic choices for these categories.

Hollow Viscus Perforation

Albeit a rare event, perforation is a complication that every therapeutic endoscopist will eventually face [38, 39]. The choice of antibiotic will depend on the location of the perforation. In analogy to surgery, microbial infections are divided into those above the diaphragm and those below the diaphragm, where *Bacteroides fragilis* is a much more common occurrence. Thus, the antibiotic choice for any small bowel or colon perforation should cover against bacteroides [38]. The recommended antibiotics for perforations of the small bowel and colon are the same as for diverticulitis and pelvic abscess, with the exception that a perforation should always be considered a serious event (i.e. equivalent to severe diverticulitis), and thus, patients should be treated in the hospital. In contrast, antibiotics used for esophageal and stomach perforations should have spectrum against oral bacteria such as peptostreptococcus.

In case of suspected or frank perforation prompt initiation of antibiotics is mandatory. Thus, appropriate antibiotics should always be available in the endoscopic suite!

References

1 Nishimura RA, Carabello BA, Faxon DP, Freed MD, Lytle BW, O'Gara PT, O'Rourke RA, Shah PM: ACC/AHA 2008 Guideline update on valvular heart disease: focused update on infective endocarditis: a report of the American College of Cardiology/American Heart Association Task Force on Practice Guidelines endorsed by the Society of Cardiovascular Anesthesiologists, Society for Cardiovascular Angiography and Interventions, and Society of Thoracic Surgeons. Am Coll Cardiol 2008;52:676–685.

2 Hirota WK, Petersen K, Baron TH, Goldstein JL, Jacobson BC, et al: Guidelines for antibiotic prophylaxis for GI endoscopy. Gastrointest Endosc 2003;58: 475–482.

3 Gilbert DN, Mollerig RC, Eliopoulos GM, Sande MA, Chambers HF, Saag MS: Recommended antimicrobial agents against selected bacteria; in Gilbert DN, Robert C, Moellering RC, Eliopoulos GM, Sande MA (eds): The Sanford Guide to Antimicrobial Therapy 2008, ed 38. Sperryville, Antimicrobial Therapy, 2008, pp 4–130.

4 Shorvon PJ, Eykyn SJ, Cotton PB: Gastrointestinal instrumentation, bacteremia, and endocarditis. Gut 1983;24: 1078–1093.

5 Baskin G: Prosthetic endocarditis after endoscopic variceal sclerotherapy: a failure of antibiotic prophylaxis. Am J Gastroenterol 1989;84:311–312.

6 Van der Meer JTM, Van Wijk W, Thompson J, Vanderbroucke JP, Valkenburg HA, Michel MF: Efficacy of antibiotic prophylaxis for prevention of native-endocarditis. Lancet 1992;339:135–139.

7 Bonow RO, Carabello B, de Leon AC, Edmunds LH Jr, Fedderly BJ, et al: ACC/AHA Guidelines for the Management of Patients with Valvular Heart Disease. Executive Summary. A report of the American College of Cardiology/American Heart Association Task Force on Practice Guidelines (Committee on Management of Patients With Valvular Heart Disease). J Heart Valve Dis 1998;7: 672–707.

8 Sharma V, Howden CW: Meta-analysis of randomized, controlled trials of antibiotic prophylaxis before percutaneous endoscopic gastrostomy. Am J Gastroenterol 2000;95:3133–3136.

9 Dormann AJ, Wigginghaus B, Risius H, Kleimann F, Kloppenborg A, Grunewald T, et al: A single dose of ceftriaxone administered 30 minutes before percutaneous endoscopic gastrostomy significantly reduces local and systemic infective complications. Am J Gastroenterol 1999;94:3220–3224.
10 Mehal WZ, Culshaw KD, Tillotson GS, Chapman RW: Antibiotic prophylaxis for ERCP: a randomized clinical trial comparing ciprofloxacin and cefuroxime in 200 patients at high risk for cholangitis. Eur J Gastroenterol Hepatol 1995;7:841–845.
11 Freeman ML, Nelson DB, Sherman S, Haber GB, Herman ME, Dorsher PJ, et al: Complications of endoscopic biliary sphincterotomy. N Engl J Med 1996;335: 909–918.
12 Thompson BF, Arguedas ME, Wilcox CM: Antibiotic prophylaxis prior to endoscopic retrograde cholangiopancreatography in patients with obstructive jaundice: is it worth the cost? Alimentary Pharmacol Ther 2002; 16:727–734.
13 Mönkemüller KE, Garcia-Gallont R, Fallon MB: Gallbladder and biliary tract disorders; in Andreoli TE (ed): Cecil's Essentials of Medicine. Philadelphia, Saunders, 2004, pp 178–182.
14 Eloubeidi MA: Antibiotics are mandatory before EUS-guided FNA in cystic or semisolid lesions of the mediastinum and the pancreas. Gastrointest Endosc 2006; 63:890.
15 Fazel A, Moezardalan K, Varadarajulu S, Draganov P, Eloubeidi MA: The utility and the safety of EUS-guided FNA in the evaluation of duplication cysts. Gastrointest Endosc 2005;62:575–580.
16 Rimola A, Bory F, Teres J, Perez-Ayuso RM, Arroyo V, Rodes J: Oral, nonabsorbable antibiotics prevent infection in cirrhotics with gastrointestinal hemorrhage. Hepatology 1985;5:463–467.
17 Bac DJ, de Marie S, Siersema Snoble J, van Buuren HR: Post-sclerotherapy bacterial peritonitis: a complication of sclerotherapy or of variceal bleeding? Am J Gastroenterol 1994;89:859–862.
18 Laine L, Cook D: Endoscopic ligation compared with sclerotherapy for treatment of esophageal variceal bleeding: a meta-analysis. Ann Intern Med 1995;123:280–287.
19 Cohen LB, Korsten MA, Scherl EJ, Velez ME, Fisse RD, Arons EJ: Bacteremia after endoscopic injection sclerosis. Gastrointest Endosc 1983;29:198–200.
20 Camara DS, Grunber M, Barde CJ, Montes M, Caruana JA, Chung RS: Transient bacteremia following endoscopic injection sclerotherapy of esophageal varices. Arch Intern Med 1983;143:1350–1352.
21 Raines DR, Branche WC, Anderson DL, Boyce HW: The occurrence of bacteremia after esophageal dilation. Gastrointest Endosc 1975;22:86–87.
22 Zuccaro G, Richter JE, Rice TW, Achkar E, Easley K, Lewis J, et al: Viridans streptococcal bacteremia after esophageal stricture dilation. Gastrointest Endosc 1998; 48:568–573.
23 Nelson DB, Sanderson SJ, Azar MM: Bacteremia with esophageal dilation. Gastrointest Endosc 1998; 48:563–567.
24 Villatoro E, Bassi C, Larvin M: Antibiotic therapy for prophylaxis against infection of pancreatic necrosis in acute pancreatitis. Cochrane Database Syst Rev 2006;4: CD002941.
25 Bai Y, Gao J, Zou DW, Li ZS: Prophylactic antibiotics cannot reduce infected pancreatic necrosis and mortality in acute necrotizing pancreatitis: evidence from a meta-analysis of randomized controlled trials. Am J Gastroenterol 2008;103:104–110.
26 Mönkemüller KE, Morgan DE, Baron TH: *Stenotrophomonas (Xanthomonas) maltophilia* infection in necrotizing pancreatitis. Int J Pancreatol 1999;25: 59–63.
27 Xu T, Cai Q: Prophylactic antibiotic treatment in acute necrotizing pancreatitis: results from a meta-analysis. Scand J Gastroenterol 2008;43:1249–1258.
28 Beger HG, Gansauge F, Poch B, Schwarz M: The use of antibiotics for acute pancreatitis: is there a role? Curr Infect Dis Rep 2009;11:101–107.
29 Banks PA: Pro: computerized tomographic fine needle aspiration (CT-FNA) is valuable in the management of infected pancreatic necrosis. Am J Gastroenterol 2005; 100:2371–2372.
30 Mönkemüller KE, Harewood GC, Curioso WH, Fry LC, Wilcox CM, Morgan DE, Baron TH: Biochemical analysis of pancreatic fluid collections predicts bacterial infection. J Gastroenterol Hepatol 2005;20:1667–1673.
31 Wilcox CM, Mönkemüller KE: Hepatobiliary diseases in patients with AIDS: focus on AIDS cholangiopathy and gallbladder disease. Dig Dis 1998;16: 205–213.
32 Pelaez-Luna M, Levy MJ, Arora AS, Baron TH, Rajan E: Mirizzi syndrome presenting as painless jaundice: a rare entity diagnosed by EUS. Gastrointest Endosc 2008; 67:974–975.
33 Yonem O, Bayraktar Y: Clinical characteristics of Caroli's syndrome. World J Gastroenterol 2007;13: 1934–1937.
34 Fry LC, Mönkemüller KE, Baron TH: Sclerosing cholangitis caused by *Clonorchis sinensis*. Gastrointest Endosc 2002;56:114.
35 Rana SS, Bhasin DK, Nanda M, Singh K: Parasitic infestations of the biliary tract. Curr Gastroenterol Rep 2007; 9:156–164.

36 Ridgway P, Latif A, Shabbir J, Ofriokuma F, Hurley MJ, Evoy D, Mahony JB, Mealy K: Randomised controlled trial of oral versus intravenous therapy for clinically diagnosed acute uncomplicated diverticulitis. Colorectal Dis 2008 [Epub ahead of print].
37 Szojda MM, Cuesta MA, Mulder CM, Felt-Bersma RJ: Review article: management of diverticulitis. Aliment Pharmacol Ther 2007;26(suppl 2):67–76.
38 Lüning TH, Keemers-Gels ME, Barendregt WB, Tan AC, Rosman C: Colonoscopic perforations: a review of 30,366 patients. Surg Endosc 2007;21:994–997.
39 Fry LC, Mönkemüller K, Neumann H, Schulz HU, Malfertheiner P: Incidence, clinical management and outcomes of esophageal perforations after endoscopic dilatation. Z Gastroenterol 2007;45:1180–1184.

Klaus Mönkemüller, MD, PhD, FASGE
Marienhospital, Bottrop
Josef-Albers-Strasse 70
DE–46236 Bottrop (Germany)
Tel. +49 2041 106 1000, Fax +49 2041 106 1009, E-Mail klaus.moenkemueller@mhb-bottrop.de

Mönkemüller K, Wilcox CM, Muñoz-Navas M (eds): Interventional and Therapeutic Gastrointestinal Endoscopy.
Front Gastrointest Res. Basel, Karger, 2010, vol 27, pp 18–36

Accessories Used for Hemostasis in Gastrointestinal Bleeding

Ivan Jovanović · Tomica Milosavljević

Clinic for Gastroenterology and Hepatology, Clinical Center of Serbia, Belgrade, Serbia

Abstract

Endoscopic hemostatic devices improve the outcome of patients bleeding from the gastrointestinal tract. They range from well-known thermal devices (multipolar and heater probes), which are efficient, safe and relatively low in cost, to novel redesigned mechanical devices such as endoscopic hemoclips that have also been widely adopted. In general, there are two basic principles of hemostasis: thermal (contact and non-contact) and non-thermal (injection and mechanical methods). Thermal hemostasis can be achieved by either contact thermal modalities: heater probe coagulation, monopolar coagulation, bipolar coagulation, or non-contact thermal modalities: argon plasma coagulation and laser photocoagulation. Their efficacies are probably more affected by personal preferences and expertise rather than minor differences between the modalities. Non-thermal modalities include injection needles, band ligators, endoclips and loops. We gathered data from various sources to describe the most commonly used hemostatic devices in everyday practice.

In general, there are two basic principles of hemostasis: thermal (contact and non-contact) and non-thermal (injection and mechanical methods) [1] (table 1; fig. 1–5).

Thermal Hemostasis

Thermal hemostasis can be achieved by either contact thermal modalities: heater probe coagulation, monopolar coagulation, bipolar coagulation, or non-contact thermal modalities such as argon plasma coagulation (APC) and laser photocoagulation. Their efficacies are probably more affected by personal preferences and expertise rather than minor differences between the modalities.

Contact Thermal Modalities

The heater probe and bipolar electrocoagulation are the most commonly used devices for contact coagulation of bleeding and non-bleeding visible vessels. Thermal hemostasis is achieved

Table 1. Methods used for hemostasis

Thermal therapy	Electrocoagulation Monopolar Multipolar/bipolar Heater probe Argon plasma coagulation Laser photocoagulation
Injection therapy	Ethanol Epinephrine Sclerosants Ethanolamine Polidocanol Thrombin
Mechanical	Endoscopic clips Detachable snare (endoloop) Endoscopic band ligation

with relatively low energy outputs and thermal heating of the tissue. All thermal devices generate heat either directly (heater probe) or by passage of electrical current through tissue (multipolar probes).

The *heater probe* consists of a Teflon-coated hollow aluminum cylinder with an inner heating coil. In addition, the heater probe has an irrigation port with flushing capabilities. The Teflon coating of the probe prevents tissue adherence to the probe tip. The mechanism of tissue coagulation is direct heat transfer. Heat application causes edema, coagulation of tissue proteins and contraction of vessels. A foot pedal controls coagulation by delivering a preselected quantity of energy in joules to the diode in the probe tip, generating coagulating heat at the tip of the catheter. The combination of pressure to co-apt the vessel walls and heat to coagulate the tissue results in effective hemostasis. During therapy, the distal tip of the heater probe is applied directly to the bleeding site. Initially, 4 or 5 pulses of 10–15 J/pulse are given. If bleeding persists, the procedure is repeated. Finally, several additional pulses can be applied, surrounding the bleeding site, to address the feeding vessel. The depth of coagulation using the heater probe is similar to that in bipolar coagulation.

Monopolar electrocoagulation requires the placement of a neutral electrode on the patient's body and the electrical current flows from the probe through the patient's body. Coagulation depth is greater than in bipolar electrocoagulation.

Repeated application of these devices can result in the build-up of coagulum at the tip, which can impede conductivity and necessitates removal of the probe and cleaning the tip.

In *bipolar electrocoagulation* an electrical current passes through the tissue between the two electrodes on the probe tip (fig. 2). In contrast to monopolar electrocoagulation, the circuit is completed locally; therefore it does not pass through the patient's body and grounding is not required. As the targeted tissue desiccates, loss of conductivity occurs. A port at the tip delivers water for irrigation, which improves overall visualization. A foot pedal controls coagulation and irrigation. Both the thermal and co-aptive components can be applied tangentially or enface to the targeted lesion. A major problem is that the probe may stick to the tissue, and removal of the probe can tear off tissue and induce bleeding. It should be kept in mind that the right colon

1 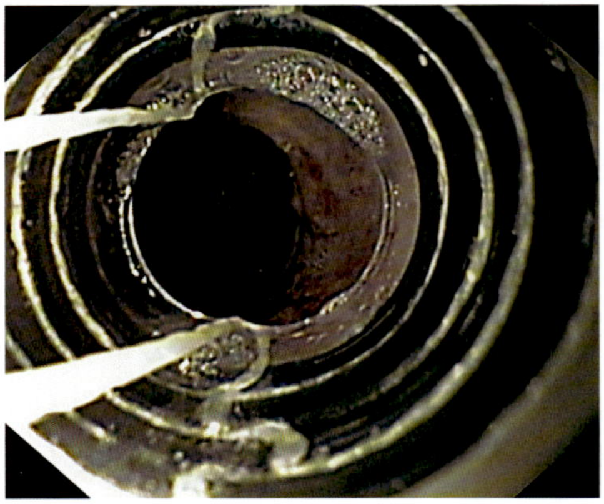

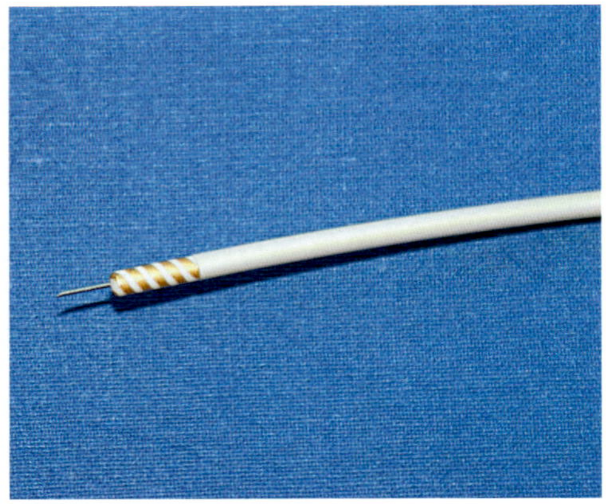 2

Fig. 1. Endoscopic band ligation is the preferred method to treat esophageal varices. However, banding can be used to treat other bleeding lesions such as hemorrhoids, Mallory-Weiss lesions and Dieulafoy's ulcer.

Fig. 2. The Gold probe is a classic thermal hemostatic method which uses bipolar electrocoagulation. Monopolar electrocoagulation is rarely used to treat bleeding lesions. The classic monopolar instrument used by endoscopists is the 'hot biopsy'. Bipolar and monopolar electrocoagulation differs from the more popular heater probe by the use of electrical current.

wall is thinner and that colonic perforation after treatment of angiodysplasia can be seen in up to 2.5% of patients in whom bipolar coagulation is performed [2]. Therefore, forceful co-aptation in this region should be avoided.

Non-Contact Thermal Modalities

Argon plasma coagulation (APC) is a non-contact electrocoagulation modality that utilizes high-frequency monopolar alternating current conducted to target tissues through ionized argon gas (argon plasma; fig. 3). Electrons flow through a channel of electrically activated, ionized argon gas from the probe electrode to the targeted tissue causing a thermal effect at the interface. The APC probe consists of a flexible Teflon tube with a tungsten electrode contained in a ceramic nozzle at its distal end. Coagulation depth depends on generator power setting, flow rate of the argon gas, duration of application and the distance of the probe tip to the target tissue which ranges from 0.8 to 3.0 mm [3] (fig. 3b). The depth of penetration is automatically limited by desiccation of the tissue. As the tissue surface loses its electrical conductivity because of desiccation, the plasma stream shifts to the adjacent non-desiccated (conductive) tissue (fig. 3c). The APC unit includes a high-frequency electrosurgical generator, automatically regulated argon gas supply unit, gas flow meter, flexible delivery catheter, grounding pad, and foot switch to activate both gas and energy (Erbe Elektromedizin GmbH, Tübingen, Germany). APC probes are available in a variety of diameters and lengths (table 2). The available probes direct plasma parallel or perpendicular to the axis of the catheter.

APC is frequently used to treat chronic, actively bleeding lesions of the gastrointestinal (GI) tract. It is especially useful when coagulation needs to be carried out over a large surface while limiting penetration depth. It provides effective, even surface coagulation with uniform hemostasis and devitalization. Major advantages are that it is non-contact procedure and enables better dosage of

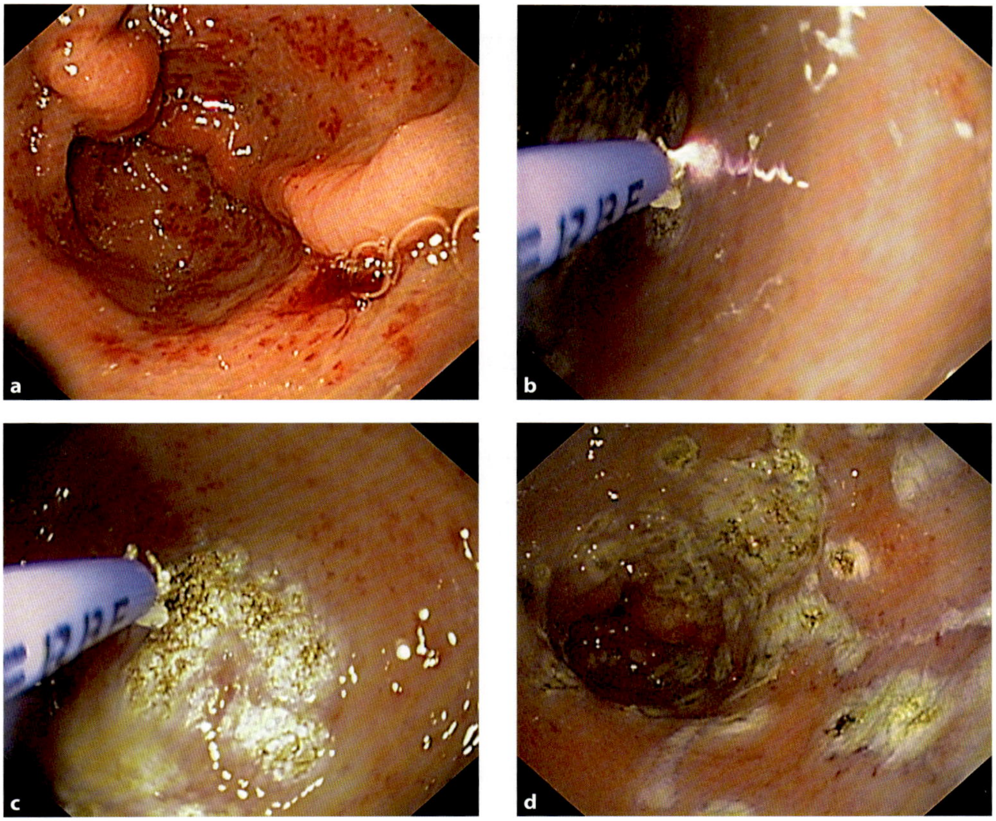

Fig. 3. a Classic endoscopic appearance of watermelon stomach or GAVE (gastric antral vascular ectasias). This condition is often missed or referred to as 'hemorrhagic gastritis'. Close inspection with standard or high definition endoscopes clearly show the submucosal vascular malformations. **b** Application of argon plasma coagulation with the Erbe device. Note that the tip of the probe should be placed about 1–2 mm above the mucosal surface. This allows the creation of a spark once electrical current is applied to the argon gas. **c** Note the fulguration of the tissue resulting from APC. The objective is to 'paint' an adequate area of mucosa. **d** End result of an APCsession. Some experts start the patient on proton pump inhibitors to accelerate the mucosal healing and prevent gastric hemorrhage. Photos with the courtesy of Klaus Mönkemüller, MD, PhD (Germany).

penetration which leads to safer application and limited risk of perforation with few complication. Nonetheless, APC carries the risk of perforation, especially in the thin-walled cecum. Although validated data regarding the rates of perforation are lacking, it is estimated that it is below 1% [4–6].

We typically use APC for ablation of solitary or multiple vascular ectasias and telangiectasias seen as a clinical spectrum of angiodysplasias, watermelon stomach (fig. 3a) and post-irradiation injury of the colon. We use APC settings of different power ranging from 50 to 60 W for the rectum, 40–50 W in the left colon, and 20–30 W for the small bowel, right colon and cecum, with a 0.8–1.5 l/min of argon flow. Care must be taken with lesions located in the small bowel and cecum as the risk of perforation is higher! However, the power can be adjusted to between 0 and 155 W, and gas flow from 0.5 to 7 l/min [3]. The operated distance between the probe and the targeted tissues depends on the power setting. At low power settings the probe must

Table 2. Flexible argon plasma coagulation (APC) probes

APC probe	Product no.	Beam forms	Flexibility	Dimension mm	Length cm	Cleaning in washer disinfector	Sterilization in autoclave	Packaging unit
1500	20132-183	A	flexible	1.5	150	max 95°C	max 138°C	1 piece
1000	20132-178	A	flexible	2.3	100	max 95°C	max 138°C	1 piece
2200	20132-177	A	flexible	2.3	220	max 95°C	max 138°C	1 piece
2200	20132-180	SW	flexible	2.3	220	max 95°C	max 138°C	1 piece
2200	20132-181	SC	flexible	2.3	220	max 95°C	max 138°C	1 piece
3000	20132-179	A	flexible	2.3	300	max 95°C	max 138°C	1 piece
2200	20132-182	A	flexible	3.2	220	max 95°C	max 138°C	1 piece
1500	20132-155	A	flexible	1.5	150	disposable	disposable	10 pieces
3000	20132-212 for DBE	A	flexible	1.5	300	disposable	disposable	10 pieces
2200	20132-156	A	flexible	2.3	220	disposable	disposable	10 pieces
2200	20132-167	SC	flexible	2.3	220	disposable	disposable	10 pieces
2200	20132-186	C	flexible	2.3	220	disposable	disposable	10 pieces
3000	20132-166	A	flexible	2.3	300	disposable	disposable	10 pieces
2200	20132-157	A	flexible	3.2	220	disposable	disposable	10 pieces

A = Axial beam; C = circumferential beam; DBE = double balloon enteroscopy; SC = side fire conical beam; SW = side fire wide beam.

be held closer to the tissue and vice versa. In general, the distance between the probe and tissue can range from 2 to 8 mm. The surface of the targeted tissue must be clear of blood and surface fluids to prevent the development of a coagulated film which leaves the tissue surface beneath inadequately treated.

Hemostasis using a laser is achieved by transmission of photoenergy to the target tissue. This method is rarely used today.

Non-Thermal Modalities

Injection Therapy

Injection Needles ('Sclerotherapy Needles')

Injection needles are used to deliver the injection solution to the intestinal wall. They are designed with outer sheath of plastic, Teflon or stainless steel, and an inner core needle. The needles are available in lengths of 200–240 cm for standard gastroscopes and colonoscopes, and 320–350 cm for the intestinoscopes. Most of the injection needles are marketed as single-use devices, but ones with a full-metal sheath can be sterilized in autoclave. Other features of injection needles include the ability to predetermine the length of the needle nose and the locking mechanism to prevent retracting [7]. The metal sheath enables needle extension with an endoscope in a looped or retroflexed position as it is kink resistant. Some needles are combined with bipolar cautery to allow injection and cauterization with the same instrument [7].

Injection Solutions

Diluted epinephrine is most often used for injection therapy. It is inexpensive and easy to learn. It is used to slow or stop bleeding by tamponade and vasoconstriction. As in treatment of a bleeding ulcer, a 1:10,000 solution is injected in 0.5-ml aliquots around but not into the bleeding lesion until hemostasis is achieved. The total injected volume of diluted epinephrine should be as low as possible (as the absorption has systemic effects) but up to 35–45 ml may be administrated to achieve hemostasis [8, 9]. Standard injection therapy of epinephrine with saline often offers transient relative hemostasis with its effects disappearing rapidly. Therefore, injection therapy can be used in combination with any thermal or mechanical modalities depending on the circumstances. Some experts prefer to first inject and then treat with contact or non-contact thermal hemostatic devices [8–10]. The bleb created with the injection may provide a safe cushion for the application of thermal energy. Other injection solutions for hemostasis include sclerosants such as absolute alcohol; fatty acid derivates (5% ethanolamine oleate and 5% sodium morrhuate; synthetic agents (1 and 3% sodium tetradecyl sulfate, 0.5–3% polidocanol); tissue adhesives (N-butyl-2-cyanoacrylate; Hystoacryl®); fibrin glue (fibrinogen + thrombin) or thrombin alone, and saline and hypertonic (50%) dextrose solutions [11–13]. The use of injection solutions other than diluted epinephrine (1:10,000–1:20,000) is declining but should still be considered applicable as they are well documented to be effective in achieving hemostasis. For the sclerosing agents, attention should be paid as they can cause transmural necrosis and carry the risk of perforation at the injection site.

Because Hystoacryl® can result in arterial embolism, most experts rarely use it, and for this reason it is not available in many countries. However, Histoacryl® is a useful method to treat bleeding gastric varices, a condition for which there are not many other endoscopic options.

Fibrin glue, although simple to use, is relatively more expensive. Its efficacy is comparable to other hemostatic injection solutions.

Endoclips

Endoclips provide mechanical hemostasis without injuring the surrounding tissue and are ideal for hemostasis when a bleeding vessel or small mucosal bleeding defect is visible, such as a bleeding peptic ulcer, post-polypectomy or diverticular bleeding [14–19] (fig. 5a–c). Clips are available in multiple sizes and some can be rotated or reopened while being deployed through the endoscope [20].

Four companies produce disposable hemoclips. (1) Olympus Corp. produces the QuickClip2, which is a rotatable clip device. These devices are produced in two sizes, 8 and 12 mm in width when opened, and 165–230 cm in length, allowing deployment through a colonoscope. (2) Boston Scientific Inc. produces the Resolution Clip which cannot be rotated but can be reopened after closure if repositioning is required. The Resolution Clip has an opening width of 11 mm and is available in lengths of 165 and 235 cm. (3) Wilson-Cook produces the TriClip, a 3-pronged endoclip. The TriClip opens to a width of 12 mm and is 205 cm long. Preliminary experience has not detected obvious advantages of this configuration. (4) Inscope (a division of Ethicon Endosurgery

4

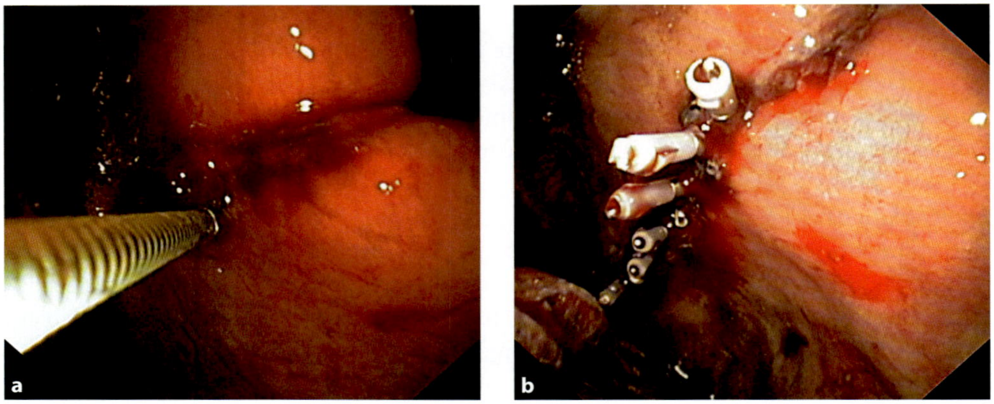

5

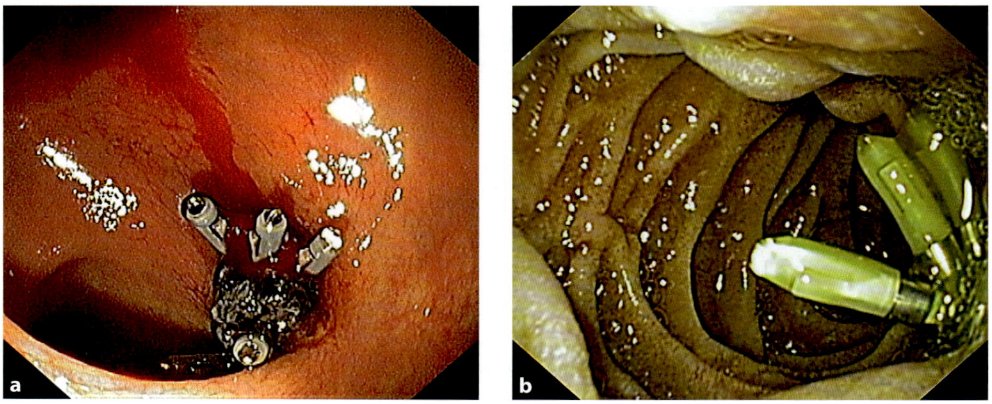

Fig. 4. a Injection of a mixture of epinephrine/saline with a sclerotherapy needle. This patient bled from a gastric lesion after resection of a submucosal tumor. **b** Multiple clips were placed to close the mucosal defect and to stop active bleeding. **Fig. 5. a** Multiple clips were placed for this bleeding duodenal ulcer located in the posterior duodenal bulb. Before placing the clips partial hemostasis had been achieved with epinephrine/ saline solution. In cases with massive gastrointestinal bleeding it is important to avoid the use of epinephrine, if the endoscopist is considering the use of angiography. Epinephrine will constrict the vessels and the radiologist will be limited in his ability to find the bleeding vessel and to apply coils or foam. Photos with the courtesy of Klaus Mönkemüller, MD, PhD (Germany). **b** Another patient with a bleeding duodenal ulcer which was controlled with combination therapy.

Inc.) introduced a multiclip applier with 4 endoclips. The jaws of this device open to a width of 14 mm; the clips are 7 mm when open and have an interlocking distal closure when placed.

Reusable clip deployment devices (EZ Clip) from Olympus are also available mostly in Europe but used infrequently in the United States mainly because they are difficult to clean and sterilize. They are available in 6 different models and sizes.

According to the FDA recommendations, the use of endoclips should be restricted to blood vessels of less than 2 mm in diameter, mucosal or submucosal defects of smaller than 3 cm in size, polyps of smaller than 1.5 cm in diameter, and intestinal perforations of smaller than 2 cm, but all of the aforementioned can be overcome by devices that have a wider span and stronger clip prongs. Loading of the hemoclip onto the applicator must be quick and proper; therefore endoscopy assistants ought to be familiar with its use. Clipping is easiest when the endoscope is

Table 3. Treatment options for acute variceal bleeding (adapted from ref. 11, 32)

	Manufacturers	Catalog No.	Bands per cap, n	Endoscope tip diameter mm
Variceal band ligators				
Stiegmann-Goff and S-G ClearVue endoscopic ligators	ConMed	100225, 200221, 000230, 000227	1	9–11
Auto-Band Ligator multiple-band ligator	Scandimed International ConMed		5, 7, 10	8.6–11.5
Speedband, Superview Super 7 multiple band ligator	Boston Scientific		7	8.6–11.5
Shooter Saeed multiband ligators	Wilson-Cook	MBL-4, MBL-6, MBL-10 (XS)	4, 6, 10	8.5–14
			Individual injection volume, ml	Total dose ml
Sclerotherapy (sclerosants)				
Ethanolamine oleat, 5%	Ethamolin QOL Medical		1.5–5	20
Sodium morrhuate, 5%	Scleromate, Glenwood LIC		0.5–5	15
Sodium tetradecyl sulfate, 1 and 3%	Sotradecol, Bioniche Life Sciences Trombovein, Omega Pharmaceuticals Ltd Fibro-vein, STD Pharmaceutical		0.5–2	10
Polidocanol, 0.5–3%	Ethoxysklerol, Kreussler Pharma Sclerovein, Resinag AG		1–2	15–20
Ethanol 99.5%			0.5–1	4
Tissue adhesives				
N-butyl-2-cyanoacrylate	Histoacryl, Braun Glubran, GEM S.r.l.			
Mechanical hemostasis				
Sengstaken-Blakemore tube				
Covered self-expandable metallic stents, SX Ella Danis	Ella Corp			

kept in a straight position with the possibility of an axial push into the tissue, but the tangential access can sometimes be used to anchor the visible blood vessel. Clips are most easily placed on small lesions where the tissue can be approximated by the clip. The proper orientation of the clip can be achieved by rotating the endoscope shaft with the right hand or, using small wheel turns, maneuvering the target lesion into the desired position. The orientation of the clip can be further adjusted by rotating the handle of the applicator. As the clip is deployed, suction should be applied to draw tissue between the prongs. If the colonoscope is flexed, pushing the clip

Table 4. Injection needles

	Manufacturers	Product No./ Order No.	Needle gauge	Usable for channel size	Catheter length cm	Needle tip extension mm	Single use
Preset variable injection needles							
AcuJect	Wilson-Cook	G22525/VIN-23	23	2.8	220	4	yes
		G22526/VIN-25	25		220	4	yes
Disposable variceal injector	Wilson-Cook	G21694/LDVI-23	23	2.8	200	4	yes
		G21866/LDVI-23-240	23	2.8	240	4	yes
Luer slip		G21697/LDVI-25	25	2.8	200	4	yes
handle		G21649/LDVI-25-240	25	2.8	240	4	yes
		G22722/LDVI-23E	23	2.8	320	4	yes
Enteroscopy		G22723/LDVI-25E	25	2.8	320	4	yes
Interject	Boston-Sci	M00518 (151, 161, 251, 261, 351, 361, 111, 301, 311)	23, 25	2.0, 2.8	200/240	4, 6	yes
Vari-Safe	US-Endoscopy	00711818, 819, 820	23	2.8	230	4, 5, 7	yes
Bipolar cautery							
Injection Gold Probe	Boston-Sci	M00560150 (160)	25	2.8, 3.7	210		
Lockable needle							
Carr-Locke	US Endoscopy	00711811	25	2.8	230	4, 5	
Click-Tip	ConMed/Bard	02-23-180 through 06-19-230	19, 22, 25	2.0, 2.8	180, 230	4, 6	
Injector Force	Olympus	NM-200L/200U/201L	21, 23, 25	2.8	165/230	4, 5, 6, 8	
Flexible tip							
FlexiTip	ConMed/Bard	000215-000138	25	2.8	160, 230	4, 5, 6	
Metal hub on tip							
With metal hub	Wilson-Cook	G22992/LDVI-23-MH	23	2.8	200	4	
		G22994/LDVI-25-MH	25	2.8	200	4	
Irrigation channel							
Injectaflow	Wilson-Cook	G22747/VINF-23	23	2.8	220	4	yes
		G22748/VINF-25	25	2.8	220	4	yes
Fully metal sheath							
Articulator	US Endoscopy	00711803, 804, 807, 808	25	2.8	160/230/ 350	4, 5	
SureShot	ConMed/Bard	100218	25	2.8	230	5	
Disposable needle	Olympus	NM-8L-1;NM-9L-1	23	2.0	165, 230	4, 6	

Adapted from Nelson et al. [7].

Table 5. Endoscopic clips

	Manufacturer	Article No.	Ready to use	Working channel mm	Working length cm	Maximum opening width, mm	Rotability/ re-opening
Rotating Clip	Olympus	HX-5LR/QR-1 HX-6UR-1	no	≥2.8 (5LR/QR >3.2 (6UR)	230 (6U) 195 (5Q) 165 (5L)	11	yes/no
Quick Clip2	Olympus	HX-201LR/UR-135	yes	≥2.8	240 (UR) 165 cm (LR)	9.5	yes/no
Quick Clip 2 Long	Olympus	HX-201LR/UR-135L	yes	≥2.8	240 (UR) 165 (LR)	11	yes/no
EZ Clip	Olympus	HX-610-090, 090L, 090S, 135, 135S, 090SC	yes	≥2.8	165 and 230	8	yes
Resolution Clip	Boston Scientific	M005226XX	yes	≥2.8	235 and 155	11	no/5 times
TriClip	Wilson Cook	TC-8-12	yes	≥2.8	205	12	no/no
TriClip	Wilson Cook	TC-7-12	yes	≥2.8	207	12	no/no
InScope Multiclip applier	InScope, Ethicon Endo-Surgery						yes/yes

Adapted from Cipoletta et al. [18], Raju et al. [19] and Yeh et al. [20].

applicator out of the working channel is difficult; therefore, it is sometimes necessary to withdraw the endoscope slightly, advance the applicator out of the endoscope in the straightened position, and then again try to reach the bleeding lesion. Prongs should always be fully opened in the lumen but not against the intestinal wall.

Band Ligation (fig. 1)
The most common indication for endoscopic band ligation is the prophylaxis and treatment of esophageal variceal bleeding. For primary prevention of esophageal variceal bleeding, endoscopic variceal banding or band ligation has been shown to be safer and possibly more effective than non-selective β-blockers (propranolol or nadolol) [21–24]. Endoscopic band ligation is also superior to sclerotherapy for secondary prevention of variceal bleeding [24].

The data on endoscopic band ligation for the management of non-variceal bleeding are scarce and mostly in the form of case reports. They include the use of band ligation to control bleeding from Mallory-Weiss tear, Dieulafoy's lesion, arteriovenous malformations, colonic diverticula, as well as from the ulcer and post-polypectomy bleeding [14, 15, 25]. Endoscopic banding devices that are commercially available include single-band and multiband devices (table 3). Single-band ligators require the placement of an overtube for repeated intubations.

Table 6. Thermal modalities

	Manu-facturer	Product No./ order No.	OD mm	Working channel mm	Working length cm	Pulses, n/pulse duration, s	Power setting
Heat probe							
	Olympus	HPU-20 + CD-110U, 120U		2.8, 3.7	230, 230	4/8–10	15–30 J
	Olympus	HPU + CD-110U, 120U		2.8, .7	300, 300	4/8–10	15–30 J
MPEC Probes							
BICAP 5, 7, 10 Fr	Circon			2.2, 2.8, 3.7		/6–10	15–20 W
Gold Probe 7, 10 Fr	Boston Scientific			>2.8, 3.7		/6–10	15–20 W
Injection Gold Probe 7, 10 Fr	Boston Scientific			>2.8, 3.7		/6–10	15–20 W
Quicksilver 7, 10 Fr	Wilson Cook			>2.8, 3.7			15–20 W
HEMArrest 7, 10 Fr	Bard			>2.8, 3.7			15–20 W
Bipolar coagulation probe dual plug	Diagmed	711841	7	2.8	350		
Bipolar coagulation probe single plug	Diagmed	711843	7	2.8	350		
Bipolar coagulation probe single plug	Diagmed	711 847	10	3.7	350		
APC probes							
1500 A	ERBE	20132-183	1.5		150	Cleaning in washer disinfector max 95°C Sterilization in autoclave max 138°C; one piece per pack; beam forms (axial, circumferential, side fire conical and side fire wide beams)	
1000 A	ERBE	20132-178	2.3		100		
2200 A	ERBE	20132-177	2.3		220		
2200 SW	ERBE	20132-180	2.3		220		
2200 SC	ERBE	20132-181	2.3		220		
3000 A	ERBE	20132-179	2.3		300		
2200 A	ERBE	20132-182	3.2		220		
1500 A	ERBE	20132-155	1.5		150		
3000 A	ERBE	20132-212 for double enteroscopy	1.5		300	Suitable for double balloon; disposable; 10 pieces/pack	

Table 6. Continued

	Manu-facturer	Product No./ order No.	OD mm	Working channel mm	Working length cm	Pulses, n/pulse duration, s	Power setting
2200 A	ERBE	20132-156	2.3		220	Disposable; 10 pieces/ pack	
2200 SC	ERBE	20132-167	2.3		220		
2200 C	ERBE	20132-186	2.3		220		
3000 A	ERBE	20132-166	2.3		300		
2200 A	ERBE	20132-157	3.2		220		
APC probe	ConMed		2.3				
APC probe	Olympus	MAJ-1012-N1034560		2.8	220	Single use; 10 pieces/ pack	
	Olympus	MAJ-1011-E0427826		3.2	220		
	Olympus	MAJ-1011-N1034460		2.8			
	Olympus	MAJ-1011-E0427825		3.2			
Hot biopsy							
Radial Jaw 3	Boston Scientific	M00515501	2.2	2.8	240		
Endobite hot	Medical Innovations	Hot1c123230		2.8–4.2		Hot oval cup insulated	
Hot biopsy forceps	MTW Endoscopie		1.8, 2.2, 2.6, 3.4	2.0–4.2	160, 230	Oval spoon-shaped mouth	
Hot biopsy forceps	Fujinon		2.3, 2.5	2.8	180, 230	Oval spoon-shaped mouth with window, coil distal tapered, Teflon-coated	
Hot biopsy forceps	Olympus	FD-1L-1 FD-1U-1	2.8	3.2	165, 230		
Hot Maxx	Cook		2.5	2.8	230	Non-spiked	
Odon	Alkapharm		2.5	2.8	220	Oval cup	
Precisor Hot	Conmed					Disposable Oval cup active	

www.omed-catalogue.com/sscategoriedes; www.endocompare.com; www.erbe-med.com/

Table 7. Electrosurgical units

ESI	Manufacturer	Product No.	Description	Cutting power W	Blended cutting	Coagulation	Bipolar
Aaron 1250™	Bovie Medical Corporation		The Aaron 1250™, by Bovie®, features cut, blend, coagulation, fulguration, and bipolar modes. Bovie incorporates automatic safety features into the Aaron 1250 such as self-test circuits, audible tones, discreet outputs, isolated circuitry, and Bovie NEM™ (neutral electrode monitoring)	120	90	80/40	30
Aaron 2250™	Bovie Medical Corporation		Large illuminated digital displays 5 output modes: cut, blend, coagulation (pinpoint and fulguration) and bipolar	200	200	120/80	80
Aaron 3250™	Bovie Medical Corporation		Nine presets large illuminated digital displays 6 output modes: cut I, cut II, blend, coagulation (pinpoint and fulguration) and bipolar	300/ 300	200	120/80	80
ICON Gi	Bovie Medical Corporation	GI120		200	100	120/80	80/50
BICAP®II	Conmed		Bipolar output. Precision timer helps regulate applications. Designed specifically for BiCap® bipolar accessories. Integral fluid pump permits irrigation 80 ml/min nominal fluid flow rate. Monopolar and bipolar capabilities				
Surgitron® Dual Frequency RF/120 IEC	Ellman		www.ellman.com/ products/medical/ radiosurgical_units.htm				
VIO 300D	ERBE		VIO Cut Modes: AUTOCUT™ Monopolar Cutting-Automated Software Power Dosing. HIGHCUT™ – unique cutting mode with broad power curve and 8 different effects for hemostasis. DRY CUT™ – intense hemostasis with slower cutting speed for cuts requiring primary hemostasis. ENDO CUT™ IQ –two different modes for spincterotomy and snare procedures. VIO Coag Modes:				

Table 7. Continued

ESI	Manufacturer	Product No.	Description	Cutting power W	Blended cutting	Coagulation	Bipolar
VIO 300D	ERBE		SWIFT COAG™ – fast coagulation for dissection with a high degree of hemostasis. SPRAY COAG™ – non-contact surface coagulation, low penetration depths. VIO Bipolar Modes: BIPOLAR CUT™ – For applications requiring cutting of a structure with restricted return pathway. BIPOLAR SOFT COAG™ – low voltage penetration based on effect level and time of activation. AUTOSTART™ – instrument activation without a foot pedal. AUTOSTOP™ – automatic end of tissue activation based on resistance. BIPOLAR FORCED COAG™ – fast Bipolar coagulation ENDO CUT IQ. The new ENDO CUT IQ offers two new procedures suitable for GI intervention: ENDO CUT IQ lets you program 4 levels of hemostasis and 8 levels of cutting speed to meet the demanding needs of your individual technique. I is the mode Used for needle electrodes and sphincterotomies. Q is the mode used for snare wire or loop electrodes				
ICC 200 E and ICC 200EA	ERBE		Power on Demand ENDO CUT™ – the physicians choice for polypectomy and sphincterotomy. FORCED COAG™ SOFT COAG™ expandable for argon use. Compatible with all accessories, including: snare wires, sphincterotomes, hemostasis probes, hot biopsy forceps				
Valleylab SurgiStat™ II	Valleylab		Includes both monopolar and bipolar outputs. Increased patient safety with a return electrode contact quality monitoring system (RECQMS). The RECQMS system continually monitors patient impedance levels and deactivates the generator if a fault in the patient/return electrode contact is detected				

www.omed-catalogue.com/sscategoriedes.

Table 8. Endoscopic methods to stop bleeding from ulcer, Mallory-Weiss tears, angiodysplasia, watermelon stomach, and Dieulafoy lesion

	Ulcer	Mallory-Weiss tear	Dieulafoy[1]	GAVE	Angiodysplasia
Injection therapy solution	Yes Epinephrine solution (1:10,000) Ethanol (99%) Hypertonic saline, thrombin, fibrin glue, polidocanol sodium tetradecyl sulfate	Yes Epinephrine solution (1:10,000) Polidocanol	Yes Epinephrine solution Polidocanol cyanoacrylate glue, sodium tetradecyl sulfate, hypertonic glucose, ethanol	No	Yes No Tetradecyl sulfate
Heater probe Probe size Power settings, J Pulses, n	Yes Large/small 15–30 4–5	Yes Large/small 20 3	Yes Large 30 4	Yes Large 30	Yes Large/small 10–20
MPEC Bipolar or Gold probe Probe size Power settings, W Pulse duration, s	 Yes Large/small 15–25 6–14	 Yes Large/small 15–20 4	 Yes Large 15–20 8–10	 Yes Large/ small 10–15 1–2	 Yes Large/small 10–15 1–2
APC Power settings, W Argon flow, liters/min	Yes	No	Yes 60–80 1–2	Yes 60–80 1–2	Yes 60–8W 1–2
Band ligators	Yes?[2]	Yes	Yes	No	Yes?[2]
Endoclips	yes	yes	yes	no	no

Adapted from Thomas et al. [26].

[1] Mechanical methods (clipping or banding) and combined therapy using injection of different solution including epinephrine (1:10,000) or 5% ethanolamine oleate solution followed by thermal coagulation is significantly better than injection methods alone [14, 27–29, 33].

[2] Limited data [15, 29–31].

Endoscopic Therapeutic Options for Various Bleeding Conditions

Acute Variceal Bleeding

Endoscopy is an essential step in the diagnosis and treatment of acute variceal bleeding. The goal of therapeutic endoscopy is to stop acute variceal bleeding by creating an intravariceal thrombus. Repeated procedures may ultimately induce variceal obliteration. Two techniques are in common use: endoscopic sclerotherapy and endoscopic variceal ligation. In endoscopic sclerotherapy, an irritant solution (e.g., sodium morrhuate, ethanolamine or polidocanol) or a dehydrating chemical (e.g., sodium tetradecyl sulfate) is injected into an esophageal varix or its adjacent supporting tissues. Variceal ligation has proved more effective and safer than

Table 9. Accessories used for hemostasis in small bowel

	Manufacturer	Catalog No.	Channel size, mm
APC probes	ERBE	20132-212	2.2
		20132-166	2.8
		20132-179 (reusable)	2.8
Lubricant	Fresenius Kabi	MCT oil	
Injection needles	Fujinon	F2EZTV1805250HP-S	2.2
	Medwork	500753	
Endoclips	Boston Sci	Resolution Clip 22612	2.8
	Olympus	Quick Clip HX-201UR-135	2.8
Hot biopsy forceps	Fujinon	F6HOPK2304250X	2.8
Fibrin glue (Beriplast®)	Various providers (Canteon, Marburg, Germany)		
Epinephrine solution			

Adapted from Schäfer and Stange [34].

sclerotherapy and is currently the endoscopic treatment of choice for esophageal varices. Besides, it is worth noting that in acute bleeding, vasoactive drugs and antibiotic prophylaxis should be started before endoscopy and maintained for 2–5 days. The efficacy of vasoactive drugs is improved when associated with emergency endoscopic therapy.

Non-Variceal Upper Gastrointestinal Hemorrhage

Acute upper non-variceal GI bleeding is a medical emergency. Peptic ulcer is the most common cause of upper non-variceal GI bleeding. Less common causes include Mallory-Weiss tears, Dieulafoy's lesions, erosive esophagitis, tumors and telangiectasias. Several endoscopic methods have been used to control GI hemorrhage. Endoscopic diagnosis and treatment of severe upper GI bleeding should be performed with therapeutic video endoscopes that have a single large suction channel (3.7–6 mm diameter) or two suction channels, if available.

A number of endoscopic methods for upper GI bleeding hemostasis have been evaluated. Because of their efficacy, safety and relatively low cost they range from well-known thermal devices (multipolar probes and heater probes) to novel redesigned mechanical devices such as endoscopic hemoclips that have also been widely adopted. Tables 4–7 are lists and information on various types of hemostatic devices.

Any of these methods can be used with or without prior injection of dilute epinephrine (1:10,000 to 1:20,000). Epinephrine injection is often used initially (before thermal coagulation or hemoclipping) to treat bleeding lesions or to prevent re-bleeding induced by clot removal or contact with accessories.

Table 10. Endoscopic modalities for lower gastrointestinal bleeding

	Diverticula	Angiectasia	Radiation proctitis	Postpolypectomy bleeding	Cancer
Injection therapy solution	Yes Epinephrine solution (1:10,00)	Yes Various sclerosants		Yes Epinephrine solution (1:10,00)	Yes Epinephrine solution (1:10 000) Ethanol (99%)
Heater probe	Yes	Yes	Yes	Yes	Yes
Probe size, Fr	7 or 10	7 or 10	7 or 10	10	10
Power settings, J	10–15	10–15	10–15	10–20	20–25
Pulses, n	Until bleeding stops		Until bleeding stops; white coagulation	Until bleeding stops	Until bleeding stops
MPEC					
Bipolar or Gold probe					
Probe size, Fr	Yes	Yes	Yes	Yes	Yes
Power settings, W	7–10	7 or 10	7 or 10	10	10
Pulse duration, s	12–16	10–16	10–16	10–20	16–20
	1–2	1	1	1–2	1–2
APC	No	Yes	Yes	Yes if diffuse after EMR	No data available
Power settings, W		15–40	15–40		
Argon flow, liters/min		1	1	40–60	
VIO technology				1–2	
Power setting, W		10–30 mode pulsed 2; thinner wall precise mode. High risk of rebleeding	10–30 mode pulsed 2; thinner wall precise mode. Retreatment often needed		
Band ligators	Yes?[1]	No	No	No	No
Endoclips	Yes	No	No	Yes	No

[1] Needs to be proven in larger case-series.

Bleeding Peptic Ulcer

Endoscopic treatment of a bleeding peptic ulcer is determined by its endoscopic appearance. The majority of bleeding from gastric and duodenal ulcers is self-limited. There is general agreement that endoscopic therapy is indicated for actively bleeding lesions as well as for high-risk stigmata of recent hemorrhage, including visible vessel, and possibly an adherent clot. Endoscopic therapies include: injection therapy, such as epinephrine or sclerosant injection; ablative therapy, such as heater probe or argon plasma coagulation, and mechanical therapy, such as endoclips or endoscopic banding. Endoscopic therapy reduces the risk of re-bleeding, the need for blood transfusions, the requirement for surgery, and patient morbidity (table 8). In achieving primary hemostasis and prevention of re-bleeding none of the methods is ideal but outcomes after endoscopic clip application alone or in combination with injection therapy seem to be advantageous but not superior over other endoscopic treatment modalities [14].

Bleeding from the Small Intestine

The double-balloon enteroscope has a working length of 200 cm and an outer diameter of 8.5 or 9.5 mm, and it has flexible overtube with a length of 145 cm and an outer diameter of 12 or 13 mm. The soft latex balloons are attached to the tips of both the enteroscope and the overtube and are inflated and deflated by a specifically designed pump. The examination can either be orally or per anally. The diagnostic yield of double balloon enteroscopy in the diagnosis of obscure GI bleeding is 43–87% and the therapeutic impact is 62–84% [34–36]. In this setting, the double balloon technique is complementary to capsule endoscopy and its therapeutic impact in achieving hemostasis is 62–84%. Despite the temporary limitation in available accessories that are sufficiently long and slim to be passed through the working channel of the enteroscope, there is an increasing range of accessories that can be used to achieve hemostasis in small intestine (table 9).

Lower Gastrointestinal Bleeding

Table 10 shows the possible endoscopic modalities for lower GI bleeding.

References

1 Nelson DB, Barkun AN, Block KP, et al: Technology status evaluation report. Endoscopic hemostatic devices. May 2001. Gastrointest Endosc 2001;54:833–840.

2 Jensen DM, Machicado GA, Cheng S, Jensen ME, Jutabha R: A randomized prospective study of endoscopic bipolar electrocoagulation and heater probe treatment of chronic rectal bleeding from radiation teleangiectasia. Gastrointest Endosc 1997;45:20–25.

3 Ginsberg GG, Barkun AN, Bosco JJ, et al: Argon plasma coagulator: February 2002. Gastrointest Endosc 2002;55:807–810.

4 Manner H, Plum N, Pech O, Ell C, Enderle M: Colon explosion during plasma coagulation. Gastrointest Endosc 2008;67:1123–1127.

5 Villavicencio RT, Rex DK, Rahmani E: Efficacy and complications of argon plasma coagulation for haematochezia related to radiation proctopathy. Gastrointest Endosc 2002;55:70–74.

6 Ben-Soussan E, Antonietti M, Savoye G, Herve S, Ducrotte P, Lerebours E: Argon plasma coagulation in the treatment of hemorrhagic radiation proctitis is efficient but requires a perfect colonic cleansing to be safe. Eur J Gastroenterol Hepatol 2004;16:1315–1318.

7 Nelson DB, Bosco JJ, Curtis WD, et al: ASGE technology status evaluation report. Injection needles. February 1999. American Society for Gastrointestinal Endoscopy. Gastrointest Endosc 1999;50:928–931.

8 Park CH, Joo YE, Kim HS, et al: A prospective, randomized trial comparing mechanical methods of hemostasis plus epinephrine injection to epinephrine injection alone for bleeding peptic ulcer. Gastrointest Endosc 2004;60:173–179.

9 Machiado GA, Jensen DM: Endoscopic hemostasis of ulcer hemorrhage with injection, thermal and combination methods. Tech Gastrointest Endosc 2005;7:124–131.

10 Bianco MA, Rotondano G, Marmo R, et al: Combined epinephrine and bipolar probe coagulation vs. bipolar probe coagulation alone for bleeding peptic ulcer: a randomized, controlled trial. Gastrointest Endosc 2004;60:910–915.

11 Croffie J, Somogyi L, Chuttani R, et al: Sclerosing agents for use in GI endoscopy. Gastrointest Endosc 2007;66:1–6.

12 Ryou M, Thompson CC: Tissue adhesives: a review. Tech Gastrointest Endosc 2006;8:33–37.

13 Gevers A, Rutgeerts P: Fibrin glue for nonvariceal hemorrhage. Tech Gastrointest Endosc 1999;1:122–125.
14 Yuan Y, Wang C, Hunt RH: Endoscopic clipping for acute nonvariceal upper-GI bleeding: a meta-analysis and critical appraisal of randomized controlled trials. Gastrointest Endosc 2008;68:339–351.
15 Misra SP, Dwivedi M, Misra V, et al: Endoscopic band ligation as salvage therapy in patients with bleeding peptic ulcers not responding to injection therapy. Endoscopy 2005;37:626–629.
16 Park CH, Sohn YH, Lee WS, et al: The usefulness of endoscopic hemoclipping for bleeding Dieulafoy's lesions. Endoscopy 2003;35:388–392.
17 Gottumukkala SR, Kaltenbach T, Soetikno R: Endoscopic mechanical hemostasis of GI arterial bleeding. Gastrointest Endosc 2007;66:774–785.
18 Cipolletta L, Rotondano G, Bianco MA, Piscopo R: Mechanical modalities of endoscopic therapy: clips, loops, and beyond. Tech Gastrointest Endosc 2005;7: 132–138.
19 Raju GS, Kaltenbach T, Soetikno R: Endoscopic mechanical hemostasis of GI arterial bleeding. Gastrointest Endosc 2007;66:774–785.
20 Yeh RW, Kaltenbach T, Soetikno R: Endoclips. Tech Gastrointest Endosc 2006;8:2–11.
21 Deschenes M, Barkun AN: Comparison of endoscopic ligation and propranolol for the primary prevention of variceal bleeding. Gastrointest Endosc 2000;51:630–633.
22 Sarin SK, Lamba GS, Kumar M, et al: Comparison of endoscopic ligation and propranolol for the primary prevention of variceal bleeding. N Engl J Med 1999; 340:988–993.
23 Lo GH, Chen WC, Chen MH, et al: Endoscopic ligation vs. nadolol in the prevention of first variceal bleeding in patients with cirrhosis. Gastrointest Endosc 2004;59:333–338.
24 Khuroo MS, Khuroo NS, Farahat KL, et al: Meta-analysis: endoscopic variceal ligation for primary prophylaxis of oesophageal variceal bleeding. Aliment Pharmacol Ther 2005;21:347–361.
25 Zapeda-Gomez S, Marcon NE: Endoscopic band ligation for nonvariceal bleeding: a review. Can J Gastroenterol 2008;22:748–752.
26 Thomas O, Kovacs G: Mallory-Weiss tears, angiodysplasia, watermelon stomach and Dieulafoy's: a potpourri. Tech Gastrointest Endosc 2005;7:139–147.
27 Cheng CL, Liu NJ, Lee CS, et al: Endoscopic management of Dieulafoy's lesions in acute nonvariceal upper gastrointestinal bleeding. Dig Dis Sci 2004; 49:1139–1144.
28 McGrath K, Mergener K, Branch S: Endoscopic band ligation of Dieulafoy's lesions: report of two cases and review of the literature. Am J Gastroenterol 1999;94:1087–1090.
29 Park CH, Joo YE, Kim HS, et al: A prospective randomized trial of endoscopic band ligation versus endoscopic hemoclip placement for bleeding gastric Dieulafoy's lesions. Endoscopy 2004;36:677–681.
30 Park CH, Lee WS, Joo YE, et al: Endoscopic band ligation for control of acute peptic ulcer bleeding. Endoscopy 2004;36:79–82.
31 Banerjee B, Trivedi MH, Swied AM: Endoscopic band ligation for gastric ulcer bleeding. Surg Laparosc Endosc Percutan Tech 2000;10:246–248.
32 ASGE Technology Committee, Liu J, Petersen BT, Tierney WM, et al: Endoscopic banding devices. Gastrointest Endosc 2008;68:217–221.
33 Mumtaz R, Shaukat M, Ramirez FC: Outcomes of endoscopic treatment of gastroduodenal Dieulafoy's lesions with rubber band ligation and thermal/injection therapy. J Clin Gastroenterol 2003;36:310–314.
34 Schäfer C, Stange EF: Therapeutic possibilities with DBE: a focus on accessories. Tech Gastrointest Endosc 2008;10:70–76.
35 Mönkemüller K, Olano C, Fry LC, Malfertheiner P: Small-bowel endoscopy. Endoscopy 2009;41:55–58.
36 Fry LC.Bellutti M, Neumann H, Malfertheiner P, Mönkemüller K: Incidence of bleeding lesions within reach of conventional upper and lower endoscopes in patients undergoing double-balloon. Aliment Pharmacol Ther 2009;29:342–349.

Ivan Jovanović, MD, PhD
Clinic for Gastroenterology and Hepatology
Clinical Center of Serbia
CS–11000 Belgrade (Serbia)
Tel./Fax + 381 11 361 5587, E-Mail ivangastro@beotel.rs

Mönkemüller K, Wilcox CM, Muñoz-Navas M (eds): Interventional and Therapeutic Gastrointestinal Endoscopy.
Front Gastrointest Res. Basel, Karger, 2010, vol 27, pp 37–54

Endoscopic Therapy for Peptic Ulcer Bleeding

Shajan Peter · C. Mel Wilcox

Division of Gastroenterology and Hepatology, University of Alabama at Birmingham, Birmingham, Ala., USA

Abstract

Among the gastrointestinal emergencies, acute upper gastrointestinal bleeding (UGIB) remains a challenging clinical problem owing to significant patient morbidity and costs involved with management. Peptic ulcer bleeding (PUB) contributes to the majority of causes of UGIB with a growing concern of its impact on the elderly and the increasing use of NSAIDs as precipitating bleeding episodes. Apart from initial critical assessment and care, endoscopy remains as the preferred initial management of PUB. Early use of high-dose proton pump inhibitor therapy is cost-effective and reduces the need for endotherapy as well as rebleed rates. Current endoscopic modalities offer a wide range of choices in high-risk PUB (active arterial bleeding or non-bleeding visible vessel). A combination of injection (epinephrine) along with thermal or endoclips therapy offers the best strategy for overall successful clinical outcomes. The role of endotherapy for adherent clots is controversial. A second-look endoscopy may be beneficial in high-risk patients. A multidisciplinary team approach should be part of all treatment protocols for the ideal management of UGIB.

Peptic ulcer bleeding (PUB) continues to account for 28–59% of all episodes of upper gastrointestinal bleeding (UGIB) [1]. Recent epidemiological estimates show incidence rates for UGIB of about 60 per 100,000 population [2]. Though the prevalence of ulcers related to *Helicobacter pylori* are steadily declining at least in the Western world, these have been overtaken by aspirin and other non-steroidal anti-inflammatory drugs (NSAIDs) as underlying causes of ulcer. The mortality rate from peptic ulcer disease has continued to rise progressively with age along with complications of perforation and hemorrhage [3]. Much of the increase in the frequency of peptic ulcer disease, particularly gastric ulcer, in the elderly is attributable to the high prevalence of NSAID use in this population. In addition to the use of NSAIDs for inflammatory conditions, increasing numbers of elderly patients take aspirin for cardiovascular and neurologic prophylaxis. Wilcox [4] reported that 65% of patients who had UGIB were taking aspirin or other NSAIDs, often administered without a prescription. In elderly patients, the risk of serious, adverse gastrointestinal events in patients taking non-selective NSAIDs is 5 times that of controls, whereas the risk in younger patients is slightly more than 1.5. Associated comorbidities in the older patient shifts the mortality rates upward approaching 7–10%, thus early diagnosis and treatment remains critical in such patients to best improve outcome [5].

Endoscopy with hemostatic therapy has clearly been shown to aid in proper diagnosis, prognosticate requirement for blood transfusions and in the majority of instances obviates the need

Table 1a. Rockall risk prediction score [12]

Variable	Score			
	0	1	2	3
Age, years	<60	60–79	>79	
Shock	BP >100 mm Hg pulse <100 bpm	BP >100 mm Hg pulse >100 bpm	BP <100 mm Hg pulse >100 bpm	
Comorbidity	none		cardiac disease, any other major comorbidity	renal failure, liver failure, disseminated malignancy
Endoscopic diagnosis	Mallory-Weiss tear, no lesion	all other diagnoses	malignancy of the upper GI tract	
Major SRH	none, or dark spots		blood in the upper GI tract, adherent clot or spurting vessel	

BP = Blood pressure; GI = gastrointestinal; SRH = stigmata of recent hemorrhage; bpm = beats per minute. Clinical score (pre-EGD) = age + shock + comorbidity; Minimal score = 0; Risk category clinical score: low = 0. Complete score (post-EGD) = clinical score + diagnosis + SRH; Maximum score (complete) = 11; Risk category (complete score): low <2, intermediate 3–4; high >5.

for surgical intervention [6–8]. In most management protocols, endoscopy is well accepted as the first-line management tool. This chapter will focus on the role of endoscopic therapy as part of the broader concept of a gastrointestinal bleeding/hemostatic-team-directed management for bleeding peptic ulcers.

Procedural Aspects

Initial Assessment, Evaluation and Preparation of the Patient

Initial assessment and evaluation of the patient starts in the emergency room or at the bedside if the patient bled during hospitalization. Hematemesis and/or melena are the commonest manifestations of UGIB. Significant bleeding results in hemodynamic alterations reflected by resting tachycardia (pulse ≥100 bpm), hypotension (systolic blood pressure <100 mm Hg), or postural changes (increase in the pulse ≥20 bpm or a drop in the systolic blood pressure of ≥20 mm Hg on standing). Clues such as dry mucous membranes, non-distensible neck veins, and decreased urinary output also point towards significant intravascular volume depletion.

Clinical assessment will best determine the fluid requirement needed for hemodynamic stabilization [9]. Large-bore intravenous (IV) access, judicial use of crystalloids; plasma expanders or

Table 1b. Glasgow-Blatchford's score risk prediction score

Admission risk marker	Score
A. Blood urea, mmol/l*	
≥25	6
10–<25	4
8–<10	3
6.5–<8	2
<6.5	0
B. H, g/l	
<100 in men and women	6
100–<120 in men only	3
100–<120 in women	1
120–<130 in men	
≥120 in women	0
≥130 in men	
C. SBP, mm Hg	
<90	3
90–99	2
100–109	1
≥110	0
D. Other markers	
Cardiac failure	2
Hepatic disease	2
Presentation with syncope	2
Presentation with melena	1

Total score: A+B+C+D. Range of scores is from 0 to 23; maximum score is 23, high risk, >0.
* Blood urea conversion: 1 mg/dl equals 0.357 mmol/l.

packed red cells can be dictated by the clinical setting. The use of nasogastric tube lavage is controversial though this might be helpful to prognosticate outcome when visualizing fresh blood and to confirm an upper gastrointestinal source for patients without hematemesis [10]. Erythromycin, a motilin receptor agonist, promotes gastric motility and thereby enhances visualization during endoscopy. A recent cost-effective analysis showed the strategy of administering erythromycin prior to endoscopy for UGIB improves overall cost saving as well as quality-adjusted life years [11].

Early and timely prediction of the outcomes of gastrointestinal hemorrhage poses a major question in clinical management. Poor clinical outcomes are consistently related to advanced age, presence of comorbidities, most notably cirrhosis, renal failure, or cardiopulmonary disease, presence of red hematemesis, hematochezia or bright red nasogastric aspirate, hemodynamic instability and laboratory abnormalities such as coagulopathy and anemia. Several independent risk factors for outcome have been established with reasonable accuracy and validated using clinical, laboratory as well as endoscopic parameters. Some of the primary outcomes measured by these scoring systems have been mortality as determined by the Rockall score (table 1a), recurrent hemorrhage for the Baylor score, and need for clinical intervention for the Glasgow-Blatchford's score (table 1b) [12, 13]. In a recent prospective study of low-risk

Table 2. Endoscopic stigmata of PUB

Endoscopic finding	Risk of rebleeding	Risk of bleeding after endoscopic therapy
High-risk lesions Active bleeding	90%	45–50%
Non-bleeding visible vessel	50%	20–30%
Adherent clot	30%	10–20%
Low-risk lesions Oozing without visible vessel	10–20%	5–8%
Flat spot	5–10%	4%
Clean base	3–5%	1–3%

patients with UGIB, the Glasgow-Blatchford's score outscored the Rockall score in predicting the need for intervention or death. Using this in clinical practice, 68% of patients could be classified as low risk and thereby managed as outpatients [14]. These risk scoring systems, however, have had variable predictive outcomes and it is questionable whether they have been accepted widely into daily clinical practice primarily relating to concerns regarding accuracy, user friendliness and clinical applicability. Nonetheless, it is increasingly recognized that such outcome predictors are needed to best triage patients to further reduce morbidity and mortality secondary to gastrointestinal bleeding.

The site of performing the endoscopy varies between each center depending on the expertise and personnel involved. In high-risk patients who are hemodynamically instable, most centers recommend the ICU setting. Some centers have facilities in the emergency room itself where endoscopy can be performed safely. The advantage of an easy-access mobile endoscopic travel-cart fully equipped with all the necessary accessories in these situations is being increasingly recognized. We prefer to perform endoscopy in the hospital endoscopy suite in low-risk patients or those who have been downgraded from a higher risk category. Further triaging for hospital admission and need for ICU monitoring can be established by the endoscopic findings and outcome of endoscopic therapy, if performed. In the patient with more severe bleeding, a double channel endoscope (therapeutic endoscope) is useful mainly for the purpose of lavage, better visualization, and ability to use the 10-Fr heater probe (HP), although there are no clear data on its advantages. In patients with ulcers located in the posterior wall of the stomach or duodenum, a colonoscope may facilitate endoscopic therapy as the working channel is located on the right side (i.e. 5-o'clock position) [15]. In addition, the channel of the colonoscope allows passing a 10-Fr HP.

Informed written consent is obtained from each patient explaining the risks, benefits, alternatives and the procedure technique including sedation and therapeutic intervention. If the patient is unable to give consent, it is obtained from the legal guardian. The standard of care should follow hospital protocols.

Sedation aims for quieter well-relaxed patients which is important for successful endoscopic therapy. The combination of a narcotic and benzodiazepine is most commonly employed for conscious sedation. Continuous hemodynamic monitoring including oxygen saturation is

Table 3. Modalities available for endoscopic therapy

1.	Injection therapy a. Epinephrine b. Hypertonic saline c. Sclerosant (absolute alcohol, polidoconol) d. Tissue adhesives: cyanoacyralate, thrombin/fibrin glue
2.	Thermal therapy a. Contact: HP, bipolar (gold probe, BICAP) b. Non-contact: APC, Nd:YAG laser
3.	Mechanical therapy a. Endoclips b. Endoscopic band ligation
4.	Dual therapy (combination of above modalities)

mandatory. The administration of conscious sedation has been usually gastroenterologist-directed; however, many centers now use the help of a nurse anesthetist. An anesthesiologist may be considered in high-risk situations where endotracheal intubation may be necessary. The growing use of propofol for moderate sedation is recognized though the role of non-anesthetist administered propofol sedation in acute UGIB is debatable and more data is needed before this can be widely recommended [16].

The stigmata of hemorrhage seen at endoscopy can be classified as (i) high-risk lesions – spurt blood (Forrest grade IA), ooze blood (grade IB), a non-bleeding visible vessel (grade IIA) or adherent clot (grade IIB), or (ii) low-risk lesions are those with a flat, pigmented spot (grade IIC) or clean base (grade III) (table 1; fig. 1–11). Those lesions with high risk (active bleeding or non-bleeding visible vessel) should receive endoscopic therapy as many studies now demonstrate a reduction in rebleeding, the major cause of morbidity and mortality in UGIB [17].

Accessories and Techniques for Endoscopic Therapy

Many techniques are available for effective endoscopic hemostatic therapy. These can be categorized based upon their mechanism of action: (a) injection therapy, (b) thermal coagulation, (c) mechanical therapy, or (d) a combination of these (table 3; fig. 1–11).

Injection Therapy

This form of therapy aims at controlling bleeding by means of hydrostatic tamponading pressure, vasoconstriction, and/or possibly a secondary inflammatory reaction. It is the simplest and commonest used technique. The advantages of this technique are that it is easy to learn and requires only a sclerotherapy needle for implementation. The disadvantages are that the area injected should be accurate for best results or, if not well placed, could mask the visible area for treatment. Also, the effects are short lasting, as the injected fluid gradually dissipates [18].

Commonly used forms of injection therapy include: (1) Epinephrine, this is diluted (1:10,000) and administered through a 25-gauge retractable sclerotherapy needle. Volumes of

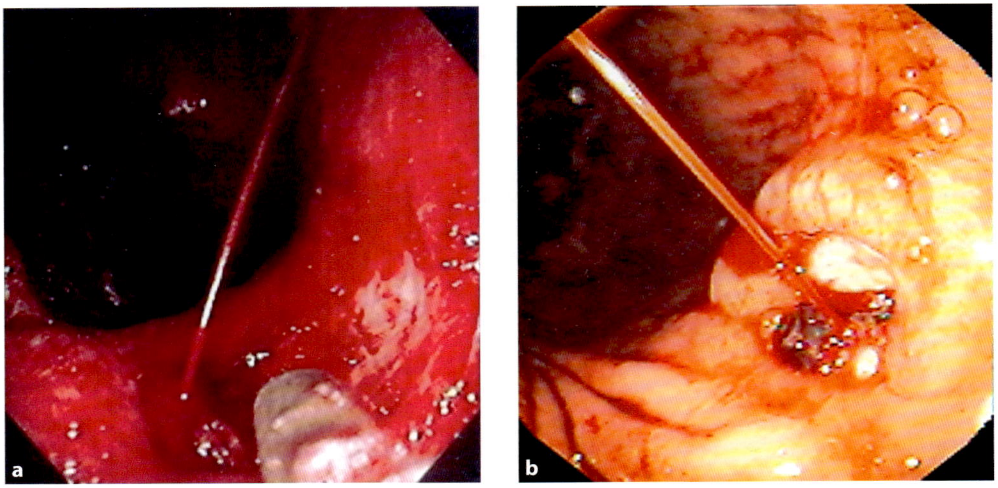

Fig. 1. Spurting ulcer. **a** Active spurting from a large ulcer on the angularis The 10-Fr HP is seen exiting the endoscope channel. **b** Active spurting from a benign-appearing gastric ulcer on the angularis.

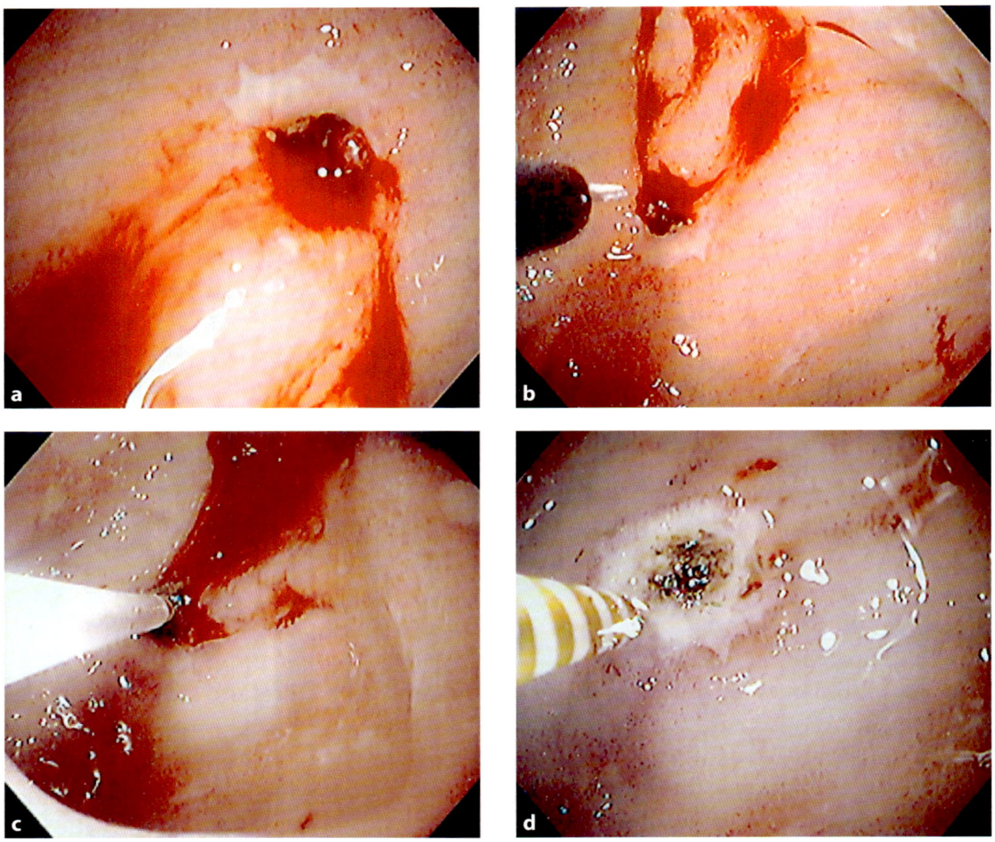

Fig. 2. Oozing visible vessel. **a** Oozing lesion seen in the anterior duodenal bulb with a fleshy component inferiorly. **b** The injection needle is exiting the channel of the diagnostic endoscope. **c** 3 cc's of dilute epinephrine are injected. **d** Black eschar (footprint) after endoscopy thermal therapy with the Bicap probe.

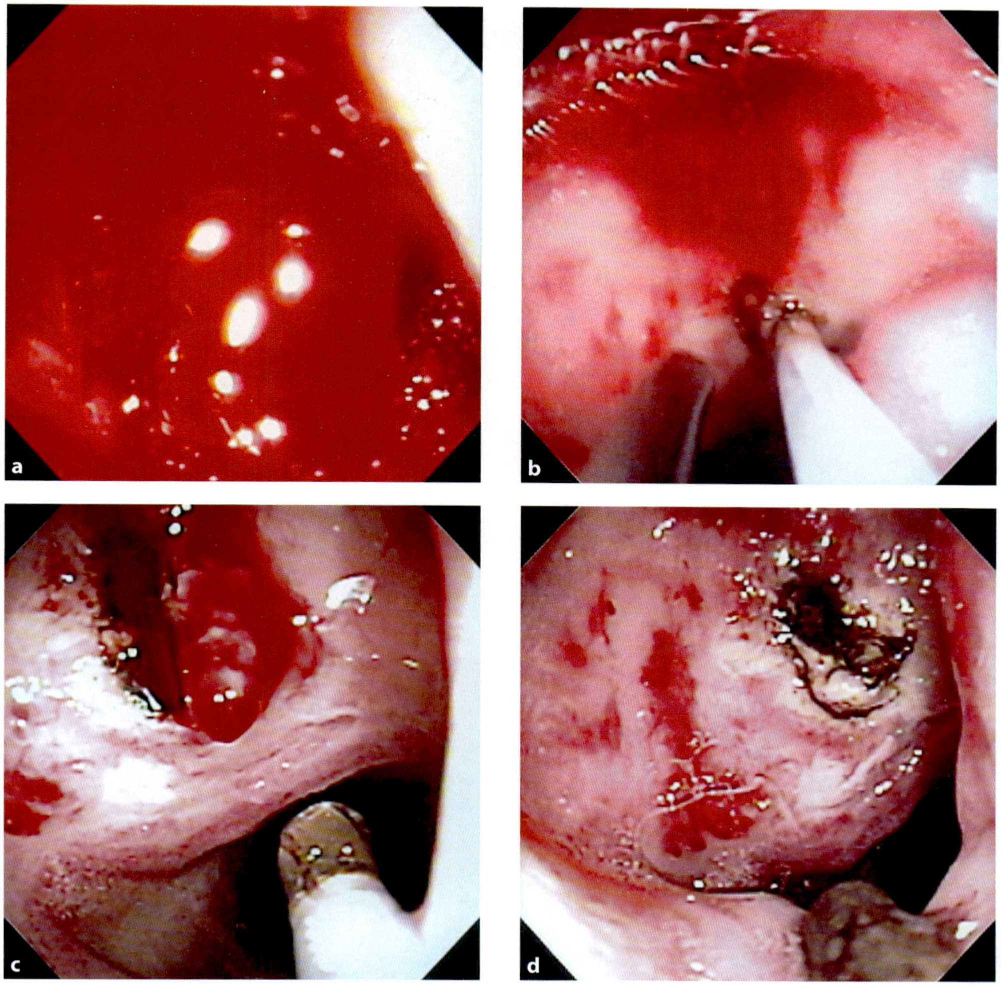

Fig. 3. Active bleeding. **a** Large amount of fresh blood in the duodenal bulb. After washing the lesion, the bleeding source was identified. **b** Both injection and endoscopic therapy are applied to arrest bleeding. **c** 10-Fr thermal probe exiting the therapeutic channel of the therapeutic endoscope. Partial therapy provided as a visible vessel is still present. **d** Further pulses of thermal therapy applied to the bleeding lesion.

up to 35–45 ml may be given in increments of 0.5 to 1.5 ml targeting four quadrants of the ulcer. Park et al. [19] showed that larger volumes (35–45 ml) were more effective in providing hemostasis as compared to standard volumes (15–25 ml) though there are no clear guidelines as to the ideal volume required. (2) Non-constrictive agents such as distilled water, normal or hypertonic saline, 50% dextrose. Studies show an initial hemostasis rate comparable to epinephrine; however, when compared to hemoclips the recurrent bleeding rates are generally higher in the injection group. These agents work by their local compressive action. (3) Other agents which include sclerosants such as ethanol and polidocanol have been used but side effects such as tissue necrosis have resulted in complications including even perforation. Tissue adhesives (cyanoacrylate) and fibrin glue are other injectable solutions which have yielded variable results.

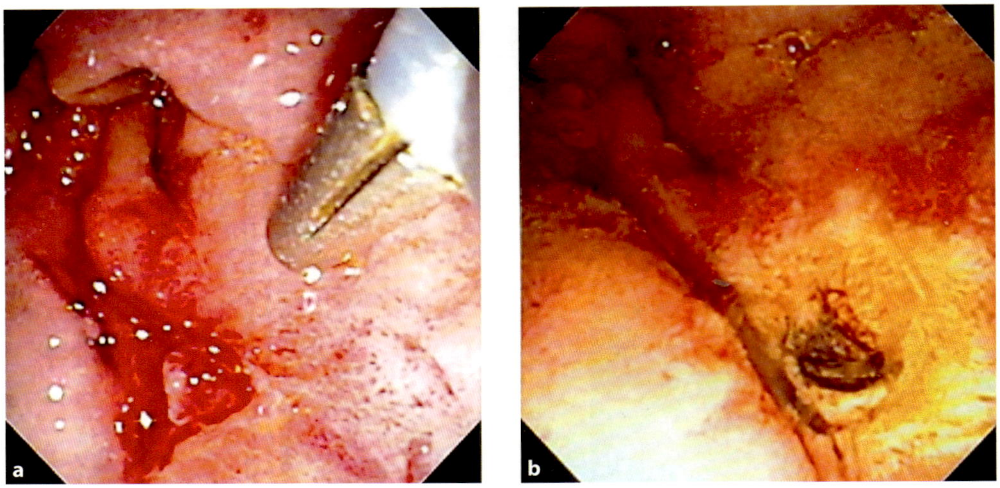

Fig. 4. Non-bleeding visible vessel on the inferior margin of a sphincterotomy site. **a** The 7-Fr probe is used to ablate the area resulting in a large footprint. **b** Mucosal depression resulting from multiple pulses with the thermal probe.

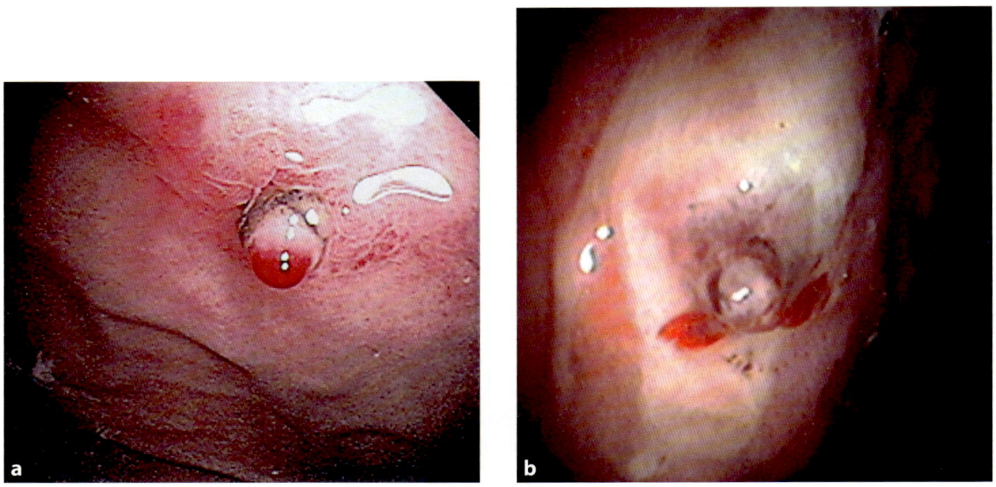

Fig. 5. Non-bleeding visible vessel. **a** Nipple-like projection on the angularis. No underlying ulcer is obvious. **b** Nipple-like projection from the base of a large gastric ulcer.

Thermal Coagulation

Thermal forms of therapy can be classified as either (a) contact or (b) non-contact.

Contact Therapies. These ensure appositional pressure resulting in a heat-sink effect in addition to tissue coagulation with contraction of blood vessels. These include the bipolar probe or the HP which can weld arteries (coaptive coagulation) as large as 2.5 mm in diameter in controlled laboratory conditions [20].

The two available bipolar probes include the Gold Probe (Microinvasive, Boston Scientific Corp., Natick, Mass., USA) and the BICAP or bipolar circumactive probe (Circon-ACMI,

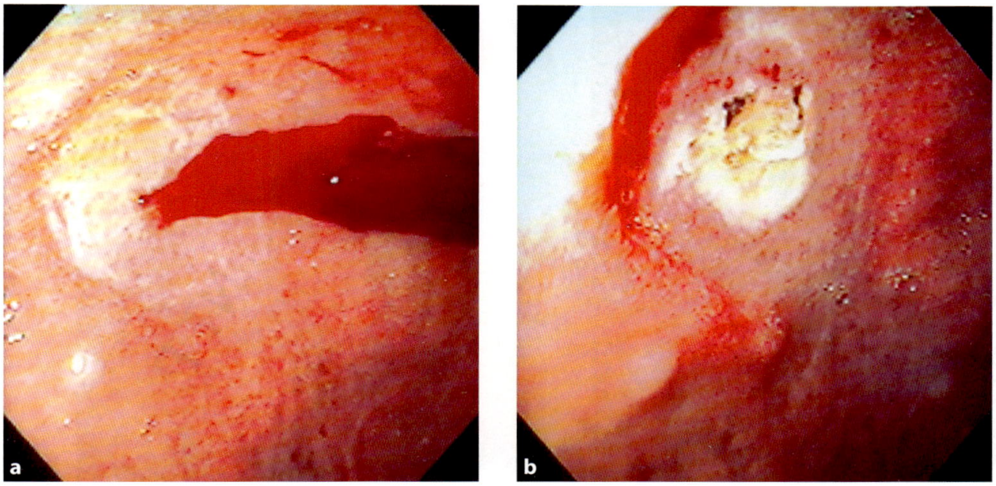

Fig. 6. Oozing lesion. **a** Oozing from a ulcer in the duodenal bulb. **b** After washing, no raised lesions are apparent. Thermal therapy was given.

7
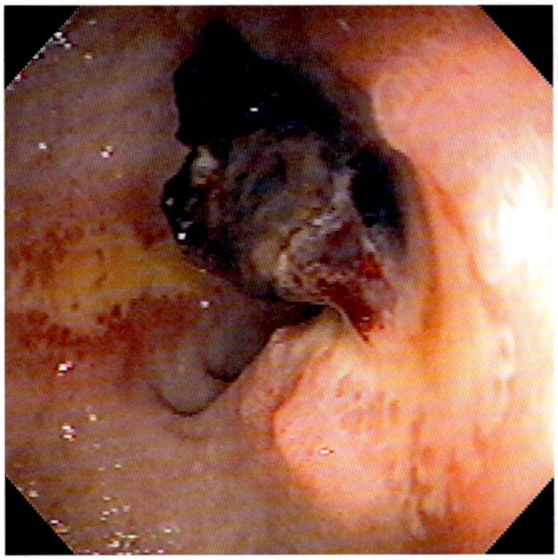

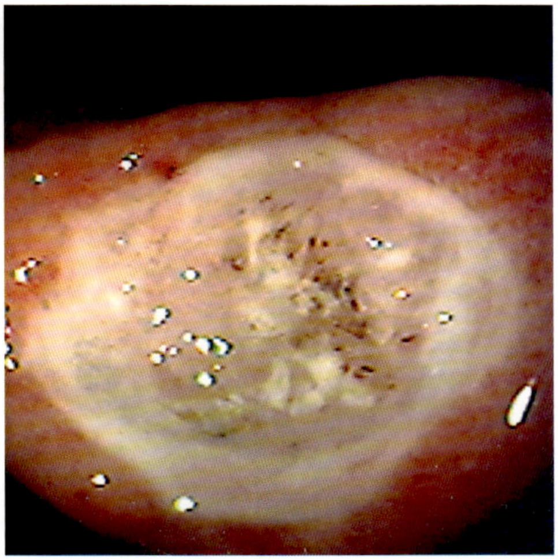
8

Fig. 7. Large clot extending from the base of a duodenal ulcer posteriorly. Small ulcers are also present in the bulb. **Fig. 8.** Multiple spots on a benign-appearing gastric ulcer.

Stamford, Conn., USA). The probes are available in diameters of 2.4–3.2 mm and have alternating positive and negative electrodes which concentrate diathermic coagulation concentrated around the tip providing lesser depth of tissue injury and lower risk for perforation. A central opening provides for working via a foot pedal-operated irrigation pump. Simultaneous injection can be provided through the same catheter. The probe is forcefully opposed directly on the major stigmata of bleeding and pulse treatment of 5–10 s with a power of 10–15 W are applied until target coagulation is achieved.

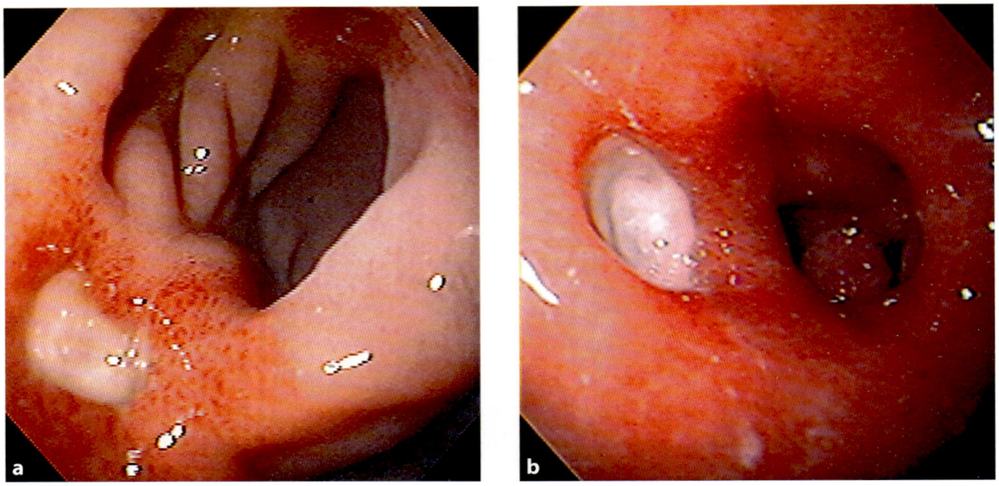

Fig. 9. Clean-based lesions. **a** Clean-based ulcer in the duodenal bulb. **b** Benign-appearing clean-based ulcer in the antrum in a patient using aspirin.

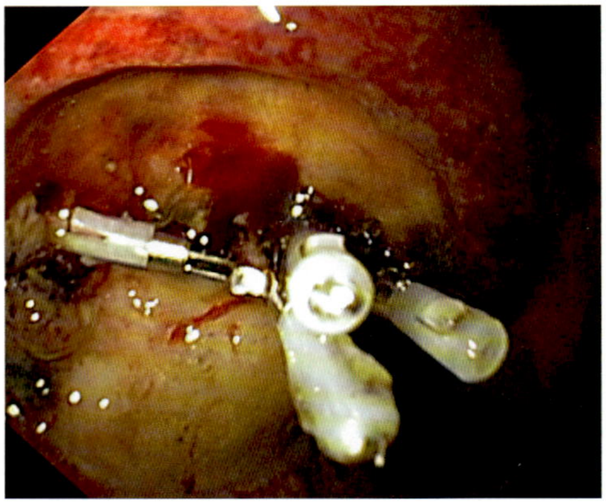

Fig. 10. Bleeding ulcer with visible vessel. Successful deployment of endoclips to achieve hemostasis.

The HP (Olympus, Tokyo, Japan) uses a simple heating device in a Teflon-coated hollow aluminum cylinder with an inner coil rather than electric current. The heat generated can be given directly or tangentially by the distal tip. Probes are available in diameters of 2.3–3.2 mm. The probe temperature can rise up to 250°C (482°F). Four to five bursts of energy of 30 J/pulse are applied for adequate coagulation.

Non-Contact Therapies. The use of Nd:YAG laser for endotherapy is rarely used today primarily owing to the increased depth of coagulation resulting in high rates of perforation as well as the excessive maintenance costs. The underlying mechanism of action is the conversion of light to heat energy by the directed beam which coagulates the bleeding site.

Argon plasma coagulation (APC) as a non-contact thermoblative technique is now available at many endoscopic units. It has advantages of being safe given the depth of penetration (<1 mm) and relative ease of use. There are disadvantages though of providing only superficial coagulation which may thus miss larger deeper vessels.

Mechanical Therapies

The endoscopic mechanical modality currently available is the hemoclip which are metallic devices designed to grasp the mucosa, seal and approximate vessels without interfering with underlying mucosal regeneration and healing [21]. They need precise deployment since inadvertent clipping of only the tip of the vessel can result in potentiating or initiating vigorous bleeding. End on clipping with axial push of surrounding tissue results in better anchoring is preferred over tangential clipping slipping on fibrotic ulcer bases. Difficult areas such as the gastric fundus, lesser curve and posterior duodenal bulb present challenging territories for effective application. Similarly, clipping in the setting of underlying coagulopathy can also aggravate bleeding. Most clips slough off within days or weeks of deployment and may vary based upon the type of clip.

Current available hemoclips available are (a) QuickClip 2, Olympus USA, Corp. which is a rotatable clip device produced in two sizes (opening width of 8 or 12 mm), (b) Resolution Clip, Boston Scientific, Inc. which cannot be rotated but can be reopened after closure if repositioning is required (opening width of 11 mm), (c) TriClip, Wilson Cook, Inc. is a three-pronged endoclip (opening width of 12 mm) and (d) Inscope (Ethicon Endosurgery Inc.) multiclip applicator with four endoclips (opening width of 14 mm). Jenson et al. [22] studied the hemostatic capability of the three aforementioned clips in a randomized canine model for bleeding ulcers and showed that all had an initial success rate of 100% with long-term retention rate higher in the resolution clip group.

Endoscopic Combination Therapy

Endoscopic therapy using a combination of the above-discussed methods is favored to monotherapy alone considering the theoretical additive effect of each modality and given the different mechanisms of action of each technique.

Outcomes of Endoscopic Therapy

In a multicenter trial, Rutgeerts et al. [23] studied the effects of single and multiple injections of fibrin glue and polidocanol. Repeated fibrin glue had more benefit in reducing the rebleed rates as compared to single injection of fibrin or polidocanol though the final outcome of rebleed was similar in all the groups. Their use has generally been declining owing to the difficulty in their administration and costs.

Comparative data between the heater and bipolar probes show different outcomes. In the study by Hui et al. [24], 91 patients were randomized to YAG laser, HP or bipolar coagulation. Recurrent bleeding rates were 10% for bipolar probe, 19% for HP and 10% for YAG laser coagulation. Need for surgery was higher in the HP group (13%) as compared to 7% in either of the other groups. In another prospective randomized study of 80 patients, Lin et al. [25] compared HP with bipolar coagulation and demonstrated a permanent hemostasis rate of 92% with the HP and 85% in the bipolar group. Chung et al. [26] compared these HP therapy with adrenaline and reported no difference between the groups with regard to transfusion requirement (4.5 vs. 3.8 units), emergency surgery (20 vs. 22%), hospital stay (8 vs. 7 days), and mortality (2 vs. 4) initial control of bleeding, rebleeding and mortality. In a randomized trail of 185 patients, APC was compared with HP (both groups received epinephrine injection). There was no significant difference between these two endoscopic techniques in achieving initial hemostasis as well as rebleeding rates, blood transfusion requirements, length of hospital stay and mortality [27]. The Cochrane review, which included this study in addition to one comparing APC with

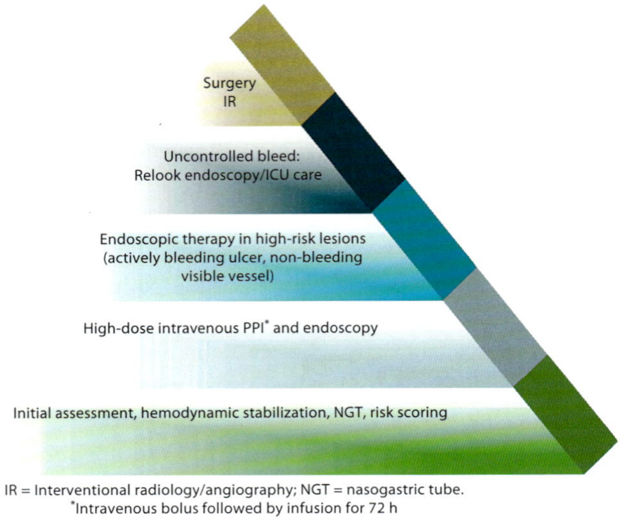

Fig. 11. The PUB pyramid [56].

sclerotherapy, concluded that there was no evidence to suggest that APC was superior to other endoscopic therapies [28].

Cipolleta et al. [29] studied the use of hemoclips initially for bleeding peptic ulcers where they were compared to HP thermocoagulation. They reported a lower risk of recurrent bleeding in the hemoclip group (1.8%) versus the heater group (21%). The efficacy of clips however was limited by difficulty in successful deployment as evidenced in separate trials by Lin et al. [30] and Gevers et al. [31]. A recent meta-analysis showed that the rate of initial hemostasis was insignificantly increased in the control group compared with the hemoclip group (92 vs. 96%) (odds ratio [OR] 0.58, 95% confidence interval [CI] 0.19–1.75). The rebleeding rate was decreased with hemoclips compared with controls (8.5 vs. 15.5%) (OR 0.56, 95% CI 0.30–1.05), though this was not statistically significant. Current evidence from meta-analyses and randomized controlled trials suggests that the hemoclip is equivalent to other endoscopic modalities in terms of initial hemostasis, rebleeding rates, emergency surgery, and mortality for treatment of PUB [32]. Newer mechanical devices such as endoscopic suturing, loops and stapling hold promise but await future trials.

The benefits of dual therapy have been studied in several trials with most studies offering an additional hemostatic therapy to epinephrine injection. The Cochrane database systematic review included 17 studies with 1,763 patients [33]. A second procedure reduced further the bleeding rate from 18.8 to 10.4% (OR 0.51), and need for emergency surgery from 10.8 to 7.1% (OR 0.63). The mortality fell by half from 5 to 2.5% (OR 0.50). They concluded that there was improvement after combination therapy with epinephrine regardless of the choice of modality. These findings were similar to a previous meta-analysis by Calvet et al. [34], though another study by Marmo et al. [35] addressing dual vs. monotherapy in high-risk ulcers suggested that single endoscopic treatment by means of thermal probes or clips (non-injection-based monotherapies) is as effective as dual treatments and probably safer. These results encourage the endoscopist to use more than one modality other than injection alone especially in high-risk ulcer bleeds.

The role of endoscopic therapy in non-bleeding ulcers with adherent clots is still controversial. The fear of dislodging a stable clot provoking bleeding has been of concern. In a meta-analysis by Kahi et al. [36] of 6 studies (240 patients) where the clot was removed, subsequently performed endoscopic therapy was shown to be superior to medical therapy alone in decreasing rebleeding rates (relative risk [RR] 0.35, 95% CI 0.14–0.83) while the results were comparable with other outcomes such length of hospital stay, need for surgery, transfusion requirements or mortality.

The recent combined meta-analysis broadly outlines the effectiveness of various therapy modalities for bleeding ulcers [37]. The authors concluded that endoscopic therapy was effective for active bleeding (RR 0.29, 95% CI 0.20–0.43) and a non-bleeding visible vessel (RR 0.49, 95% CI 0.40–0.59). Clearly, dual therapy was more beneficial than epinephrine alone (table 4). These results are echoed by another systematic review [38].

Limitations and Complications

Complications of endoscopic therapy are limited including aspiration pneumonia and perforation. A pooled analysis for all these modalities revealed a complication rate of 0.5% (95% CI 0.4–0.8) [37]. Clips and epinephrine had the lowest rates of perforations while the HP group had the highest. Endoscopic therapy is limited by factors such as an unstable patient, poor sedation, inadequate visualization due to blood, difficult areas of reach such as the posterior wall of duodenum, junction between the first and second part of duodenum, and lesser curve.

Post-Procedure Care

Patients with hemodynamic unstable acute gastrointestinal bleeding are usually managed in the ICU till they are stabilized. Close monitoring with serial hemoglobin levels are required thereby assessing the patient for downgrading to onward transfer to the ward and then on for discharge. Despite initial success, rebleeding occurs in 10–20% of patients, directly or indirectly related to the size or site of ulcer, associated comorbidities, technical difficulties and endoscopic expertise. Further rebleeding is documented by any further changes in stools and color, vital signs and hematocrit keeping in mind laboratory variability. The benefit of a second-look endoscopy was evaluated by Chiu et al. [39]. They found several predictors for peptic ulcer rebleeding by logistic regression analysis including: American Society of Anesthesiologists (ASA) grade III or grade IV status (OR 3.81, 95% CI 1.27–11.44), ulcer size >1.0 cm (OR 4.69, 95% CI 1.60–13.80), and a finding of persistent stigmata of recent hemorrhage at the scheduled second endoscopy (OR 6.65, 95% CI 2.11–20.98). In the meta-analysis by Marmo et al. [40], they concluded that a systematic second-look endoscopy with retreatment significantly reduced the risk of recurrent bleeding compared to controls, although such an approach did not substantially reduce the need for subsequent surgery or mortality.

The role of Doppler ultrasound has been shown to help in guiding the use and predicting the failure of endoscopic therapy of PUB especially in high-risk patients [41]. Further studies are required to show the beneficial cost-effectiveness of these endoscopic tools and such trials are underway.

Acute PUB in anticoagulated patients requires optimal management even though there are no clear guidelines available due to lack of prospective trials. Therapy should therefore be addressed on an individual case-by-case basis requiring normalizing or targeting the INR to <1.6 with fresh-frozen plasma and/or vitamin K. This includes discontinuing the anticoagulant such as warfarin, coumadin, aspirin or antiplatelet agents. A combination endoscopic therapy will be preferred than a monotherapy. The timing of resuming anticoagulation is controversial due to lack of clear data and would have to be decided depending on the underlying medical condition and the overall patient's clinical and endoscopic characteristics [42].

Concurrent Medical Therapy

Acid Suppression

The rationale for acid suppression stems from the fact that gastric juice is an anticoagulant by decreasing platelet aggregation (even disintegration), promoting clot lysis due to pepsin activating by acid, and further increasing the fibrinolytic activity that is impaired. Based on in vitro and animal data, a pH of 6–6.5 is targeted to reverse these effects and maintain clot stability. Proton pump inhibitors (PPI) are effective in maintaining the gastric pH above 4.0 though recent studies cast doubt on their ability to maintain a gastric pH of 6 or more [43]. Khuroo et al. [44] initially showed the efficacy of oral omeprazole (40 mg twice daily for 5 days) compared to placebo in a randomized trial of 220 patients from India. Acid suppression prevented recurrent bleeding in patients with ulcers who had stopped bleeding spontaneously. Lau et al. [45] randomized patients to receive high-dose IV omeprazole (bolus of 80 mg followed by an infusion 8 mg/h). Rebleeding rates within the first 3 days were 4.2% in the omeprazole group compared to 20% in the placebo group, while rebleeding within 30 days was 6.7 vs. 22.5% respectively ($p < 0.001$). Similarly, the need for surgery and 30-day mortality were significantly reduced in the PPI group. Sung et al. [46] clearly demonstrated that a combination of endoscopic therapy with omeprazole IV infusion was better than omeprazole alone with regard to 30-day rebleeding rates, requirement for blood transfusions and 30-day mortality. Current data shows that IV PPI provides more rapid increase in gastrin pH, reaching a mean pH of 6 approximately 1 h sooner than oral PPI [47]. The Cochrane meta-analysis which included 24 trials (4,373 patients) concludes that the use of PPI significantly decreased rebleeding (OR 0.40, 95% CI 0.24–0.67), need for urgent surgery (OR 0.50, 95% CI 0.33–0.76), and the risk of death (OR 0.53, 95% CI 0.31–0.91) [48].

Timing of Acid Suppression

The use of PPI prior to endoscopy accelerates resolution of signs of bleeding in ulcers [32, 39]. In a randomized trial of 638 patients [49], one group received a high-dose IV bolus followed by omeprazole infusion, while the other group, placebo was followed by endoscopy the next morning. The infusion group had a significantly lower number of patients who required endoscopic therapy than placebo (23 vs. 37% $p = 0.007$) though there were no differences in outcomes of rebleeding rates, requirement of blood transfusions or mortality. These findings were supported by a Cochrane meta-analysis by Dorward et al. [50] showing the usefulness of early PPI therapy in downstaging stigmata of recent hemorrhage at index endoscopy. In a cost-effective analysis, PPI reduced the need for endoscopic therapy by 7.4% and resulted in a lower cost-effectiveness ratio per endoscopic therapy averted (USD 3,561) than placebo (USD 4,117) [51]. In the meta-analysis by Laine and McQuaid [37], PPI therapy as an adjunct after endoscopic hemostatic therapy was examined in three groups: (1) IV PPI (bolus + continuous infusion) vs. placebo, (2) IV PPI (bolus + continuous infusion) vs. H_2 receptor antagonists, and (3) oral or intermittent IV bolus vs. placebo. They concluded that PPI after endoscopic therapy reduced rebleeding, need for surgery, need for urgent intervention and mortality. The results were most consistent for bolus followed by continuous IV PPI infusion for 72 h. This data is further corroborated by

Table 4. Summary of meta-analyses of randomized controlled trials for endoscopic therapy in PUB (adapted from Laine et al. [37])

Study description	Endoscopic hemostatic technique	Number of studies compared for meta-analyses	Outcomes, RR (95% CI)			
			further bleeding	surgery	urgent Intervention	mortality
Meta-analyses for endoscopic hemostatic therapy versus no endoscopic therapy						
Thermal (HP, BPEC) vs. no endoscopic therapy	thermal therapy	2–3	0.44 (0.36–0.54)	0.39 (0.27–0.55)	0.50 (0.37–0.66)	0.58 (0.34–0.98)
Epinephrine + thermal contact vs. no endoscopic therapy	injection + thermal therapy	13–15	0.10 (0.03–0.40)	0.71 (0.19–2.62)	0.16 (0.04–0.69)	0.80 (0.27–2.37)
Sclerosant vs. no endoscopic therapy	injection therapy	3	0.56 (0.38–0.83)	0.24 (0.09–0.64)	0.65 (0.43–0.98)	0.18 (0.05–0.68)
Epinephrine + Sclerosant vs. no endoscopic therapy	injection therapy	6	0.60 (0.36–1.00)	0.61 (0.22–1.73)	0.62 (0.45–0.86)	0.80 (0.40–1.61)
Meta-analyses for epinephrine only versus other monotherapy and epinephrine dual therapy						
Monotherapy (BIPEC, fibrin glue, clip) vs. epinephrine	injection, thermal, mechanical	2–3	0.58 (0.36–0.93)	0.44 (0.20–0.98)	0.73 (0.44–1.21)	0.37 (0.10–1.37)
Epinephrine + second therapy (HP, BPEC, sclerosant, thrombin, clip vs. epiphrine	injection, thermal, mechanical	4–7	0.34 (0.23–0.50)	0.33 (0.17–0.66)	0.39 (0.24–0.62)	0.52 (0.23–1.16)
Clips vs. epinephrine	mechanical, injection	2	0.22 (0.09–0.55)	0.22 (0.06–0.83)	NA	1.68 (0.23–12.45)
Clips vs. other therapy (HP, epinephrine + BPEC, sclerosants, epinephrine)	mechanical, thermal, injection	2–4	1.312 (0.36–4.75)	0.85 (0.32–2.26)	1.17 (0.09–14.46)	1.16 (0.38–3.52)

HP = Heater probe; BPEC = bipolar electrocoagulation.

a recent multicenter worldwide study examining the use of IV esomeprazole bolus 80 mg followed by 8 mg/h infusion over a 72-hour period versus placebo in patients following successful endoscopic hemostasis for PUB. At 72 h, fewer patients receiving IV esomeprazole had recurrent bleeding compared to placebo (5.9 vs. 10.3%), and the difference in rebleeding remained significant at 7 days. Endoscopic retreatment was also reduced from 11.6 to 6.4% significantly within 30 days of primary therapy. The data may be slightly skewed for more patients being *H. pylori* positive (approximately 70% of the treated group) and therefore further studies should confirm the similar efficacy in *H. pylori*-negative patients [52].

H. pylori Eradication
Several studies have conclusively shown the benefit of *H. pylori* eradication in reducing the rate of bleeding peptic ulcer [53]. Appropriate testing is and treatment is a cost-effective strategy despite the low prevalence in the developed world. The rapid urease test in the setting of active bleeding has a lower sensitivity as compared to other tests such as the ^{13}C breath test, serology or histology. The use of PPI also decreases the sensitivity of the CLO test, breath test and stool antigen test [54]. It is unknown how many days of PPI treatment are needed before the tests become less accurate [55]. Histology examining for chronic active gastritis is a reliable marker *H. pylori* infection which is not influenced by PPI therapy.

Conclusion

Endoscopy has clearly defined its role in the primary management of acute PUB which is by far the most important cause of UGIB. Initial triage and assessment obtained at the time of endoscopy form the base for initiating further treatment. We can to a large extent predict the outcomes and risk stratify by using clinical and endoscopic information. Early endoscopy is indicated in all high-risk patients. Empiric early use of PPI therapy with high-dose bolus and subsequent infusion prior to endoscopy may decrease bleeding stigmata and need for endoscopic therapy. A combination of PPI therapy along with endoscopic therapy offers the best hemostatic results. Endoscopic therapy should be used for all ulcers with active bleeding and non-bleeding vessels. Among the endoscopic therapies, epinephrine should not be used alone, while other treatments including thermal, injection or mechanical clips have all shown efficacy in controlling bleeding. Combinations of epinephrine injection along with either mechanical or thermal methods may be preferable to a single therapy approach although further studies may be needed. The role of endoscopic therapy in adherent clots is still uncertain, although intensive PPI therapy may be sufficient in this setting. PPI infusion must be continued after endoscopic therapy for at least 72 h before switching to oral therapy. *H. pylori* should be sought for, treated, and eradication confirmed by subsequent testing.

Recent advances in pharmacotherapy as well as endotherapy have favorably changed the management strategies for PUB. Endotherapy forms the basis for any further intervention, be it surgery or interventional radiology, thereby stressing the importance of a multidisciplinary targeted approach. All of these improvements together pave the way for future newer modalities and trials to help further improve outcomes while reducing costs in UGIB treatment.

References

1 Van Leerdam ME: Epidemiology of acute upper gastrointestinal bleeding. Best Pract Res Clin Gastroenterol 2008;22:209–224.
2 Lassen A, Hallas J, Schaffalitzky de Muckadell OB: Complicated and uncomplicated peptic ulcers in a Danish county 1993–2002: a population-based cohort study. Am J Gastroenterol 2006;101:945–953.
3 Laine L, Peterson WL: Bleeding peptic ulcer. N Engl J Med 1994;331:717–727.
4 Wilcox CM Jr: Gastrointestinal considerations in patients with cardiovascular disease using non-opioid analgesics for mild-to-moderate pain or cardioprotection. Am J Cardiol 2006;97:17–22.
5 Lim CH, Vani D, Shah SG, Everett SM, Rembacken BJ: The outcome of suspected upper gastrointestinal bleeding with 24-hour access to upper gastrointestinal endoscopy: a prospective cohort study. Endoscopy 2006;38: 581–585.
6 Aabakken L: Current endoscopic and pharmacological therapy of peptic ulcer bleeding. Best Pract Res Clin Gastroenterol 2008;22:243–259.
7 Cappell MS, Friedel D: Acute nonvariceal upper gastrointestinal bleeding: endoscopic diagnosis and therapy. Med Clin North Am 2008;92:511–550, vii–viii.

8 Sung J: Current management of peptic ulcer bleeding. Nat Clin Pract 2006;3:24–32.
9 Baradarian R, Ramdhaney S, Chapalamadugu R, Skoczylas L, Wang K, Rivilis S, Remus K, Mayer I, Iswara K, Tenner S: Early intensive resuscitation of patients with upper gastrointestinal bleeding decreases mortality. Am J Gastroenterol 2004;99: 619–622.
10 Aljebreen AM, Fallone CA, Barkun AN: Nasogastric aspirate predicts high-risk endoscopic lesions in patients with acute upper-GI bleeding. Gastrointest Endosc 2004; 59:172–178.
11 Winstead NS, Wilcox CM: Erythromycin prior to endoscopy for acute upper gastrointestinal haemorrhage: a cost-effectiveness analysis. Aliment Pharmacol Ther 2007;26: 1371–1377.
12 Rockall TA, Logan RF, Devlin HB, Northfield TC: Risk assessment after acute upper gastrointestinal haemorrhage. Gut 1996;38:316–321.
13 Blatchford O, Murray WR, Blatchford M: A risk score to predict need for treatment for upper gastrointestinal haemorrhage. Lancet 2000;356:1318–1321.
14 Stanley A, Ashley D, Dalton H, Mowat C, Gaya D, Thompson E, Warshow U, Groome M, Cahill A, Benson G, Blatchford O, Murray W: Outpatient management of patients with low-risk upper gastrointestinal haemorrhage: multicentre validation and prospective evaluation. Lancet 2009;373:42–47.
15 Mönkemüller K, Neumann H, Bellutti M, Malfertheiner P, Fry LC: Use of a colonoscope to perform endoscopic therapy in patients with active bleeding from posterior duodenal and gastric ulcers. Endoscopy 2009;41:93–94.
16 Lichtenstein DR, Jagannath S, Baron TH, Anderson MA, Banerjee S, Dominitz JA, Fanelli RD, Gan SI, Harrison ME, Ikenberry SO, Shen B, Stewart L, Khan K, Vargo JJ: Sedation and anesthesia in GI endoscopy. Gastrointest Endosc 2008;68:205–216.
17 Forrest JA, Finlayson ND, Shearman DJ: Endoscopy in gastrointestinal bleeding. Lancet 1974;2:394–397.
18 Park WG, Yeh RW, Triadafilopoulos G: Injection therapies for nonvariceal bleeding disorders of the GI tract. Gastrointest Endosc 2007;66:343–354.
19 Park CH, Lee SJ, Park JH, Park JH, Lee WS, Joo YE, Kim HS, Choi SK, Rew JS, Kim SJ: Optimal injection volume of epinephrine for endoscopic prevention of recurrent peptic ulcer bleeding. Gastrointest Endosc 2004;60:875–880.
20 Johnston JH, Jensen DM, Auth D: Experimental comparison of endoscopic yttrium-aluminum-garnet laser, electrosurgery, and heater probe for canine gut arterial coagulation. Importance of compression and avoidance of erosion. Gastroenterology 1987; 92:1101–1108.
21 Anastassiades CP, Baron TH, Wong Kee Song LM: Endoscopic clipping for the management of gastrointestinal bleeding. Nat Clin Pract 2008;5:559–568.
22 Jensen DM, Machicado GA, Hirabayashi K: Randomized controlled study of three different types of hemoclips for hemostasis of bleeding canine acute gastric ulcers. Gastrointest Endosc 2006;64:768–773.
23 Rutgeerts P, Rauws E, Wara P, Swain P, Hoos A, Solleder E, Halttunen J, Dobrilla G, Richter G, Prassler R: Randomised trial of single and repeated fibrin glue compared with injection of polidocanol in treatment of bleeding peptic ulcer. Lancet 1997;350:692–696.
24 Hui WM, Ng MM, Lok AS, Lai CL, Lau YN, Lam SK: A randomized comparative study of laser photocoagulation, heater probe, and bipolar electrocoagulation in the treatment of actively bleeding ulcers. Gastrointest Endosc 1991;37:299–304.
25 Lin HJ, Wang K, Perng CL, Lee CH, Lee SD: Heater probe thermocoagulation and multipolar electrocoagulation for arrest of peptic ulcer bleeding. A prospective, randomized comparative trial. J Clin Gastroenterol 1995;21:99–102.
26 Chung SC, Leung JW, Sung JY, Lo KK, Li AK: Injection or heat probe for bleeding ulcer. Gastroenterology 1991; 100:33–37.
27 Chau CH, Siu WT, Law BK, Tang CN, Kwok SY, Luk YW, Lao WC, Li MK: Randomized controlled trial comparing epinephrine injection plus heat probe coagulation versus epinephrine injection plus argon plasma coagulation for bleeding peptic ulcers. Gastrointest Endosc 2003;57:455–461.
28 Havanond C, Havanond P: Argon plasma coagulation therapy for acute non-variceal upper gastrointestinal bleeding. Cochrane Database of Systematic Reviews (Online) 2005:CD003791.
29 Cipolletta L, Bianco MA, Marmo R, Rotondano G, Piscopo R, Vingiani AM, Meucci C: Endoclips versus heater probe in preventing early recurrent bleeding from peptic ulcer: a prospective and randomized trial. Gastrointest Endosc 2001;53:147–151.
30 Lin HJ, Hsieh YH, Tseng GY, Perng CL, Chang FY, Lee SD: A prospective, randomized trial of endoscopic hemoclip versus heater probe thermocoagulation for peptic ulcer bleeding. Am J Gastroenterol 2002;97:2250–2254.
31 Gevers AM, De Goede E, Simoens M, Hiele M, Rutgeerts P: A randomized trial comparing injection therapy with hemoclip and with injection combined with hemoclip for bleeding ulcers. Gastrointest Endosc 2002;55:466–469.
32 Yuan Y, Wang C, Hunt RH: Endoscopic clipping for acute nonvariceal upper-GI bleeding: a meta-analysis and critical appraisal of randomized controlled trials. Gastrointest Endosc 2008;68:339–351.
33 Vergara M, Calvet X, Gisbert JP: Epinephrine injection versus epinephrine injection and a second endoscopic method in high-risk bleeding ulcers. Cochrane Database of Systematic Reviews (Online) 2007:CD005584.
34 Calvet X, Vergara M, Brullet E, Gisbert JP, Campo R: Addition of a second endoscopic treatment following epinephrine injection improves outcome in high-risk bleeding ulcers. Gastroenterology 2004; 126:441–450.

35 Marmo R, Rotondano G, Piscopo R, Bianco MA, D'Angella R, Cipolletta L: Dual therapy versus monotherapy in the endoscopic treatment of high-risk bleeding ulcers: a meta-analysis of controlled trials. Am J Gastroenterol 2007;102:279–289.
36 Kahi CJ, Jensen DM, Sung JJ, Bleau BL, Jung HK, Eckert G, Imperiale TF: Endoscopic therapy versus medical therapy for bleeding peptic ulcer with adherent clot: a meta-analysis. Gastroenterology 2005;129:855–862.
37 Laine L, McQuaid K: Endoscopic therapy for bleeding ulcers: an evidence-based approach based on meta-analyses of randomized controlled trials. Clin Gastroenterol Hepatol 2009;7:33–47.
38 Barkun A, Martel M, Toubouti Y, Rahme E, Bardou M: Endoscopic hemostasis in peptic ulcer bleeding for patients with high-risk lesions: a series of meta-analyses. Gastrointest Endosc 2009;69:786–799.
39 Chiu PW, Joeng HK, Choi CL, Kwong KH, Ng EK, Lam SH: Predictors of peptic ulcer rebleeding after scheduled second endoscopy: clinical or endoscopic factors? Endoscopy 2006;38:726–729.
40 Marmo R, Rotondano G, Bianco MA, Piscopo R, Prisco A, Cipolletta L: Outcome of endoscopic treatment for peptic ulcer bleeding: is a second look necessary? A meta-analysis. Gastrointest Endosc 2003;57:62–67.
41 Chen VK, Wong RC: Endoscopic Doppler ultrasound versus endoscopic stigmata-directed management of acute peptic ulcer hemorrhage: a multimodel cost analysis. Dig Dis Sci 2007;52:149–160.
42 Makar GA, Ginsberg GG: Therapy insight: approaching endoscopy in anticoagulated patients. Nat Clin Pract 2006;3:43–52.
43 Metz DC, Amer F, Hunt B, Vakily M, Kukulka MJ, Samra N: Lansoprazole regimens that sustain intragastric pH >6.0: an evaluation of intermittent oral and continuous intravenous infusion dosages. Aliment Pharmacol Ther 2006;23:985–995.
44 Khuroo MS, Yattoo GN, Javid G, Khan BA, Shah AA, Gulzar GM, Sodi JS: A comparison of omeprazole and placebo for bleeding peptic ulcer. N Engl J Med 1997;336:1054–1058.
45 Lau JY, Sung JJ, Lee KK, Yung MY, Wong SK, Wu JC, Chan FK, Ng EK, You JH, Lee CW, Chan AC, Chung SC: Effect of intravenous omeprazole on recurrent bleeding after endoscopic treatment of bleeding peptic ulcers. N Engl J Med 2000;343:310–316.
46 Sung JJ, Chan FK, Lau JY, Yung MY, Leung WK, Wu JC, Ng EK, Chung SC: The effect of endoscopic therapy in patients receiving omeprazole for bleeding ulcers with nonbleeding visible vessels or adherent clots: a randomized comparison. Ann Intern Med 2003;139:237–243.
47 Laine L, Shah A, Bemanian S: Intragastric pH with oral vs. intravenous bolus plus infusion proton-pump inhibitor therapy in patients with bleeding ulcers. Gastroenterology 2008;134:1836–1841.
48 Leontiadis GI, Sharma VK, Howden CW: Proton pump inhibitor treatment for acute peptic ulcer bleeding. Cochrane Database of Systematic Reviews (Online) 2006:CD002094.
49 Lau JY, Leung WK, Wu JC, Chan FK, Wong VW, Chiu PW, Lee VW, Lee KK, Cheung FK, Siu P, Ng EK, Sung JJ: Omeprazole before endoscopy in patients with gastrointestinal bleeding. N Engl J Med 2007;356:1631–1640.
50 Dorward S, Sreedharan A, Leontiadis GI, Howden CW, Moayyedi P, Forman D: Proton pump inhibitor treatment initiated prior to endoscopic diagnosis in upper gastrointestinal bleeding. Cochrane Database of Systematic Reviews (Online) 2006:CD005415.
51 Tsoi KK, Lau JY, Sung JJ: Cost-effectiveness analysis of high-dose omeprazole infusion before endoscopy for patients with upper-GI bleeding. Gastrointest Endosc 2008;67:1056–1063.
52 Sung J, Barkun A, Kuipers E, Mössner J, Jensen D, Stuart R, Lau J, Ahlbom H, Kilhamn J, Lind T: Intravenous esomeprazole for prevention of recurrent peptic ulcer bleeding: a randomized trial. Ann Intern Med 2009;150:455–464.
53 Pohl H, Finlayson SR, Sonnenberg A, Robertson DJ: *Helicobacter pylori*-associated ulcer bleeding: should we test for eradication after treatment? Aliment Pharmacol Ther 2005;22:529–537.
54 Grino P, Pascual S, Such J, Casellas JA, Niveiro M, Andreu M, Saez J, Aparicio JR, Grino E, Company L, Laveda R, Perez-Mateo M: Comparison of stool immunoassay with standard methods for detection of *Helicobacter pylori* infection in patients with upper gastrointestinal bleeding of peptic origin. Eur J Gastroenterol Hepatol 2003;15:525–529.
55 Holtmann G, Howden CW: Management of peptic ulcer bleeding-the roles of proton pump inhibitors and *Helicobacter pylori* eradication. Aliment Pharmacol Ther 2004;19(suppl 1):66–70.
56 Peter S, Wilcox C: Modern endoscopic therapy of peptic ulcer bleeding. Dig Dis 2008;26:291–299.

C. Mel Wilcox, MD
Division of Gastroenterology and Hepatology
University of Alabama at Birmingham
Birmingham, AL 35294 (USA)
Tel. +1 205 975 4958, Fax +1 205 934 1546, E-Mail melw@uab.edu

Mönkemüller K, Wilcox CM, Muñoz-Navas M (eds): Interventional and Therapeutic Gastrointestinal Endoscopy.
Front Gastrointest Res. Basel, Karger, 2010, vol 27, pp 55–63

Endoscopic Therapy for Esophageal Varices

R. Cestari · L. Minelli · G. Cengia · G. Missale · D. Moneghini

Department of Surgery, Digestive Endoscopy Unit, University of Brescia, Spedali Civili, Brescia, Italy

Abstract

Among therapeutic endoscopic options for esophageal varices (EV), endoscopic variceal ligation (EVL) has proven more effectiveness and safety compared with endoscopic sclerotherapy and is currently considered as the first choice. In acute EV bleeding, vasoactive therapy (either with terlipressin or somatostatin) prior to endoscopy improves outcomes; moreover, antibiotic prophylaxis has to be generally adopted. Variceal glue injection (cyanoacrylates) seems to be effective in the treatment of esophageal as well as in gastric varices. Prevention of rebleeding can be provided both by EVL alone or combined with non-selective β-blockers. Moreover, EVL can be adopted for primary prophylaxis, with no differences in mortality compared with drugs, in subjects with large varices and unfit for a β-blocker regimen.

Esophageal varices (EV) affect about 50% of patients with liver cirrhosis and formation rate is about 5% per year. The current most reliable predictor of EV development in cirrhosis is an increased hepatic vein pressure gradient (HVPG) >12 mm Hg [1], an indirect method for portal vein pressure measurement and therapy response assessment. In the last decade, however, intravascular esophageal variceal pressure by direct variceal puncture has been used for this purpose, although there is a risk of complications [2].

The overall incidence of bleeding from EV ranges from 25 to 30% at 2 years from the diagnosis and both the variceal size and red color signs are the most important endoscopic parameters to predict the risk of hemorrhage, as well as the severity of liver dysfunction, according to the NIEC Index [3]. Mortality rate from the initial EV bleeding can still rise up to 30% in patients with advanced liver disease and large varices and it seems to be related to several factors such as torrential bleeding with shock, compromised hepatic function, coagulopathy, infections and the time required for bleeding control. Many treatment options, such as vasoactive drugs, endoscopic therapy, balloon tamponade, surgical and more recently radiological shunt (TIPS) can be helpful to stop EV bleeding in order to prevent recurrence and complications. A multimodality approach would be adopted according to clinical presentation and the choice for the optimal treatment is dependent on availability of expertise and local resources. Emergency endoscopy (within 12 h from admission) is the main method to detect EV and to rule out different sources (15% of hemorrhages in cirrhotic patients are not related to portal hypertension) and has gained a primary role in the management of EV bleeding, through different techniques, such as sclerotherapy, ligation and obliteration.

Procedural Aspects

Patient Preparation

In patients with active EV bleeding, appropriate maneuvers including secure venous access for colloids and administration of blood products must initially be conducted to stabilize the patient; cardiovascular and other complications related to the degree of estimated volume loss and comorbidities should also be assessed. Moreover, reversal of coagulation defects improves the successful of initial hemostasis and reduces the risk of rebleeding after therapeutic endoscopic procedures. Timing of endoscopy is still controversial and few studies actually address this issue directly. While endoscopy with the intent of a therapeutic intervention is intuitively expected to improve short-term medical outcomes, 'early' endoscopy is difficult to define, since the majority of studies generally evaluated endoscopy within 24 h of presentation. Emergency endoscopy is generally performed for patients hemodynamically unstable or with signs of continued bleeding and hemostasis can be achieved with therapeutic endoscopic intervention. Otherwise, endoscopy may be performed within 24 h after hemodynamic stabilization in patients with no evidence of persistent bleeding.

Accessories (Instruments and Materials Used, Preferences)

A large-channel endoscope (3.8 mm) and a powerful suction unit are required and an additional water irrigation pump may be very helpful. Injection needles should have a small diameter (23–25 gauge) to minimize the risk of back bleeding from the injection site and no longer than 5 mm to avoid extravisceral injection and bacteriemia; otherwise, for tissue adhesives injection (cyanoacrylate), greater calibers (19–21 gauge) are preferable in order to enhance needle patency. Ligation devices consist of a single-use system counting a transparent friction fit adapter (similar to transparent cap) attached to the tip of the scope, preloaded rubber band(s) (1, 4, 5, 6, 7 or 10) and a release trigger-like mechanism which deploys elastic bands after the tissue is suctioned into the hollow chamber of the adapter.

Techniques

Endoscopic Sclerotherapy (EST)
Endoscopic injection of sclerosants results in chemical variceal obliteration through rapid vascular thrombosis. Technical differences in EST include the type, concentration and volume of the agent injected, the interval between sessions, and number of sessions needed to eradicate varices. The most widely used sclerosants are polidocanol 1–3% or ethanolamine oleate 5% (in Europe and Asia), sodium morrhuate or sodium tetradecyl sulfate (in the USA), none of which has demonstrated superiority [4]. The *'free-hand'* technique of injection, with flexible scopes, is gaining popularity due to the high risk of complications with overtube adoption.

Currently, there is no accepted standard technique for the injection of sclerosants, and most of the controversies lie between intra- and paravariceal injection. In the *intravariceal technique*, the agent is injected directly into the varix. In our experience, the first injection (polidocanol 2%

in active bleeding) 1–2 ml is placed 1 cm below the bleeding source, if visible (fig. 1). All visible varices are then injected with 1–2 ml of sclerosant at the gastroesophageal junction. More proximally, injections are placed in 3- to 5-cm intervals up to 10 cm from the gastroesophageal junction. Approximately 10–20 ml of sclerosant is used per session, based on the size and number of varices. Ethanol is an exception in that injection of no more than a 4-ml volume is recommended in an intravariceal fashion.

In the *paravariceal technique*, 1–2 ml of sclerosant is injected in the submucosa bordering the visible varices. The first injection starts at the gastroesophageal junction and can be repeated circumferentially and proximally up to 10 cm. The subsequent inflammation and fibrosis around the vessel wall provides bleeding control while allowing for portal decompression by preserving vessel patency.

The eradication period (time for complete variceal obliteration) takes usually 6–8 EST sessions scheduled at a 1- to 3-week interval time; in our experience, polidocanol 1.5% is usually adopted for injection in this setting. Successful EST is generally demonstrated by superficial variceal ulcerations resulting from tissue necrosis, arising in 90% of patients on day 1 after EST and in 70% after 1 week. EST is a highly individualized technique, as demonstrated by different results in EV management, with an overall success rate in acute bleeding control ranging from 70 to 100% in experienced hands. Nevertheless, EST is associated with frequent local or systemic complications, such as chest pain, pleural effusion, dysphagia, and fever. Severe complications include deep ulcers through the esophageal wall, which predispose to hemorrhage, stricture formation and perforation, with an overall mortality rate of 15% [5].

While rebleeding from EV occurs most frequently before obliteration, variceal recurrence can affect 20–50% in the long-term period after eradication, therefore surveillance and, eventually, EST retreatment every 6–12 months should be recommended. [6].

Endoscopic Variceal Ligation (EVL)

EVL is performed by the positioning of rubber rings on the variceal columns previously sucked into a plastic, transparent cap distally attached to the endoscope, achieving mechanical vessel occlusion. Since the introduction of multiple-shot devices, the procedure has become safer, faster and easier to apply compared with single ligators, due to the absence of severe complications from overtube insertion.

The procedure usually starts at the gastroesophageal junction proximally for 6–8 cm in a helical manner to avoid circumferential ligation (fig. 2); otherwise, in active hemorrhage, banding is usually started at the source of bleeding. Up to 10 bands for each procedure can be deployed and sessions are conventionally repeated at 2- to 4-week intervals until variceal obliteration (2–4 sessions required) (fig. 3); moreover, eradication can be considered when either varices disappear or cannot be sucked for banding and occurs in about 90% of patients, although recurrence is not uncommon. Similarly with EST, endoscopic surveillance should be scheduled and recurrent varices should be treated with new EVL sessions. EVL has been revealed to be as effective as EST in bleeding control, but is associated with a significant lower complication rate. Minor complaints, including transient dysphagia and chest discomfort or pain, are not uncommon (up to 45%); otherwise, superficial ulcers at the banding site are frequent and bleeding is rare; bacteriemia and infections, such as spontaneous bacterial peritonitis, occur less frequently after EVL compared with EST [7].

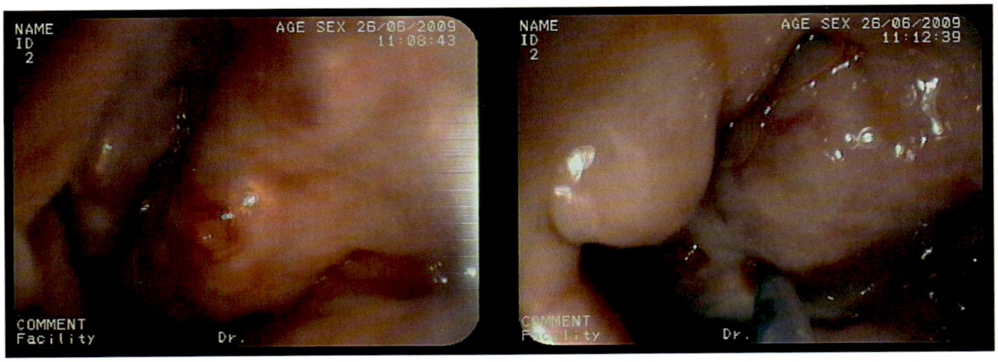

Fig. 1. Intravariceal EST for bleeding EV ('white nipple') with polidocanol 2%.

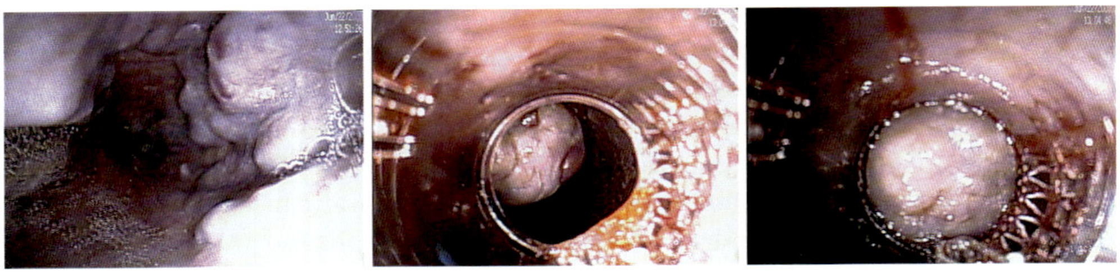

Fig. 2. EBL (7 bands) for bleeding EV ('white nipple').

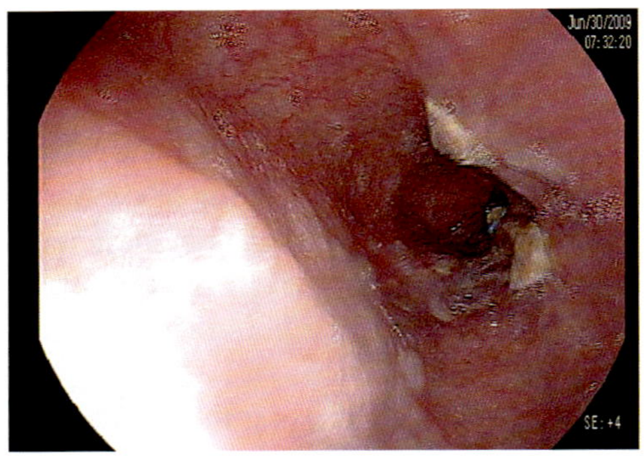

Fig. 3. Follow-up 7 days after EBL: single band persistence and dual esophageal scar on banding sites.

Glue injection

Emerging glue clot after injection

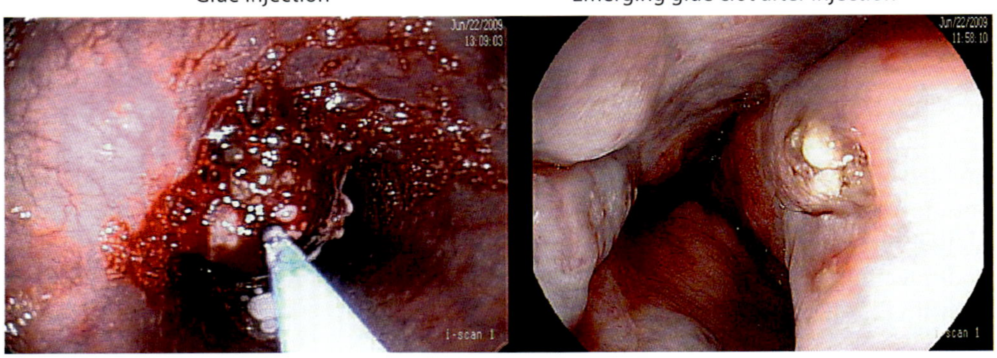

Fig. 4. EST for active EV with Glubran 2® (2 ml).

Endoscopic Variceal Obliteration (EVO)
Intravariceal injection of synthetic glues (cyanoacrylates) provides rapid (within a few seconds) occlusion of the vessel due to the adhesive consolidation at the blood contact.

Glubran 2® (*N*-butyl-cyanoacrylate + metacrylossisulfolane; GEM Srl, Viareggio, Italy), officially approved for endoscopic use in Europe, is currently the optimal agent to gain faster and easier VO compared with Histoacryl® (*N*-butyl-2-cyanoacrylate; B. Braun, Melsungen, Germany) which necessitated addicted lipiodol for dilution to avoid rapid hardening. In our experience, the injection technique, in a 'free-hand' fashion, is similar to EST except for the greater needle caliber (19–20 gauge), as follows: Glubran 2® injection is performed just below the bleeding site with 0.5–1.0 ml, rapidly followed by distilled water or normal saline solution to fill the varix (visible by foaming outside the puncture site) (fig. 4) and to flush out any remaining cyanoacrylate in the injection catheter. Suctioning should be avoided for 20 s after injection to prevent glue adherence to the instrument and the scope should be rapidly withdrawn (with the tip of the needle on the outside of the channel). A second injection, with a new needle, if necessary, can be performed until bleeding control.

Differently from EST, glue injection must be executed intravariceally, due to the risk of deep ulceration with parietal necrosis and perforation; therefore, a small amount of saline could be injected prior to Glubran 2® to verify the appropriateness of the site of needle insertion. Endoscopists should be concerned with some warnings dealing with Glubran 2® use: the glue is ready to use, the glue is for single use only, and the product should be stored at temperature not exceeding +4°C.

The optimal results (high efficacy and safety) with synthetic glues for treatment of gastric varices have gained this technique a primary role in active bleeding control from EV, however significant data from controlled studies are still lacking [8, 9]. In our personal experience (since 1999), among 275 patients with active bleeding from EV, 144 (52.36%) have been treated by endoscopic variceal obliteration with cyanoacrylates and 53 (19.2%) by combined polidocanol 2% and cyanoacrylate injection; recurrence of bleeding occurred in only 4 cases (2.03%) within 30 days from the treatment; neither glue-related nor systemic complications have been reported.

Human and bovine thrombin have been applied to provide hemorrhage control from gastric varices, but limited data and preliminary results suggest the use in further controlled, randomized studies to define the role of these agents in the treatment of EV [4, 6].

Outcomes
Data from the literature and guidelines of different societies have demonstrated well that endoscopic techniques play a significant role in the management of patients with portal hypertension who developed EV only as a component of a multimodality treatment, combined with medical therapy in any phase of the disease, in order to achieve active bleeding control, to prevent recurrences and for the prophylaxis of the first bleeding episode. Randomized trials comparing emergency EST and EVL for active EV bleeding stated the potential difficulties of EVL, due to the poor vision during the procedure; however, multiple-band ligators with transparent caps may overcome these limits [10, 11]. Positive issues include the superior local hemostatic effect of EVL (mechanical) on varices, compared with EST, as supported by the smaller number of sessions and the shorter time needed for eradication with EVL; furthermore, in acute bleeding, sclerosing agents might overincrease portal pressure, which may be unfavorable for a successful treatment.

Acute Bleeding from Esophageal Varices

General Management

Although current treatment strategies have significantly improved prognosis after acute EV bleeding, this event is still associated with high mortality rates (≥20% at 6 weeks) [12]. The aims of initial management are the correction of hemodynamic abnormalities, the prevention of complications (bacterial infections or acute renal failure), the control of acute bleeding and the prevention of early recurrences which drastically make the outcome worse. [13]. Antibiotic prophylaxis plays a significant role in cirrhotic patients (with or without ascites) with variceal bleeding and leads to improvement of survival as demonstrated by the real reduction of bacterial infection rate and incidence of early rebleeding [14]. Oral, when possible, norfloxacin is the agent of first choice, otherwise intravenous ceftriaxone seems to be more effective in patients with advanced liver dysfunction (fig. 5) [15].

Vasoactive Drugs

In suspected variceal hemorrhage, vasoactive drugs should be started as soon as possible (and maintained for 2–5 days), before diagnostic endoscopy, to achieve reduction in active bleeding rate by improvement of endoscopic performance with lower acute mortality; moreover, the incidence of active bleeding during the endoscopy decreases from up to 50% to only 20–25% [16, 17]. The efficacy of vasoactive drugs can be significantly improved when emergency EST is associated [18].

Terlipressin or somatostatin are considered the first choice, regarding the efficacy and safety [5, 16]; but only terlipressin has been showed to improve survival. Furthermore, somatostatin (started before endoscopy and maintained for 5 days) added with EVL significantly improved outcomes when compared with EST, therefore demonstrating the combination of vasoactive drugs and emergency EVL as the first-line therapy for acute variceal bleeding [19]. This recommended combined treatment can be further enhanced by the addition of antibiotic prophylaxis as demonstrated by the 5-day failure rate in only 10–15% of cases [20]. Balloon tamponade (Sengstaken probe) should be adopted only in torrential hemorrhage, as a salvage option until optimal treatment can be instituted (maximum for 24 h and in ICU) [21].

Prevention of Recurrent Variceal Bleeding

Prevention of EV rebleeding can be successfully managed by EST compared with untreated controls. However, EST shows a higher rate of side effects as demonstrated by several comparative trials. Conversely, EVL (and non-selective β-blockers) showed higher safety and effectiveness, as reported by the meta-analysis of 13 randomized trials (>1,000 patients), by significant reduction of rebleeding rate and time for eradication, as well as complications even if survival does not significantly increase. Therefore, EVL can be assumed as the current endoscopic treatment of choice in the prevention of EV rebleeding (fig. 6) [21, 22].

TIPS is strongly indicated in non-surgical patients who failed endoscopic and pharmacological therapies as well as the 'bridge' to liver transplantation in Child class B/C patients. Surgical

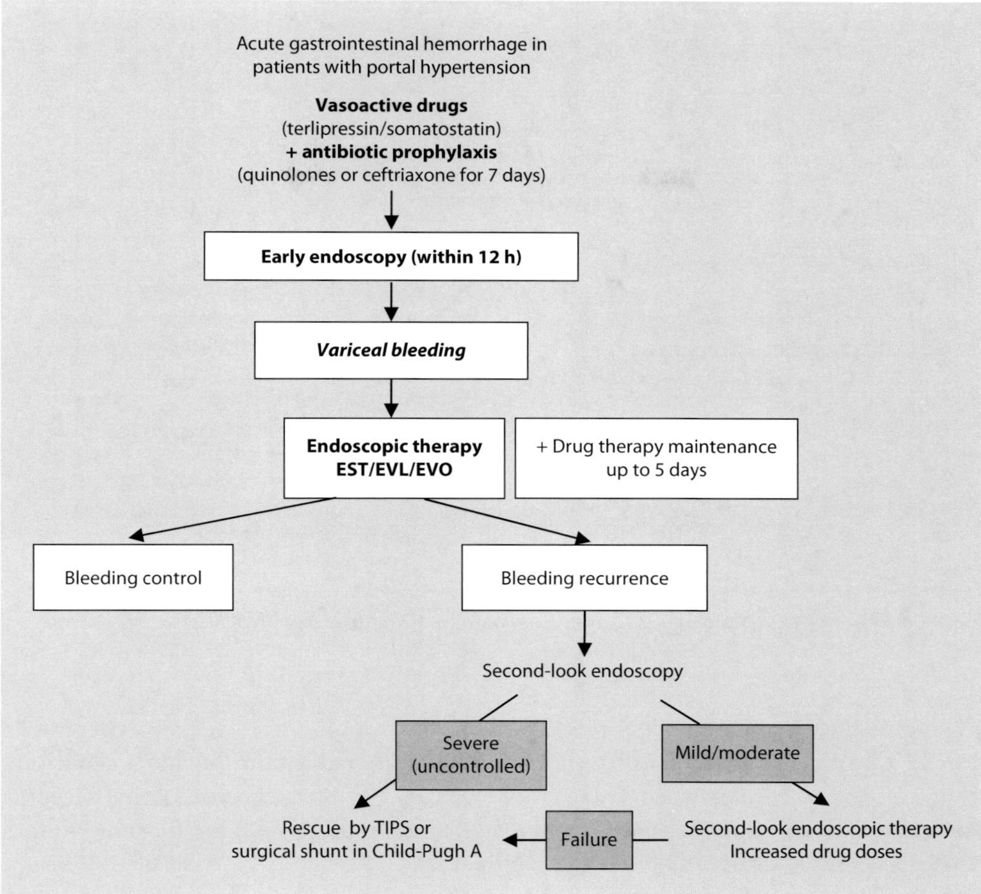

Fig. 5. Management algorithm for acute variceal bleeding [modified from 24].

shunts (distal splenorenal shunt or 8-mm H-graft) can be assumed for subjects with Child class A/B cirrhosis [23].

Summary

Compared with EST, EVL has proven more effectiveness and safety, and is currently the first choice among endoscopic treatments for EV; furthermore, no beneficial effects can be obtained by addition of EST.

In acute EV hemorrhage, early administration of vasoactive drugs (either terlipressin or somatostatin) before diagnostic endoscopy improves emergency endoscopic performances; in this setting, antibiotic prophylaxis has to be generally adopted. In acute variceal hemorrhage, both EST and EVL can achieve bleeding control, although sclerotherapy may expose to a higher complication rate. Variceal glue injection (cyanoacrylates) seems to be effective in the treatment of esophageal as well as in gastric varices. Secondary prevention can be achieved both by EVL

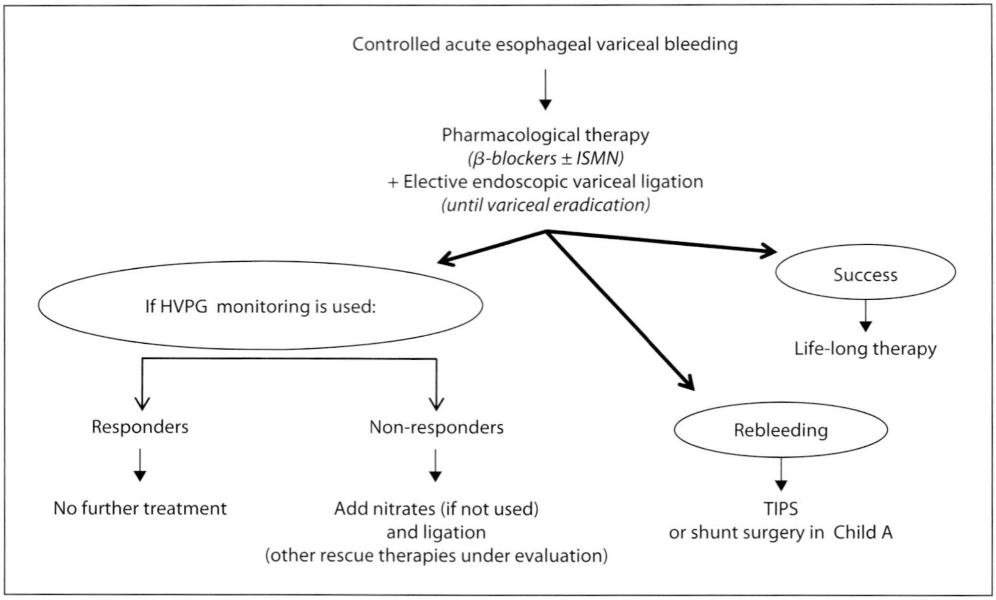

Fig. 6. Management algorithm for variceal bleeding prevention [modified from 24].

alone or combined with non-selective β-blockers. Both the response to β-blockers (decrease in HVPG to <12 mm Hg or by >20% of baseline) and variceal eradication provide a significant reduction in the risk of hemorrhage (<10%). Moreover, EVL reduces the risk of first bleeding with no differences in mortality, compared with drugs, and should be reserved for subjects with large varices and who are unfit for a β-blocker regimen.

Practical Management Issues in Acute Variceal Bleeding

To conclude: (1) antibiotic prophylaxis (quinolones or ceftriaxone) and vasoactive drugs (terlipressin and somatostatin) should be administered after admission and maintained for 2–5 days; (2) endoscopic examination should be performed as soon as possible (within 12 h), especially in cirrhotic patients with severe bleeding; (3) EVL is more effective than EST as emergency endoscopic therapy associated with vasoactive drugs; (4) EVL can be considered the endoscopic method of choice for treating EV, and (5) multimodality treatment (EVL + vasoactive drugs + antibiotics) failures occur in 10–15% and can be best managed by TIPS.

References

1 Escorsell A, Bosch J: Pathophysiology of variceal rupture; in Groszmann RJ, Bosch J (eds): Portal Hypertension in the 21st Century. Dordrecht, Kluwer Academics, 2004, pp 155–166.

2 Cestari R, Missale G, Burroughs AK, et al: Haemodynamic effect of triglycyl-lysine-vasopressin (glypressin) on intravascular oesophageal pressure in patients with cirrhosis. J Hepatol 1990;10:205–210.

3 North Italian Endoscopic Club for The study and Treatment of Esophageal Varices: Prediction of the first variceal hemorrhage in patients with cirrhosis of the liver and esophageal varices. A prospective multicenter study. N Engl J Med 1988;319:983–989.

4 Helmy A, Hayes PC: Current endoscopic therapeutic options in the management of variceal bleeding. Aliment Pharmacol Ther 2001;15:575–594.

5 Baillie J, Yudelman P: Complications of endoscopic sclerotherapy of esophageal varices. Endoscopy 1992;24:284–291.

6 De Franchis R, Primignani M: Endoscopic treatments for portal hypertension. Semin Liver Dis 1999;19:439–455.

7 Garcia-Pagan JC, Bosch J: Endoscopic band ligation in the treatment of portal hypertension. Nat Clin Pract Gastroenterol Hepatol 2005;2:526–535.

8 Tan PC, Hou MC, Lin HC, et al. A randomized trial of endoscopic treatment of acute gastric variceal hemorrhage: *N*-butyl-2-cyanoacrylate injection versus band ligation. Hepatology 2006;43:690–697.

9 Lo GH, Lai KH, Cheng JS, et al: A prospective, randomized trial of butyl cyanoacrylate injection versus band ligation in the management of bleeding gastric varices. Hepatology 2001;33:1060–1064.

10 Laine L: Ligation: endoscopic treatment of choice for patients with bleeding esophageal varices. Hepatology 1995; 22:663–665.

11 Lo GH, Lai KH, Cheng JS, et al: Emergency banding ligation versus sclerotherapy for the control of active bleeding from esophageal varices. Hepatology 1997; 25: 1101–1104.

12 D'Amico G, De Franchis R, and Cooperative Study Group: Upper digestive bleeding in cirrhosis. Post-therapeutic outcome and prognostic indicators. Hepatology 2003;38:599–612.

13 Chalasani N, Kahi C, Francois F, et al: Improved patient survival after acute variceal bleeding: a multicenter, cohort study. Am J Gastroenterol 2003;98: 653–659.

14 Bernard B, Grange JD, Khac EN, et al: Antibiotic prophylaxis for the prevention of bacterial infections in cirrhotic patients with gastrointestinal bleeding: a meta-analysis. Hepatology 1999;29:1655–1661.

15 Hou MC, Lin HC, Liu TT, et al: Antibiotic prophylaxis after endoscopic therapy prevents rebleeding in acute variceal hemorrhage: a randomized trial. Hepatology 2004;39:746–753.

16 Feu F, Ruiz del Arbol L, Banares R, et al: Double-blind randomized controlled trial comparing terlipressin and somatostatin for acute variceal hemorrhage. Gastroenterology 1996;111:1291–1299.

17 Avgerinos A, Nevens F, Raptis S, et al: Early administration of somatostatin and efficacy of sclerotherapy in acute oesophageal variceal bleeds: the European Acute Bleeding Oesophageal Variceal Episodes (ABOVE) randomised trial. Lancet 1997;350:1495–1499.

18 Villanueva C, Ortiz J, Sabat M, et al: Somatostatin alone or combined with emergency sclerotherapy in the treatment of acute esophageal variceal bleeding: a prospective randomized trial. Hepatology 1999; 30:384–389.

19 Villanueva C, Piqueras M, Aracil C, et al: A randomized controlled trial comparing ligation and sclerotherapy as emergency endoscopic treatment added to somatostatin in acute variceal bleeding. J Hepatol 2006;45:560–567.

20 Banares R, Albillos A, Rincon D, et al: Endoscopic treatment versus endoscopic plus pharmacologic treatment for acute variceal bleeding: a meta-analysis. Hepatology 2002;35:609–615.

21 De Franchis R: Evolving consensus in portal hypertension. Report of the Baveno IV consensus workshop on methodology of diagnosis and therapy in portal hypertension. J Hepatol 2005;43:167–176.

22 Garcia-Tsao G, Sanyal A, Grace ND, et al: Prevention and management of gastroesophageal varices and variceal hemorrhage in cirrhosis. Hepatology 2007; 46:922–938.

23 Henderson JM, Boyer TD, Kutner MH, et al: Distal splenorenal shunt versus transjugular intrahepatic portal systematic shunt for variceal bleeding: a randomized trial. Gastroenterology 2006;130:1643– 1651.

24 Villanueva C, Colomo A, Aracil C, et al: Current endoscopic therapy of variceal bleeding. Best Pract Res Clin Gastroenterol 2008;22:261–278.

Renzo Cestari, MD
Digestive Endoscopy Unit, A.O. Spedali Civili di Brescia
Piazzale Spedali Civili, 1, IT–25123 Brescia (Italy)
Tel. +39 030 3995539, Fax +39 030 398276, E-Mail cestari@med.unibs.it

Mönkemüller K, Wilcox CM, Muñoz-Navas M (eds): Interventional and Therapeutic Gastrointestinal Endoscopy.
Front Gastrointest Res. Basel, Karger, 2010, vol 27, pp 64–69

Endoscopic Therapy for Gastric Varices

Klaus Mönkemüller[a,b] · Lucia C. Fry[a,b]

[a]Department of Internal Medicine, Gastroenterology, Hepatology and Infectious Diseases, Marienhospital, Bottrop, and [b]Divison of Gastroenterology, Hepatology and Infectious Diseases, Otto von Guericke University, Magdeburg, Germany

Abstract

Gastric varices occur in about 20% of patients with portal hypertension. Although bleeding from gastric varices occurs less frequently than from esophageal varices, it is usually more severe and more difficult to treat. There are multiple treatment options for bleeding gastric varices including placement of the Sengstaken-Blakemore tube, endoscopic sclerotherapy, performing a transjugular intrahepatic portosystemic shunt (TIPSS) and balloon-occluded retrograde transvenous obliteration (B-RTO). However, B-RTO is only possible to perform in the presence of splenorenal shunts. The Sengstaken is a measure of last resort, not used by most experts anymore. TIPSS should mainly be used if there is chance for liver transplantation. Of the available endoscocpic options, injection of *N*-butyl-2-cyanoacrylate sclerotherapy is highly effective for the obliteration and treatment of active bleeding gastric varices. This article describes the endoscopic approach to gastric varices.

Gastric varices occur in 20% of patients with portal hypertension [1]. Although bleeding from gastric varices occurs less frequently than from esophageal varices, it is usually more severe and more difficult to treat [1–3]. There are multiple treatment options for bleeding gastric varices including placement of the Sengstaken-Blakemore tube, endoscopic sclerotherapy, performing a transjugular intrahepatic portosystemic shunt (TIPSS) and balloon-occluded retrograde transvenous obliteration (B-RTO). Of note, B-RTO is only possible to perform in the presence of splenorenal shunts [3–7]. Of the available endoscocpic options, injection of *N*-butyl-2-cyanoacrylate sclerotherapy is highly effective for the obliteration and treatment of active bleeding gastric varices [6–12].

Procedural Aspects

Patient Preparation

Generally, endoscopic therapy for gastric varices is performed in patients who have significant bleeding and is rarely used on elective basis (fig. 1). It is of paramount importance that the

Part of this article was published in *Digestive Diseases* in 2008, and is reproduced with permission of Karger Publishers.

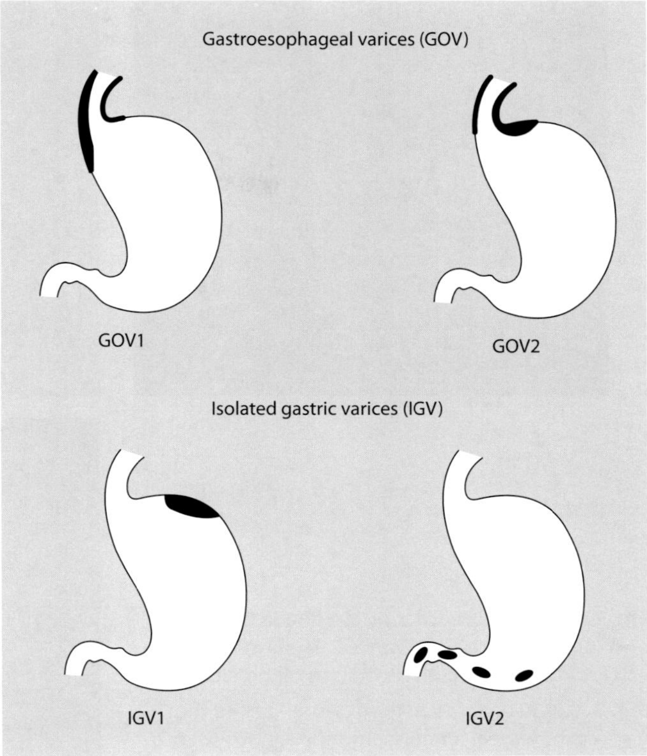

Fig. 1. Endoscopic classification of gastric varices (classification of Sarin and Kumar [9]).

patient is hemodynamically stable and adequate airway protection can be warranted. In cases of massive bleeding, patients should undergo endotracheal intubation to protect the airways. If the patient is hemodynamically stable the endoscopy is performed either in the shock room of the emergency room or in the endoscopy suite under constant monitoring of their vital signs. In cases of hemodynamic instability the endoscopy should always be performed in the intensive care unit. If present, correction of a bleeding diathesis is mandatory. We do not transfuse with platelets unless the total count is <20,000. In patients with advanced cirrhosis of the liver, we routinely administer intravenous vitamin K for at least 3 days. Antibiotic prophylaxis is mandatory as it associated with less variceal rebleeding and may also prevent spontaneous bacterial peritonitis in patients with ascites. The preferred antibiotics are ceftriaxone or levofloxacin.

Accessories

Endoscopy. Endoscopy is performed using a forward-viewing endoscope. Gastric varices are categorized according to the classification of Sarin and Kumar [9] into two main categories. The first category includes varices which extend from the gastroesophageal junction into the stomach (GOV). The varices which extend from the esophagus into the lesser curvature of the stomach are GOV type 1 (GOV1). GOV1 appear as a continuation of esophageal varices and extend for 2–5 cm below the gastroesophageal junction into the lesser curvature. Frequently such varices can and should be treated using endoscopic band ligation, in the same way as esophageal varices, especially if they extend <3 cm into the lesser curvature. GOV type 2 (GOV2) varices extend beyond the gastroesophageal junction into the fundus of the stomach (fig. 1–4) [9]. The second category,

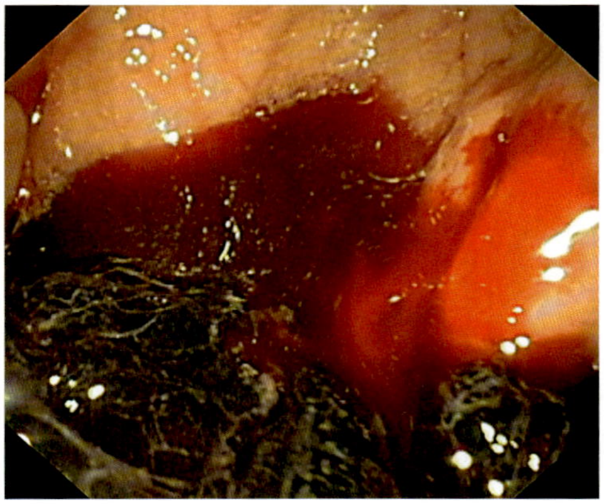

2

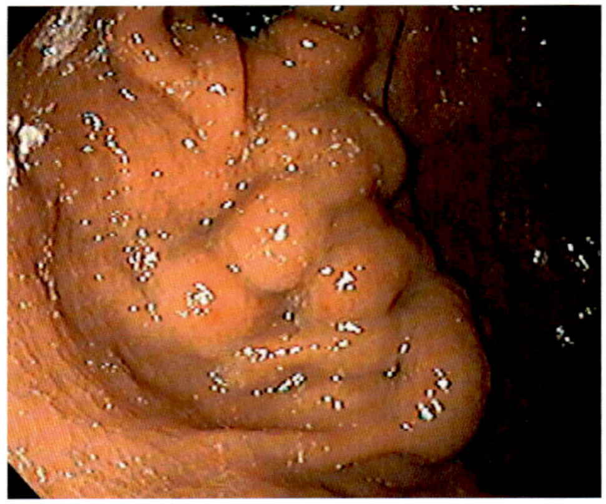

3

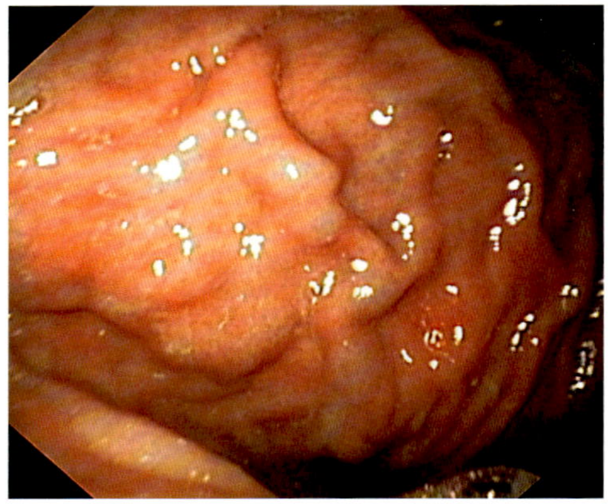

4

Fig. 2. Common endoscopic finding in the presence of bleeding gastric varices. Usually the stomach fundus is filled with blood and blood clots.

Fig. 3. Large gastric varices extending from the gastroesophageal junction into the fundus (GOV2). They have the appearance of a bunch of grapes.

Fig. 4. Isolated fundic varices (IGV1).

isolated gastric varices (IGV), includes two types: fundic (IGV1) or those located anywhere else in the stomach (IGV2). Active bleeding is defined as active blood spurting or oozing from a varix and evidence of recent bleeding was defined as the presence of nipple or red whale signs.

Potential complications from the procedure include aspiration, fever, worsening hemorrhage due to the sclerotherapy and systemic embolization of cyanoacrylate.

Materials Used for Sclerotherapy. There are two major cynaoacrylates (*N*-butyl-2-cyanoacrylate and 2-octyl-cyanoacrylate, Dermabond®). Histoacryl® (*N*-butyl-2-cyanoacrylate (B. Braun, Aesculap AG, Tuttlingen, Germany) is prepared as follows: the injection needle is primed with water, followed by the mixture of Histoacryl (0.5 ml) and lipiodol (1.5 ml) (Lipidol Ultra-Fluid, Guerbet GmbH, Sulzbach, Germany). Sclerotherapy should always be performed using a disposable sclerotherapy needle (e.g. sclerotherapy needle, 2.3 mm diameter, MTW Endoskopie, Wesel, Germany).

Technique

The catheter is introduced into the working channel of the endoscope and advanced. Once the bleeding varix is localized, the needle is exposed and inserted into the base of the varix and the assistant injects the Histoacryl-lipiodol mixture. The injection is done slowly, lasting about 10 s. The need for further injection is determined by probing the varix with the catheter. In the presence of a 'cushion sign' (i.e. soft varix filled with blood) there is a need for further injections [11].

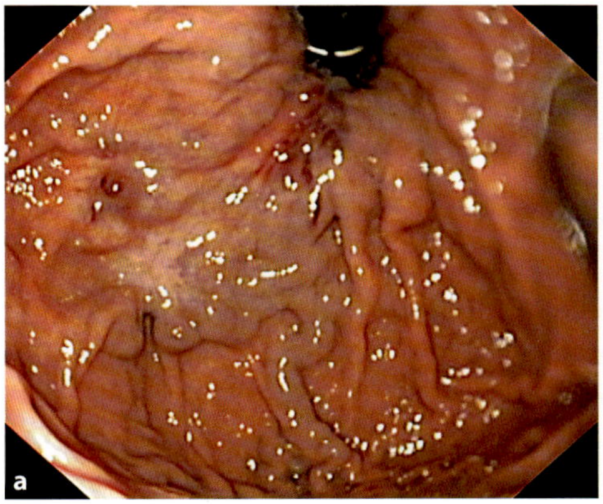

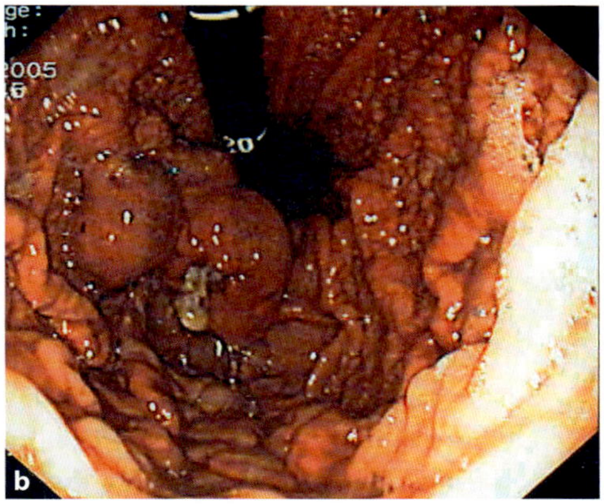

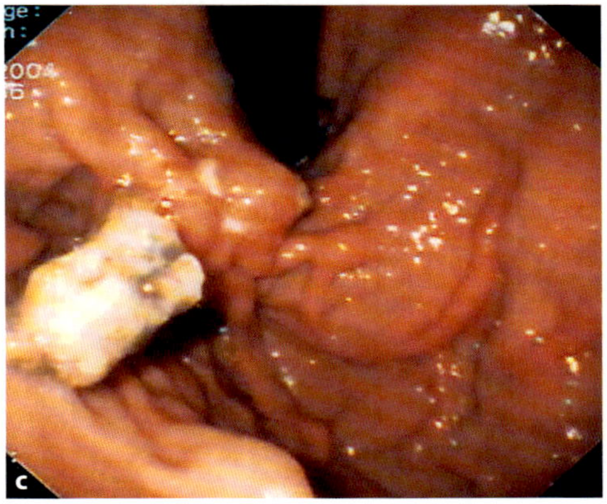

Fig. 5. **a** Note the mucosal fibrosis as a result from Histoacryl injection into fundic varices. This varix has been successfully obliterated. **b** This varix was obliterated with Histoacryl 1 month earlier. **c** Three months later a Histoacryl plug is being extruded from the varix. Never pull on this plug as it may result in catastrophic bleeding.

However, we recommended not to inject more than 1 ml Histoacryl per session as this may be associated with a higher risk of thromboembolism. Upon removing the needle from the varix, the assistant injects normal saline to flush the remaining glue from the catheter. In order to prevent damage to the endoscope, the needle catheter is not retrieved out of the working channel. Instead, the endoscope and the catheter are removed in toto. Both the endoscopist and endoscopy assistant should use goggles as part of the universal precautions guidelines, but also to decrease the likelihood of accidental sprinkling and glue-induced damage to the eyes. Eradication of gastric varices can be accomplished in two thirds of treated patients (fig. 5). Please remember that GOV1 can often be treated using band ligation, as they behave more like esophageal varices.

Post-Procedure Care

Patients with bleeding gastric varices should be managed in the intensive care unit. The patient should remain NPO and receive adequate intravenous fluid volume and electrolyte substitution. Transfusion of fresh-frozen plasma is recommended when the INR remains > 1.6, despite adequate vitamin K supplementation. All patients should also receive either intravenous octreotide or terlipressin. Unless there is no further bleeding, a repeat or second-look endoscopy is not necessary.

Outcomes

Therapy of bleeding gastric varices is a therapeutic challenge. Thus, it is important to have methods that can be helpful in such situations [3]. Most patients with bleeding gastric varices receive medical therapy with octreotide or terlipressin with the aim of reducing portal pressure by inducing splanchnic vasodilation [13–15]. Whereas this approach has been validated for bleeding esophageal varices, its use has not been confirmed for gastric varices. Nevertheless, we always use any of these agents in the treatment algorithm of patients with bleeding gastric varices with the hope of reducing the pressure of the varix. Similar to patients with esophageal varices, we also recommend using β-blockers in patients with IGV.

Many endoscopists, especially outside Europe, are wary of using tissue adhesives such as cyanoacrylate to treat gastric varices because of the reported complications including embolization, increased bleeding and bacteremia [16–18]. This fear is not unfounded. Nevertheless, endoscopic therapy of gastric varices with band ligation is also associated with complications [19–22]. Furthermore, when treating patients with a catastrophic event such as gastric variceal bleeding, the endoscopist needs to take into consideration the higher benefit of stopping the bleeding in relation to the lower risk of complications. The hemostatic success of rates Histoacryl ranges from 55 to 90% [7–19]. Furthermore, it is important to emphasize that there are currently very few other options to treat patients with gastric variceal bleeding [23, 24]. The use of TIPSS is limited if there is portal vein thrombosis, a small portal vein or awkward anatomy [25, 26]. The use of endoloops to obliterate gastric varices appears promising, but there are only few data documenting its efficacy [27]. The use of the Sengstaken-Blakemore tube is considered by many a futile exercise and is generally used as a last resort [28]. However, if a patient is a good candidate to receive a TIPSS, then temporary use of the Sengstaken-Blakemore tube may be beneficial.

To summarize, *N*-butyl-2-cyanoacrylate sclerotherapy is highly effective for the treatment of active bleeding gastric varices, with 15% complications occurring both acutely and long term.

References

1 Kind R, Guglielmi A, Rodella L, Lombardo F, Catalano F, Ruzzenente A, Borzellino G, Girlanda R, Leopardi F, Patticò F, Cordiano C: Bucrylate treatment of bleeding gastric varices: 12 years' experience. Endoscopy 2000;32: 512–519.

2 Fry LC, Neumann H, Olano C, Malfertheiner P, Mönkemüller K: Endoscopic treatment of bleeding gastric varices by *N*-butyl-2-cyanoacrylate (Histoacryl) injection. Dig Dis 2008;26:300–303.

3 Tripathi D, Ferguson JW, Therapondos G, Plevris JN, Hayes PC: Recent advances in the management of bleeding gastric varices. Aliment Pharmacol Ther 2006;24:1–17.

4 Gerke H: Glue for gastric varices: why are we so reluctant in the United States? Gastrointest Endosc 2006;63: 735.

5 Qureshi W, Adler DG, Davila R, Egan J, Hirota W, Leighton J, Rajan E, Zuckerman MJ, Fanelli R, Wheeler-Harbaugh J, Baron TH, Faigel DO, Standards of Practice Committee: ASGE Guideline: the role of endoscopy in the management of variceal hemorrhage, updated July 2005. Gastrointest Endosc 2005;625:651–655.

6 Bhasin DK, Siyad I: Variceal bleeding and portal hypertension: new lights on old horizon. Endoscopy 2004;36: 120–129.

7 Lo GH, Liang HL, Chen WC, Chen MH, Lai KH, Hsu PI, Lin CK, Chan HH, Pan HB: A prospective, randomized controlled trial of transjugular intrahepatic portosystemic shunt versus cyanoacrylate injection in the prevention of gastric variceal rebleeding. Endoscopy 2007;39:679–685.

8 Rengstorff DS, Binmoeller KF: A pilot study of 2-octyl-cyanoacrylate injection for treatment of gastric fundal varices in humans. Gastrointest Endosc 2004;59:553–558.

9 Sarin SK, Kumar A: Gastric varices: profile, classification, and management. Am J Gastroenterol 1989; 84: 1244–1249.

10 Shi B, Wu W, Zhu H, Wu YL: Successful endoscopic sclerotherapy for bleeding gastric varices with combined cyanoacrylate and aethoxysklerol. World J Gastroenterol 2008;14:3598–601.

11 Seewald S, Sriram PV, Naga M, Fennerty MB, Boyer J, Oberti F, Soehendra N: Cyanoacrylate glue in gastric variceal bleeding. Endoscopy 2002;34:926–932.
12 Spaander VM, van Buuren HR, Janssen HL: The management of non-cirrhotic non-malignant portal vein thrombosis and concurrent portal hypertension in adults. Aliment Pharmacol Ther 2007;26: 203–209.
13 Dell'Era A, de Franchis R, Iannuzzi F: Acute variceal bleeding: pharmacological treatment and primary/secondary prophylaxis. Best Pract Res Clin Gastroenterol 2008;22:279–294.
14 Baik SK, Jeong PH, Ji SW, Yoo BS, Kim HS, Lee DK, Kwon SO, Kim YJ, Park JW, Chang SJ, Lee SS: Acute hemodynamic effects of octreotide and terlipressin in patients with cirrhosis: a randomized comparison. Am J Gastroenterol 2005;100:631–635.
15 D'Amico G, Pietrosi G, Tarantino I, Pagliaro L: Emergency sclerotherapy versus vasoactive drugs for variceal bleeding in cirrhosis: a Cochrane meta-analysis. Gastroenterology 2003;124:1277–1291.
16 Martins Santos MM, Correia LP, Rodrigues RA, Lenz Tolentino LH, Ferrari AP, Della Libera E: Splenic artery embolization and infarction after cyanoacrylate injection for esophageal varices. Gastrointest Endosc 2007;65:1088–1090.
17 Dhiman RK, Chawla Y, Taneja S, Biswas R, Sharma TR, Dilawari JB: Endoscopic sclerotherapy of gastric variceal bleeding with *N*-butyl-2-cyanoacrylate. J Clin Gastroenterol 2002;35:222–227.
18 Wahl P, Lammer F, Conen D, Schlumpf R, Bock A: Septic complications after injection of *N*-butyl-2-cyanoacrylate: report of two cases and review. Gastrointest Endosc 2004;59:911–916.
19 Chey WD, Elta GH: Natural history of gastric varices. Gastroenterology 1993;105:599–602.
20 Helmy A, Hayes PC: Review article: current endoscopic therapeutic options in the management of variceal bleeding. Aliment Pharmacol Ther 2001; 15:575–594.
21 Shiha G, El-Sayed SS: Gastric variceal ligation: a new technique. Gastrointest Endosc 1999;49:437–441.
22 Moitinho E, Escorsell A, Bandi JC, Salmerón JM, García-Pagán JC, Rodés J, Bosch J: Prognostic value of early measurements of portal pressure in acute variceal bleeding. Gastroenterology 1999;117:626–631.
23 Abraldes JG, Bosch J: The treatment of acute variceal bleeding. J Clin Gastroenterol 2007;41:312–317.
24 Ryan BM, Stockbrugger RW, Ryan JM: A pathophysiologic, gastroenterologic, and radiologic approach to the management of gastric varices. Gastroenterology 2004;126:1175–1189.
25 Van Buuren HR, ter Borg PC: Transjugular intrahepatic portosystemic shunt: indications and long-term patency. Scand J Gastroenterol 2003;239: 100–104.
26 Ferguson JW, Tripathi D, Hayes PC: The management of acute variceal bleeding. Aliment Pharmacol Ther 2003; 18:253–262.
27 Rácz I, Kárász T, Saleh H: Endoscopic hemostasis of bleeding gastric ulcer with a combination of multiple hemoclips and endoloops. Gastrointest Endosc 2009;69: 580–583.
28 Terés J, Cecilia A, Bordas JM, Rimola A, Bru C, Rodés J: Esophageal tamponade for bleeding varices. Controlled trial between the Sengstaken-Blakemore tube and the Linton-Nachlas tube. Gastroenterology 1978;75:566–569.

Klaus Mönkemüller
Marienhospital, Bottrop, Josef-Albers-Strasse 70
DE–46236 Bottrop (Germany)
Tel. +49 2041 106 1000, Fax +49 2041 106 1009
E-Mail klaus.moenkemueller@mhb-bottrop.de

Mönkemüller K, Wilcox CM, Muñoz-Navas M (eds): Interventional and Therapeutic Gastrointestinal Endoscopy.
Front Gastrointest Res. Basel, Karger, 2010, vol 27, pp 70–78

Portal Hypertensive Gastropathy

R. Cestari · G. Missale · G. Cengia · L. Minelli · D. Moneghini

Department of Surgery, Digestive Endoscopy Unit, University of Brescia, Spedali Civili, Brescia, Italy

Abstract

Portal hypertensive gastropathy (PHG) and gastric antral vascular ectasia (GAVE), frequently combined, are responsible for acute and chronic bleeding in patients with liver cirrhosis and portal hypertension. Endoscopy is basic for detection of typical features and histological examination can enhance diagnostic accuracy. PHG is frequently responsible for chronic bleeding/anemia and the first treatment option is medical therapy; otherwise, failures can be managed by shunting procedures, such as transjugular intrahepatic portosystemic shunt or surgery. Vasoactive drugs (terlipressin or somatostatin and analogues) can be effectively adopted in less common acute bleeding episodes and additional endoscopic therapy can be performed. Endoscopic hemostatic techniques, like argon plasma coagulation, heater probe and laser, are the first-line treatment for both acute and chronic bleeding from GAVE; preliminary data supported the effectiveness of cryotherapy, radiofrequency and banding ligation as appropriate management options.

Portal hypertensive gastropathy (PHG) can be considered as a portal hypertension-related syndrome which affects patients with liver cirrhosis (32.7%), liver fibrosis (23.4%) or extrahepatic portal obstruction (43%) and is frequently associated with esophageal and/or gastric varices [1]. PHG, uncommon in cirrhotic patients, can however be considered as a predictor of bleeding from esophageal varices when associated with gastric varices [2], and accounts for 8% of obscure non-variceal hemorrhages in chronic liver disease, along with chronic iron deficiency anemia and high blood transfusion, with an overall mortality rate of 12.5% [3].

Pathophysiology. The mechanisms involved in the pathogenesis of PHG have not been fully elucidated, however increased gastric total blood flow, with reduction in the mucosal component and enhancement in the submucosal and muscular layers, has been demonstrated [4]. Moreover, reduction in the mucus secretion, abnormalities in gastric nitric oxide regulation as well as anomalous production of prostaglandins [4, 5], tumor necrosis factor (TNF-α), and epidermal growth factor may be involved [6]. All these elements can explain the high sensitivity of the gastric mucosa to NSAIDs and the likelihood of developing non-*Helicobacter coli*-related peptic disease [7].

Furthermore, esophageal and associated gastric varices, as well as previous endoscopic treatments (sclerotherapy 20.5%, ligation 2.3%), have been recognized as risk factors for the development of PHG [1, 8]. Anyway, the natural history of PHG, precisely defined in two prospective trials (cirrhotic patients followed for 3 years at 6-month intervals) correlates well with the severity and duration of liver disease [9]; PHG affects 80% of patients, with different evolution patterns

1

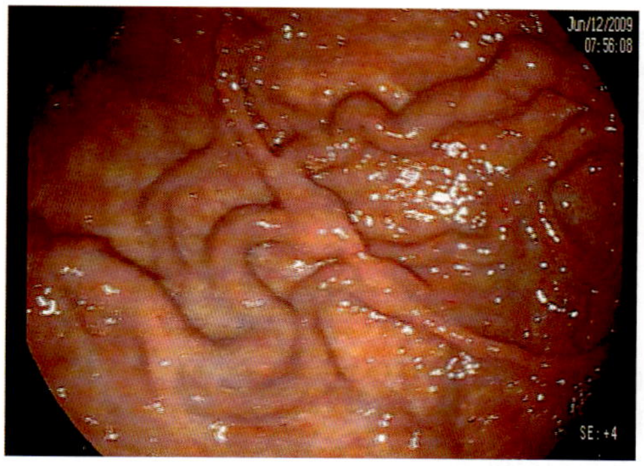

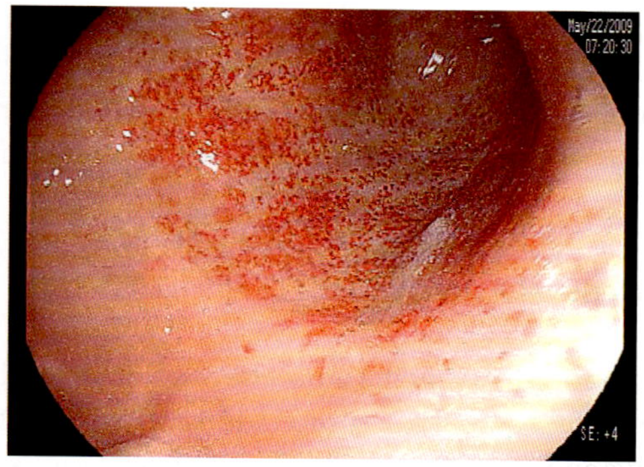

3

2

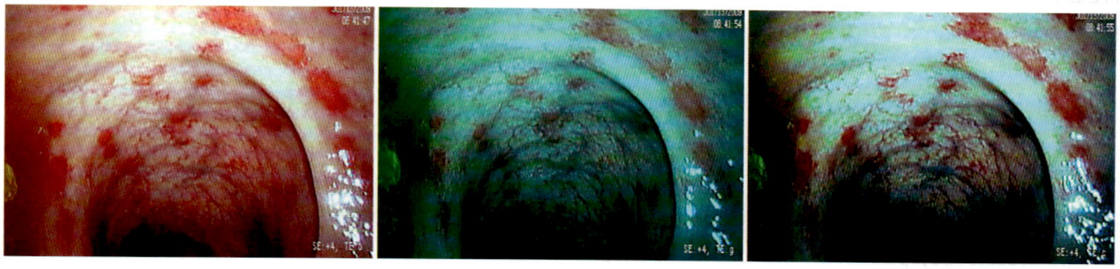

Fig. 1. Fundic 'red point' mild grade PHG (with associated varices). **Fig. 2.** Portal hypertensive colopathy with different enhancement filters (by Pentax EPK-i Processor®). **Fig. 3.** Non-hemorrhagic GAVE.

(worsening 23%, stationary 29%, improvement 23%, variable 25%), with acute (2.5%) or chronic bleeding (10.8%) and a mortality rate of 12.5% [10]; otherwise, both the worsening (9.4 vs. 18%) and bleeding risks can be lower (4.7 vs. 32%) when PHG develops after variceal eradication [11].

Diagnosis can be correctly made by endoscopic examination and severity is usually scored by the presence of typical features such as mosaic-like pattern, red-point lesions, cherry-red and black-brown spots (fig. 1) [12]. Mild lesions are present in 29–57%, while severe stigmata can be detected in 9–46% of patients [13]. Mucosal lesions usually affect fundic and corporal gastric mucosa; however, PHG-like abnormalities can be detected elsewhere in the gastrointestinal tract, from the duodenum toward the colon and rectum [14] (fig. 2).

PHG with Gastric Antral Vascular Ectasia (GAVE). Initially reported by Rider in 1953, GAVE consists of hypertrophic prepyloric antral folds affected by evident tortuous vascular ectasia with a red color very similar to the 'watermelon stomach' (fig. 3). Histological examination shows typical abnormalities such as intramucosal microvascular ectasia, thrombosis, fibromuscular hyperplasia, fibrohyalinosis and spindle cell proliferation detectable in focal as well as diffuse patterns and a diagnostic accuracy of up to 85% [15]. Differential diagnosis with PHG can sometimes be demanding although it may improve by portal hypertension reduction. Moreover, GAVE can be suspected by the predominant gastric location (fundus and corpus), the more severe liver disease, higher frequency of bleeding episodes, hypogastrinemia, and the history of variceal sclerotherapy; similarly, histological evaluation has shown to be accurate in GAVE confirmation by antral microvascular thromboses, fibrohyalinosis and spindle cell proliferation detection [16] (table 1).

The natural history of GAVE is still controversial, with significant differences among patients with or without cirrhosis; in such cases it can be detected more frequently in females with autoimmune diseases (62%) (scleroderma) [17] as well as in subjects with chronic renal failure, primary biliary cirrhosis, hypothyroidism and after bone marrow transplantation. In all these cases, GAVE is usually confined to the antral region, while in cirrhotic patients it can affect the entire gastric surface. Anyway, liver dysfunction, more than portal hypertension, can be considered the main cause, as demonstrated by the relative low prevalence in cirrhosis (30–83%) [18] and the poor response after the correction of portal hypertension as well as after liver transplantation [19, 20].

Procedural Aspects

Endoscopic treatment cannot be considered as the first option in case of bleeding from PHG, due to the low entity and the spread source of the hemorrhage. Conversely, when the source of bleeding is active and focal, such as in GAVE-related lesions, endoscopy plays a primary role in bleeding control, by the following techniques: (a) *contact thermal*: heater probe (HP), multipolar electrocoagulation (MPEC), radiofrequency (RF); (b) *non-contact thermal:* argon plasma coagulation (APC), cryotherapy; (c) *photocoagulative:* Nd:YAG laser, and (d) *mechanical:* elastic banding ligation (EBL).

APC, HP and Nd:YAG laser can be effective in bleeding control as well as in focal vascular lesion treatment [21, 22]; more recently, EBL [23, 24] seems to be a promising option for wide vascular ectasia, even recurrent after APC treatment, since the significant lower complication rate. Furthermore, preliminary data from pilot studies with cryotherapy [25–27] and RF are available [28, 29].

Patient Preparation

In cirrhotic patients with portal hypertension, medical therapy (propranolol, somatostatin and octreotide, vasopressin and terlipressin) can be considered the first option in order to decrease portal pressure in PHG; additionally, rebamide, tranexamic acid, steroids, estrogens, progesterone and octreotide are currently adopted in experimental trials for bleeding control in GAVE. Invasive procedures, however, such as antrectomy/gastrectomy for GAVE and shunts (transjugular intrahepatic portosystemic shunt vs. surgical) or liver transplantation sustain a role in the management of patients with PHG. Losartan, talidomide, and steroids in PHG are currently under investigation [16].

Technique and Accessories

In active bleeding, examination should be performed with large channel (≥3.2 mm) scopes, in order to improve visualization of source and type of the lesions.

Thermal hemostatic treatment is based on the effects of high temperature on the tissues (edema, protein denaturation, vascular constriction and subsequent coagulation bond) and can be achieved by direct heating (HP) as well as by electrocautery devices (MPEC, APC).

Heater Probe. HP consists of a Teflon-coated hollow aluminum catheter and an inner-heating coil. A thermocoupling device at the tip of the probe keeps the temperature constant. The mechanism of tissue coagulation is direct heat transfer, but coactive pressure is also used with HP therapy; an irrigation distal port is combined. Preselected quantity of energy deployment to the diode in the probe tip is actionable by foot pedal. Therefore, once the pulse has been initiated the duration of activation is predetermined [30].

Table 1. Differentiation of severe PHG from GAVE in the setting of cirrhosis and portal hypertension [adapted from 39]

	PHG	GAVE	p value
Clinical features			
Child-Pugh score	6.9±1.9	8.6±2.3	<0.05
Blood loss, ml/day	8.9±1.6	21.6±35	<0.05
Previous sclerotherapy	42.8%	0%	<0.02
Hemoglobin level, g/dl	13±3.1	10.8±2.4	<0.05
Histological features (antrum)			
Microvascular thrombi	0%	50%	0.006
Vascular ectasia	64%	100%	0.04
Spindle cell proliferation	29%	86%	<0.01
Fibrohyalinosis	36%	92%	0.004

Multipolar Electrocoagulation. Contact probes provide tissue exsiccation and reduction in electric conductivity, leading to a decrease in the maximal temperature (100°C) and the depth of the effect. The MPEC generator is preset at 20–50 W and a port at the tip delivers water for irrigation, with improvement in visualization.

Argon Plasma Coagulation. APC is a non-contact electrocoagulative technique based on high-frequency monopolar current conducted to the tissues through ionized argon gas (argon plasma). Coagulation depth is dependent upon several factors such as generator power setting, gas flow rate, duration of application, and distance of the tissue closest to the electrode allowing for en-face or tangential coagulation (depth and diameter of the coagulation zone increased with duration of application and increase in power settings). The APC unit includes a high-frequency monopolar electrosurgical generator, a source of argon gas and gas flow meter. Disposable probes for endoscopic application consists of a flexible Teflon tube with a tungsten monopolar electrode enclosed in a ceramic nozzle located close to its distal end. APC probes are available in different shapes (linear, radial or spherical) diameters and lengths (2.3 mm OD [220 cm, and 440 cm length], and 3.2 mm OD [220 cm length]).

A foot switch synchronizes argon gas release with the delivery of electrical current. Generators deliver an output voltage of 5,000–6,500 V; the power can be adjusted between 0 and 155 W. Argon gas flow may be adjusted from 0.5 to 7 l/min. In general, low power and low argon flow rates are used for hemostasis of superficial vascular lesions with settings of 40–50 W and 0.8 l/min and the probe tip must be close to the tissue to allow the argon plasma to contact the targeted tissue; conversely, higher output settings are used for the tissue ablation with settings up to 70–90 W and 1 l/min. Very high flow rates may result in prompt gaseous distention and patient discomfort, as well as gas penetration through the wall (pneumatosis) or outside the organ. The operative distance between the probe and tissue ranges from 2 to 8 mm [31]. The surface of the targeted tissue should be free of liquid (including blood), to avoid a coagulated film leaving the tissue surface beneath inadequately treated, reducing efficacy in active hemorrhage. APC is generally performed with applications of 0.5–3 s duration [32] and the probe tip can be directed to 'paint' confluent or near-confluent surface areas, avoiding tissue contact (such as a monopolar fashion).

Nd:YAG Laser. Laser photocoagulation provides light energy of a characteristic wavelength emission and focus into a coherent monochromatic beam, which may result in coagulation or vaporization of the targeted tissue. A flexible optical fiber transmits the laser beam, which can be used in a contact or non-contact fashion. The distal tip (sapphire or ceramic) of the probe must be maintained at 1 cm from targeted area, with a preset power of 40–90 W and 0.5–1 s in duration time application.

Elastic Banding Ligation. Ligation devices consist of a single-use system counting a transparent friction fit adapter (similar to transparent cap) attached to the tip of the scope, preloaded rubber band(s) [1, 4–7, 10] and a release trigger-like mechanism which deploys elastic bands after the tissue is suctioned into the hollow chamber of the adapter. Tissue ligation results in direct hemostatic effect and through necrosis and sloughing [30]. GAVE treatment is generally performed by ligation of the vascular ectasia from the pylorus to the corpus with proximal estension until the normal appearance of gastric tissue with 12.7 bands per session (SD 4.6, range 9–23) (fig. 4).

Cryotherapy. Cryotherapy is a non-contact method for tissue disruption by application of refrigerated gas onto the target mucosa (nitrous oxide, CO_2) and the use in the gastrointestinal tract is still limited, as reported by several pilot studies [33]. Two different methods are suitable for this purpose: one consists of an insulating coated catheter, which releases liquid nitrogen, at –196°C, and the second applies pressurized CO_2 through a 6-french, 200-cm long, single-use catheter. Application is conducted 2–3 cm away from the targeted tissue and the effect is visible after 3–4 s by tissue whitening and ice formation; the procedure can be repeated after 2–3 days to achieve treatment completion [25].

Radiofrequency. RF has recently been applied for GAVE treatment by using the HALO90 (Barrx Medical), consisting of 24 alternate-polarity microelectrodes, which applies energy in up to 3 cm^2 wide areas; the probe, mounted on the distal tip of the scope (in the 12 o'clock position), must be used with 2.8- to 3.4-mm channel instruments. The RF generator is usually preset at 40 W/cm^2 with 12 J/cm^2 of energy density (fig. 5). Treatment consists of four applications for each area, leading ablation uniformly concerning the surface and depth of the effect, which is dependent on the deployed energy density [29].

Personal Experience

Between 2000 and 2008, 43 patients with GAVE were observed at our department. Of these, 21 (48.8%) underwent 54 endoscopic treatments with APC for bleeding. The mean number of therapeutic procedures in each patient was 1.55. More than half of the patients (52.4%) required at least two treatments; in 23.8%, three or more therapeutic endoscopies were needed and 19% of cases were treated 5 times. No patients had more than six examinations. In all cases the endoscopic procedures allowed bleeding control and reduced blood transfusion requirement. Because of the high number of endoscopies needed per patient, in 2009 we introduced EBL in our clinical practice. This initial experience seems to be very effective: we achieved bleeding control in all patients with a single treatment and mucosal healing was faster, reducing the risk of rebleeding from the treated area.

Outcomes

The main goals of GAVE endoscopic treatment are the prevention and control of bleeding, as well as the reduction in blood transfusion requirement; moreover, the choice of the appropriate technique is strictly dependent upon the confidence with the method itself as well as the local expertise and resource availability.

Argon Plasma Coagulation. The effectiveness of this technique is well demonstrated by the abolition in blood transfusion in 77% of patients [21] with subsequent improvement in portal encephalopathy [34] (fig. 6).

Multipolar Electrocoagulation. The depth of tissue injury is dependent upon the power setting, the duration of the contact and the degree of pressure applied to the targeted area (1 mm in depth for slight pressure of 2 s)

Nd:YAG Laser. The hemostatic effect has been shown to be earlier compared with APC and the long-term results are similar [35]. A thermal effect can reach 4–6 mm in depth on the targeted tissue.

Cryotherapy and RF. These techniques have been demonstrated effective for the treatment of lesions that are large and recurrent after APC [26]. Limited available data reported the absence of active bleeding in 71% of patients after 3.6 sessions, with a significant reduction for the need of blood transfusion and an increase in hemoglobin and hematocrit levels, without hematemesis; furthermore, both healing of erosive lesions and complete epithelial restoration were found at 2–4 weeks and 3 months respectively [27, 29].

Radiofrequency. Standardized RF (4 applications at 14 J/cm^2) has shown to be effective in ablating the superficial part of the submucosal layer (1,000 μm), as reported in 6 patients (66.6% APC-resistant) treated with 10 ablative sessions (33 applications for each session; electrode cleaning up to 2.5 times/session; mean duration time 26 min) with technical success in 83.3% [29].

Elastic Banding Ligation. As demonstrated for esophageal varices and compared with thermal treatment, ligation provides vascular ectasia interruption in GAVE, with a significant reduction in the number of blood units transfused (0.9 ± 2.0 vs. 5.7 ± 13.7), the number of hospital admissions for bleeding (0.1 ± 0.3 vs. 1.2 ± 1.7), the number of sessions required for treatment (1.9 ± 0.6, range 1–3 vs. 4.7 ± 4.7, range 1–14), the need for rebleeding prevention after treatment (33 ± 50 vs. 82 ± 41) and, finally, the number of overall blood transfusions after therapy (0.89 ± 2.03 vs. 6.45 ± 14.87) [23]. The mean healing time was about 4 weeks, with mild persistent lesions. The superiority of EBL seems to be related to the higher efficacy in the obliteration of vascular abnormalities affecting mucosal and submucosal layers, as confirmed by results in patients refractory to thermal treatments [24, 36].

Need for retreatment (4–6 weeks later) is based on technical success (efficacy in bleeding control), clinical outcome (recurrent bleeding episodes, hemodynamic instability, blood transfusion requirement) and endoscopic features. Total costs for endoscopic therapy have been demonstrated to be lower for APC compared with Nd:YAG laser; no data about the cost-effectiveness of APC, HP, Nd:YAG laser and cryotherapy are currently available.

Limitations and Complications

The depth of the thermal effect and coagulation are the main predictors of complications, such as perforations and strictures, and dependent upon the technique (lower with APC, mild with MPEC, higher with laser) and the power settings applied; nevertheless, all these methods equally predispose to bleeding and perforation through ulcer and scar formation on the gastric surface as result of treatment.

HP is limited by the small areas treatable in one single session, with a perforation rate of 1.8–3% and intraprocedural bleeding in 5% [37]. APC demonstrated a wide range of complication rates (0–24%), including pneumoperitoneum, pneumomediastinum, visceral perforation,

4
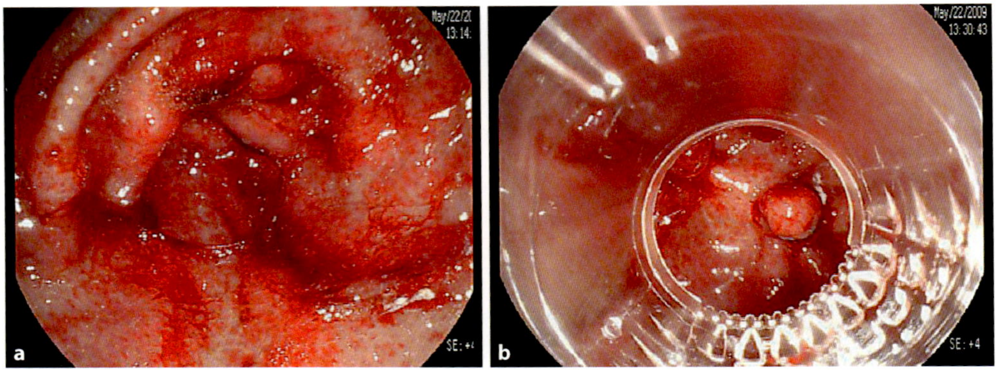

Fig. 4. **a** Hemorrhagic GAVE. **b** After ligation with 5 bands.

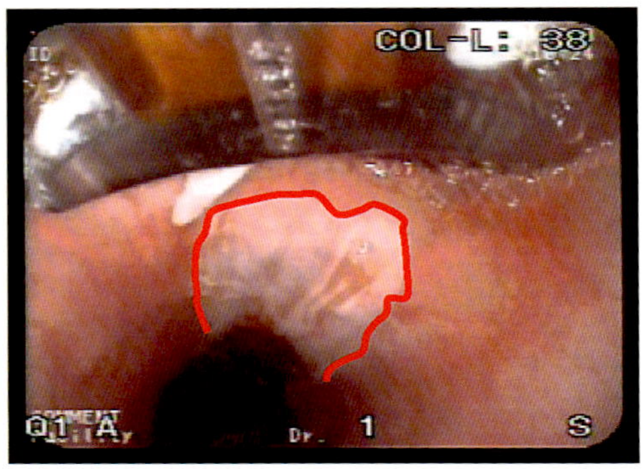

5

Fig. 5. RF ablation with HALO90 system (ablated area delimited by red line).

6
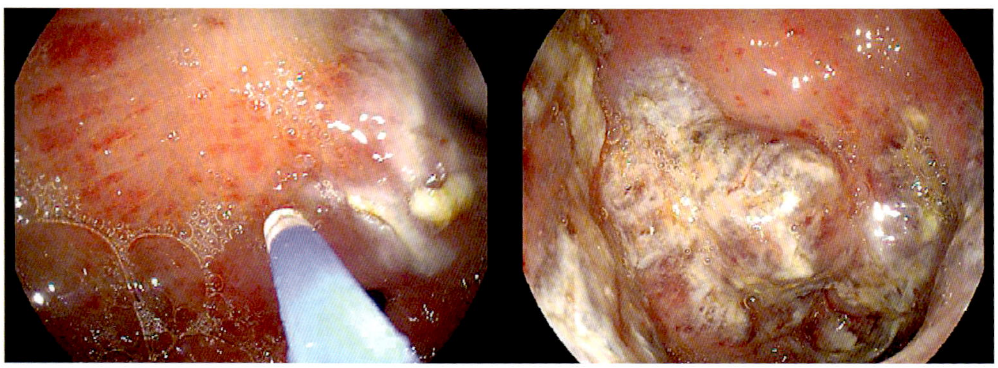

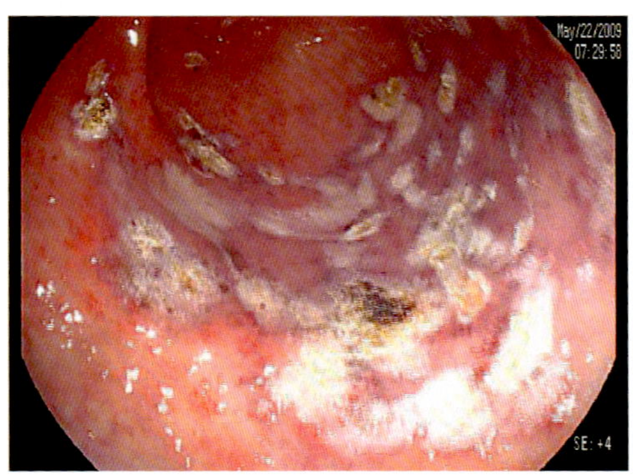

7

Fig. 6. Hemorrhagic GAVE treated by the APC-VIO II system (30 W; pulse mode; end-side probe).

Fig. 7. Follow-up endoscopy after APC treatment of hemorrhagic GAVE (1 week later).

subcutaneous emphysema, burning wall syndrome, chronic ulcerations (fig. 7), local pain and bleeding. For analogous power settings, duration and operative distance, APC showed significantly lower perforation rates compared to Nd:YAG laser [32], while the overall number of sessions needed to eradicate lesions is higher. In one single patient, a 74-year-old male, gastric antral stricture has been described after 7 APC sessions [38]. Nd:YAG laser: the risk of perforation (9%) and bleeding (29%) is strictly related to the power adopted; other reported complications include strictures, fistulas, abscesses, fever and pain. Finally, risk for complications seems to be lower with cryotherapy (2.2%) [25], RF (0.25%) and EBL (0%) [23].

Post-Procedure Care Algorithm. Once endoscopic treatment has been considered complete, re examination should be scheduled at 2–4 weeks, at 3 and 6 months interval time.

To summarize: PHG and GAVE can be considered as two different pathological entities, frequently combined, affecting patients with liver cirrhosis and portal hypertension and responsible for acute and chronic bleeding. Differential diagnosis can sometimes be challenging, but endoscopy is basic for the detection of typical features (mosaic-like with or without 'red points' in the proximal stomach versus confluent linear 'red points' with no mosaic-like lesions in the distal stomach) and histological examination can enhance diagnostic accuracy. PHG is frequently responsible for chronic bleeding/anemia and the first treatment option is medical therapy with non-selective β-blockers; failures can be managed by shunting procedures, such as transjugular intrahepatic portosystemic shunt or surgery. Vasoactive drugs, such as terlipressin or somatostatin and analogues, can be effectively adopted in less common acute bleeding episodes; in such cases additional endoscopic therapy can be performed, with a lower successful rate however. Traditional endoscopic hemostatic techniques, like APC, HP and laser are the first-line treatment for both acute and chronic bleeding from GAVE; preliminary data supported the effectiveness of cryotherapy, radiofrequency and banding ligation as appropriate management options.

References

1 Sarin SK, Sreenivas DV, Lahoti D, et al: Factors influencing development of portal hypertensive gastropathy in patients with portal hypertension. Gastroenterology 1992;102:994–999.

2 Zoli M, Merkel C, Magalotti D, et al: Evaluation of a new endoscopic index to predict first bleeding from the upper gastrointestinal tract in patients with cirrhosis. Hepatology 1996;24:1047–1052.

3 Primignani M, Carpinelli L, Sarin SK, et al: Portal Hypertensive Gastropathy in Portal Hypertension III. Proc 3rd Baveno International Consensus Workshop on Definitions, Methodology and Therapeutic Strategies. Oxford, Blackwell Science, 2001, pp 65–75.

4 Beck PL, McKnight W, Lee SS, et al: Prostaglandin modulation of the gastric vasculature and mucosal integrity in cirrhotic rats. Am J Physiol 1993;265: G453–G458.

5 Arakawa T, Satoh H, Fukuda T, et al: Endogenous prostaglandin E_2 in gastric mucosa of patients with alcoholic cirrhosis and portal hypertension. Gastroenterology 1987;93:135–140.

6 Romano M, Meise KS, Suozzo R, et al: Regional distribution of transforming growth factor-α and epidermal growth factor in normal and portal hypertensive gastric mucosa in humans. Dig Dis Sci 1995;40:263–267.

7 Balan KK, Jones AT, Roberts NB, et al: The effects of *Helicobacter pylori* colonization on gastric function and the incidence of portal hypertensive gastropathy in patients with cirrhosis of the liver. Am J Gastroenterol 1996;91:1400–1406.

8 Sarin SK, Govil A, Jain AK, et al: Prospective randomized trial of endoscopic sclerotherapy versus variceal band ligation for esophageal varices: influence on gastropathy, gastric varices and variceal recurrence. J Hepatol 1997;26:826–832.

9 Merli M, Nicolini G, Angeloni S, et al: The natural history of portal hypertensive gastropathy in patients with liver cirrhosis and mild portal hypertension. Am J Gastroenterol 2004;99:1959–1965.

10 Primignani M, Carpinelli L, Preatoni P, et al: Natural history of portal hypertensive gastropathy in patients with liver cirrhosis. The New Italian Endoscopic Club for the study and treatment of esophageal varices. Gastroenterology 2000;119:181–187.

11 Sarin SK, Shahi HM, Jain M, et al: The natural history of portal hypertensive gastropathy: influence of variceal eradication. Am J Gastroenterol 2000;95: 2888–2893.

12 Carpinelli L, Primignani M, Preatoni P, et al: Portal hypertensive gastropathy: reproducibility of a classification, prevalence of elementary lesions, sensitivity and specificity in the diagnosis of cirrhosis of the liver. A NIEC multicentre study. New Italian Endoscopic Club. Ital J Gastroenterol Hepatol 1997; 29:533–540.

13 Pique JM: Portal hypertensive gastropathy. Baillieres Clin Gastroenterol 1997;11:257–270.

14 Gupta R, Saraswat VA, Kumar M, et al: Frequency and factors influencing portal hypertensive gastropathy and duodenopathy in cirrhotic portal hypertension. J Gastroenterol Hepatol 1996;11:728–733.

15 Jabbari M, Cherry R, Lough JO, et al: Gastric antral vascular ectasia: the watermelon stomach. Gastroenterology 1984;87:1165–1170.

16 Burak KW, Beck PL: Portal hypertensive gastropathy and gastric antral vascular ectasia (GAVE) syndrome. Gut 2001;49:866–872.

17 Murphy FT, Enzenauer RJ, Cheney CP: Watermelon stomach. Arthritis Rheum 1999;42:573.

18 Ito M, Uchida Y, Kamano S, et al: Clinical comparisons between two subsets of gastric antral vascular ectasia. Gastrointest Endosc 2001;53:764–770.

19 Spahr L, Villeneuve JP, Dufresne MP, et al: Gastric antral vascular ectasia in cirrhotic patients: absence of relation with portal hypertension. Gut 1999;44: 739–742.

20 Vinvent C, Pomier-Layrargues G, Dagenais M, et al: Cure of gastric antral vascular ectasia by liver transplantation despite persistent portal hypertension: a clue for pathogenesis. Liver Transplant 2002;8:717–720.

21 Kwan V, Bourke MJ, Williams SJ, et al: Argon plasma coagulation in the management of symptomatic gastrointestinal vascular lesions: experience in 100 consecutive patients with long-term follow-up. Am J Gastroenterol 2006;101:58–63.

22 Mathou NG, Lovat LB, Thorpe SM, et al: Nd:YAG laser induces long-term remission in transfusion-dependent patients with watermelon stomach. Lasers Med Sci 2004; 18:213–218.

23 Wells CD, Harrison ME, Gurudu SR, et al: Treatment of gastric antral vascular ectasia (watermelon stomach) with endoscopic band ligation. Gastrointest Endosc 2008; 68:231–236.

24 Sinha SK, Udawat HP, Varma S, et al: Watermelon stomach treated with endoscopic band ligation. Gastrointest Endosc 2006;64:1028–1031.

25 Kantsevoy SV, Cruz-Correa MR, Vaughn CA, et al: Endoscopic cryotherapy for the treatment of bleeding mucosal vascular lesions of the gastrointestinal tract: a pilot study. Gastrointest Endosc 2003;57:403–406.

26 Cho S, Yong E, Zanati S, et al: Endoscopic cryotherapy for the management of gastric antral vascular ectasia: a pilot study (abstract). Gastrointest Endosc 2006;63:AB81.

27 Cho S, Zanati S, Yong E, et al: Endoscopic cryotherapy for the management of gastric antral vascular ectasia. Gastrointest Endosc 2008;68:895–902.

28 Rodriguez SA, Adler DG, Chand B, et al: Mucosal ablation devices: status evaluation report. Gastrointest Endosc 2008;68:1031–1042.

29 Gross SA, Al-Haddad M, Gill KR, et al: Endoscopic mucosal ablation for the treatment of gastric antral vascular ectasia with the HALO90 system: a pilot study. Gastrointest Endosc 2008;67:324–327.

30 ASGE Technology Status Evaluation Report: Mucosal ablation device. Gastrointest Endosc 2008;68:1031–1042.

31 Wahab PJ, Mulder CJ, den Hartog G, et al: Argon plasma coagulation in flexible gastrointestinal endoscopy: pilot experiences. Endoscopy 1997;29:176–181.

32 Watson JP, Bennett MK, Griffin SM, et al: The tissue effect of argon plasma coagulation on gastric and esophageal mucosa. Gastrointest Endosc 2000;52: 342–345.

33 Pasricha PJ, Hill S, Wadwa KS, et al: Endoscopic cryotherapy: experimental results and first clinical use. Gastrointest Endosc 1999;49:627–31.

34 Zushi S, Imai Y, Fukuda K, et al: Endoscopic coagulation therapy is useful for improving encephalopathy in cirrhotic patients with gastric antral vascular ectasia. Dig Endosc 2005;17:32–35.

35 Bjorkman DJ, Buchi KN: Endoscopic laser therapy of the watermelon stomach. Lasers Surg Med 1992; 12:478–481.

36 Kumar R, Mohindra S, Pruthi HS: Endoscopic band ligation: a novel therapy for bleeding gastric antral vascular ectasia. Endoscopy 2007;39(suppl 1):E56–E57.

37 Cook DJ, Guyatt GH, Salena BJ, et al: Endoscopic therapy for acute non-variceal upper gastrointestinal hemorrhage: a meta-analysis. Gastroenterology 1992;102:139–148.

38 Farooq FT, Wong RC, Yang P, et al: Gastric outlet obstruction as a complication of argon plasma coagulation for watermelon stomach. Gastrointest Endosc 2007;65:1090–1092.

39 Payen JL, Calès P, Voigt JJ, et al: Severe portal hypertensive gastropathy and antral vascular ectasia are distinct entities in patients with cirrhosis. Gastroenterology 1995;108:138–144.

Renzo Cestari, MD
Digestive Endoscopy Unit, A.O. Spedali Civili di Brescia
Piazzale Spedali Civili, 1, IT–25123 Brescia (Italy)
Tel. +39 030 3995539, Fax +39 030 398276
E-Mail cestari@med.unibs.it

Mönkemüller K, Wilcox CM, Muñoz-Navas M (eds): Interventional and Therapeutic Gastrointestinal Endoscopy.
Front Gastrointest Res. Basel, Karger, 2010, vol 27, pp 79–90

Removal of Gastrointestinal Foreign Bodies

Josep M. Bordas[a] · Josep Llach[a] · Miguel Muñoz-Navas[b]

[a]Endoscopy S., Gastroenterology Department, Institut de Malalties Digestives, Hospital Clinic, Barcelona, and [b]Gastroenterology Department, Clínica Universitaria de Navarra, Pamplona, Spain

Abstract

More than 80–95% of the ingested foreign bodies pass spontaneously through the gastrointestinal (GI) tract without or with few complications; it is considered that 10–20% require medical intervention. In the great majority of the cases, endoscopy solves the problem and in around 1% of the cases surgery is required for exploration and extraction. Although foreign body ingestion can induce severe complications and even death, in recent years, deaths caused by foreign bodies have rarely been reported. The greatest incidence of foreign body ingestion occurs in children, psychiatric patients and prisoners and, in general, foreign bodies are found in previously healthy patients. It is mandatory to spend some time to acquire an accurate history followed by front and profile x-rays. The most common foreign bodies are ingested foreign bodies. The risks are related to sharp and long objects, button batteries and magnets. A number of rectal foreign bodies may be retained inside the rectum or sigmoid. When endoscopy fails, surgery is mandatory. Nowadays some medical therapies may introduce foreign bodies in the digestive tract that must be retrieved. After retrieval, 24-hour admission should be only considered when complications or possible complications are suspected or when surgery is considered. All patients with foreign bodies are admitted to hospital after surgery if required. It is very important to recognize a significant complication induced by a foreign body even before any active medical intervention or after retrieval, since it is known that early treatment greatly influences the outcome.

Foreign bodies are a recurrent problem and a challenge in gastrointestinal (GI) endoscopy. Ingested foreign bodies are the most frequent foreign bodies in the digestive tract. However, rectal introduction may also be considered and nowadays another source of digestive foreign bodies may be due to GI medical therapy or the migration of foreign medical objects from other parts of the body.

This subject has had a great impact in medical journals and for many years nearly 200 papers on foreign bodies have been published every year in journals submitted for peer review. Most are case reports and only a few are retrospective series.

The greatest incidence of foreign body ingestion occurs in children, psychiatric patients and prisoners and, in general, swallowed or rectal foreign bodies are found in previously healthy patients [1, 2]. The management of this situation sometimes involves risks of which both the patient and relatives must be aware. After assessing that a foreign body is present and ruling out the presence

Table 1. Foreign body work-up

1. History	In some patients the presence of a foreign body is only suspected In children this situation is more frequent
2. Physical examination	Presence, location, shape and relationship with surrounding organs
3. Assessing suspected diagnosis	X-ray study (front and lateral study) other imaging studies
4. Diagnosis	Presence, location, shape and relationship with surrounding organs
5. Plan foreign body extraction	Observation, endoscopic treatment, surgery
6. Searching for endoscopic material, personnel	Location, nature and shape of the foreign body determine the method for retrieval When an endoscopic method is decided, adequate sedation facilities, scope and ancillary devices must be selected and ready to use before starting the treatment It is also convenient to try the best method in hanging similar objects when possible
7. To prevent solution for the side effects (admission and surgical facilities)	Surgery department should be contacted in difficult cases
8. Explanation of the procedure and informed consent	It is mandatory to inform the patient of the usual risk involved with the location, nature and shape of the foreign body
9. Endoscopic procedure	Sometimes endoscopy is used as a diagnostic tool mainly in the hypopharynx and in esophageal foreign bodies
10. Post-procedure care	Decision as to hospital admission

Table 2. Material for foreign body retrieval

Endoscopic devices	
Flexible scopes	Rigid scopes
Ancillary devices Endoscopic scissors Dormia basket (different sizes) Lithotriptor Retrieval net Atraumatic grasping forceps Special forceps Alligator Rat-tooth Rubber-covered forceps Polypectomy snares Magnetic catheter Forcep hooks	Magill forceps Standard forceps
Special ancillary devices Overtube Soft rubber funnel hood attached to the tip of the scope Finger part of a latex hand globe attached to the tip of the scope TTS balloon dilators	

of severe side effects needing more invasive management, endoscopy can be applied in the great majority of patients experiencing symptoms in the upper GI tract and in those with potentially dangerous foreign bodies.

Procedural Aspects (table 1)

It is mandatory to spend some time to acquire an accurate history followed by some basic instrumental diagnostic procedures. Front and profile x-rays are sometimes very useful, mainly when the suspected foreign body can be visualized by this method. Nonetheless, in these cases the x-ray reading must be accurate since, in some cases, the images of the foreign body may be difficult to assess. Nonetheless, even in negative readings, these documents may be useful in relation to any legal problem [3].

The aim of the x-ray examination is: (1) to confirm the presence of a foreign body [4]; (2) to know the size and shape; (3) to diagnose a preexisting perforation; (4) to know its location and avoid unexpected perforation, and (5) to have some idea of the method and possible risk involved in extraction.

After evaluating the foreign body or having a high suspicion of its presence, the following are necessary: (1) to obtain written informed consent; (2) to establish the work-up plan, and (3) prepare the adequate material/personnel (tables 2, 3).

Patient Preparation

Only a few scientific societies have published guidelines on this subject. These documents are important because they are the procedural basis and inform the society on the difficulties and risks involved [5]. It is necessary to decide if foreign body retrieval maneuvers should start immediately or if it would be convenient to wait for the stomach to be empty or the colon prepared.

Patients with esophageal foreign bodies can be explored by endoscopy immediately if appropriate. The endoscopy of patients with stomach and intestinal foreign bodies may wait for the cavity to be empty which facilitates the search and diminishes the risk of aspiration. The colon needs adequate cleansing (prograde in non-obstructive cases) if perforation has been ruled out and endoscopy is considered the procedure of choice.

Treatment for Specific Foreign Bodies

Ingested Foreign Bodies (table 3)

Impacted Food Bolus

Most ingested foreign bodies occur in children with a maximal incidence between 6 months and 3 years of age. In adults, patients with an increased risk are those wearing dental prostheses because of the lesser sensitivity during swallowing, overall if they do not wear their glasses for eating. These circumstances facilitate the ingestion of bone, some hard food pieces or shellfish such as cockles. Other medical situations that facilitate food impaction in the esophagus are

Table 3. Foreign body treatment

Decision			
Observation without admission	Minimal invasive treatment (retrieval, destruction dissolution/digestion, dislodge)	Admission for observation	Surgery
For small blunt foreign body in stomach In 90% of cases, foreign bodies reach stomach	Flexible endoscopes are used in most cases Rigid endoscopes can be used for objects in a hypopharyngeal location Different ancillary devices can be used but the most frequently used are: – Rat-tooth grasping forceps – Atraumatic three-arm forceps – Dormia basket – Polypectomy snare – Retrieval net – Magnetic retriever – Overtube – Soft rubber protector hood attached to the endoscope tip These devices facilitate retrieval of some sharp objects	Complications or possible complications are suspected Some complex foreign bodies Foreign body in which previous endoscopic retrieval failed	Must be considered – In free abdominal perforation – When vascular involvement is suspected – Complex foreign bodies with high risk of perforation during retrieval maneuvers

esophageal motor disturbances (achalasia, sclerodermia, diffuse spasm) strictures (Schatzki's ring, peptic strictures, tumors and membranes) and diverticulae.

Most of the patients with food impaction require endoscopic (95%) or surgical intervention. The most important information in this group of patients who need endoscopic (95%) or surgical intervention in a high percentage of cases is to obtain knowledge on the type of foreign body by: (1) clinical history to determine whether a fish or meat bone may be included in the ingested foreign body; (2) the second most important information is the length of time from the ingestion to the appearance of symptoms; (3) the clinical manifestations are also important, and (4) exploration and data obtained by x-ray examination are convenient and in some cases are necessary.

These data allow a decision to be made in selecting the best treatment: observation, endoscopy or surgery. When there is high probability that no bone is included in the impacted bolus, minimal invasive treatment using flexible endoscopy is usually the best procedure. Unchewed meat or large meat fragments may be removed using different types of grasping forceps, snare or Dormia basket (fig. 1), after dislodging. When the foreign body is soft in absence of bone or sharp objects, endoscopy provides knowledge on the nature of the foreign body. Agglomerated food debris usually needs patience to progressively disaggregate retained food allowing the debris to be broken down little by little. This action reduces the size of the foreign body allowing the main part of the retained bolus to pass through the cardia/stricture to the stomach. This action usually

Table 4. Digestive tract foreign bodies

Upper GI tract	Food	– Bone – Fish bone – Pieces of meat or other (hard/solid) consistent food – Pills – Almonds and other consistent fruits or seeds
	Foreign bodies with poisoning risk	– Batteries – Mercury thermometers – Metals
	Magnets	
	Unclassified objects with risk of perforation	– Nails – Glass fragments – Toys and objects with sharp and potentially cutting edges – Dental prostheses – Tooth stick
	Unclassified objects without risk of perforation	– Coins and toys – Hair – Toothbrush/spoons/springs and other metallic devices
	Medical devices	– Prostheses – Lost material
	Other	– Large biliary stones
Biliary tract		– Prostheses (plastic and expandable), guidewire fragments
Small bowel		– Prostheses – Migrated gastric balloons – Magnets
Colon	Non-medical devices	– Migrated from upper GI tract – Cylinders and round objects
	Medical devices	– Prostheses (stenosis treatment) – Lost material

requires multiple passages of the endoscope and the use of atraumatic grasping forceps. In these cases the overtube is useful. The use of the retrieval basket or devices used to hook the varices to perform elastic band ligation can facilitate the retrieval of retained material.

In most of the cases, esophageal stricture or Schatzki ring induces the impaction. Intubation is rarely considered and success of foreign body retrieval is achieved in nearly 100% of the cases with scarce need for surgery or development of side effects [6, 7]. In some cases, mainly when hard foreign bodies are present, glucagon or other spasmolytics are an important help.

Other Foreign Bodies Retained in the Hypopharynx and the Esophagus

Meat bones and shellfish may be seen using an adequate radiologic technique. Fish bones are difficult to assess by radiology and endoscopy may be considered the best diagnostic method in

Fig. 1. The main flexible endoscopic tools used for retrieval of foreign bodies.

Fig. 2. a, b. A soft rubber hood which is automatically reversed when the endoscope is pulled back onto the cardia.

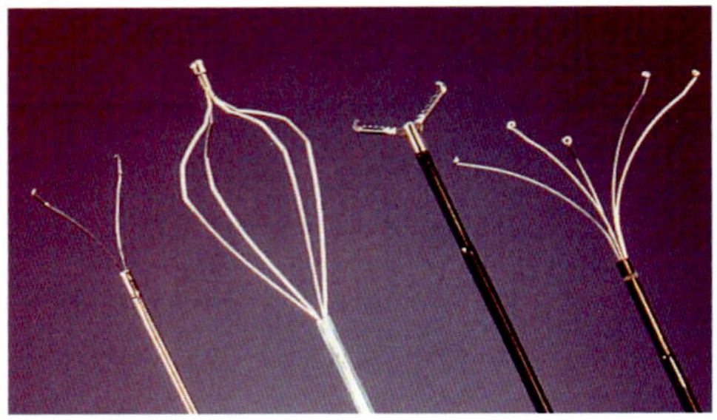

1

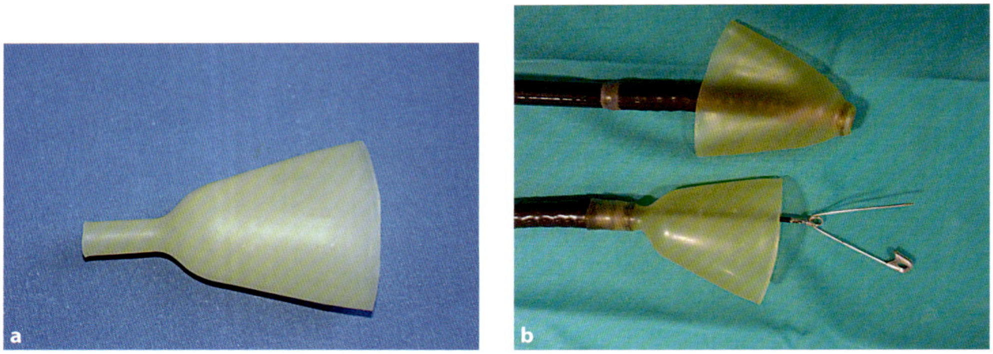

2

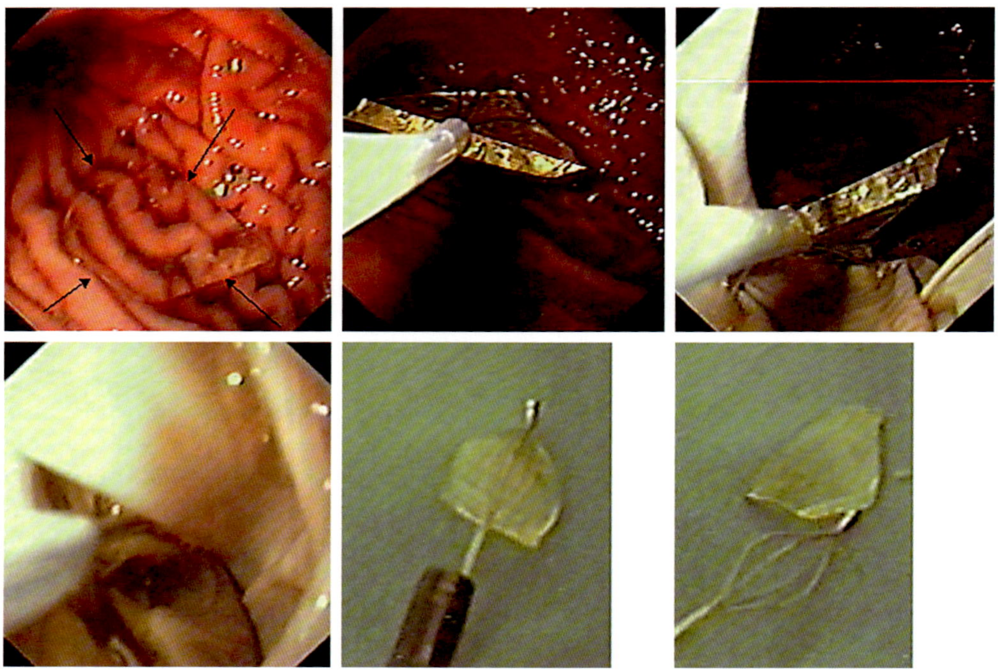

Fig. 3. Sharp foreign body (glass fragment) retrieved with the use of latex glove attached to the endoscope tip. Glass fragment in the great curve of the stomach. The foreign body is caught by Dormia basket and retrieved into the latex glove attached to the tip of the endoscope. The glove hood protects the esophageal wall during retrieval. The glass fragment firmly caught in the Dormia basket. The foreign body obtained was 2.5 × 3.2 cm.

these patients. Bone retrieval should be carried out with caution to avoid perforation and tears. A spasmolytic may facilitate the maneuvers. Grasping forceps are the best endoscopic ancillary device used and the policy for removal requires the best position and direction of these tools to be obtained. Sometimes the overtube or latex protector hood is useful (fig. 2). It is mandatory to carefully explore the esophagus immediately after foreign body removal, in order to avoid perforation and assess what may have precipitated the event.

Sharp and Long Objects
Sharp and pointed objects lodged in the esophagus represent a medical emergency. Independently of whether the foreign body is retained in the esophagus or the stomach, the system to grasp this type of foreign body is similar and must be performed in association with stomach and esophagus wall protection. The overtube and the latex protector hood (fig. 2, 3) attached to the end of endoscope are very efficient ancillary devices in protecting the esophageal and the pharyngeal walls [8, 9]. Safety and efficacy in retrieval depends mainly on the size and the shape of the object. The final treatment decision is sometimes made during endoscopy and is related to the inability to grasp, impossibility to mobilize or the high risk involved in retrieving the ingested foreign body.

Coins and Button Batteries
Coins usually pass through the GI tract. Progress control is usually easy with the use of x-ray. In most cases in adults, these foreign bodies pass through the digestive tract. When they remain in the esophagus or in the stomach, endoscopic maneuvers are needed. The main problem with coins is to obtain adequate apprehension, although the rat-tooth grasping forceps is usually adequate. In other cases, overtube or the Roth basket is the best method. Batteries may induce a chemical risk and must therefore be retrieved as soon as possible. Regular cylinder-shaped batteries can usually be retrieved using polypectomy snares. Button batteries must be retrieved using a net.

Magnets
When only one magnet is present in the digestive tract the action depends on the size and shape. All objects <2.5 cm in size pass through the pylorus and observation is considered the best treatment. If more than one magnet is present in the digestive tract, retrieval maneuvers are needed. If left in the gut the magnets may be attracted to each other and induce gut perforation. When such foreign bodies are in the stomach the method for retrieval is similar as that for other types of foreign bodies. When they are in the gut, balloon enteroscopy or surgery may be considered [10, 11].

Bezoars
Bezoars are foreign material which are compacted and retained in the stomach and sometimes in the upper part of the duodenum, e.g. vegetable fiber (phytobezoar) or ingested hair (trichobezoar). Delayed emptying or partial gastrectomy facilitates phytobezoar. The best treatment is enzymatic dissolution, but sometimes endoscopy facilitates the disaggregation and retrieval using the overtube because of the need for multiple passages of the endoscope [12].

Trichobezoar usually needs surgery. Sometimes the phytobezoar is hard and rupture can be achieved with the lithotriptor basket or with polypectomy snares. If digestion or fragmentation is difficult or fails, laparoscopic surgery is the treatment option [13, 14].

Rectal Foreign Bodies

Some foreign bodies reach the colon after passing through the stomach and small intestine and remain in the cecum. Colonoscopy can be used for retrieval using standard devices, mainly polypectomy snare forceps, retrieval net or Dormia basket. A number of rectal foreign bodies are related to sexual play and may be retained inside the rectum or sigmoid colon and sometimes even proximal migration is observed. Most of these objects are cylindrical or long and are difficult to be efficiently grasped, managed and retrieved. The work-up includes x-ray planes to rule out perforation and establish the position of the foreign body before any manipulation. Often only small objects may be grasped and retrieved. Large or impacted objects usually need surgery because of the risk of perforation and the great difficulties in retrieval [15–18].

Medical Foreign Bodies

Cholelithiasis may induce direct pass of the biliary stones to the duodenal bulb or to proximal duodenum. Large stones may induce obstruction (biliary ileus and Bouveret syndrome). The main problem in these cases is to adequately grasp the stone with the lithotriptor Dormia basket. To crush the stone or to retrieve it from the duodenum to the stomach is the first main aim, which may not always be accomplished. Afterwards, fragmentation and retrieval is usually a minor problem. When endoscopy fails, surgery is mandatory.

Foreign Bodies-Related Medical Therapy

Nowadays some medical therapies may introduce foreign bodies in the digestive tract and must be retrieved after a period of time. Mainly esophageal enteral and biliary plastic or metallic expandable prosthesis are now used for stricture dilation or for closing leaks and fistulas.

(1) Plastic biliary prostheses are easily retrieved using polypectomy snares. The distal tip or lateral flap of the plastic tube is taken by the snare. Sometimes the use of grasping forceps is necessary for mobilization, when the distal prostheses tip remains closely in contact with the mucosa in front of the papilla. Proximal migrated plastic biliary prostheses may be held using the Dormia basket in the majority of cases [19]. In some cases, prostheses cannulation by dilation or stone retrieval balloon or by biopsy forceps allow the problem to be solved, inflating the balloon or opening the forceps. In other cases we can use the Soehendra stent retriever [19] or an ultrathin endoscope introduced in the biliary tract through the papilla, which will allow to use different pediatrics accessories. The choice of a retrieval technique depends on several factors including biliary ductal dilation, depth of stent migration, distal stent impaction and biliary stricture distal to the migrated stent. The placement of an additional stent alongside an irretrievable stent is a satisfactory alternative to retrieval [19]. Biliary totally or partially covered expandable prostheses may be retrieved using polypectomy snare or rat-tooth grasping forceps. If there is some difficulty in mobilizing the prostheses, the introduction of a biliary dilation balloon into the prostheses makes mobilization and retrieval easier [20].

(2) Temporary esophageal expandable prostheses are mainly used for treating leaks or fistulas and to manage difficult strictures. Partial or total cover prostheses are used and retrieval

is convenient 2–4 weeks after introduction. Now most of the prostheses have a retrieval system using grasping forceps. The mechanism is a loop in both tips of the prostheses which may be easily grasped by rat-tooth forceps allowing closure of the proximal part of the expandable prostheses and facilitating the retrieval maneuvers. Although this mechanism is useful immediately just after the introduction, some weeks later the loop often breaks during the retrieval maneuvers. In these cases, rat-tooth forceps allow patient detachment of the proximal part of the prostheses from the esophageal wall and the prostheses can be held and removed by rat-tooth forceps attached to the proximal edge of the prostheses. Even after detaching the proximal part of the prostheses, mesh mobilization is sometimes difficult. One solution is to introduce the scope, grasping the caudal edge of the mesh with the foreign body forceps in an attempt to mobilize the prostheses in the caudal direction by introducing the scope. Mobilization in the caudal direction then makes it easier to retrieve the prostheses holding it from the cephalic edge. The use of polypectomy devices can also be used, but it is usually difficult to adequately snare the proximal part of the prostheses. If these maneuvers fail, the prostheses can reportedly be retrieved from the distal part holding it by foreign body forceps, inverting the mesh. Radiology facilitates the retrieval maneuvers.

Other tricks have been described for retrieval of partial cover prostheses when the uncovered part remains firmly included in the digestive wall. The most common mechanism is new prostheses introduction into that which needs to be retrieved. After 4–7 days the new prostheses pressure induces necroses to the imbibed part of the old prostheses. Immediately after new mesh retrieval, the old one can be more easily mobilized.

There is a new device for retrieving metallic expandable covered mesh designed to manage acute esophageal variceal hemorrhage (SX-Ella Stent Danis). The stent has a proximal loop thus elongating and narrowing the mesh, meanwhile an overtube may be synchronically advanced in the esophagus and the stent may be progressively and easily introduced in the overtube [21]. This maneuver can also be used by retrieving other expandable stents.

Distally migrated expandable stents are usually retrieved with a polypectomy snare but can also be retrieved with the use of a dilation balloon introduced into the expanded prostheses making it easier to reposition the mesh in the distal esophagus and grasp the proximal part with other retrieval tools. Some authors have used a mechanical lithotripsy device [22], or some endoloops to collapse the metallic stent [23, 24]. It is very helpful to have a soft rubber protector hood attached to the distal part of the endoscope (fig. 2) or to use an overtube in order to ease the passing of the grasped stent through the cardiac sphincter, the esophagus and the pharynx [24].

In the digestive tract some objects used during surgery may induce external pressure to the digestive wall and finally migrate into the lumen [25, 26]. Most of these foreign bodies require surgery for retrieval because of their size and relationship with the surrounding structures. In these cases, CT scan facilitates establishment of the size, shape and situation of the foreign body for making a decision regarding the best treatment.

Body Packing

The introduction of packed illicit drugs into the digestive tract is well known (swallowed or inserted into the rectum). Radiology is the method to detect their presence being characterized by an induced radiolucent halo or 'double condom' sign. These foreign bodies can sometimes be retrieved, but the risk of acute intoxication must be considered and even if complications are not present, surgical treatment is often applied [27–29].

Admission Decision

All patients with foreign bodies are admitted to hospital after surgery if required. In other cases, 24-hour admission should be only considered when: (1) complications or possible complications are suspected; (2) if retrieval of multiple or complex foreign bodies has been difficult, and (3) when retrieval is not possible and a new attempt or surgery is considered.

Results

Although foreign body ingestion may be considered as a banal accident, it can induce severe complications and even death. In recent years, deaths caused by foreign bodies have rarely been reported, with related mortality being considered extremely low [30]. Although more than 80–95% of the ingested foreign bodies pass spontaneously through the GI tract without or with few complications [31–33], it is considered that 10–20% require medical intervention. In the great majority of the cases, GI or OHN (OTL) endoscopy solve the problem and in around 1% of the cases surgery is required for exploration and extraction [34]. However, in the Palta study [35] reporting the experience obtained in an urban county hospital during 7 years and including 262 cases with 92% intentional foreign body ingestion, surgery was needed in 11% of the cases. In this group of patients needing surgery, foreign objects beyond the pylorus was more frequent and was treated with a significant great delay from ingestion to clinical presentation. In the Chaves prospective study [34], the efficacy in retrieval of foreign bodies was 99%. Another retrospective study reported a success rate of 96% [36]. Other studies have reported success rates from 83 to 98% with flexible endoscopes. In the Bergreen study [36], the use of flexible endoscopes described a success rate of 96%, being 100% with the rigid scope, although the difference was not significant. Nevertheless, these data suggest that the use of rigid scopes should be considered the second option when the flexible scope fails on deciding the need for endoscopic treatment. A study conducted by Ciriza et al. [37] indicated that dysphagia is the best parameter for emergency GI endoscopy.

Complications

Severe complications due to retrieval are uncommon [38]. The most frequent complication is perforation related to the extraction of esophageal foreign bodies. Other complications are bleeding, aspiration and sedation-related side effects. It must be taken in account that some severe complications occur before any active medical intervention, mainly due to perforation. In this situation it is convenient to consider surgery. Progressive pain, fever dysphagia, gagging, vomiting or sensation of choking to induce oral secretion, complex foreign bodies and the time elapsed from the ingestion and clinical manifestations are the clinical data for this potentially severe condition. The complication rate varies when the total number of patients with foreign bodies ingestion requiring medical care or all those endoscopically treated is considered. In the

Chaves study [34] the complication rate was 38%, but only 9% occurred during the removal procedure (laceration, perforation and hematoma). The remaining complications were related to direct injury in the esophagus (27%) and injury of the stomach wall (2%) by the foreign body before removal was attempted. In the literature the total incidence of complications due to foreign bodies in the upper GI tract varies from 15 to 42%. In the Palta study [35] the total complication rate was 6% but these complications were detected before endoscopy in 10 out of 262 cases (4%).

It is very important to recognize a significant complication related to foreign body or after retrieval early since it is known that early treatment greatly influences the outcome [39]. If a complication is suspected, an x-ray can show air around the esophageal lumen. The clinical signs of complication are crackling post-procedure, progressive chest or abdominal pain, fever, tachycardia and shortness of breath. In this situation, front and lateral x-ray planes and radiography may show the presence of extraluminal air and the use of a hydrosoluble contrast study may facilitate the localization of perforation when the existing CT scan is a very sensitive method to assess extraluminal inflammation or perforation. In these cases the diagnostic work-up must be associated with surgical consultation.

References

1 Yalçin S, Karnak I, Ciftci AO, Senocak ME, et al: Foreign body ingestion in children: an analysis of pediatric surgical practice. Pediatr Surg Int 2007;23: 755–761.

2 Lee TH, Kang YW, Kim HJ, et al: Foreign objects in Korean prisoners. Korean J Intern Med 2007;22:275–278.

3 Lee SC, Ebert CS Jr, Fordham L, Rose AS: Plain films in the evaluation of batteries as esophageal foreign bodies. Int J Pediatr Otorhinolaryngol 2008; 72:1487–1491.

4 Karnwal A, Ho EC, Hall A, Molony N: Lateral soft tissue neck X-rays: are they useful in management of upper aero-digestive tract foreign bodies? J Laryngol Otol 2008;122:845–847.

5 Eisen GM, Baron TH, Dominitz JA, et al: Guidelines for the management of ingested foreign bodies. Gastrointest Endosc 2002;55:802–806.

6 Güitrón A, Adalid R, Huerta F, et al: Extracción de cuerpos extraños en el esófago. Experiencia en 215 casos. Rev Gastroenterol Mex 1996;61:19–26.

7 Prasad GA, Reddy JG, Boyd-Enders FT, et al: Predictors of recurrent esophageal food impaction: a case-control study. J Clin Gastroenterol 2008;42: 771–775.

8 Bertoni G, Sassatelli R, Conigliaro R, et al: A simple latex protector hood for safe endoscopic removal of sharp-pointed gastroesophageal foreign bodies. Gastrointest Endosc 1996;44:458–461.

9 Patel NC, Fry LC, Mönkemüller KE: Modified suction cap technique for endoscopic management of esophageal food impaction. Endoscopy 2003;35:548.

10 Baliga SK, Hussain D, Sarfraz SL, Hartung RU: Magnetic attraction: dual complications in a single case. J Coll Physicians Surg Pak 2008;18:440–441.

11 Fenton SJ, Torgenson M, Holsti M, Black RE: Magnetic attraction leading to a small bowel obstruction in a child. Pediatr Surg Int 2007;23:1245–1247.

12 Matsushita M, Fukui T, Uchida K, et al: Effective 'Coca-Cola' therapy for phytobezoars. Intern Med 2008;47: 1161.

13 Shami SB, Jararaa AA, Hamade A, Ammori BJ: Laparoscopic removal of a huge gastric trichobezoar in a patient with trichotillomania. Surg Laparosc Endosc Percutan Tech 2007;17:197–200.

14 Naik S, Gupta V, Naik S, et al: Rapunzel syndrome reviewed and redefined. Dig Surg 2007;24:157–161.

15 Singaporewalla RM, Tan DE, Tan TK: Use of endoscopic snare to extract a large rectosigmoid foreign body with review of literature. Surg Laparosc Percutan Tech 2007; 17:145–148.

16 Cirocco WC: Anesthesia facilitates the extraction of rectal foreign bodies. Gastrointest Endosc 2000;52: 452–453.

17 Koornstra JJ, Weersma RK: Management of rectal foreign bodies: description of a new technique and clinical practice guidelines. World J Gastroenterol 2008;14:4403–4406.

18 Rodríguez-Hermosa JI, Codina-Cazador A, Ruiz B, et al: Management of foreign bodies in the rectum. Colorectal Dis 2007;9:543–548.

19 Chaurasia OP, Rauws EA, Fockens P, Huibregtse K: Endoscopic techniques for retrieval of proximally migrated biliary stents: the Amsterdam experience. Gastrointest Endosc 1999;50:780–785.

20 Matsushita M, Uchida K, Okazaki K: Open-biopsy-forceps technique for removing biliary metallic stents that have migrated distally and wedged transversely in the duodenum. Endoscopy 2007;39:570.
21 Hubmann R, Bodlaj G, Czompo M, et al: The use of self-expanding metal stents to treat acute esophageal variceal bleeding. Endoscopy 2006;38:896–901.
22 May A, Gossner L, Fees G, et al: Extraction of migrated self-expanding esophageal metal stents. Gastrointest Endosc 1999;49:524–527.
23 Seitz U, Thonke F, Bohnacker S, et al: Endoscopic extraction of a covered Z-stent with the aid of endoloops. Endoscopy 1998;30:S91–S92.
24 De Ronde T, Martinet JP, Melange M: Easy removal of migrated self-expanding esophageal metal stent using an endoloop device. Gastrointest Endosc 2000;52:125–127.
25 Fernandez-Esparrach G, Ginès A, Garcia P, et al: Vertebral prosthetic arthrodesis migration to the esophageal lumen: a rare cause of dysphagia. Endoscopy 2007(suppl 1):E188.
26 Nathan S, Piccione W Jr, Kumar A, et al: Erosion of an extrapericardial implantable cardioverter defibrillator patch through the gastric fundus with fistulous tract formation Cardiol Rev 2006;14:21–23.
27 Luburich P, Santamaría G, Tomás X, et al: The gastrointestinal concealment of illegal drugs. Rev Esp Enf Dig 1991;79:190–195.
28 De Jesus-Monge WE: Electronic clinical challenges and Images in GI. Illegal drug body packing. Gastroenterology 2008;135:e1–2.
29 Veyrie N, Servajean S, Aissat A, et al: Value of a systematic operative protocol for cocaine body packers. World J Surg 2008;32:1432–1437.
30 Webb WA: Management of foreign bodies of the upper gastrointestinal tract: update. Gastrointest Endosc 1995;41:39–51.
31 Urkciyan I, Frossard M, Kettenbach, et al: Conservative management of foreign bodies in the gastrointestinal tract. Z Gastroenterol 1996;34: 173–177.
32 Weiland ST, Schurr MJ: Conservative management of ingested foreign bodies. J Gastrointest Surg 2002; 6:496–500.
33 Smith MT, Wong RKH: Esophageal foreign bodies: types and techniques for removal. Curr Treat Options Gastroenterol 2006;9:75–84.
34 Chaves MD, Ishioka S, Felix VN, et al: Removal of foreign body from the upper gastrointestinal tract with flexible endoscope: a prospective study. Endoscopy 2004; 36:887–892.
35 Palta R, Sahota A, Benmarki A, et al: Foreign-body ingestion: characteristics and outcomes in lower socioeconomic population with predominantly intentional ingestion. Gastrointest Endosc 2009;69: 426–433.
36 Bergreen PJ, Harrison E, Sanowski RA, et al: Techniques and complications of esophageal foreign body extraction in children and adults. Gastrointest Endosc 1996;39:626–630.
37 Ciriza C, Garcia L, Suarez P, et al: What predictive parameter best indicate the need for emergency gastrointestinal endoscopy after foreign body ingestion? J Clin Gastroenterol 2000;31:23–28.
38 O'Sullivan ST, McGreal GT, Reardon CM, et al: Selective endoscopy in management of ingested foreign bodies of the upper gastrointestinal tract: is it safe? Int J Clin Pract 1997;51:289–292.
39 Webb WA: Management of foreign bodies of the upper gastrointestinal tract: update. Gastrointestinal Endosc 1995;41:39–51.

Josep M. Bordas, MD, PhD
GI Endoscopy, Gastroenterology Department
Institut de Malalties Digestives, Hospital Clinic
C/Villarroel, 170, ES–08022 Barcelona (Spain)
Tel. +34 93 227 55 23, Fax +34 93 227 98 50, E-Mail jbordas@adam.es

Mönkemüller K, Wilcox CM, Muñoz-Navas M (eds): Interventional and Therapeutic Gastrointestinal Endoscopy.
Front Gastrointest Res. Basel, Karger, 2010, vol 27, pp 91–105

Endoscopic Dilation of Benign and Malignant Esophageal Strictures

Klaus Mönkemüller[a,b] · Mirjana Kalauz[c] · Lucía C. Fry[a,b]

[a]Department of Internal Medicine, Gastroenterology and Infectious Diseases, Marienhospital, Bottrop and [b]Division of Gastroenterology, Hepatology and Infectious Diseases, Otto von Guericke University, Magdeburg, Germany, and [c]Divison of Gastroenterology, Department of Internal Medicine, University Hospital Rebro, Zagreb, Croatia

Abstract

The main indication for esophageal dilation is to relieve benign or malignant dysphagia. Endoscopic dilation of malignant strictures is also performed to facilitate the completion of endoscopic procedures, such as endoscopic ultrasonographic tumor staging and to permit the placement of esophageal stents or to place a percutaneous endoscopic gastrostomy for feeding purposes. Esophageal strictures are structurally categorized into two groups: complex and simple. Complex strictures are those that are asymmetric, irregular or angulated with diameter <12 mm. Simple strictures are symmetric or concentric with a diameter of ≥12 mm or those that easily allow passage of a diagnostic upper endoscope. Dilation can be accomplished through several steps using a variety of dilating devices and adjunctive techniques. The approach to management of esophageal strictures is reviewed with a focus on dilation technique.

Esophageal dilation is performed for the treatment of anatomic and sometimes functional narrowing of the esophageal lumen caused by a variety of benign and malignant conditions (table 1) [1–3]. Until the late 1980s, nearly 80% of esophageal strictures were due to gastroesophageal reflux, but at present the incidence of peptic strictures may be decreasing due to the widespread use of proton pump inhibitors (PPIs) [2] (fig. 1). Currently, malignant disorders, post-anastomotic or radiation-induced stenosis constitute common causes of esophageal strictures [1, 3–6] (fig. 2, 3).

Most patients with esophageal stenosis present with dysphagia. Dysphagia is a subjective sensation that suggests the presence of an organic abnormality in the passage of liquids or solids from the oral cavity to the stomach (fig. 4). Patient's complaints range from the inability to initiate a swallow (oropharyngeal dysphagia) to the sensation of solids or liquids being hindered during their passage through the esophagus into the stomach (esophageal dysphagia). Table 1 presents a list of differential diagnosis of dysphagia. The term 'odynophagia' refers to painful swallowing.

The main indication for esophageal dilation is to relieve benign or malignant dysphagia [2–5]. Endoscopic dilation of malignant strictures is also performed to facilitate the completion of endoscopic procedures, such as endoscopic ultrasonographic tumor staging, to permit the

Table 1. Differential diagnosis of dysphagia

Oropharyngeal	Esophageal
Neuromuscular disorders	Motility disorders
Cerebrovascular accident, dementia	*Primary*
Brainstem tumors	Achalasia
Head trauma	Diffuse esophageal spasm
Parkinson's disease	Hypertensive LES
Multiple sclerosis	Non-specific esophageal motility disorder
Amyotrophic lateral sclerosis	Nutcracker esophagus
Idiopathic UES dysfunction	*Secondary*
Manometric dysfunction of the UES or pharynx	Reflux-related dysmotility
Metabolic encephalopathies	Scleroderma and other connective tissue
Wilson's disease	Disorders
Guillain-Barré syndrome	Chagas' disease
Myopathic disorders	Structural disorders
Connective tissue disease	*Intrinsic*
Polymyositis	Benign stricture (peptic, radiation, post-surgery, PDT, corrosive)
Dermatomyositis	Schatzki ring
Myasthenia gravis	Benign tumors
Myotonic dystrophy	Malignancy
Oculopharyngeal dystrophy	Eosinophilic esophagitis
Metabolic myopathy	Pill esophagitis
Sarcoidosis	Esophageal diverticula
Paraneoplastic syndrome	Crohn's disease
	Extrinsic
Infectious diseases	Vascular compression (enlarged aorta, left
Mucositis (herpes, cytomegalovirus, *Candida*)	atrium or aberrant subclavian artery)
Lymes disease	Mediastinal mass (lymphadenopathy,
Diphtheria	abscess, lung cancer)
	Cervical osteophytes
Structural lesions	Iatrogenic causes
Tumors	Pill injury

Table 1. Continued

Oropharyngeal	Esophageal
Zenker diverticulum	Medication side effects (chemotherapy, neuroleptics, etc.)
Cricopharyngeal bar	Postsurgical muscular or neurogenic
Cervical webs	Radiation
Congenital abnormalities	
Miscellaneous	
Depression, Alzheimer's disease	Functional
Decreased saliva (Sy-Sjögren)	Functional dysphagia

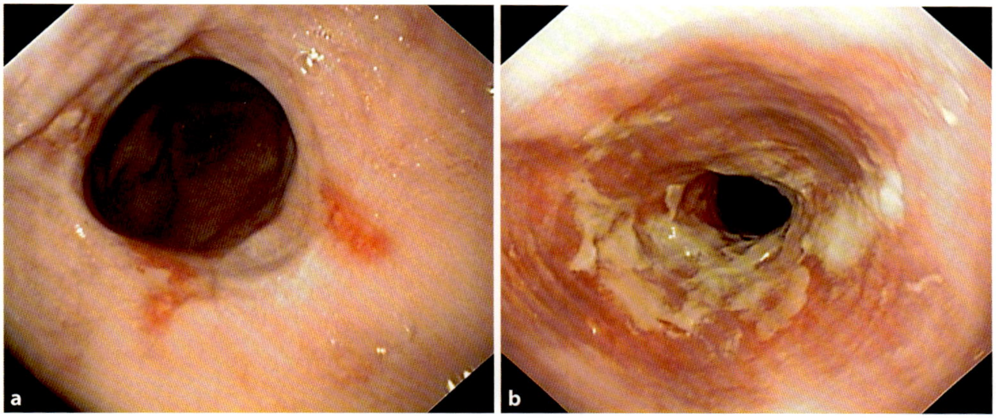

Fig. 1. Peptic strictures may be decreasing due to the widespread use of PPIs. **a** A Schatzki ring. **b** Severe esophagitis with stricture. Despite having a lesser degree of esophagitis, this patient also has a peptic stricture. This example shows that the Los Angeles classification is still an imperfect classification for gastroesophageal reflux disease.

placement of esophageal stents or to place a percutaneous endoscopic gastrostomy for feeding purposes [6–8]. Figure 4 provides a useful algorithm for the endoscopic approach of patients with esophageal stenosis. However, not all patients with dysphagia will require an endoscopic intervention. Note that most patients with dysphagia or odynophagia have conditions that can be managed medically, such as gastroesophageal reflux disease, infectious ulcers and eosinophilic esophagitis [9] (fig. 5).

Esophageal strictures can be structurally categorized into two groups: complex and simple. Complex strictures are those that are asymmetric, irregular or angulated with diameter <12 mm (malignant, anastomotic, post-radiation) (fig. 6). Simple strictures are symmetric or concentric with a diameter of ≥12 mm or those that easily allow passage of a diagnostic upper endoscope [1, 3, 10] (fig. 7). Esophageal strictures from a variety of benign and malignant causes require

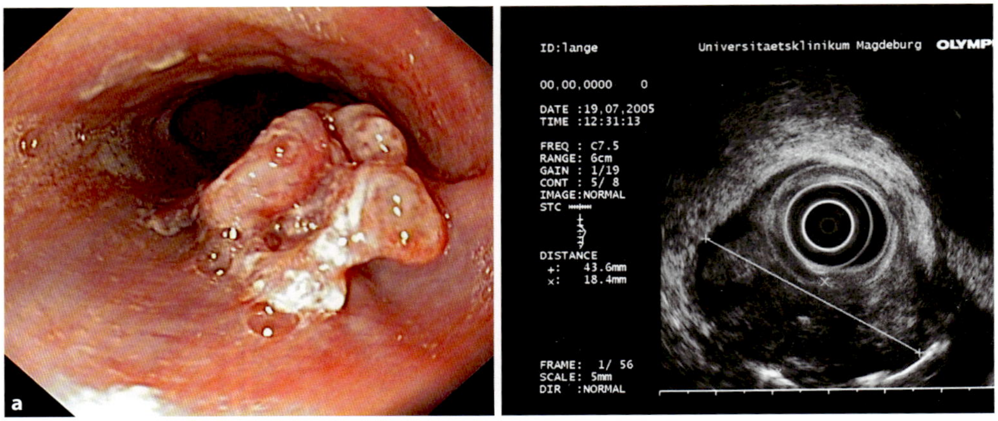

Fig. 2. **a** An adenocarcinoma of the distal esophagus presenting as a partially obstructing mass. **b** Endoscopic ultrasound. The tumor is very large and has spread into the mediastinum (T4).

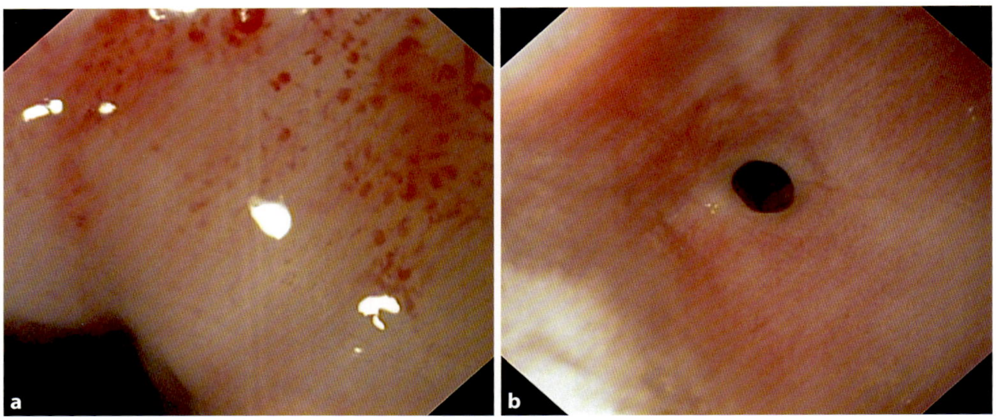

Fig. 3. **a** Radiation-induced stricture. **b** Using magnification endoscopy it is easy to see the proliferation of submucosal vessels that is characteristically seen in radiation esophagitis.

dilation therapy when patients develop symptoms of dysphagia. Dilation can be accomplished through several steps using a variety of dilating devices and adjunctive techniques (table 2). The approach to management of esophageal strictures is reviewed with a focus on dilation technique and special consideration for various stricture types and complications of the method.

Procedural Aspects

Patient Preparation

Patient preparation will depend upon the main cause of dysphagia. Patients with achalasia may require prolonged fasting and removal of food rests using a nasoesophageal tube (see also chapter on therapy of achalasia). Besides remaining NPO, laboratory tests may be warranted in patients

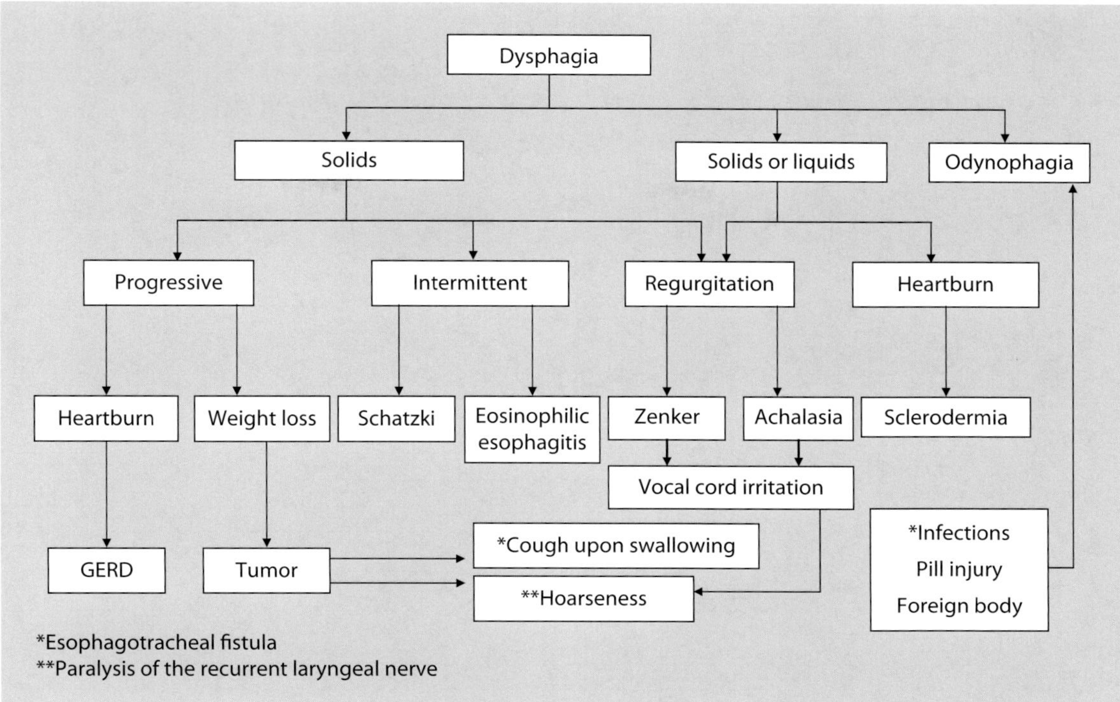

Fig. 4. Diagnostic algorithm for the assessment of a patient with dysphagia.

with blood dyscrasias or those taking anticoagulant therapy. Prior to endoscopy all patients have to provide written informed consent, also with written information about the risk of perforation (i.e. 1%) and the possible need for surgery. Endoscopies and dilations are carried out in the morning after an overnight fast and as an outpatient procedure, with the exception of patients with complex strictures, who should be observed for 24 h after the procedure. Radiographic contrast examination is not performed routinely before dilation, but it is performed after dilation of achalasia or complex strictures to exclude perforation.

As dilation is an invasive and uncomfortable procedure, conscious sedation is generally used. Esophageal dilations should always be performed or closely supervised by experienced endoscopists. Antibiotics are not used routinely before dilation; endocarditis prophylaxis guidelines should be followed [11]. Anticoagulants should be discontinued [12].

Accessories

Most esophageal dilations can be performed without the use of fluoroscopy [13]. However, some endoscopists working in open-access or fast-track endoscopy units prefer to have the patients placed in the fluoroscopy room (fig. 8). This is to avoid the unpleasant, and not infrequent situation in which a contrast imaging of the esophagus is needed either before or after the procedure and when a stent placement is planned or anticipated. The worst case scenario is to have a perforation and suddenly have to move with the patient to an appropriate room with x-ray capabilities in order to be able to place an emergent covered metal stent. In addition, currently, most esophageal strictures treated at some tertiary centers are complex, and their dilation may be facilitated

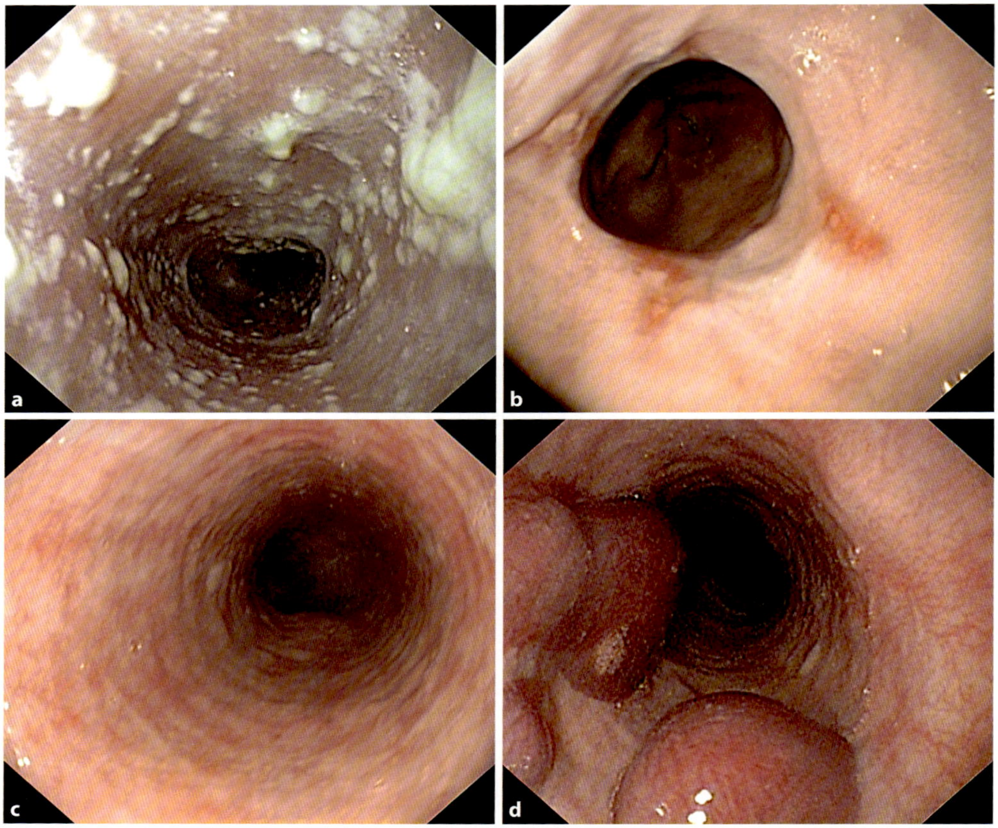

Fig. 5. Most patients with dysphagia or odynophagia have conditions that can be managed medically, *Candida* esophagitis (**a**), such as gastroesophageal reflux (**b**) disease, eosinophilic esophagitis (**c**) and pemphigoid (**d**).

by the use of fluoroscopy [14]. Furthermore, one study showed that fluoroscopy may lead to better functional results and fewer adverse events [15]. Regardless of the existing and controversial data, we believe that all patients with complex strictures should be dilated under radiographic control. Figure 9 is a practical algorithm for the management of esophageal strictures.

Technique
Esophageal dilation is currently performed using either bougies or balloons (table 3) (fig. 10–12) [1–4, 16, 17]. The word *bougie* comes from the French and means 'candle'. Formerly, esophageal dilation was performed using large candles. The words 'bougienage' and dilation mean the same, but we prefer to use the word 'dilation' and specify whether this was performed using a bougie or a balloon.

Historically, there are a large variety of bougies that have been used to perform esophageal dilation. However, currently two main types of bougies are used: mercury or tungsten-filled bougies (Maloney or Hurst) and over-the-wire (OTW) polyvinyl bougies (Savary-Gilliard® or American, Wilson-Cook Medical, Inc., Winston-Salem, N.C., USA) [4] (fig. 10). The Maloney type bougies have a tapered tip and are passed either blindly or under fluoroscopic control [18].

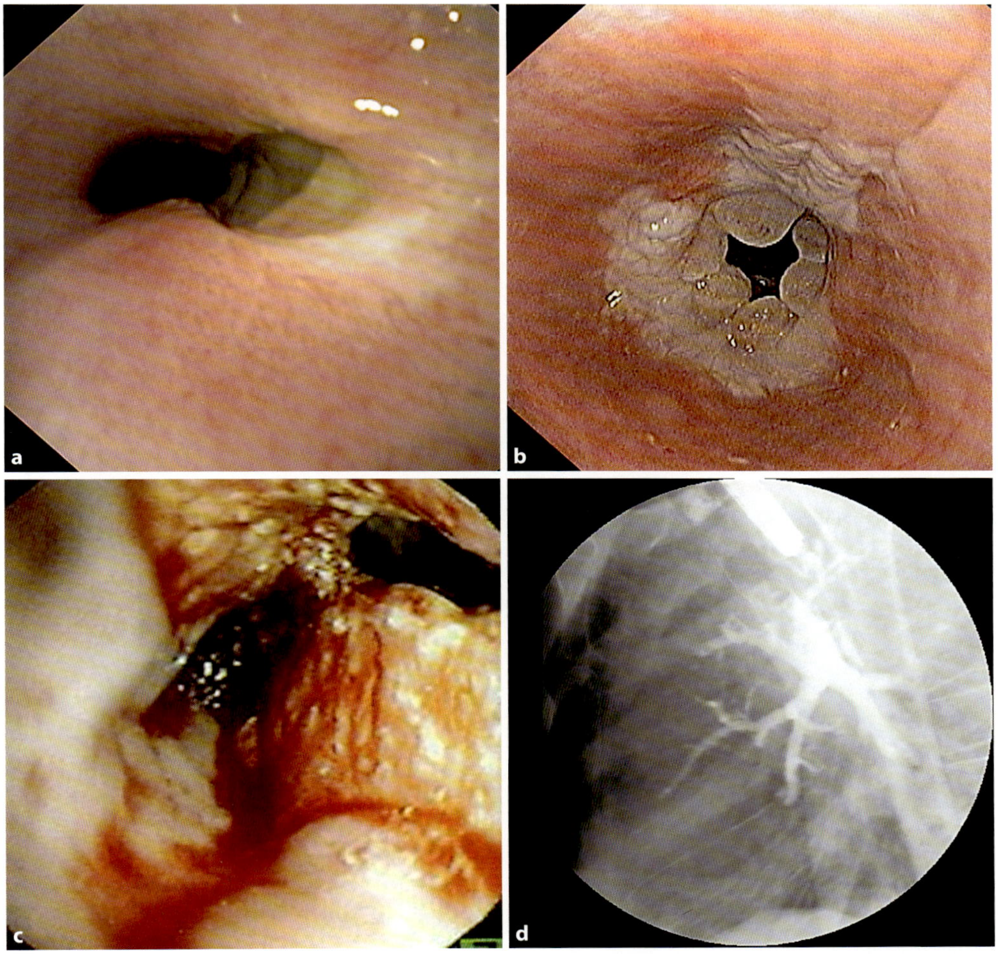

6

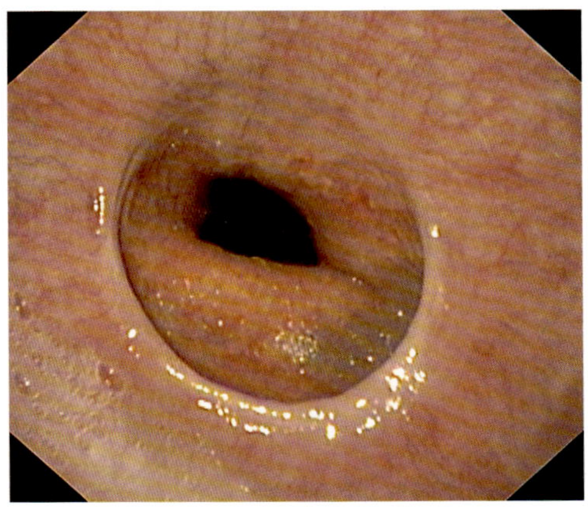

7

Fig. 6. Complex esophageal strictures are those that are (**a**) asymmetric or ulcerated, (**b**) irregular or angulated or (**c**, **d**) associated with a fistula.

Fig. 7. Simple esophageal strictures are symmetric or concentric with a diameter of ≥12 mm or those that easily allow passage of a diagnostic upper endoscope.

This type of dilator is used for simple strictures with a diameter of 12–14 mm. The risk of esophageal perforation may be higher with blind passage of the Maloney dilators than with OTW Savary or TTS (through-the-scope) balloons, particularly in patients with a large hiatal hernia, a

Table 2. Steps in esophageal dilation

Patient preparation	
	Informed consent, fasting overnight, anticoagulants discontinued, sedation
Evaluate diameter and length of stenosis	
Choose method	
	Bougie vs. balloon
If complex stricture or achalasia	
	Use fluoroscopy
	When using balloon use wire (Jagwire) Observe for 24 h
Fluoroscopy: not needed for most stenosis	

Table 3. Type of dilators

Mercury or tungsten-filled bougies	
	Maloney
	Hurst
Wire-guided polyvinyl dilators (OTW)	
	Savary-Gilliard
	American
Balloons	
TTS dilation balloons	
	Without wire guidance
	With wire guidance (Jagwire)

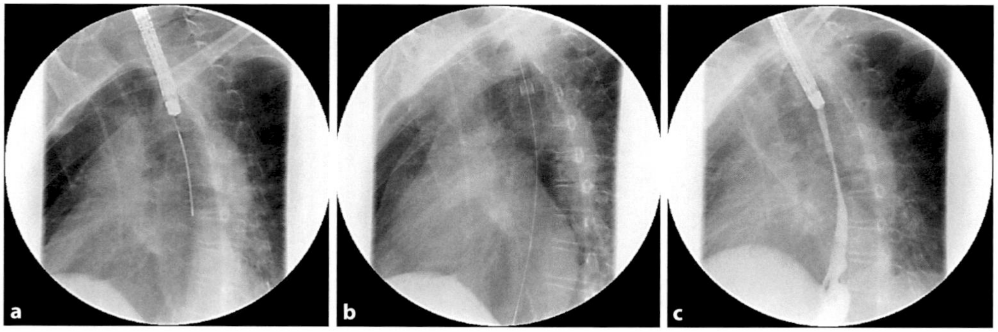

Fig. 8. Some endoscopists working in open-access or fast-track endoscopy units prefer to dilate esophageal strictures under fluoroscopy. This allows for a precise advancement and placement of a guidewire (**a**, **b**), especially when the stricture is very tight or irregular. In addition, contrast can be applied after the dilation, and thus rule out (**c**) or discover a perforation.

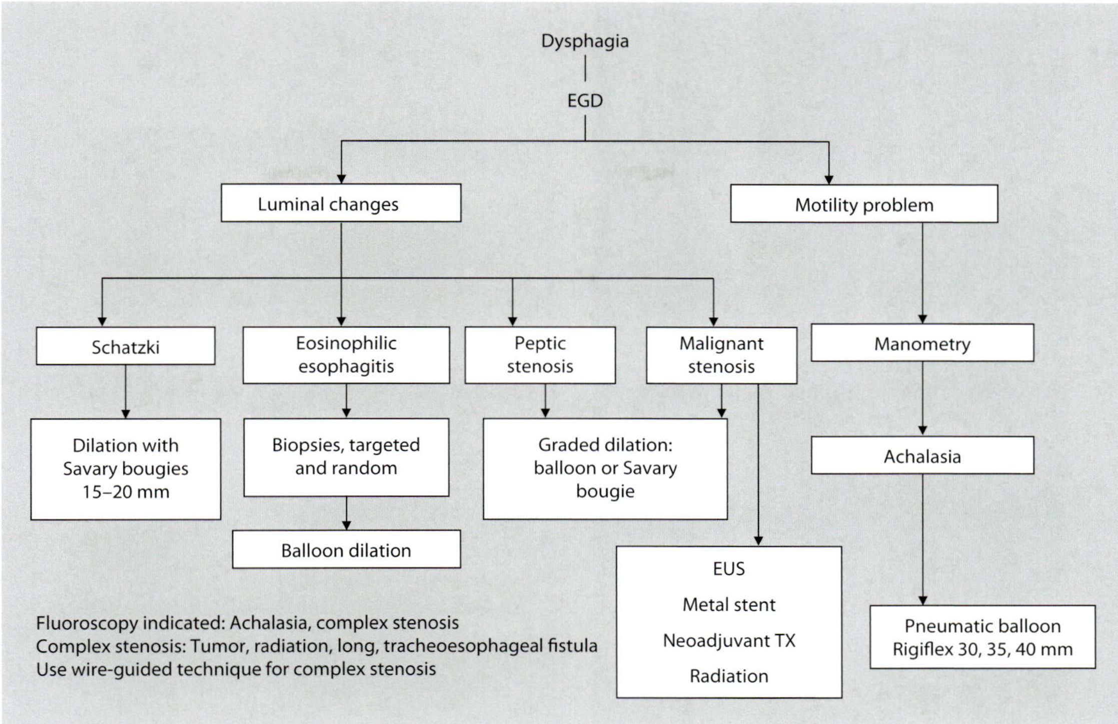

Fig. 9. Practical algorithm for the management of esophageal strictures.

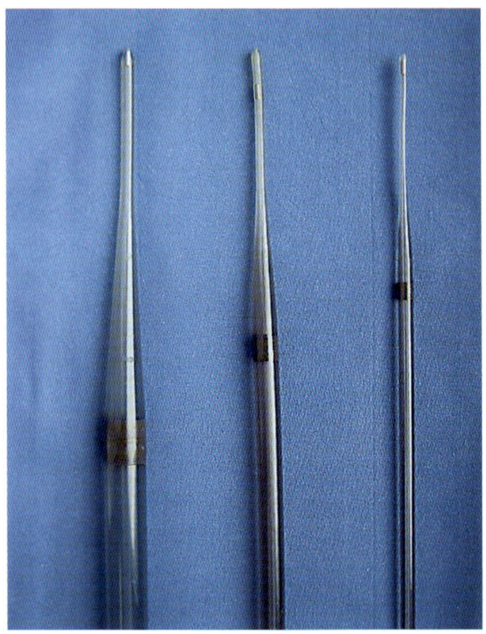

Fig. 10. Classic Savary or American dilators. Dilators are also called bougies, which originates from the French word 'candle'. Formerly, esophageal dilations were performed with wax candles. American dilators are advanced OTW, usually the spring-tipped hard Savary wire. However, any soft wire, such as a 'Jagwire', can be sued to advance the Savary dilator.

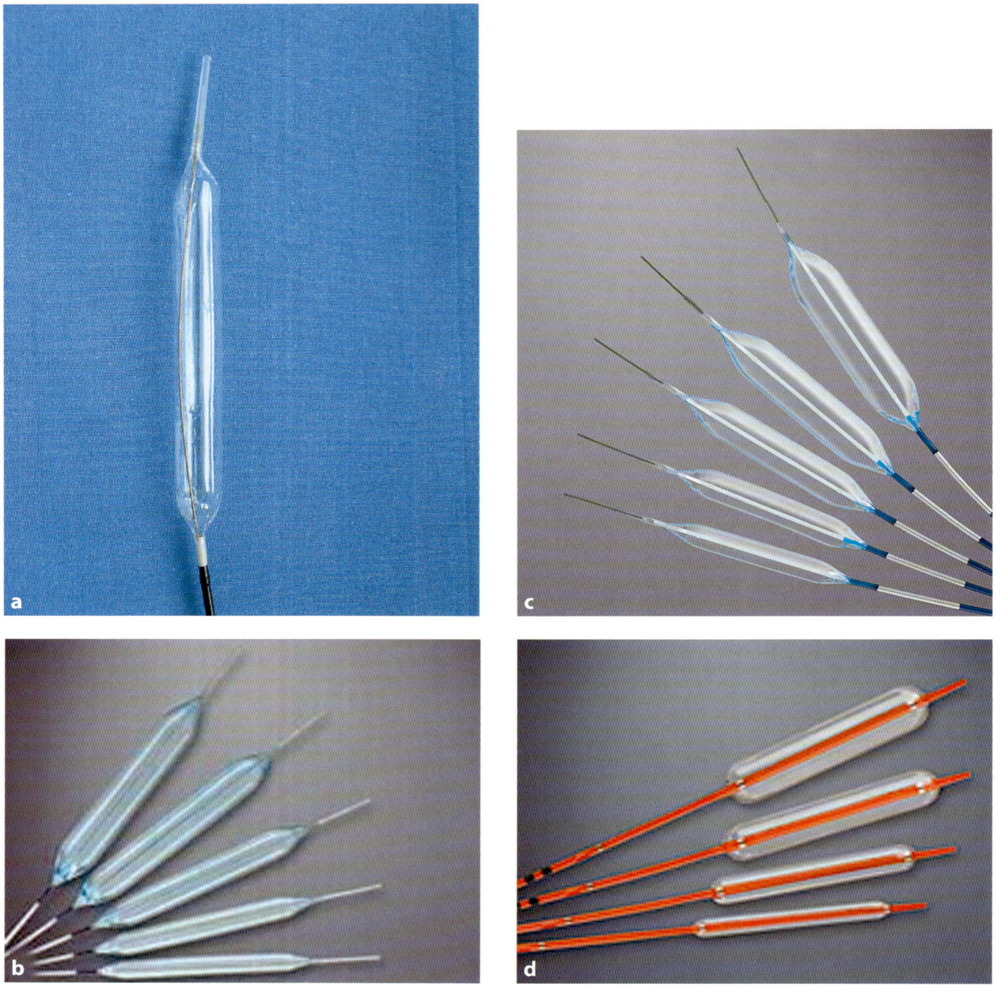

Fig. 11. Balloons used for esophageal dilation are advanced TTS and can be standard or OTW. If the stricture is tight, irregular or high risk it is always better to advance OTW. **a** Standard TTS balloon. **b** The Hercules® 3 Stage Balloon Dilator (Cook, USA) is available in various sizes, the smallest being 8 mm. The advantage of this balloon is its three-stage capability, which means that it can dilate a stricture in three different inflation diameters, thus following the classic 'rule-of-three'. The smallest balloon can dilate 8–9–10 mm (24–27–30 Fr), whereas the largest balloon goes from 18 to 20 (54–57–60 Fr). **c** If the stricture is irregular, tight or high risk, it is always better to perform the dilation with OTW balloons. **d** Titan® biliary balloon (Cook). Although this balloon is used to dilate biliary strictures, we have also found it very useful to dilate very tight esophageal stenosis (permission for image reproduction granted by Cook Medical Inc., Bloomington, Ind., USA).

tortuous esophagus, or those with complex strictures [1, 3, 4, 10] (fig. 11). Savary and American dilators are passed over a guidewire that has been positioned with a tip in the gastric antrum, with or without fluoroscopic guidance [19].

Various types of balloons are available to dilate the esophagus. We have accumulated a large experience using two main types of balloons: (CRE™, Controlled Radial Expansion, Boston Scientific Cork Ltd, Cork, Ireland, and Eclipse® Wire Guided Balloon Dilators Cook Ireland Ltd,

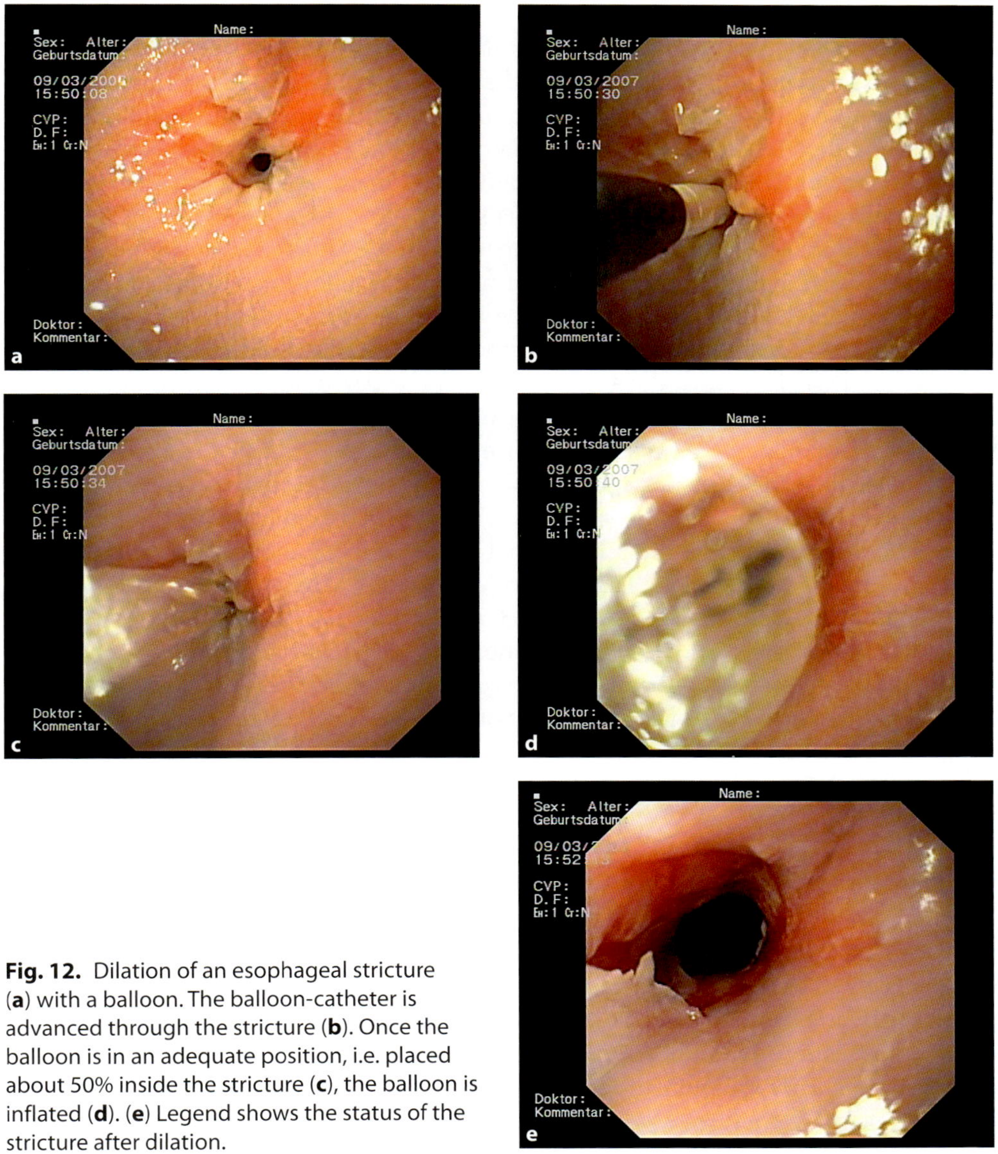

Fig. 12. Dilation of an esophageal stricture (**a**) with a balloon. The balloon-catheter is advanced through the stricture (**b**). Once the balloon is in an adequate position, i.e. placed about 50% inside the stricture (**c**), the balloon is inflated (**d**). (**e**) Legend shows the status of the stricture after dilation.

Limerick, Ireland). Balloons for esophageal stricture dilation come in various shapes and sizes. Because these balloons can be advanced through the accessory channel of the endoscope they are also referred to as 'through-the-scope' or TTS balloons [20] (fig. 11). One of the most important aspects to consider when choosing these balloons is the ability to further advance them OTW. These wires generally refer to any wire ≤0.035 inch (e.g. Jagwire, Microvasive, Boston Scientific). These TTS OTW balloons are particularly useful for complex, large, angulated, irregular, very tight strictures or if the luminal diameter of the stricture is <3 mm (fig. 12). In the presence of complex strictures the wire can be advanced under fluoroscopic guidance across the stricture and then, under direct endoscopic vision, the balloon can be advanced OTW (fig. 8). Advancing a 'plain'

TTS balloon without wire guidance in such strictures can lead to perforation, as the tip, even when it is floppy, can take a bend through the fibrosed or ulcerated stenosis and result in direct perforation or create a false passage, which after inflating the balloon, results in a large perforation.

It is important to clearly differentiate these balloons from the pneumatic balloons used to treat achalasia (Rigiflex® II Achalasia Balloon Dilators, Boston Scientific Corp., Natick, Mass., USA; Witzel Pneumatic Dilator, M-T-W-W Buderich, Germany, see achalasia chapter). The achalasia balloons can reach large diameters (30–40 mm).

Although the choice of dilatation device is left to the individual endoscopist, dilations in patients with tumors are mainly performed with Savary dilators following the conventional technique, using incremental diameters of the bougies, but no more than three per session ('rule-of-three'), and always under fluoroscopic monitoring. The 'rule of three' has been the standard for bougie dilation [21]. The initial dilator chosen should be based on the known or estimated stricture diameter. After moderate resistance is encountered with the bougie dilator, no greater than three consecutive dilations in increments of 1 mm should be performed in a single session [21, 22]. Although this rule does not apply to balloon dilators, a recent study suggested that inflation of a single large-diameter dilator (>15 mm) or incremental dilation of >3 mm may be safe in simple esophageal strictures [23]. Interestingly, most balloons allow a three-step inflation process, each of 1 mm, practically paralleling the 'rule-of-three'. Current AGA recommendations for management of peptic esophageal stricture include consideration that steroid injection into benign strictures immediately before or after dilation has been advocated to improve outcome by decreasing the need for repeat dilations [4]. A recent randomized trial of intralesional steroid injection with PPI therapy versus sham injection with PPI therapy in patients with recalcitrant peptic esophageal strictures showed that the need for repeat dilation was significantly diminished in the steroid group [24].

Limitations and Complications

Regardless of the specific method of dilation, early improvement in the ability to swallow is achieved in virtually all patients. Longer-term outcomes are influenced by the underlying pathology. For peptic strictures, smaller lumen diameter, presence of a hiatal hernia >5 cm, persistence of heartburn after dilation, and number of dilations needed for initial dysphagia relief were significant predictors of early symptomatic recurrence [25]. A multivariate analysis revealed that a non-peptic etiology of strictures was a significant predictor of early symptomatic recurrence within 1 year of initial dilation [26]. Patients with peptic strictures should be treated with PPI therapy. Compared with histamine receptor antagonist therapy, PPI use decreases stricture recurrence and the need for repeat stricture dilation [27, 28].

Esophageal perforation is the major complication associated with endoscopic dilation [4, 29–32]. The perforation rate for esophageal strictures after dilation has been reported to be 0.1–1% [11]. A United Kingdom regional audit reported an overall perforation rate of 2.6% with a mortality of 1% [32]. In that study, perforation was less common following dilatation of benign strictures (1.1%) than following dilatation of malignant strictures (6.4%) [31]. In older studies, perforation was most commonly associated with the blind passage of Maloney or non-wire-guided bougies into complex strictures [10, 31]. In another study from England the incidence of iatrogenic perforation for endoscopic treatment of tumors of the esophagus and cardia was 3.3% [32]. A common practice in England at that time was the use of single-sized bougies. Whilst data were not available as to the caliber of dilators routinely used in that region, it was commonplace in the early 1990s to use large dilators (18–20 mm). Therefore, it appears that perforations are common when using a single bougie size dilator, irrespective of stricture diameter [32].

Perforation after esophageal dilation usually occurs at the site of the stricture, either intraabdominally or intrathoracically. Some experts recommend endoscopic reinspection immediately upon completion of the dilatation procedure as the appearances may raise the possibility of perforation and prompt early treatment. Perforation should be suspected if severe or persistent pain, dyspnea, tachycardia, or fever develops. Physical examination may reveal subcutaneous crepitus of the chest or cervical region. Although a chest radiograph may indicate a perforation, a normal study result does not exclude this diagnosis and a water-soluble contrast esophagram or contrast computed tomogram of the chest may be necessary to disclose a perforation [33].

When using bougies we prefer to use OTW Savary dilators. Bougie-type dilators exert not only radial forces as they are passed but also longitudinal forces as the result of a shearing effect [34]. Therefore, it is possible that the risk of perforation is less when using balloon dilators. In contrast, longitudinal forces are not transmitted with balloon dilators because the entire dilating force is delivered radially and simultaneously over the entire length of the stenosis rather than progressively from its proximal to distal extent [34]. However, this has not been shown yet by clinical studies and no clear advantage has been demonstrated between the two dilator types [29, 35, 36].

Data from the literature also confirm that the risk of perforation is higher in complex strictures and lower in simple strictures [10]. In a retrospective study performed at our endoscopy unit, we found that the perforation rate for malignant strictures was higher than for peptic strictures [14]. Some authors also suggest that perforation may be more common and severe with radiation-induced strictures [37]. Nevertheless, this was not observed in our study. Although we did not observe any overt perforations associated with radiation-induced strictures, we had two possible microperforations [14]. The perforation rate may also be influenced by the endoscopist's level of experience; one study indicated that the perforation rate was four times greater when the operator had performed fewer than 500 previous diagnostic upper endoscopic examinations [31]. Therefore, in small hospitals where thoracic surgeons are not routinely available, arrangements should be made in order to have available a surgeon capable of repairing an esophageal perforation.

The use of large-diameter covered metal stents and the use of expandable, removable plastic stents have been shown to be effective in the management of perforations after dilation of benign and malignant esophageal strictures [38, 39].

To summarize, endoscopic esophageal dilation is a safe procedure for the management of benign strictures, for the palliation of malignant strictures, and to expand malignant strictures previous to the placement of a self-expanding metal stent. A thorough clinical knowledge of dysphagia and its management is paramount for the interventional endoscopist, as only a minority of patients will require endoscopic therapy. The endoscopist should be well versed and trained with all the available accessories used for esophageal dilation, including wires, bougies and balloons. As perforation occurs in about 0.5–1.5% of esophageal dilations, identification of patients at higher risk and with complex strictures is crucial to prevent iatrogenic perforation. In addition, knowledge and skills on placement of self-expanding covered metal stents and close collaboration with the surgeon is mandatory. As with any other therapeutic endoscopic procedure, esophageal dilation should only be performed by endoscopists well trained in interventional endoscopy.

References

1 Lew RJ, Kochman ML: A review of endoscopic methods of esophageal dilation. J Clin Gastroenterol 2002;35:117–126.

2 Richter JE: Peptic strictures of the esophagus. Gastroenterol Clin North Am 1999;28:875–891.

3 Riley SA, Attwood SE: Guidelines on the use of oesophageal dilatation in clinical practice. Gut 2004; 53:i1–i6.

4 Egan JV, Baron TH, Adler DG, Davila R, Faigel DO, Gan SL, Hirota WK, Leighton JA, Lichtenstein D, Qureshi WA, Rajan E, Shen B, Zuckerman MJ, VanGuilder T, Fanelli RD, Standards of Practice Committee: Esophageal dilation. Gastrointest Endosc 2006;63:755–760.

5 Lavu K, Mathew TP, Minocha A: Effectiveness of esophageal dilation in relieving nonobstructive esophageal dysphagia and improving quality of life. South Med J 2004;97:137–140.

6 Adler DG, Baron TH: Endoscopic palliation of malignant dysphagia. Mayo Clin Proc 2001;76:731–738.

7 Pfau PR, Ginsberg GG, Lew RJ, et al: Esophageal dilation for endosonographic evaluation of malignant esophageal strictures is safe and effective. Am J Gastroenterol 2000;95:2813–2815.

8 Adler DG, Baron TH, Geels W, et al: Placement of PEG tubes through previously placed self-expanding esophageal metal stents. Gastrointest Endosc 2001;54:237–241.

9 Mönkemüller KE, Wilcox CM: Diagnosis of esophageal ulcers in acquired immunodeficiency syndrome. Semin Gastrointest Dis 1999;10:85–92.

10 Hernandez LV, Jacobson JW, Harris MS: Comparison among the perforation rates of Maloney, balloon, and Savary dilation of esophageal strictures. Gastrointest Endosc 2000;51:460–462.

11 Hirota K, Petersen K, Baron TH, et al: Antibiotic prophylaxis for GI endoscopy. Gastointest Endosc 2003; 58:475–482.

12 Eisen GM, Baron TH, Dominitz JA, et al: Guideline on the management of anticoagulation and antiplatelet therapy for endoscopic procedures. Gastrointest Endosc 2002;55:775–779.

13 Marshall JB, Afridi SA, King PD, Barthel JS, Butt JH: Esophageal dilation with polyvinyl (American) dilators over a marked guidewire: practice and safety at one center over a 5-year period. Am J Gastroenterol 1996;91: 1503–1506

14 Fry LC, Mönkemüller K, Neumann H, Schulz HU, Malfertheiner P: Incidence, clinical management and outcomes of esophageal perforations after endoscopic dilatation. Z Gastroenterol 2007;45:1180–1184.

15 McClave SA, Brady PG, Wright RA, et al: Does fluoroscopic guidance for Maloney esophageal dilation impact on the clinical endpoint of therapy: relief of dysphagia and achievement of luminal patency. Gastrointest Endosc 1996;43:93–97.

16 Vaezi MF, Richter JE: Current therapies for achalasia: comparison and efficacy. J Clin Gastroenterol 1998;27: 21–35.

17 Mikaeli J, Bishehsari F, Montazeri G, et al: Pneumatic balloon dilation in achalasia: a prospective comparison of safety and efficacy with different balloon diameters. Aliment Pharmacol Ther 2004;15:431–436.

18 Ho SB, Cass O, Katsman RJ, et al: Fluoroscopy is not necessary for Maloney dilation of chronic esophageal strictures. Gastrointest Endosc 1995;42:11–14.

19 Wang YG, Tio TL, Soehendra N: Endoscopic dilation of esophageal stricture without fluoroscopy is safe and effective. World J Gastroenterol 2002;8:766–768.

20 Goldstein JA, Barkin JS: Comparison of the diameter consistency and dilating force of the controlled radial expansion balloon catheter to the conventional balloon dilators. Am J Gastroenterol 2000;95: 3423–3427.

21 Langdon DF: The rule of three in esophageal dilation. Gastrointest Endosc 1997;45:111.

22 Vaezi MF, Richter JE: Diagnosis and management of achalasia. American College of Gastroenterology Practice Parameter Committee. Am J Gastroenterol 1999;94: 3406–3412.

23 Kozarek RA, Patterson DJ, Ball TJ, et al: Esophageal dilation can be done safely using selective fluoroscopy and single dilating sessions. J Clin Gastroenterol 1995;20: 184–188.

24 Ramage JI Jr, Rumalla A, Baron TH, et al: A prospective, randomized, double-blind, placebo-controlled trial of endoscopic steroid injection therapy for recalcitrant esophageal strictures. Am J Gastroenterol 2005;100:2419–2425.

25 Said A, Brust DJ, Gaumnitz EA, et al: Predictors of early recurrence of benign esophageal strictures. Am J Gastroenterol 2003;98:1252–1256.

26 Chiu YC, Hsu CC, Chiu KW, et al: Factors influencing clinical applications of endoscopic balloon dilation for benign esophageal strictures. Endoscopy 2004;36:595–600.

27 Barbezat GO, Schlup M, Lubcke R: Omeprazole therapy decreases the need for dilatation of peptic esophageal strictures. Aliment Pharmacol Ther 1999;13:1041–1045.

28 Marks RD, Richter JE, Rizzo J, et al: Omeprazole versus H_2-receptor antagonists in treating patients with peptic stricture and esophagitis. Gastroenterology 1994;106: 907–915.

29 Portale G, Costantini M, Rizzetto C, Guirroli E, Ceolin M, Salvador R, Ancona E, Zaninotto G: Long-term outcome of laparoscopic Heller-Dor surgery for esophageal achalasia: possible detrimental role of previous endoscopic treatment. J Gastrointest Surg 2005;9:1332–1339.

30 Metman EH, Lagasse JP, d'Alteroche L, et al: Risk factors for immediate complications after progressive pneumatic dilation for achalasia. Am J Gastroenterol 1999;94: 1179–1185.

31 Quine MA, Bell GD, McCloy RF, et al: Prospective audit of perforation rates following upper gastrointestinal endoscopy in two regions of England. Br J Surg 1995; 82:530–533.
32 Jethwa P, Lala A, Powell J, et al: A regional audit of iatrogenic perforation of tumours of the oesophagus and cardia. Aliment Pharmacol Ther 2005;21: 479–484.
33 Fadoo F, Ruiz DE, Dawn SK, et al: Helical CT esophagography for the evaluation of suspected esophageal perforation or rupture: Am J Roentgenol 2004;182: 1177–1179
34 McLean GK, LeVeen RF: Shear stress in the performance of esophageal dilation: comparison of balloon dilation and bougienage. Radiology 1989;172: 983–986.
35 Saeed ZA, Winchester CB, Ferro PS, et al: Prospective randomized comparison of polyvinyl bougies and through-the-scope balloons for dilation of peptic strictures of the esophagus. Gastrointest Endosc 1995;41:189–195.
36 Scolapio JS, Pasha TM, Gostout CJ, et al: A randomized prospective study comparing rigid to balloon dilators for benign esophageal strictures and rings. Gastrointest Endosc 1999;50:13–17.
37 Clouse RE: Complications of endoscopic gastrointestinal dilation techniques. Gastrointest Endosc Clin North Am 1996;6:323–341.
38 Siersema PD, Homs MY, Haringsma J, et al: Use of large-diameter metallic stents to seal traumatic non-malignant perforations of the esophagus. Gastrointest Endosc 2003;58:356–361.
39 Gelbmann CM, Ratiu NL, Rath HC, et al: Use of self-expandable plastic stents for the treatment of esophageal perforations and symptomatic anastomotic leaks. Endoscopy 2004;36:695–699.

Klaus Mönkemüller, MD, PhD, FASGE
Marienhospital, Bottrop, Josef-Albers-Strasse 70
DE–46236 Bottrop (Germany)
Tel. +49 2041 106 1000, Fax +49 2041 106 1009
E-Mail klaus.moenkemueller@mhb-bottrop.de

Mönkemüller K, Wilcox CM, Muñoz-Navas M (eds): Interventional and Therapeutic Gastrointestinal Endoscopy.
Front Gastrointest Res. Basel, Karger, 2010, vol 27, pp 106–114

Self-Expanding Metallic Stents for the Palliation of Malignant Esophageal Obstruction

Klaus Mönkemüller[a,b] · Lars Zimmermann[a,b]

[a]Department of Internal Medicine, Gastroenterology, Hepatology and Infectious Diseases, Marienhospital, Bottrop, and [b]Divison of Gastroenterology, Hepatology and Infectious Diseases, Otto von Guericke University, Magdeburg, Germany

Abstract

Every endoscopist will encounter patients with malignant dysphagia that will require some sort of palliative therapy. Self-expanding metallic stents (SEMS) are a major mode of palliative therapy in esophageal cancer. SEMS have become increasingly popular as a result of improvement in design and the availability of different models. Hence, the use of SEMS for the palliation of malignant dysphagia has increased dramatically over the last few years. When choosing stents as palliative therapy, several aspects need to be taken into consideration such as patient condition, tumor location and characteristics, presence of fistula and previous or planned treatments such as chemo- or radiation therapy. This chapter reviews the indications, technique, complications and outcome of expandable metal stents for malignant dysphagia.

Esophageal cancer accounts for approximately 7% of all gastrointestinal (GI) malignancies and is currently the leading cause of malignant dysphagia (fig. 1a). However, malignant dysphagia can also result from extrinsic compression due to lung cancer or malignant lymphadenopathy (fig. 1b) [1, 2]. Despite advances in its diagnosis and treatment, up to 70% of patients with malignant dysphagia have incurable disease at presentation [3]. Most of these tumors are not amenable to resection for cure. The goal of therapy in these patients with unresectable esophageal or paraesophageal tumors is to palliate the accompanying symptoms and complications such as dysphagia, tracheoesophageal (TE) fistulas, malnutrition, aspiration and pain and hence improve their quality of life [4].

SEMS are one of the pillars for the palliative therapy of patients with malignant esophageal stenosis. They are useful for patients with poor functional status who cannot tolerate radiation or chemotherapy, who have advanced metastatic disease, or in whom previous therapy has failed [1]. The main indication for placement of SEMS is malignant dysphagia. Further indications include cough and aspiration due to a TE fistula and malnutrition. The type and location of the stenosis may indicate the type of stent that needs to be used. In the presence of TE fistula, covered SEMS are preferred. A SEMS should not be placed in patients with very poor survival chances. In addition, the presence of coagulopathy, uncooperative or clinically unstable patients, recent myocardial infarction, presence of a fixed cervical spine or cervical arthritis and active infection are relative contraindications. There is still controversy regarding the use of stents before

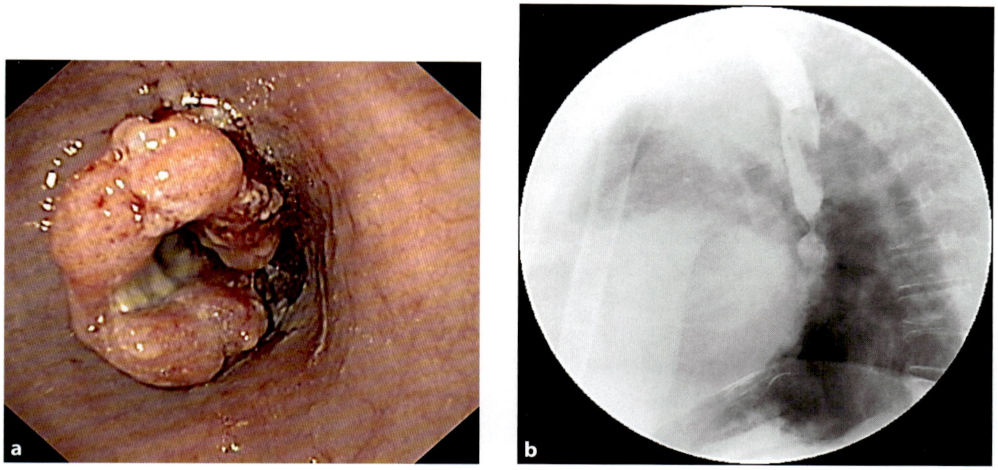

Fig. 1. **a** Endoscopic view of a squamous epithelial esophageal carcinoma in the mid-esophagus leading to partial obstruction. **b** Malignant esophageal stricture caused by external compression due to metastasis in the mediastinum.

or after radiochemotherapy, as some studies have shown a higher risk of complications such as perforation, GI bleeding and stent migration [5, 6]. If a patient is deemed a surgical candidate, no attempt should be made to place a SEMS.

Procedural Aspects

Besides remaining NPO, laboratory tests may be warranted in patients with blood dyscrasias or those taking anticoagulant therapy. Prior to endoscopy, all patients have to provide written informed consent, also with written information about the risk of perforation (i.e. 2–3%) and the possible need for surgery and/or prolonged hospitalization Endoscopies and SEMS placement are carried out in the morning after an overnight fast and as an inpatient procedure, as all patients should be observed for 24 h after the procedure. We routinely perform stent placement in the fluoroscopy room, using either endoscopic or radiologic guidance. Sometimes we perform radiographic contrast examination before SEMS placement, but almost always after the procedure. Esophageal SEMS placement should always be performed or closely supervised by experienced endoscopists. Antibiotics are not used routinely before dilation; endocarditis prophylaxis guidelines should be followed [7]. Anticoagulants should be discontinued [8].

Adequate venous access is of paramount importance as all SEMS should be placed using conscious sedation.

Types of Stents

Expandable metal stents are made of metal alloys and have varying shapes and sizes, depending on the manufacturer [1, 4] (fig. 2). *Wallstents* are prosthesis woven in the form of a tubular mesh

2

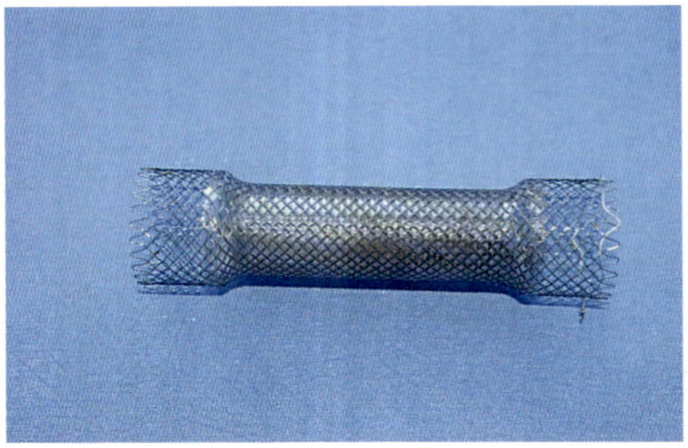

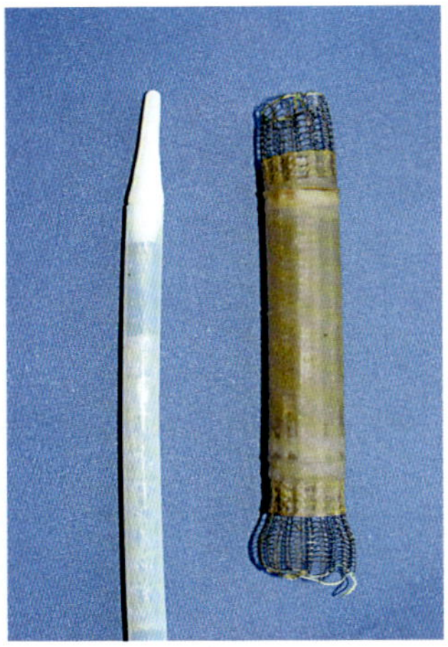

3

Fig. 2. Example of a commercially available SEMS. **Fig. 3.** A fully released SEMS is placed besides a SEMS which is still mounted within its delivery device. Note the relatively small diameter of the delivery catheter, which holds the compressed stent inside.

made from surgical-grade stainless steel alloy filaments. These stents are pliable, self-expanding and flexible in the longitudinal axis. The stent is kept in its compressed from by an invaginated rolling membrane with an 18-Fr diameter, and it can be loaded on a 0.035-in guidewire [9, 10]. The *Z-stent* is a self-expanding tubular prosthesis. The basic structure consists of a variable number of interconnected cages of 2 cm length. Each cage is composed of Z-shaped stainless steel wire. It can be compressed and placed inside a delivery catheter. The stent is available in several lengths (6, 8, 10 and 12 cm), with an 18-mm diameter. There are several modifications that evolved from the original uncovered prototype. It has been coated with a silicone membrane. In order to avoid dislodgement or migration (due to the silicone coating), special anchoring hooks ('barbs') have been placed on the external surface (European model). The radial force exerted by the stent is considerable, making it suitable for tight strictures. The presence of barbs theoretically decreases the incidence of migration. However, not all Z-stents have barbs. Because of this, it is easier to extract if its migrated into the stomach. In order to prevent migration, most SEMS have flared distal and proximal ends 25 mm for greater anchoring (fig. 2, 3).The silicone covering decreases the exposure of the metal to tissue and hence decreases granulation and potential occlusion. It also prohibits tumor ingrowth.

The *Ultraflex* stent, which is knitted from a single wire of elastic alloy of nickel-titanium, is made of nitinol embedded in gelatin to keep it in a compressed state [10, 11]. When released, the gelatin dissolves slowly and the stent expands, but deployment may take as long as 9 min while the gelatin dissolves to free the stent. Injecting warm water through the biopsy channel accelerates the process, but carries the risk of aspiration [10]. The expanded stent varies in length (7, 10, or 15 cm) [10, 11]. Incomplete expansion is a significant problem and is due to low radial expansile force exerted by the stent. Thus, balloon dilation of the stent may be needed to achieve full expansion. It is delivered mounted in a stabilizer with an outer diameter of 8 mm. Within the stabilizer, the stent is localized by four radiopaque markers. The two outer markers indicate the length of the stent in the compressed state; the two inner markers indicate the position of the ends of the stent after expansion (shortened) [11].

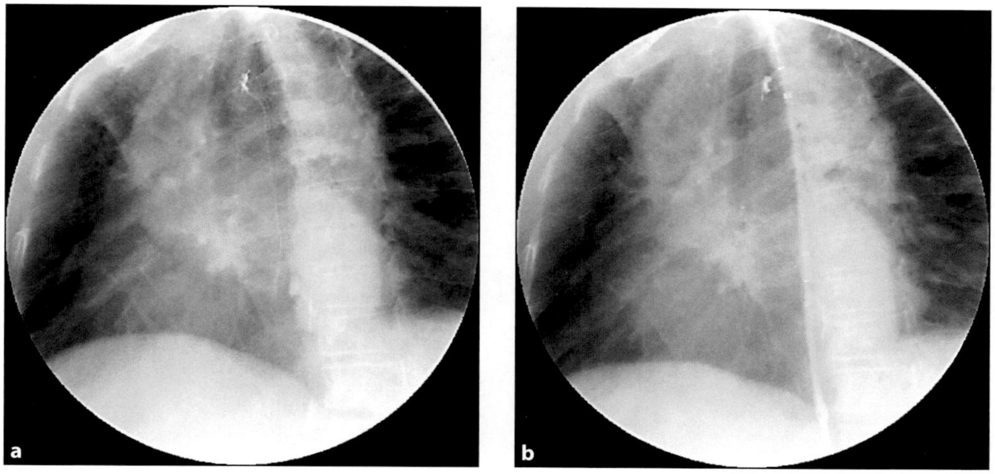

Fig. 4. **a** The lipiodol marking is easily seen in the distal part of the stricture (or distal part of the fully deployed stent). **b** Note the markings of the delivery device. These serve to place the stent into a correct deploying position.

This *Esophacoil* stent is rarely used today. This SEMS consists of a single-coiled flat wire made of nickel-titanium alloy [12, 13]. This SEMS is unique in that it is a simple coil with tight loop. It has a high radial force and almost no dilation is necessary prior to implantation. The ends of the stent are wide to prevent migration. Its soft spherical wire ends avoid epithelial injury. The stent's flexibility allows adaptation to the wall of the tumor, diminishing significantly retrosternal pain and foreign body sensation. The very close loops of the spring prevent tumor ingrowth and impart appropriate wall permeability. For these reasons this stent has also been used to palliate TE fistula [13].

Technique of SEMS Placement

Each stent has its own characteristics, delivery devices and placement technique. The radial expansile forces and the degree of shortening differ among different types of stents [1]. However, all SEMS are mounted in a preloaded constrained position on a delivery catheter (fig. 3). Furthermore, there are some general guidelines for placement of most SEMS. It is important to have fluoroscopic equipment available. The placement of a stent should to be performed by an experienced therapeutic endoscopist or interventional radiologist.

Analysis of the Stricture
The success of esophageal SEMS placement requires precise knowledge of the location and length of the anatomical disruption to be palliated. Several methods are used to accomplish this. We always determine the proximal location of the stricture endoscopically. If the endoscope can be passed through the stenosis, then the distal end of the stricture is analyzed and documented as well. If the stricture is impassable, then we perform an endoscopic-assisted contrast esophagography to measure the stricture's length. If the stenosis is tight and precludes the

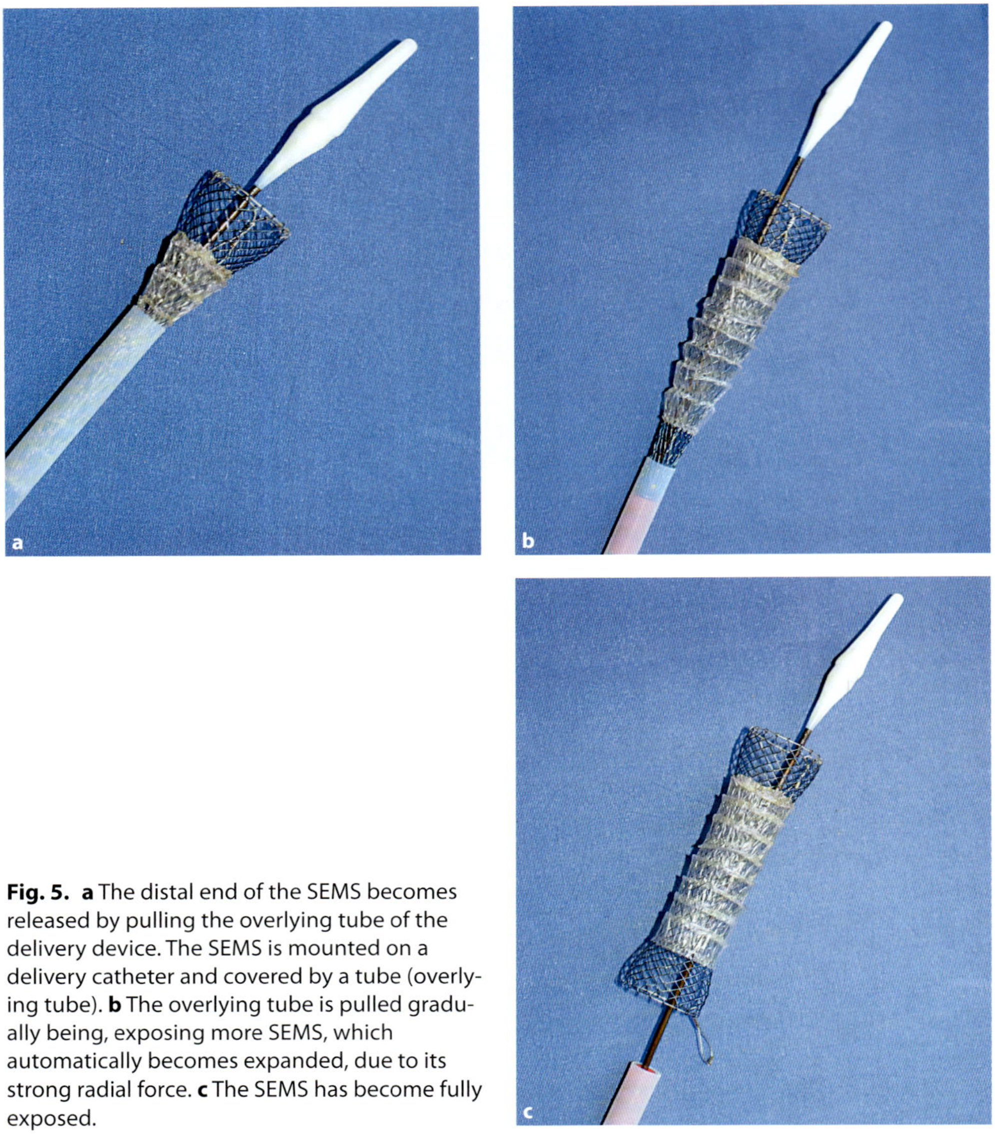

Fig. 5. a The distal end of the SEMS becomes released by pulling the overlying tube of the delivery device. The SEMS is mounted on a delivery catheter and covered by a tube (overlying tube). **b** The overlying tube is pulled gradually being, exposing more SEMS, which automatically becomes expanded, due to its strong radial force. **c** The SEMS has become fully exposed.

passage of the delivery system, we dilate the stricture using either through-the-scope balloons or Savary-Gillard dilators (please refer to the chapter on esophageal dilation). The endoscope is then passed into the stomach. However, the small diameter of the delivery devices of current SEMS before deployment makes aggressive dilation of the esophagus before or after deployment unnecessary [1].

Demarcation of the Stricture

It is essential to define the stricture limits to appropriately select an SEMS. The stricture margins can be marked in several ways. The most common method consists of placing external markings on the patient's chest wall to correspond with the end of stricture as pointed out with the endoscope during fluoroscopy. Although easy to perform, this method has the major disadvantage of being prone to moving artifacts (respiration, body movement) or miscalculation, because the external markers are only an approximation of where the stricture is. The bowing of the pusher tube against a tight tumor may also make markings less reliable. Therefore, we prefer to inject lipiodol (1.5 ml) (Lipiodol Ultra-Fluid, Guerbet GmbH, Sulzbach, Germany) (fig. 4a). Other endoscopists inject radiocontrast (meglumine iothalamate, Conray; May & Baker Ltd, Dagenham, UK, and diatrizoate, Hypaque 50%) into the upper and lower margins of the stricture. However, contrast dissipates rapidly from the submucosa. Another effective way of marking the margins of the stricture consists of the intraluminal placement of marking clips (HX-3l clip fixing device; Olympus Europe, Hamburg, Germany). In addition, most stent-delivery devices have their own markers to guide the prosthesis into the correct position.

SEMS Deployment

A biliary (0.035 in) or Savary-Gilliard wire is placed through the stricture into the stomach under endoscopic control. After withdrawing the endoscope, the delivery system (with the mounted stent) is inserted over the guidewire and passed over the obstruction, across the stricture. The collapsed stent is visible by radiopaque markers placed on the shaft of the delivery device (fig. 4b). The prosthesis is manipulated until it is positioned so that the shortened stent would extend 2 cm beyond the markings that represent the proximal and distal ends of the tumor. Nitinol stents are less clearly visualized than stainless steel stents, and thicker stents (Esophacoil) are easier to visualize than thinner ones (Ultraflex) [10, 14, 15]. Then the constraining mechanism is released, which causes the length of the stent to decrease and its diameter to increase. Nowadays there are several delivery methods (fig. 4). Most stents are released form its distal end (fig. 5a–c). What happens is that the overlying catheter is pushed back, allowing the SEMS to be freed and expand. In other SEMS delivery systems a string which holds the stent tight in compressed position is removed gradually. If the process of pulling back the 'overtube' or string release is done to fast, the SEMS can open to fast and migrate distally. Therefore, caution should be paid when retrieving the overlying catheter or pulling on the string. One easy method is the one used by the Evolution system of SEMS (Cook, Ireland and USA). With this method the SEMS is released by pressing on a release mechanism located proximally, on a handle that resembles a pistol. Due to its design it allows manipulation and relocation of the SEMS. Using this method we have been able to perfectly place a SEMS in perfect position in <1–2 min. This is especially useful in patients who do not tolerate sedation well. After the SEMS is fully expanded, the introducing catheter and the guidewire are then retrieved (fig. 6). A radiocontrast swallow may need to be done immediately if a perforation is suspected. Figures 7 and 8 show fully expanded SEMS. Partially or fully covered SEMS are preferred in patients with TE fistulas (fig. 9) [16]. Covered metal stents have a membrane to prevent reobstruction due to ingrowth of tumor through the mesh wall (Baron). However, proximal and distal obstruction can occur also occur with these stents (fig. 10).

Post-Procedure Care

Patients with esophageal stents must modify their diet to prevent large boluses of food from becoming impacted within the stent. Fiber poor diets are recommended. Avoidance of food

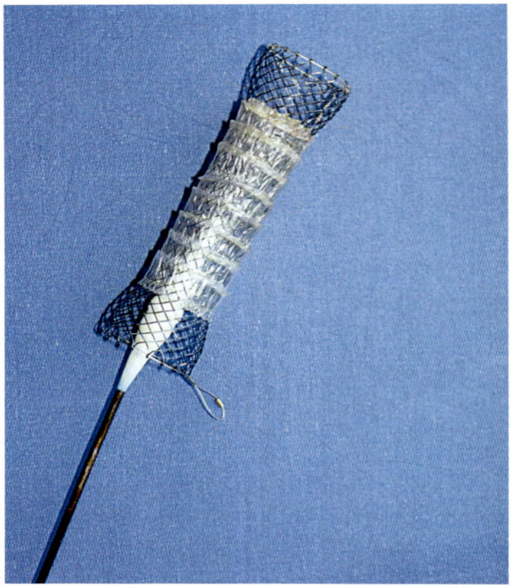

6

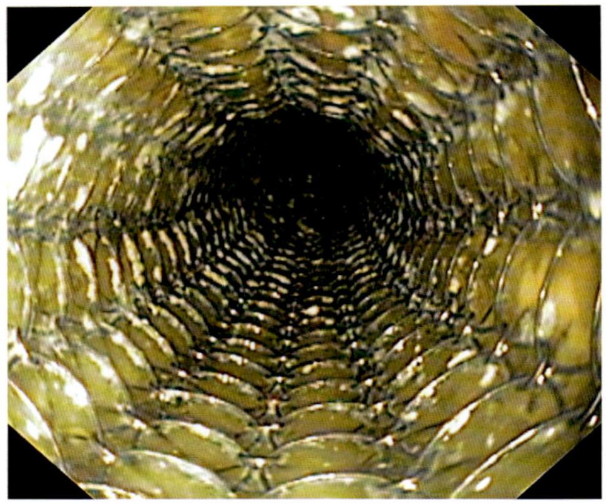

7

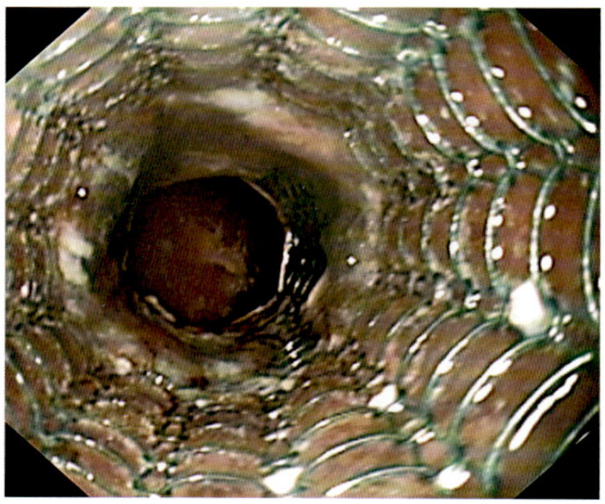

8

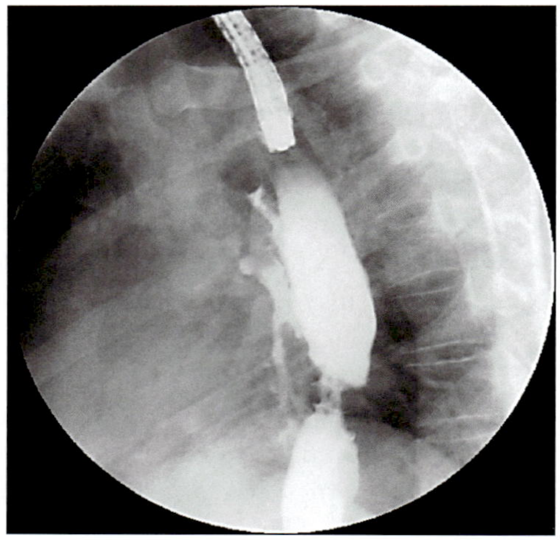

9

Fig. 6. By doing soft to-and-fro wiggly movements, the endoscopist can retract the inner catheter once the stent has been fully deployed. Make sure the SEMS has expanded some before pulling, as the distal tip can occasionally get entrapped at a stenotic area or at worst, move the stent proximally (migration!).
Fig. 7. Endoscopic view of a fully expanded covered SEMS. **Fig. 8.** Endoscopic view of a fully expanded standard SEMS. **Fig. 9.** Malignant stricture associated with an esophagobronchial fistula.

that is difficult to digest or sausages with 'skin' is also recommended. In addition, we advise patients not to drink cold drinks for 36–48 h after stent placement, as cold water can 'constrain' the expanded stent and cause migration. Indeed, if there is an emergent need to remove a malpositioned stent, endoscopic instillation of cold water can improve stent removal. However, on a long-term basis, we advise the patient to drink some carbonated water during and after each meal and also to regularly drink fruit juices containing digestive enzymes such as papaya and pineapple. The carbonated water will help 'push' the food down the stent, and the juices containing digestive enzymes may help 'digest' some of the food that normally gets attached to the inner part of the stent. There is no worse situation than the removal of hot dogs or

Table 1. Complications associated with esophageal SEMS placement

Intraprocedural	Early (<30 days)	Late (>30 days)
Problems associated with conscious sedation	Pain	Tumor ingrowth
Aspiration	Food impaction	Bleeding
Malpositioning of the SEMS	Tumor ingrowth	Food impaction
Bleeding	Bleeding	Pain
Esophageal perforation	Fistulae	Fistulae
	Stridor	Gastroesophageal reflux
	Esophageal ulceration	Migration
	Esophageal erosion	Foreign body sensation
	Gastroesophageal reflux	
	Migration	
	Foreign body sensation	
	Perforation	

SEMS = Self-expanding metal stent.

10
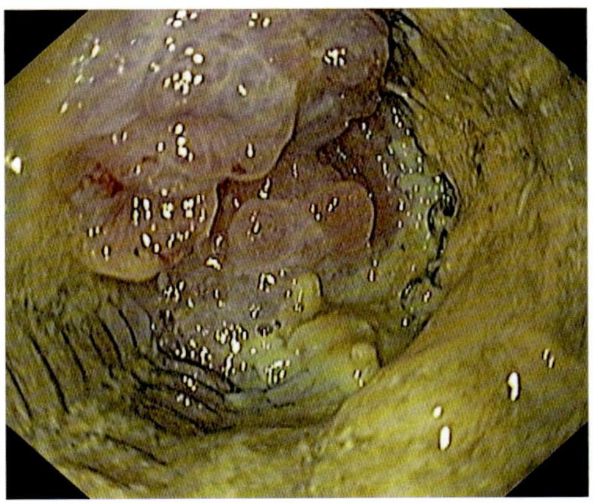

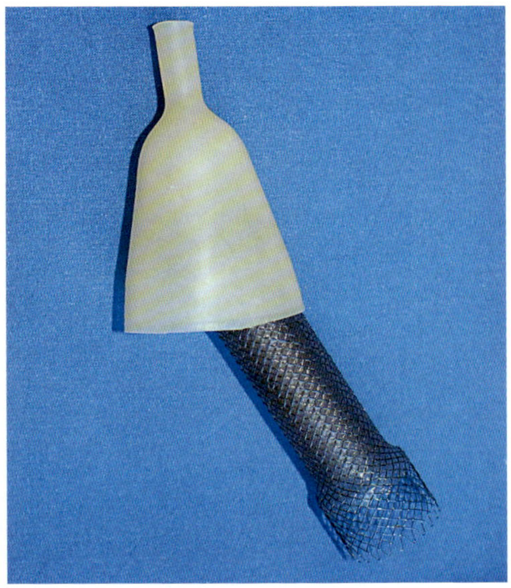
11

Fig. 10. Tumor ingrowth inside of the distal part of a SEMS. **Fig. 11.** By placing a Capuchon® on the distal part of the scope it is possible to pull the migrated SEMS into towards the tip of the scope, and then pull it up through the esophagus, without the risk of lacerating the mucosa or getting the stent trapped in the esophagus.

large amounts of fibered food from an occluded SEMS! If a stent without an antireflux valve crosses the gastroesophageal junction, strict antireflux precautions and aggressive acid suppression therapy using proton pump inhibitors are needed to prevent gastroesophageal reflux and aspiration.

Limitations and Complications

Table 1 lists the possible complications associated with SEMS placement [1, 4, 16–19]. It is important to remember that approximately 0.5–2% of patients who undergo the procedure die as a direct result of placement of an expandable metal stent [1]. If the stent lumen becomes occluded by tissue ingrowth, overgrowth, or hyperplasia, a second stent may be placed through the first stent with good results. Alternatively, endoscopic laser therapy, electrocautery, or photodynamic therapy may be used to treat stent occlusion. If a stent migrates into the stomach then we retrieve it using the Capuchon® retriever (fig. 11).

References

1 Baron TH: Expandable metal stents for the treatment of cancerous obstruction of the gastrointestinal tract. N Engl J Med 2001;344:1681–1687.
2 Fleischer DE, Bull-Henry K: A new coated self-expanding metal stent for malignant esophageal strictures. Gastrointest Endosc 1992;38:494–496.
3 Khandelwal M: Palliative therapy for carcinoma of the esophagus. Compr Ther 1995;21:177–183.
4 Mönkemüller K, Wilcox CM: The options for palliation of esophageal adenocarcinoma; in Sharma P, Sampliner R (eds): Barrett's Esophagus and Esophageal Adenocarcinoma. Philadelphia, Lippincott Raven, 2001, vol 20, pp 208–217.
5 Kinsman KJ, DeGregorio BT, Katon RM, Morrison K, Saxon RR, Keller FS, Rösch J: Prior radiation and chemotherapy increase the risk of life-threatening complications after insertion of metallic stents for esophagogastric malignancy. Gastrointest Endosc 1996; 43:196–203.
6 Kozarek RA, Ball TJ, Brandabur JJ, Patterson DJ, Low D, Hill L, Raltz S: Expandable versus conventional esophageal prostheses: easier insertion may not preclude subsequent stent-related problems. Gastrointest Endosc 1996; 43:204–208.
7 Hirota K, Petersen K, Baron TH, et al: Antibiotic prophylaxis for GI endoscopy. Gastrointest Endosc 2003; 58:475–482.
8 Eisen GM, Baron TH, Dominitz JA, et al: Guideline on the management of anticoagulation and antiplatelet therapy for endoscopic procedures. Gastrointest Endosc 2002;55:775–779.
9 Vermeijden JR, Bartelsman JFWM, Fockens P, Meijer RC, Tytgat GNJ: Self-expanding metal stents for palliation of esophagocardial malignancies. Gastrointest Endosc 1995;41:58–63.
10 Bethge N, Sommer A, Vakil N: Palliation of malignant esophageal obstruction due to intrinsic and extrinsic lesions with expandable metal stents. Am J Gastroenterol 1998;93:1829–1832.
11 Raijman I, Siddique I, Ajani J, Lynch P: Palliation of malignant dysphagia and fistulae with coated expandable metal stents: experience with 101 patients. Gastrointest Endosc 1998;48:172–179.
12 Axelrad AM, Fleischer DE, Gomes M: Nitinol coil esophageal prosthesis: advantages of removable self-expanding metallic stents. Gastrointest Endosc 1996; 43:155–160.
13 Fiorini AB, Goldin E, Valero JL, Bloom A, Beyar M, Pfeffer RP, Globerma n O: Expandable metal coil stent for treatment of bronchoesophageal fistula. Gastrointest Endosc 1995;42:81–83.
14 Siersema PD, Marcon N, Vakil N: Endoscopy metal stents for tumors of the distal esophagus and gastric cardia. Endoscopy 2003;35:79–85.
15 Kozarek RA: Endoscopic palliation of esophageal malignancy. Endoscopy 2003;35:S9–S13.
16 Silva RA, Mesquita N, Brandão C, Dinis-Ribeiro M, Fernandes N, Moreira Dias L: Safety and efficacy of large-diameter esophageal metal stents. Endoscopy 2006; 38:756.
17 Furlong H, Nasr A, Walsh TN: Gastropleural fistula: a complication of esophageal self-expanding metallic stent migration. Endoscopy 2009;41:E38–E39.
18 Siersema PD, Homs MY, Kuipers EJ: Large-diameter metal stents are associated with stent-related esophageal complications. Endoscopy 2005;37:600.
19 Modi P, Rahamim J: Use of coronary angiography wires as guidewires to avoid iatrogenic perforation during stenting of oesophageal cancers. Endoscopy 2006;38: 292.

Klaus Mönkemüller, MD, PhD, FASGE
Marienhospital, Bottrop, Josef-Albers-Strasse 70
DE–46236 Bottrop (Germany)
Tel. +49 2041 106 1000, Fax +49 2041 106 1009
E-Mail klaus.moenkemueller@mhb-bottrop.de

Mönkemüller K, Wilcox CM, Muñoz-Navas M (eds): Interventional and Therapeutic Gastrointestinal Endoscopy.
Front Gastrointest Res. Basel, Karger, 2010, vol 27, pp 115–121

Endoscopic Therapy of Zenker's Diverticulum

Fábio Yuji Hondo · Atul Kumar · Paulo Sakai

Gastrointestinal Endoscopy Unit, Department of Surgery, Medical School University of São Paulo, São Paulo, Brazil

Abstract

Zenker's diverticulum (ZD) is an upper esophageal diverticulum that results from evagination of the hypopharyngeal mucosa in the Killian's triangle. The defect lies in an area between the oblique fibers of the inferior pharyngeal constrictor muscle and the transverse fibers of the cricopharyngeal muscle. Symptoms range from transient dysphagia to frequent regurgitation complicated by aspiration pneumonia. Diagnosis is usually made at endoscopy or barium imaging. Surgical treatment of ZD is a well-established modality being effective in 80–100% of patients. However, patients with ZD are often old with several comorbidities which increases the procedural risks. The development of several accessories, such as an oblique transparent cap, a diverticuloscope which facilitates electrodissection of the septum using a needle-knife, argon plasma coagulation or a harmonic scalpel, has led to an increasing use of flexible endoscopic approaches. Development of novel accessories and techniques along with better animal/computer training models are likely to help improve outcomes following treatment of ZD using flexible endoscopes.

Zenker's diverticulum (ZD) results from evagination of the hypopharyngeal mucosa in the Killian's triangle, an area between the oblique fibers of the inferior pharyngeal constrictor muscle and the transverse fibers of the cricopharyngeal muscle. The condition is generally acquired and has a male predominance. While first described by Ludlow in 1767, Zenker and Ziemssen published the first review in 1877, hence its name [1]. It is believed that motor dysfunction in the upper esophagus leads to evagination of an area of weakness immediately above the posterior aspect of the upper esophageal sphincter, more commonly on the left side [1]. In early stages, these outpouchings spontaneously reverse in the relaxed state. However, in later stages, the diverticulum progressively enlarges and descends into the neck, occasionally extending down into the superior mediastinum.

The size of ZD may be measured by endoscopically or radiologically. Conventionally the lesion is considered small when the size is <2.0 cm in length, medium when the size is between 2.0 and 4.0 cm, and large when the size >4.0 cm. The size of the vertebra may be used as a reference; small being <1, medium up to 3, and large >3 vertebrae.

Clinical Symptoms and Diagnosis

Symptoms depend on the size of the ZD. Transient dysphagia may be the only complaint early-on. When the pouch becomes large and starts to retain sputum and food, patients may complain of regurgitation and develop aspiration pneumonia. This usually results when the opening of a large ZD is aligned with the pharyngeal sac. Patients usually do not present until their sixth or seventh decade and often have had symptoms for months to years preceding clinical presentation. Diagnosis is usually made at endoscopy or barium imaging in a patient presenting with dysphagia. Small diverticula can often be missed, and require a rotated film to prevent overlap of ZD with the esophageal column of barium. Manometry has no role as studies evaluating upper esophageal sphincter pressures in such patients have been inconsistent and are conclusive.

Treatment

Surgical Treatment. Surgical treatment of ZD is a well-established modality and effective in 80–100% of patients. In a technical review, The American Gastroenterological Association reported surgery as the treatment of choice [2]. While there are several variations of the procedure, the preferred approach involves resection of the pouch (diverticulectomy) in conjunction with cricopharyngeal myotomy through a left cervicotomy [2]. Other methods include mobilization and excision of the ZD, cricopharyngeal myotomy leaving the ZD undisturbed. Any surgical intervention carries a high morbidity and mortality rate mainly due to the advanced age of the patients and presence of several comorbidities. Complications include mediastinitis, vocal cord paralysis, pharyngocutaneous fistula, esophageal stenosis and recurrent or persistent ZD.

Endoscopic Treatment. An alternate modality using the endoscopic approach was first reported in the early 1900s. This modality often achieves the same clinical results as surgical treatment while reducing the incidence of complications and mortality [3–6]. Endoscopic modality has been increasingly used in Europe and South America.

The first human trials describing endoscopic myotomy through a flexible endoscope were published simultaneously by Ishioka et al. [3] and Mulder et al. [4]. Following placement of a nasogastric tube as a guide, the septum was incised using pure cut/coagulation electrical current. The endoscopic technique involves sectioning the bridge of the ZD which is mainly constituted by the cricopharyngeal muscle, lying in between the esophagus and the diverticulum. This eliminates the anterior wall, resulting in an overflow of contents from the ZD into the esophagus. We believe that cutting the septum in one stage for a small or medium-sized ZD and in two or more stages for a large ZD limits the complication rate. Several accessories have been developed to facilitate visualization during this procedure, including a hood attached to the endoscope [7] and a flexible overtube called diverticuloscope [8].

In 1917, Mosher first described an endoscopic approach to treatment of ZD. The technique was later popularized by Dohlman and Mattson [9] in the 1960s. They devised a rigid, double-lipped laryngoscope to facilitate electrocoagulation of the bridge using an insulated forceps with a diathermic knife. In 1984, Van Overbeek et al. [10] used the CO_2 laser via a rigid laryngoscope. Endoscopic stapler-assisted esophagodiverticulostomy has been shown by Collard et al. [11] to be safe and effective, but requires general anesthesia along with a specialized long and rigid laryngoscope. The procedure is unsuitable for patients with a small diverticulum and may also

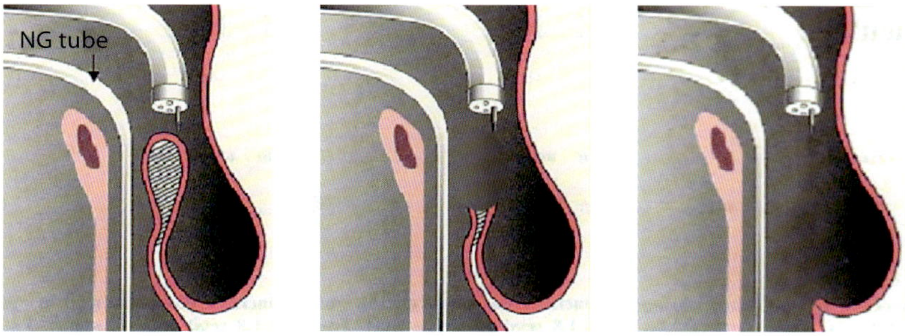

Fig. 1. Schematic sequence of endoscopic diverticulostomy by needle-knife.

result in cervical injuries in elderly patients with spondyloarthroses. Several studies utilizing the stapler-assisted method have reported short-term effectiveness with shortened hospital stays. For larger diverticulum, the residual cavity may be large enough, even following two applications and not completely empty with inadequate symptom relief.

Endoscopic treatment of ZD using a flexible endoscope is a feasible and practical alternative to surgical intervention. A monopolar forceps or a needle-knife is utilized to cut the septum/bridge in patients with ZD. Argon plasma coagulation (APC) has also been reported for this purpose. More recently, we have utilized the harmonic scalpel [unpubl. data].

Indications for Endoscopic Treatment

Endoscopic treatment of ZD is mainly indicated for older and debilitated patients who are often at high risk for general anesthesia and surgical intervention. Although this condition mainly afflicts the elderly, younger patients under 50–60 years with symptoms are referred for treatment. We offer these patients both surgical and endoscopic alternatives. An important advantage of the endoscopic procedure is that it is easier to repeat in case of treatment failure.

Technique for Endoscopic Dissection

Adequate sedation facilitates the procedure and general anesthesia with orotracheal intubation is preferable in order to prevent aspiration. A standard upper endoscope is introduced with the patient in the left lateral position. Contents of the pouch are aspirated and the esophageal orifice is outlined by insertion of a nasogastric tube (fig. 1), which is additionally used for enteral feeding following the procedure.

The attachment of an oblique cap or hood [10] is useful to obtain an adequate wide view of the septum which separates the diverticulum from the esophageal lumen (fig. 2). A flexible overtube, also termed a diverticuloscope [11], has a double-lipped extremity which fits the anterior esophageal wall and the posterior wall of the diverticulum, leaving the septum in the center of the endoscopic field (fig. 3). While this device helps maintain stability during the procedure, it often is unsuitable for a small ZD.

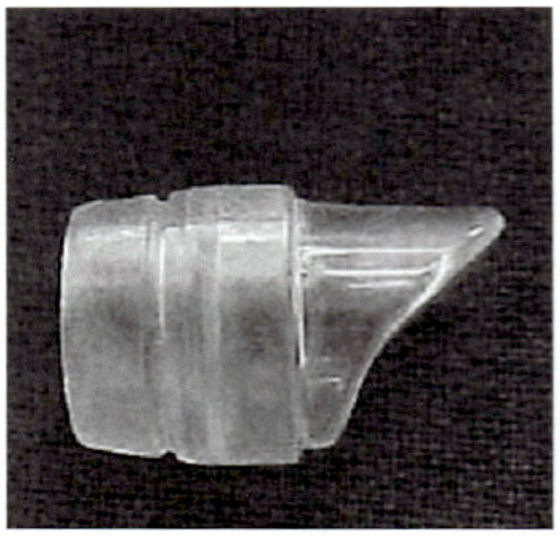

2

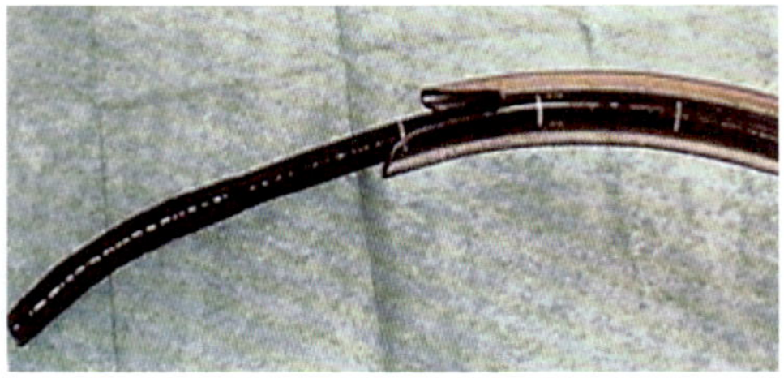

3

Fig. 2. The hood that attaches to a flexible endoscope (Olympus). **Fig. 3.** Diverticuloscope with distal end to facilitate (ZDO overtube – Wilson-Cook).

Electrodissection of the septum using a needle-knife is performed using monopolar cautery with blended or pure coagulation current (fig. 1). Occasionally pure coagulation current provides an adequate cut. Dissection is performed in the mid-section of the septum in a craniocaudal approach from the esophageal side. The aim of the procedure is to completely section the septum along the diverticular pouch downwards close to the bottom, thus achieving a wide communication between the diverticulum and the esophagus. It is important to not dissect all the way to the bottom of the diverticulum, rather to leave a 5-mm lip in order to avoid the risk of perforation into the mediastinum.

Argon beam equipment has also been utilized as a 'knife', but in our personal experience it is difficult to use and has not been effective. It may however be utilized as rescue therapy for excessive bleeding with needle-knife or other techniques.

A 5-mm harmonic scalpel may alternatively be utilized for endoscopic dissection of ZD. Following insertion of a flexible overtube (diverticuloscope), the septum is identified and isolated and the harmonic scalpel 'scissors' is then applied to the mid-portion under full endoscopic view. A pediatric endoscope is preferable for this procedure alongside which the harmonic scalpel is deployed. Activation of the scalpel blade leads to coaptive coagulation of the septum along with the vessels and tissue [12].

If repeated endoscopic interventions are required, 2 or 3 weeks should be allowed to elapse before reintervening. A nasogastric tube is left in situ for enteral feeding for 48–72 h following the procedure as patients often complain of dysphagia. Oral feeding may be gradually resumed thereafter. In event of perforation, pneumomediastinum may often present as subcutaneous emphysema palpable in the neck or alternatively be visualized on CT scan. Perforation can often be managed conservatively by leaving a nasogastric tube for 1 week followed by a contrast study of the upper airway esophagus to evaluate for leakage of contrast. Prophylactic antibiotics may be administered intravenously, just prior to the procedure and continued if perforation occurs.

Results and Complications

The primary indication for endoscopic therapy is an older patient with comorbidities [3]. Over 90% of patients report relief of dysphagia and 5–15% will report recurrence usually as a result of residual diverticulum. Repeat endoscopic intervention is feasible in such cases [13]. Complications include cervical or mediastinal emphysema in up to 23% of patients and

Table 1. Outcomes of flexible endoscopic treatment of ZD

Author	Year	n	Endoscopic device	Incision	Sessions	Emphysema	Bleeding	Recurrence	Clinical resolution
Ishioka	1995	20	none	forceps coagulation	1.8	1 (2%)	1 (2.4%)	3 (7.1%)	92.80%
Mulder	1995	42	none	needle-knife	3 (1–12)	none	none	n.a.	n.a.
Sakai	2001	10	hood	needle-knife	1	none	none	none	100%
Hashiba	1999	47	none	needle-knife	(1–4)	6 (13%)	1 (2.1%)	n.a.	96%
Mulder	1999	125	none	APC	1.8 (1–12)	19 (15%)	2 (1.6%)	n.a.	100%
Costamagna	2007	28	cap	needle-knife	n.a.	5 (18%)	4 (14%)	8 (2.9%)	43%
Costamagna	2007	11	diverticulo-scope	needle-knife	n.a.	none	none	1 (9%)	91%
Rabenstein	2007	41	cap	APC	3 (2–10)	1 (3%)	none	17%	95%
Christaens	2007	21	hood	monopolar forceps	1.1 (1–2)	1 (4.8%)	none	10%	100%
Vogelsang	2007	31	cap	needle-knife	1.4 (1–3)	7 (23%)	1 (3.3%)	35%	84%
Hondo	2009	13	diverticulo-scope	harmonic scalpel	1.07 (1–2)	1 (7.7%)	none	1 (7.7%)	100%

bleeding in up to 10% following endoscopic cricopharyngeal myotomy [14]. Mortality is usually related to complications unrelated to the procedure itself [13–22]. An overview of the results and complications is presented in table 1. Included are preliminary results using the harmonic scalpel in humans [unpubl. data] with complications mainly related to neck hyperextension (fig. 4).

Conclusion

Endoscopic treatment of patients with ZD is best performed in centers with sufficient local expertise and experience. The primary indication for endoscopic intervention is in an older patient with co-morbidities, although younger patients may also be considered depending on operator expertise. Surgical intervention is a well established procedure with excellent results and is usually definitive with low recurrence rates [23]. In our own practice, patients are offered surgical and endoscopic alternatives. The major advantages of the flexible endoscopic approach are its minimally invasive nature, shorter postoperative course, lack of inpatient stays, early

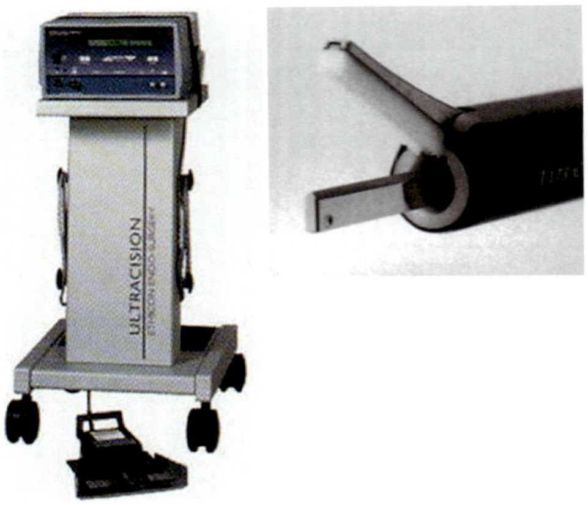

4

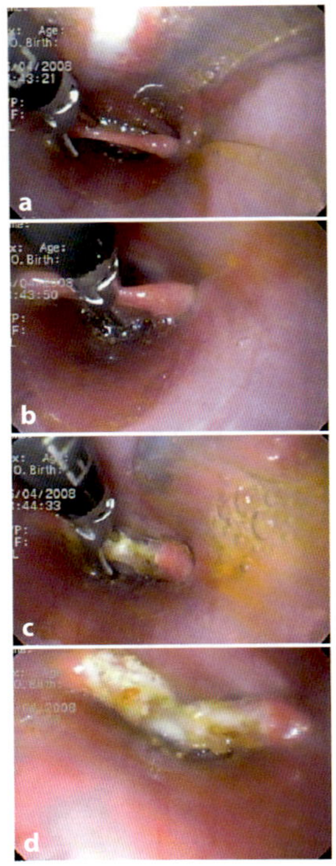

5

Fig. 4. Harmonic scissors and the generator of Ultracision® (Ethicon-Johnson).

Fig. 5. Endoscopic view sequence of the procedure: (**a**) harmonic scissors are placed over the septum; (**b**) initiating cut using harmonic scissors; (**c**) diverticulum bridge is cut, and (**d**) final results.

resumption of oral intake, with the possibility of repeat intervention if ZD recurs. Given the incidence of ZD, the opportunity to train and gain adequate experience for endoscopic treatment of ZD is difficult. The swine model offers an excellent alternative for training and development of new techniques and accessories [15]. In our own experimental laboratory, the harmonic scissors through a flexible overtube facilitated the procedure and reduced the risk of bleeding with an excellent visualization of the bottom of the diverticulum (fig. 5). An articulated stapler has also been evaluated in feasibility studies [16]. Animal models are being further utilized to develop new and novel ZD treatment techniques and accessories, such as the flexible stapler and a flexible harmonic scalpel.

References

1 Veenker EA, Andersen PE, Cohen JI: Cricopharyngeal spasm and Zenker's diverticulum. Head Neck 2003;25:681–693.

2 Cook IJ, Kahrilas PJ: AGA Technical review on the management of oropharyngeal dysphagia. Gastroenterology 1999;116:455–478.

3 Ishioka S, Sakai P, Maluf-Filho F, et al: Endoscopic incision of Zenker's diverticulum: a new approach. Endoscopy 1995;27:433–437.

4 Mulder CJ, den Hartog G, Robijn RJ, et al: Flexible endoscopic treatment of Zenker's diverticulum: a new approach. Endoscopy 1995;27:438–442.

5 Hashiba K, de Paula AL, da Silva JGN, et al: Endoscopic treatment of Zenker's diverticulum. Gastrointest Endosc 1999;49:93–96.

6 Waye JD, Sakai P, Belsaguy AF, et al: Treatment of Zenker's diverticulum. Gastrointest Endosc 2001;54:135–137.

7 Sakai P, Ishioka S, Maluf F, et al: Endoscopic treatment of Zenker's diverticulum with an oblique-end hood attached to the endoscope. Gastrointest Endosc 2001;54:760–763.
8 Evrard S, Le Moine O, Hassid S, et al: Zenker's diverticulum: a new endoscopic treatment with a soft diverticuloscope. Gastrointest Endosc 2003;58: 116–120.
9 Dohlman G, Mattson O: The endoscopic operation for hypopharyngeal diverticula: a roentgen-cinematographic study. Arch Otolaryngol 1960;71:744–752.
10 Van Overbeek JJM, Hoeksema PE, Edens ET: Microendoscopic surgery of the hypopharyngeal diverticulum using electrocoagulation or carbon dioxide laser. Ann Otol Rhinol Laryngol 1984;93:34–36.
11 Collard JM, Otte JB, Kestens PJ: Endoscopic stapling technique of esophagodiverticulostomy for Zenker's diverticulum. Ann Thorac Surg 1993;56: 573–576.
12 Hondo FY, Maluf-Filho F, Giordano-Nappi JH, et al: Endoscopic diverticulotomy by harmonic scalpel (ultracision): an experimental model. Endoscopy 2009; 41(suppl 2):E104–E105.
13 Mulder CJ, Costamagna G, Sakai P: Zenker's diverticulum: treatment using a flexible endoscope. Endoscopy 2001;33:991–997.
14 Ferreira LE, Simmons DT, Baron TH: Zenker's diverticula: pathophysiology, clinical presentation, and flexible endoscopic management. Dis Esophagus 2008;21:1–8.
15 Seaman DL, de la Mora Levy J, Gostout CJ, et al: An animal training model for endoscopic treatment of Zenker's diverticulum. Gastrointest Endosc 2007; 65:1050–1053.
16 Hondo FY, Giordano-Nappi JH; Maluf-Filho F, et al: Experimental model for endoscopic stapled diverticulotomy. Gastrointest Endosc 2008;67:AB-189.
17 Christiaens P, De Roock W, Van Olmen A, Moons V, D'Haens G: Treatment of Zenker's diverticulum through a flexible endoscope with a transparent oblique-end hood attached to the tip and a monopolar forceps. Endoscopy 2007;39:137–140.
18 Vogelsang A, Preiss C, Neuhaus H, Schumacher B: Endotherapy of Zenker's diverticulum using the needle-knife technique: long-term follow-up. Endoscopy 2007; 39:131–136.
19 Rabenstein T, May A, Michel J, Manner H, Pech O, Gossner L, Ell C: Argon plasma coagulation for flexible endoscopic Zenker's diverticulotomy. Endoscopy 2007; 39:141–145.
20 Rösch T: Summary of the four articles on Zenker's diverticulum endotherapy. Endoscopy 2007;39:153.
21 Feussner H: Endoscopic therapy for Zenker diverticulum – the good and the bad. Endoscopy 2007; 39:154–155.
22 Costamagna G, Iacopini F, Tringali A, Marchese M, Spada C, Familiari P, Mutignani M, Bella A: Flexible endoscopic Zenker's diverticulotomy: cap-assisted technique vs. diverticuloscope-assisted technique. Endoscopy 2007;39:146–152.
23 Aggerholm K, Illum P: Surgical treatment of Zenker's diverticulum. J Laryngol Otol 1990;104:312–314.

Fabio Y. Hondo, MD
Gastrointestinal Endoscopy Unit
Clinics Hospital of Medical School of University of São Paulo
São Paulo (Brazil)
Tel. +55 11 8249 8672, Fax +55 11 3069 7579, E-Mail fyhondo@uol.com.br

Mönkemüller K, Wilcox CM, Muñoz-Navas M (eds): Interventional and Therapeutic Gastrointestinal Endoscopy.
Front Gastrointest Res. Basel, Karger, 2010, vol 27, pp 122–127

Endoscopic Ablation of Barrett's Esophagus Using Argon Plasma Coagulation

Júlio C. Pereira-Lima · César Vivian Lopes

Department of Gastroenterology and Endoscopy Unit of the Santa Casa University Hospital/University of Health Sciences of Porto Alegre, UFCSPA, Medical School, Porto Alegre, Brazil

Abstract

Barrett's esophagus (BE) is a complication of gastroesophageal reflux disease (GERD), and GERD symptoms, as well as fear of cancer, are the most disturbing concerns for BE patients. The vast majority of BE patients should be treated as ordinary GERD patients, except for periodical surveillance endoscopies. Ablation trials should not even be contemplated in BE patients without dysplasia. BE with low-grade dysplasia follows the same rules as for BE without dysplasia, but with more frequent surveillance esophagogastroduodenoscopies. These patients could be included in ablation trials. In BE with visible areas of high-grade intraepithelial neoplasia or intramucosal cancer, resection and adjuvant thermal ablation seems to be the most reasonable therapy. In BE with high-grade intraepithelial neoplasia without visible lesions, thermal ablation alone appears to demonstrate the best results.

Barrett's esophagus (BE) is a premalignant complication of gastroesophageal reflux disease (GERD) and possesses a potential for neoplastic transformation ranging from 2 to 40%, according to several risk factors such as extension of the metaplastic tissue, grade of dysplasia, duration of disease and mutation-induced gene alterations [1, 2]. Esophageal adenocarcinoma arising in BE has one of the most rapidly increasing incidence rates of any malignancy over the last 30 years [2]. Since antireflux surgery and longstanding acid-reducing therapies by pharmacological means did not show a consistent fashion either to reduce the metaplastic epithelium extent or to halt the evolution to cancer in this population [3, 4], a myriad of endoscopic ablation techniques have been developed, although the vast majority of BE patients will never develop adenocarcinoma or die of this cancer [5].

BE patients with high-grade dysplasia (HGD) (high-grade intraepithelial neoplasia (HGIN)) or intramucosal adenocarcinoma are those with indications for endoscopic treatment in clinical practice. In the past, esophagectomy was the standard therapy for such patients. However, surgery carries high mortality and morbidity rates (about 5 and 30–40%, respectively), even when performed in referral centers [6]. Thus, as it occurs in the colon and stomach, surgery is no longer the treatment of choice for esophageal HGIN. Endoscopic methods that have been developed in the last decade include thermal ablation techniques: argon plasma coagulation (APC), photodynamic therapy (PDT), laser, multipolar electrocoagulation, heater probe, cryotherapy and radiofrequency ablation (RFA) [2, 7], and total or partial endoscopic resection or a combination of these methods [8, 9].

Technique of Endoscopic Ablation with APC

Each patient received supplementary medical therapy with high-dose proton pump inhibitors (60 mg omeprazole, 80 mg esomeprazole, 120 mg pantoprazole), commencing 2 days before the first APC session. This high-dose regimen is indicated until BE is considered ablated; thereafter, antireflux surgery or prolonged medical therapy is recommended according to the patient's life expectancy and wish.

APC is carried out using an argon beamer device (APC300; Erbe Medizintechnik, Tübingen, Germany) and 3.2-mm catheters with a monopolar electrode contained in a ceramic nozzle located close to the catheter distal tip. We do not employ catheters with a lateral opening. The use of a double-channel endoscope is preferable, although not obligatory, since during the procedure a large amount of gas in the upper gastrointestinal tract is insufflated, and with one-channel endoscopes, the APC probe has to be withdrawn many times in order to aspirate the argon gas. In our protocol, Barrett's mucosa is cauterized hemicircumferentially, beginning at its proximal end and continuing distally up to the cranial borders of the hiatal hernia folds or up to a maximum of 4 cm per session. Side effects (pain, fever, pleural effusion, stricture) are related to the extent of the cauterized area [10] (fig. 1, 2).

The operative distance between the probe tip and the tissue should be about 2–3 mm – the probe should not touch the tissue, otherwise high-pressure gas will be insufflated into the submucosa and/or deeper layers. Each application should be in a paintbrush manner in confluent areas and the probe should be maintained in the same area for about 8–10 s, or until the area is fully coagulated, and then advanced. Usually, 3–5 passes are necessary in each area to deeply coagulate Barrett's mucosa. Barrett's mucosa has a depth of about 1.5 mm [11] and APC can reach depths of 3 mm, according to power setting (at least 65 W – we use 69 W), gas flow (we employ 2 l/min) and contact time [12] The worst mistake is to pinpoint Barrett's mucosa. With this technique, BE will be ablated until the submucosa, no Barrett's glands will be left underneath the necrotic tissue and the adjacent squamous epithelium will repopulate the area [10, 13].

At the present time, we perform local endoscopic mucosal resection (EMR) for intramucosal cancer, dysplasia-associated lesions or masses (DALM) with the lift-and-cut technique and APC ablation of the rest of Barrett's epithelium (fig. 3–5).

Accessories

APC ablation is performed with a high-frequency monopolar electrosurgical generator source of argon gas, gas flow meter, APC delivery catheters, grounding pad and footswitch. Probes that deliver the energy either perpendicular or at the extremity of the catheter are available. EMR could be performed using band ligator – without submucosal saline injection – or with the lift-and-cut technique with submucosal saline injection (injection needle, grasping forceps or alligator forceps and a large snare).

Outcomes

Once BE is established (fig. 6), the possibility of malignant transformation does not depend on the elimination of acid reflux [1], thus the only mean of eliminating this higher risk of malignization

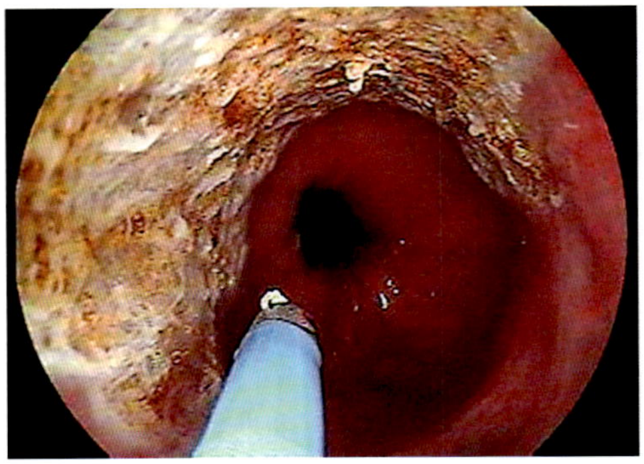

1

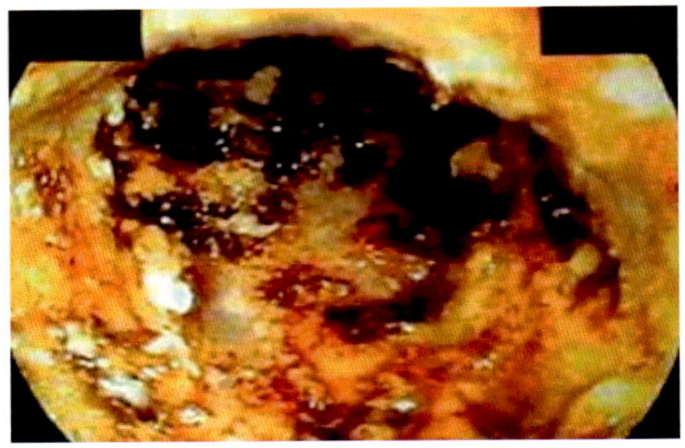

2

Fig. 1. Hemicircumferential cauterization of a BE with APC. **Fig. 2.** Circumferential ablation of a HGD BE with APC. Side effects are associated with the extent of the ablated area.

would be resection (endoscopic or surgical) or by endoscopic thermal ablation. Endoscopic ablation is based on the hypothesis that Barrett's epithelium is a healing process induced by multipotential stem cells from the basal layer of the squamous epithelium in response to acid injury [14]. Once the mucosa is destroyed by endoscopic techniques and reflux is effectively controlled, stem cells from the contiguous normal squamous epithelium repopulate this area and the distal esophagus turns again to become a squamous mucosa [13].

Endoscopic ablation is reported to reduce the incidence of Barrett's cancer in a study using weighted-average rates derived from pooled data taken from various studies [7]. The cancer incidence would be reduced from 5.98/1,000 patients-years to 1.63/1,000 in non-dysplastic BE; from 16.98/1,000 to 1.58/1,000 patient-years in low-grade dysplasia BE and from 65.8 to 16.76/1,000 patient-years in HGD patients.

The greatest concerns with ablation therapy for BE are the lack of histologic specimens, and the risk of 'development' of Barrett's tissue underneath the new squamous epithelium. This 'new' BE tissue, with or without dysplasia, does not develop beneath the new squamous mucosa during repopulation of the distal esophagus after ablation. These Barrett's glands remained undestroyed during the thermal ablation due to an inadequate technique. This flaw is reported to occur with all thermal ablative modalities [15]. In the case of APC, it is reported in up to 40% of the cases [15]. Since the depth of tissue destruction depends on the gas flow rate, power setting, duration of application and the distance from the mucosa, inappropriate power setting or contact time would produce a shallow depth of tissue injury, and hence insufficient ablation of all Barrett's epithelium. Inappropriate power settings to reach the submucosa are reported in many studies [16–18] and even low doses of omeprazole, such as 10 mg, have been used by some groups [17, 18].

A high-power setting with a long contact time successfully ablates BE without intramucosal cancer [10, 19, 20]. After a follow-up of 5 years in 79 patients, there were no cases of buried glands in more than 5,000 biopsy specimens. There were 5 cases of BE recurrence. These patients developed BE after ablation had been confirmed, since they presented with normal squamous mucosa 6 months after ablation, erosive esophagitis in another follow-up endoscopy and finally a de novo BE. This was due to 4 surgical failures in controlling reflux and 1 case of medication non-compliance [20].

The most severe side effect of mucosal ablation with APC is not stenosis, fever, or chest pain that occurs in up to 20% of the patients, but the development of adenocarcinoma underneath the new squamous epithelium after inadequately performed ablation as reported by some authors

Fig. 3. Patient with long segment BE and DALM. Note the ablation of the metaplastic epithelium close to the DALM (arrow), which was submitted to EMR in the same procedure.

Fig. 4. An intramucosal adenocarcinoma in a patient with a long segment BE with previous anti-reflux surgery.

Fig. 5. Same case as in figure 4. The muscularis propria is visible after EMR. This patient underwent APC ablation in a following procedure.

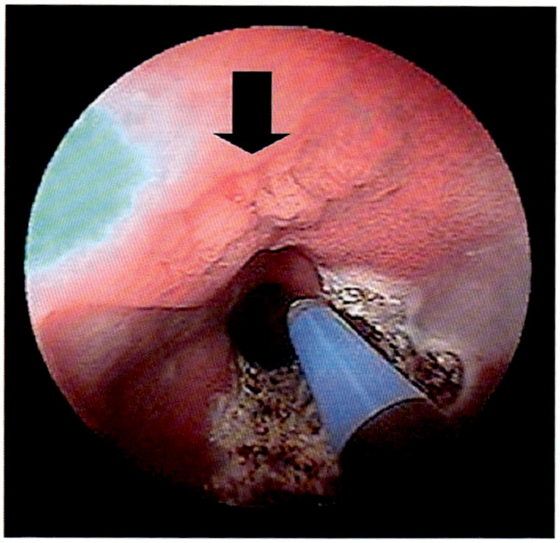

3

4

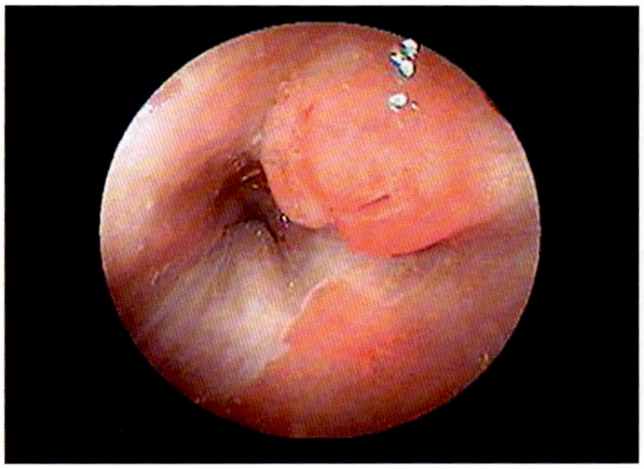

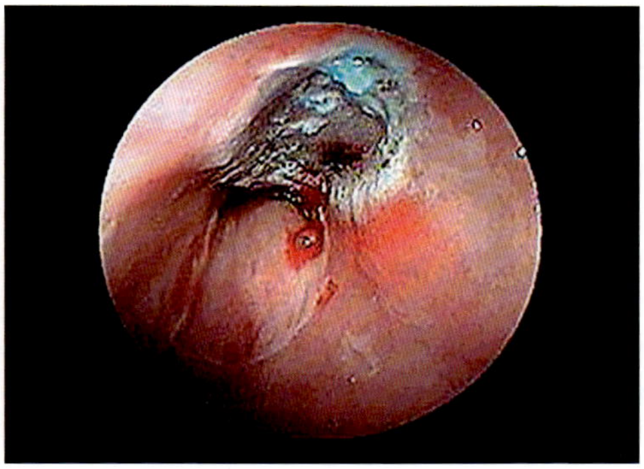

5

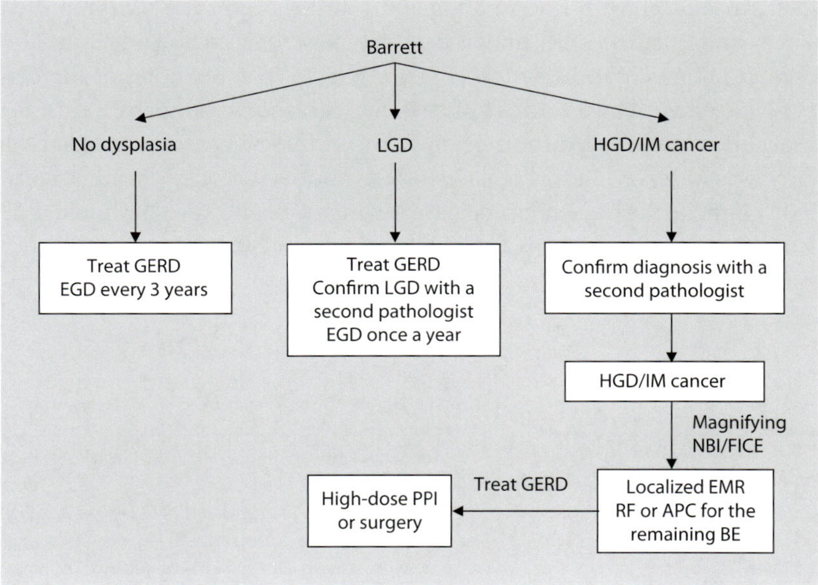

Fig. 6. Algorithm for Barrett's esophagus.

[21, 22]. Direct contact techniques (heat probe, multipolar electrocoagulation) have the drawback of not being particularly suitable for large areas of mucosa and also have difficulty in regulating the depth of tissue damage [15]. PDT is reported to have plenty of major side effects, such as strictures (one-third of patients) and photosensitivity for up to 3 months, and HGD ablation occurs in 78–95%, with a 15% cancer occurrence being reported over a 5-year follow-up period [15, 23]. In one study, PDT was as effective as APC, but the latter is cheaper and safer [24].

RFA is the newest of endoscopic ablative techniques and offers as its greatest advantage (in opposite to APC) uniformity of results in all the targeted mucosa at a given power setting. At the present time, RFA is the thermal technique that should be propagated throughout the world (especially in non-referral centers), despite its costs. RFA enables similar results by all operators in contrast to APC and EMR. In fact, RFA could be compared to the results of fast-food chains sandwiches – they are all the same thing around the globe and APC is like French cooking. RFA alone or combined with EMR for focal lesions achieved excellent results, with 98% of BE eradication (with HGD or intramucosal cancer) [8, 25].

EMR offers significant advantages over thermal ablation in the treatment of BE. EMR supplies histological specimens which provide accurate pathologic analysis in terms of disease differentiation and invasion. Localized resection of HGIN/intramucosal carcinoma in BE leaving the rest of Barrett's mucosa untouched counts with a rate of metachronous lesions of 21.5–31% in a German series, according to the length of BE and follow-up [26]. It seems logical that a BE that contains chromosomal abnormalities (that had already produced a cancer) cannot be left untreated, otherwise new cancers will develop in this metaplastic segment. In total, Barrett's EMR, both the HGIN/intramucosal cancer and all underlying Barrett's segments are theoretically completely removed. This technique would resect all at-risk zones, addressing the pitfalls of missing synchronic lesions, as well as possible future metachronic tumors. However, total BE-EMR is performed in a piecemeal fashion and can leave ridges of Barrett's epithelium within the resected zones. In a large French series, Lopes et al. [27] reported a 12% recurrence rate at 32 months. Soehendra et al. [28] analyzed 10 patients who underwent total BE-EMR with a ligator device. These authors reported the development of stricture in 7 (70%) with 1 perforation and 1 death. Larghi et al. [29] reported 1 (4%) intramucosal cancer and 2 cases of BE underneath the new squamous epithelium at a 2-year follow-up. Endoscopic submucosal dissection (ESD) offers en bloc resection of the diseased area. Yoshinaga et al. [30] described 15 cases (14 of them with short-segment BE) of ESD due to Barrett's cancer. Specimen sizes ranged from 2.5 to 6 cm. Of these 15 cases, 4 invaded the submucosa. No recurrence was observed in the 11 cases of intramucosal cancer during a mean follow-up of 2.5 years. ESD might be the best endoscopic treatment for BE, however it should only be performed by endoscopists experienced in this field. Do they exist outside of Japan?

References

1 Sharma P, McQuaid K, Dent J, et al: A critical review of the diagnosis and management of Barrett's esophagus: the AGA Chicago Workshop. Gastroenterology 2004; 127:310–330.

2 Fennerty MB: Endoscopic ablation of Barrett's-related neoplasia: what is the evidence supporting its use? Gastrointest Endosc 2003;58:246–249.

3 Gurski RR, Peters JH, Hagen JA, et al: Barrett's esophagus can and does regress after antireflux surgery: a study of prevalence and predictive features. J Am Coll Surg 2003;196:706–713.

4 Corey KE, Schmitz SM, Shaheen NT: Does a surgical antireflux procedure decrease the incidence of esophageal adenocarcinoma in Barrett's esophagus? A meta-analysis. Am J Gastroenterol 2003;98:2390–2394.

5 Rastogi A, Puli S, El-Serag HB, et al: Incidence of esophageal adenocarcinoma in patients with Barrett's esophagus and high-grade dysplasia: a meta-analysis. Gastrointest Endosc 2008;67:394–398.

6 Hulscher JB, van Sandick JW, de Boer AG, et al: Extended transthoracic resection compared with limited transhiatal resection for adenocarcinoma of the esophagus. N Engl J Med 2002;347:1662–1669.

7 Wani S, Puli SR, Shaheen NJ, et al: Esophageal adenocarcinoma in Barrett's esophagus after endoscopic ablative therapy: a meta-analysis and systematic review. Am J Gastroenterol 2009;104:502–513.

8 Pouw RE, Gondrie JJ, Sondermeijer CM, et al: Eradication of Barrett's esophagus with early neoplasia by radiofrequency ablation, with or without endoscopic resection. J Gastrointest Surg 2008;12: 1627–1636.

9 Seewald S, Ang TL, Gotoda T, et al: Total endoscopic resection of Barrett esophagus. Endoscopy 2008;40:1016–1020.

10 Pereira-Lima JC, Busnello JV, Saul C, et al: High power setting argon plasma coagulation for the eradication of Barrett's esophagus. Am J Gastroenterol 2000;95:1661–1668.

11 Sampliner RE: Ablative therapies for the columnar-lined esophagus. Gastroenterol Clin North Am 1997; 26:685–694.

12 Johanns W, Luis W, Jansen J, et al: Argon plasma coagulation in gastroenterology: experimental and clinical experiences. Eur J Gastroenterol Hepatol 1997;9:581–587.

13 Lopes CV, Pereira-Lima J, Hartmann AA: p53 immunohistochemical expression in Barrett's esophagus before and after endoscopic ablation by argon plasma coagulation. Scand J Gastroenterol 2005;40:259–263.

14 Bright T, Watson D, Tam W, et al: Randomized trial of argon plasma coagulation versus endoscopic surveillance for Barrett's esophagus after antireflux surgery: late results. Ann Surg 2007;246:1016–1020.

15 Rodriguez SA, Adler DG, Chand B, et al: Mucosal ablation devices. Gastrointest Endosc 2008;68:1031–1042.

16 Martin WR, Jakobs R, Spiethoff A, et al: Treatment of Barrett's esophagus with argon plasma coagulation with acid suppression – a prospective study. Z Gastroenterol 1999;37:779–784.

17 Byrne J, Armstrong G, Atwood S: Restoration of the normal squamous lining in Barrett's esophagus by argon beam plasma coagulation Am J Gastroenterol 1998;93: 1810–1815.

18 Van Laethem J, Cremer M, Peny MO, et al: Eradication of Barrett's mucosa with argon plasma coagulation and acid suppression: immediate and mid term results. Gut 1998;43:747–751.

19 Schulz H, Miehlke S, Antos D, et al: Ablation of Barrett's epithelium by endoscopic argon plasma coagulation in combination with high-dose omeprazole. Gastrointest Endosc 2000;51:659–663.

20 Pereira-Lima JC, Hornos AP, Lopes CV, et al: Tratamento Endoscópico do Esôfago de Barrett por Ablação (Plasma de Argônio); in Parada AA et al (eds): Esôfago de Barrett, ed 1. Ribeirão Preto, Tecmedd Editora, 2006, pp 202–211.

21 Maas S, Martin WR, Spiethoff A, et al: Barrett's esophagus with severe dysplasia in argon beam therapy. Z Gastroenterol 1998;36:301–306.

22 Van Laethem JL, Jagodzinski R, Peny MO, et al: Argon plasma coagulation in the treatment of Barrett's high-grade dysplasia and in situ adenocarcinoma. Endoscopy 2001;33:257–261.

23 Overholt B, Wang K, Burdick S, et al: Five-year efficacy and safety of photodynamic therapy with Photofrin in Barrett's high-grade dysplasia. Gastrointest Endosc 2007;66:460–468.

24 Kelty CJ, Ackroyd R, Brown NJ, et al: Endoscopic ablation of Barrett's esophagus: a randomized-controlled trial of photodynamic therapy vs. argon plasma coagulation. Aliment Pharmacol Ther 2004; 20:1289–1296.

25 Ganz RA, Overholt BF, Sharma VK, et al: Circumferential ablation of Barrett's esophagus that contains high-grade dysplasia: a US multicenter registry. Gastrointest Endosc 2008;68:35–40.

26 Pech O, Behrens A, May A, et al: Long-term results and risk factor analysis for recurrence after curative endoscopic therapy in 349 patients with high-grade intraepithelial neoplasia and mucosal adenocarcinoma in Barrett's esophagus. Gut 2008;57:1200–1206.

27 Lopes CV, Hela M, Pesenti C, et al: Circumferential endoscopic resection of Barrett's esophagus with high-grade dysplasia or early adenocarcinoma. Surg Endosc 2007;21:820–824.

28 Soehendra N, Seewald S, Grath S, et al: Use of modified multiband ligator facilitates circumferential endoscopic mucosal resection in Barrett's esophagus. Gastrointest Endosc 2006;63:847–852.

29 Larghi A, Lightgale CJ, Ross AS, et al: Long-term follow-up of complete Barrett's eradication endoscopic mucosal resection for the treatment of high-grade dysplasia and intramucosal carcinoma. Endoscopy 2007;39:1086–1091.

30 Yoshinaga S, Gotoda T, Kusano C, et al: Clinical impact of endoscopic submucosal dissection for superficial adenocarcinoma located at the esophagogastric junction. Gastrointest Endosc 2008;67: 202–209.

Júlio C. Pereira-Lima
Rua Com. Rheingantz 910/801
90450-020 Porto Alegre (Brazil)
Tel. +55 51 30225794, Fax +55 51 30225791, E-Mail jpereiralima@terra.com.br

Mönkemüller K, Wilcox CM, Muñoz-Navas M (eds): Interventional and Therapeutic Gastrointestinal Endoscopy.
Front Gastrointest Res. Basel, Karger, 2010, vol 27, pp 128–139

Photodynamic Therapy for Barrett's Esophagus

Masoud Panjehpour · Bergein F. Overholt

Center of Excellence for Treatment of Barrett's Esophagus, Thompson Cancer Survival Center, Knoxville, Tenn., USA

Abstract

Barrett's esophagus is a premalignant condition associated with gastroesophageal reflux disease where the normal squamous lining is replaced by specialized columnar mucosa. For many years, esophagectomy was the standard treatment for Barrett's patients with high-grade dysplasia or early cancer. Photodynamic therapy (PDT) offers an alternative outpatient endoscopic procedure that eliminates dysplasia and superficial cancer while reducing the risks of complications compared to esophagectomy. Guidelines for the application of PDT in the management of Barrett's esophagus with high grade dysplasia are provided. Detailed discussion is provided on patient selection, treatment delivery techniques, follow-up endoscopy strategies for efficacy evaluation, potential side effects and complications, and management of post-PDT strictures. A brief discussion of clinical outcomes in single-center and multicenter studies is presented.

Barrett's esophagus (BE) is a precancerous condition associated with gastroesophageal reflux disease where the normal squamous lining is replaced by specialized columnar mucosa. BE is associated with an increased risk of mucosal dysplasia and cancer with a 30- to 120-fold increase in the occurrence of adenocarcinoma compared to the normal population [1–3].

For many years, esophagectomy was the standard treatment for Barrett's patients with high-grade dysplasia (HGD) or early cancer. Esophagectomy is associated with a 40–50% risk of major complications and a mortality rate of 3–5% at high-volume centers and up to 20% at low-volume hospitals [4–10]. Photodynamic therapy (PDT) offers an alternative outpatient endoscopic procedure that eliminates dysplasia and superficial cancer and reduces the length of Barrett's mucosa while reducing risks compared to esophagectomy [11–16]. PDT utilizes the photochemical reaction between a photosensitizing drug, light and tissue oxygen. Interaction of the three components results is production of singlet oxygen and free radicals that are highly cytotoxic, resulting in the ablation of illuminated tissue. Porfimer sodium is a photosensitizer that has been used effectively for PDT of HGD and early cancer in BE when delivered concurrently with effective acid-suppression therapy [15–17].

This chapter will provide the technique and guidelines for the application of PDT for management of BE with HGD. Special emphasis will be made by providing information on the technique that has been approved by the FDA [15]. Throughout the chapter, we will provide comparisons between the FDA-approved technique and the relevant data published during phases of the development to clarify any confusion.

Techniques

Patient Selection

All patients must have an endoscopy with 4 quadrant large-particle biopsies every 1–2 cm. Biopsy results should be confirmed by an expert GI pathologist trained in Barrett's diagnosis. Patients with nodular disease should have endoscopic ultrasound (EUS) for evaluation of esophageal wall layers (either intact or thickened) as well as examination of adjacent lymph nodes. Patients with abnormal appearing nodes or nodes larger than 1 cm should undergo fine needle aspiration. Patients with T1 mucosal lesions should have an endoscopic mucosal resection (EMR) [18] followed in 4–8 weeks with PDT to treat the remaining Barrett's mucosa. Pathological evaluation of lesions removed during EMR is a valuable tool for planning treatment strategy. Patients with lesions extending into the submucosa or deeper layers should be referred for surgical intervention. If patients are denied esophagectomy, they may be treated with PDT. Prior to availability of EMR, T1 mucosal lesions received an extra light dose using a small cylindrical diffuser before the entire area was treated using the balloon for 'field PDT'. If EMR is not performed, an extra light dose targeted to the nodular area is recommended [12, 15]. This will be discussed in more detail later.

Photodynamic Therapy

Before delivery of PDT, a thorough history and physical examination including laboratory work, chest X-ray and ECG should be performed. Patients with known porphyria or known hypersensitivity to porphyrins should not be treated.

Administration of Porfimer Sodium and Application of PDT

Patients may be treated as outpatient. All patients receive an intravenous (2 mg/kg) injection of porfimer sodium (Photofrin®, Axcan Pharma, Mont-Saint-Hilaire, Que., Canada). Two to three days after drug injection, 630 nm light from a KTP/dye laser (Laserscope, San Jose, Calif., USA), a diode laser (Diomed, Andover, Mass., USA) (fig. 1) or an argon-pumped dye-laser (Lumenis, (previously Coherent), Santa Clara, Calif., USA) is delivered using an Xcell PDT balloon (Wilson-Cook Medical, Winston Salem, N.C., USA). This is a 25-mm diameter esophageal PDT balloon that is provided with window lengths of 3, 5 and 7 cm. These balloons come with a matching cylindrical diffuser to be inserted into the balloon. The length of the cylindrical diffuser is always 2 cm longer than the window length (fig. 2). Therefore, 3-, 5- and 7-cm windowed balloons are used with 5-, 7- or 9-cm cylindrical diffusers, respectively. The balloon is positioned in the esophagus over a guide wire. The position of the balloon window should be monitored using an endoscope passed along side the shaft of the balloon (fig. 3). A yellow marker on the balloon shaft (located 3 cm proximal to the edge of the window) allows proper positioning of the window where treatment is to be delivered.

The Xcell PDT balloon has a reflective inner surface which was used in the multicenter study and subsequently approved by the FDA for treatment of HGD in BE [15]. The reflective balloon was developed to improve the uniformity of the light along the length of the window. A comprehensive discussion of different light-delivery devices has been published elsewhere [19].

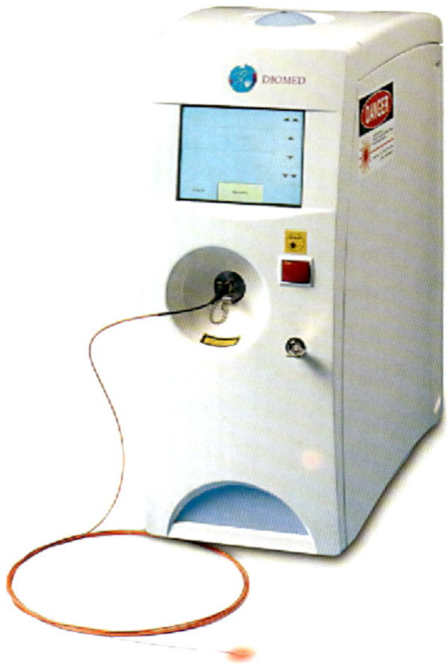

1

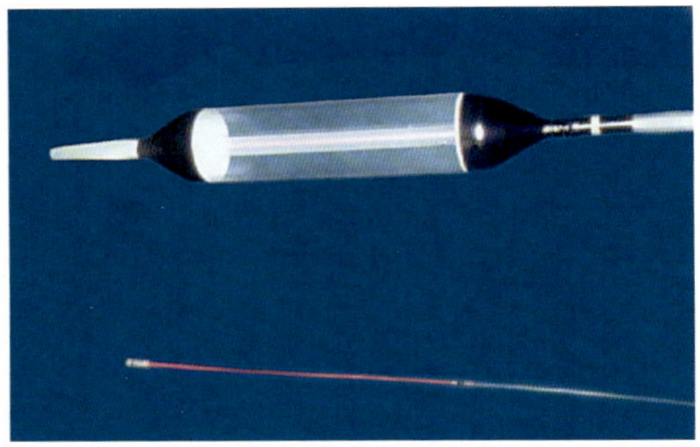

2

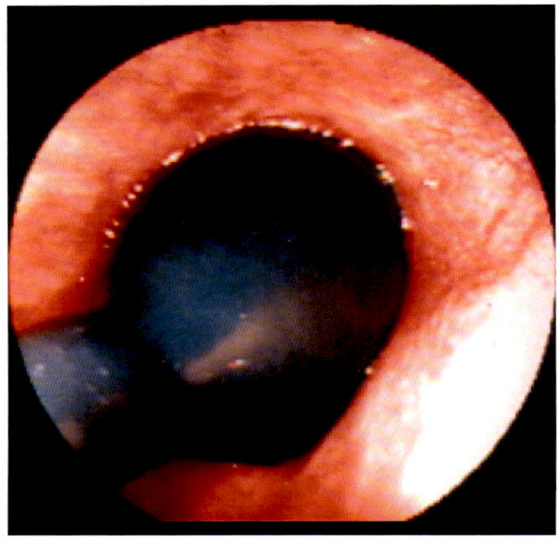

3

Fig. 1. Diomed PDT laser.

Fig. 2. Xcell PDT balloon (top) and cylindrical diffuser (bottom).

Fig. 3. Endoscopic monitoring of PDT balloon during treatment.

Handling of the Balloon for PDT

When choosing the length of balloon window, at least 0.5–1 cm of normal tissue should be included in the treatment field at both the proximal and distal margin of BE to assure proper targeting of the affected mucosa. This is important due to inadvertent movement of the balloon in the esophagus during treatment. The 5- and 7-cm balloons are most commonly used for treatment. Due to the length of a typical Barrett's segment and constant movement, a 3-cm windowed balloon is used infrequently. A maximum of 7 cm of Barrett's mucosa may be treated in one session.

The balloon inflation should start with a pressure of 80–100 mm Hg to fully inflate and flatten the esophageal folds, followed by reduction to 20 mm Hg immediately before initiation of laser treatment. While high balloon pressure is desired to keep the balloon fully inflated, it has the potential to press against the esophageal wall, affecting blood flow to the treatment area. The reduction in blood flow lowers the oxygen concentration in tissue, which in turn reduces the PDT injury [20]. In our earlier studies, we used higher balloon pressures which frequently resulted in areas of mild injury (called skipped areas). Gradual reduction of the inflation pressure in subsequent patients proved effective in eliminating the majority of skip areas [11].

Calculation of Energy Density

Patients should be treated using an energy density dose of 130 J/cm. If possible, the power density should be set at 270 mW/cm of cylindrical diffuser length. This would mean that a total power of 2,430 mW is required when using a 9-cm cylindrical diffuser in a 7-cm balloon (270 mW/

4 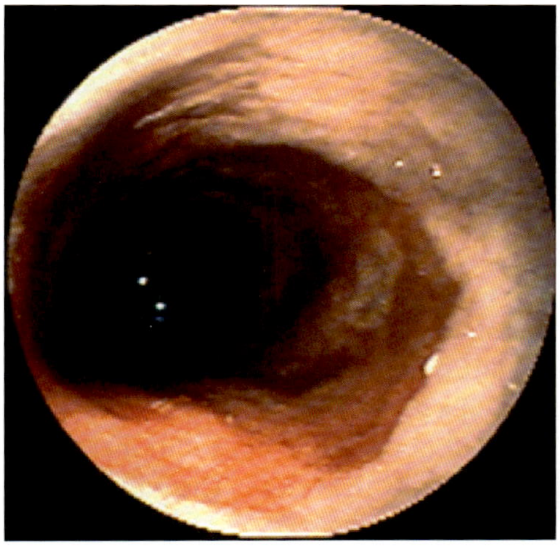 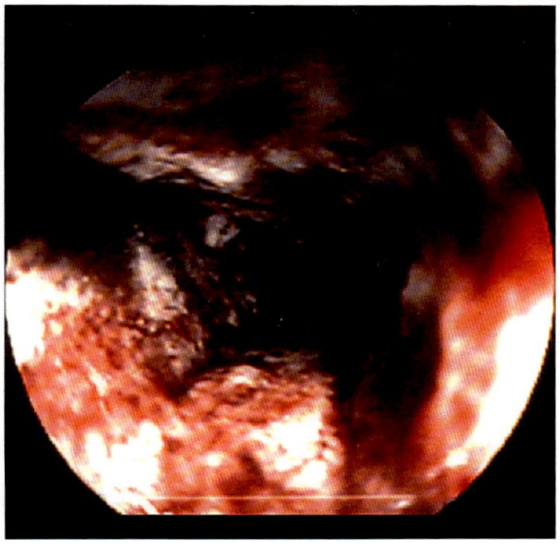 5

Fig. 4. Barrett's esophagus at the level of squamo-columnar junction before PDT. **Fig. 5.** Barrett's esophagus 48 h after PDT showing severe hemorrhagic necrosis.

cm × 9 cm). The illumination time is calculated by dividing the energy density (in J/cm) by the power density (in W/cm). For example, using the power density of 270 mW/cm, it requires 480 s to deliver a light dose of 130 J/cm (130 J/cm ÷ 0.27 W/cm). Some lasers (such as Diomed Laser) do not provide sufficient output power to deliver 2,430 mW from a 9-cm cylindrical diffuser. In such cases, the power density of 200 mW/cm may be used. Therefore, the total power from a 9-cm diffuser is reduced to 1,800 mW (200 mW/cm × 9 cm). Using a power density of 200 mW/cm, a 650-second illumination is required to deliver 130 J/cm. Power densities lower than 200 mW/cm require illumination times that become impractical. For example, using a power density of 150 mW/cm (or 0.15 W/cm), it requires 866 s to deliver 130 J/cm (130 J/cm ÷ 0.15 W/cm).

It should be noted that light dosimetry, associated with the non-reflective balloon [11, 12, 16] used in previous phases of protocol development, was different from that used with the Xcell reflective PDT balloon and should not be confused. The optimum energy density delivered using the non-reflective balloon was 200 J/cm. The power density was 400 mW/cm which required 500 s to deliver a treatment. The equivalency studies to compare non-reflective and reflective balloons were performed in canine esophagus by measuring the actual light dose delivered to the mucosa using isotropic probes attached to the outside of the balloon window (unpublished preclinical studies).

Prior to EMR or in patients not suitable for EMR, patients with a nodular area within the BE should be treated with an extra 50 J/cm targeted to the nodule using a short cylindrical diffuser before 'field' delivery of 130 J/cm using the Xcell PDT balloon. The power density from short cylindrical diffusers should be set at 400 mW/cm. For example, using a 2.5-cm diffuser, the total power will be 1,000 mW (2.5 cm × 400 mW/cm) from the diffuser. Delivery of 50 J/cm at the power density of 400 mW/cm, requires 125 s of illumination time (50 J/cm ÷ 0.4 W/cm). The dose of 50 J/cm was selected and tested during protocol development and proved to be a safe dose as a boost to the balloon treatment [12, 15].

Proper light dosimetry requires accurate measurement of laser power. When using the Diomed laser, an internal power meter is provided which must be used for calibration of the fiber and setting the power. An external integrating sphere power meter (with a large-diameter sphere) should be used when using Laserscope or Lumenis lasers. Currently, UDT Instruments (Model 371, Baltimore, Md., USA) manufactures a power meter that is specifically designed for PDT. One should be aware that the power meter provided with the Laserscope PDT system is not recommend for use with a cylindrical diffuser longer than 3 cm.

Post-PDT EGD

Two days after laser treatment, the mucosal injury should be evaluated endoscopically. Figures 4 and 5 show endoscopic views of Barrett's esophagus prior to and 48 hrs after PDT, respectively. A supplemental dose of 50 J/cm (or more at the discretion of physician) [12, 15] may be delivered to areas with mild response using a short cylindrical diffuser inserted through the biopsy channel of the scope. Also at the discretion of the physician, if a patient with Barrett's segment longer than 6–7 cm is doing well and is clinically stable at the 48-hour follow-up, additional treatment may be delivered to the untreated segment using the standard light dose. The additional treatment will likely produce more post-procedure discomfort. Treatment overlap should be avoided to reduce the risk of excessive treatment of the previously treated area, which may increase the risk of stricture development. Since the diffuser is used for most of the retreatments, the physician should recognize that the diffuser light extends distally from the tip of the diffuser and will create a treatment effect for an additional 0.5–1.0 cm from the end of the diffuser.

Special Precautions

After the treatment, most patients experience some chest pain, nausea and low-grade fever for 3–7 days. Following PDT, oral narcotics may be given to control chest discomfort in addition to antiemetics for nausea. Acetaminophen may be taken for low-grade fever as needed.

Prophylactic intravenous hydration over the first 12–24 h should be considered to prevent dehydration in some patients. Typically, patients remain on liquids and soft foods for several days after laser treatment. Patients may return to a normal diet as tolerated. Most patients return to a normal diet within 2–3 weeks.

An effective acid-suppression protocol is extremely important after endoscopic ablation of Barrett's mucosa [15, 21]. Patients should use high-dose proton pump inhibitor (PPI) therapy twice daily beginning several days before PDT and for at least 3 months after the treatment. On the day of laser treatment, gastric pH can be checked. If the pH is 4 or less, the dose of PPI should be doubled and pH checked during the 48-hour follow-up endoscopy to assess the effectiveness of PPI therapy. We recommend that patients remain on high-dose PPI therapy for at least 1 year after they have been fully cleared of Barrett's mucosa. Thereafter, patients may reduce their dose to once daily. If their symptoms are controlled, they may continue with daily PPI medication. We recommend long-term PPI treatment for all patients. If a patient is an operative candidate, surgical (laparoscopic) repair of a hiatal hernia may be recommended.

Evaluation of Treatment Efficacy

All patients should undergo surveillance EGD 3 months after PDT to allow complete healing of the treated area. The 3-month follow-up consists of 2 endoscopy procedures. The first endoscopy should include visual examination of the treated area: Lugol's, Fujinon intelligent color enhancement or narrow-banding imaging chromoendoscopy to detect small islands of Barrett's mucosa, and 4 quadrant large-particle biopsies every 2 cm of the treated and untreated areas, if any. Large-particle biopsies are preferable to detect any subsquamous Barrett's. A second endoscopy with thermal ablation may be performed in patients who have residual Barrett's mucosa. Endoscopy with biopsies (and possible ablation) should be repeated at 6-month intervals for at least 2 years. When possible, patients should be followed for at least 5 years [16].

Supplemental Treatments during Follow-Up Endoscopies

On follow-up endoscopies, residual small islands of Barrett's mucosa may be found within the treated area. These islands should be biopsied carefully. Thermal ablation techniques such as Nd:YAG contact laser [11] and argon plasma coagulation [14] may be used to ablate the residual Barrett's mucosa. In our institution, we use a contact Nd:YAG laser which allows accurate targeted treatment of small islands of residual Barrett's mucosa within the treated field or untreated Barrett's mucosa (outside the treated field). If the residual segment does not contain HGD, then thermal ablation may be used to treat that area during subsequent visits. If HGD is present, additional PDT, mucosal resection or, in some cases, aggressive thermal ablation should be considered. We repeat PDT a maximum of three times.

When a second PDT is delivered, overlapping of the first and second fields should be avoided, if possible. This strategy would reduce the risk of stricture development seen with overlapping of the PDT fields [11].

Management of Esophageal Strictures after PDT

One of the complications after PDT for BE is formation of strictures which occur more frequently in long-segment Barrett's or in areas of treatment overlap. Thus, patients should be contacted by phone weekly. Dysphagia may be diagnosed by persistent difficulty in swallowing solid foods over several days. Those with documented dysphagia should be assessed by endoscopy for the presence of a stricture. In some patients, dysphagia may be due to transient esophageal spasms. While others have reported [22] abnormal esophageal motility following PDT, we consider persistent solid food dysphagia a symptom highly suggestive of stricture formation. The length of strictures are typically short, ranging from 1–2 cm. Esophageal strictures typically occur 3–4 weeks after PDT. If a stricture is present, dilations should be performed twice a week, starting with Savary 33 or 36 until Savary 48–51 is reached, then weekly for several weeks with Savary 51 or 54, then monthly for several months. Methylprednisolone acetate (Depo-medrol, Pharmacia & Upjohn Company) may be injected (20 mg in 4 sites) into the inflamed stricture weekly during each of the first 3 weeks [23].

Clinical Outcomes

Efficacy Results of Multicenter Randomized Study

PDT for BE with HGD received regulatory approval in the US based on the results of a multicenter randomized trial [15] using the techniques described here. This was a report on a minimum 2-year follow-up of a 2:1 randomized controlled trial of Ps-PDT plus omeprazole (treatment arm) versus omeprazole only (control arm) in the treatment of Barrett's HGD. The study enrolled 208 patients with 138 in the PDT treatment arm and 70 in the control arm. At the end of a minimum 24-month follow-up, PDT plus omeprazole showed statistically significant improvement in elimination of HGD and in the reduction of the incidence of adenocarcinoma compared to the control arm. Ablation of all HGD was noted in 77% of patients in the PDT arm versus 39% in the control arm. Complete ablation of all Barrett's epithelium and dysplasia was achieved in 52% of patients in the PDT group vs. 7% in the control arm. A reduction in the progression to cancer from 28% in the control arm to 13% in the PDT arm was found. It is noted that during the follow-up biopsies, any pathologic interpretation that raised any suggestion of cancer, e.g. 'cannot rule out adenocarcinoma', was classified as progression to cancer in these patients. It should also be noted that no adjuvant therapy such as Nd:YAG laser or argon plasma coagulation was used to treat residual Barrett's mucosa upon follow-up endoscopy during the study. The landmark 5-year follow-up study confirmed the 2-year results [24]. This study demonstrated the long-term durability of the treatment results found at the 2-year follow-up. At 5 years, PDT was still significantly more effective than PPI alone in eliminating HGD (77 vs. 39%). Similarly, the reduction in progression to cancer remained similar to that reported at the 2-year follow-up. There was a 15% likelihood of cancer occurring in the PDT arm versus 29% in those receiving PPI alone. There was also a significantly longer time in progression to cancer in the PDT group.

It is noted that at the time of this writing, PDT is the only ablation treatment for Barrett's HGD that has been evaluated in a 5-year randomized controlled multicenter trial.

Squamous overgrowth in Barrett's patients receiving PDT under the multicenter randomized study was evaluated in 33,658 biopsy samples at the 5-year follow-up [25]. This study demonstrated no significant difference in squamous overgrowth comparing patients receiving PDT/PPI versus those received PPI alone. In no patient was the worst follow-up pathology located in subsquamous Barrett's.

Efficacy Results in Single-Center Studies

While results of the multicenter randomized study best represent the expected outcome from the technique described here, one should be familiar with the relevant publications on porfimer sodium PDT for BE [11–14].

Overholt et al. [11] reported on the treatment of 100 patients with Barrett's dysplasia including 13 with superficial cancers using porfimer sodium PDT. They used either a non-reflective balloon or cylindrical diffusers alone to deliver a light dose of 100–250 J/cm. All patients were on long-term PPI therapy. The Nd:YAG laser was used to ablate small residual areas of Barrett's mucosa. Patients were followed for 4–84 (mean 19) months. Conversion of approximately 75–80% of treated Barrett's mucosa to normal squamous epithelium was found in all patients with complete elimination in 43 patients. Dysplasia was eliminated in 78 patients. Ten of the 13 malignancies were ablated. Of clinical importance, in their initial work PDT was directed only to the dysplastic segment of Barrett's mucosa. Dysplasia developed during follow-up in 11 of 48 patients in *untreated* Barrett's mucosa requiring additional therapy, indicating the need for complete ablation of Barrett's mucosa in such patients.

Panjehpour et al. [12] used a 5- or 7-cm non-reflective PDT balloon and Nd:YAG thermal ablation in 60 patients with BE with low-grade dysplasia, HGD and early cancer. Patients were followed for 3–18 (mean 9.8) months. While the protocol was designed to deliver 175 J/cm for low-grade dysplasia and 200 J/cm for HGD, the majority of patients received 200 J/cm due to a history of high grade or the presence of nodular disease. Nodular areas received an extra light dose of 50–75 J/cm using a short diffuser prior to balloon treatment. Balloon pressure was maintained between 20 and 30 mm Hg during laser delivery. They reported ablation of cancer in all patients, and elimination of HGD in 96% of patients. Cancer and dysplasia were eliminated in 77% of patients. Barrett's mucosa was totally eliminated in 42% of patients. The overall length of Barrett's segment was reduced by 5.22 cm. Wang [13] used a hematoporphyrin derivative as the photosensitizer and short cylindrical diffusers passed through the biopsy channel of the endoscope. Using a light dose of 200 J/cm, they treated 26 patients and achieved elimination of HGD in 88%. Elimination of Barrett's mucosa was seen in 35% of patients. Wolfsen et al. [14] reported results of porfimer sodium PDT in 102 patients with HGD and mucosal adenocarcinoma. The median follow-up was 1.6 years. They used 2.5- to 5.0-cm cylindrical diffusers passed through the endoscope and delivered a light dose of 150–225 J/cm. Using a single dose of PDT, complete ablation of Barrett's epithelium was obtained in 56% of patients. They used an argon plasma coagulator to ablate the residual Barrett's mucosa in the remaining patients. Four patients (4%) had incomplete ablation of Barrett's mucosa. In 3 patients, subsquamous HGD and carcinoma were detected. Esophagectomy was used to successfully resect the intramucosal cancer without any evidence of submucosal or lymph involvements. The 4th patient had previously undergone EMR documenting intramucosal carcinoma with an extensive thermal effect limiting evaluation of deeper tissue layers. CT and EUS demonstrated abnormal lymphadenopathy. Despite radiation and chemotherapy, the patient developed metastatic adenocarcinoma.

Long-term results of single-center studies for BE have also been reported. Overholt et al. [16] reported on 103 patients in a phase I/II study evaluating porfimer-PDT in the treatment of Barrett's dysplasia or early cancer using cylindrical diffusers or non-reflective balloon. 82 patients completed a mean follow-up of 58.5 (range 41–132) months. Following PDT, the length of Barrett's mucosa decreased by a mean 6.92 (range 1–22) cm. 56 of 82 patients (68%) had elimination of Barrett's mucosa. Of the 65 patients with HGD followed for the entire 5-year follow-up, 60 (94%) had elimination of HGD.

Three (4.6%) patients developed subsquamous adenocarcinoma. The first case was diagnosed 6 months after PDT. The authors believe the cancer was preexisting and that the initial PDT did not clear the lesion. The patient was non-operative and was therefore treated with PDT a second time. The lesion was cleared and the patient remained free of disease when last seen 3 years after the second PDT session. In 2 patients, subsquamous cancer was found 5 years after PDT. Both patients had initially been cleared of all Barrett's as determined by biopsies on their previous 2 annual examinations. Interestingly, both cancers were 1–3 mm in size, were endoscopically visualized as small submucosal nodules and both occurred within 1–2 cm of the neo-squamo-columnar junction. Both patients had reduced their PPI medications over the preceding 1–2 years. One was retreated with PDT and was clear 2 years after retreatment. The 3rd patient was treated with brachytherapy but died 6 months later. Based on the medical and surgical literature, an expected incidence of cancer in these 65 patients with HGD followed over a 5-year period after treatment would be expected to be between 16 and 32, indicating a significant reduction in the incidence of cancer in patients with HGD treated with PDT, thermal ablation and PPI therapy. Subsquamous, non-dysplastic metaplastic epithelium was found in 4 patients (4.9%). It should be noted that these patients were treated at different stages of protocol development which included optimization of different treatment parameters such as light dose and balloon pressure, two very important parameters.

Table 1. Side effects and complications of PDT

Side effects	Incidence, %
Chest pain	20
Nausea	11
Vomiting	32
Constipation	13
Dysphagia	19
Dehydration	12
Hiccups	10
Atrial fibrillation	1–3
Photosensitivity reaction	7–18
Esophageal perforation	<1[a]
Pleural effusion	2[b]
Esophageal strictures	36[c]

Data are based mainly on the results of a large multicenter study [15].
[a] Not reported in the multicenter study [15]. One esophageal perforation reported by Wolfosn et al. [14] possibly due to vomiting.
[b] Pleural effusions typically clear spontaneously over several weeks [11].
[c] 12% after 1 PDT, 32% after 2 treatments and 9% after a 3rd treatment.

Potential Side Effects/Complications

The side effects and complications reported in the multicenter study best represent the expected incidences using the PDT techniques described here [15] (table 1).

During the multicenter randomized study [15], patients reported chest pain (20%), nausea (11%), vomiting (32%), constipation (13%), dysphagia (19%), dehydration (12%), and hiccups (10%). While not reported in the multicenter study, we also typically see patients running a low-grade fever following PDT. Chest pain, nausea and vomiting and dysphagia were transient and were controlled with medications. Overall, 36% of patients developed strictures which were managed successfully with dilations. 12% of patients developed strictures after 1 PDT as opposed to 32% from 2 treatments and 9% after a 3rd treatment [15]. Others have reported different incidence rates for esophageal strictures in single-center studies. Overholt et al. [11] reported overall esophageal strictures in 34% of patients.

The incidence of strictures appears to be dependent on the delivery technique of PDT, such as type and length of balloons, as well as the number of PDT sessions applied. Overholt et al. [16] reported that use of longer centering balloons reduced the incidence of strictures possibly due to elimination of treatment overlaps when using sequential PDTs using short balloons. In another publication, Overholt et al. [16] reported strictures in 18% of patients who received 1 PDT and 50% of those who received 2 PDT treatments, 30% overall. Using a light dose of 200 J/cm, Panjehpour et al. [12] reported an overall 31% esophageal strictures using 7-cm and 7% strictures using 5-cm non-reflective balloons. Additionally, they reported no improvement in the rate of stricture formation when oral steroids were administered after PDT. Wang [13] reported strictures in 27% of patients treated with a hematoporphyrin derivative and cylindrical diffusers. Wolfsen et al. [14] reported strictures requiring dilations in 20% of patients. A median of 5 dilation procedures were needed to restore stable lumen patency.

Photosensitivity reaction is the main drawback of porfimer sodium PDT. In the multicenter study [15], sunburn-like reactions affected mostly the skin of the face, hands and neck. The majority of reactions were mild and resolved without any medical intervention. 7% of cases had severe reactions. Wolfsen et al. [14] reported skin phototoxicity in 18% of patients due to inadvertent exposure to sun light. Severe reactions may require treatment including steroids to reduce the symptoms. Patients receiving porfimer sodium must protect their skin and eyes from sun and bright lights for at least 30 and up to 90 days. The importance of proper patient education on photosensitivity cannot be overemphasized.

Other complications have been reported in publications prior to the multicenter trial. There is a small (1–3%) risk of atrial fibrillation after PDT. No atrial fibrillations were reported in the 138 patients treated during the multicenter study [15]. In a series of 100 patients treated during the initial phase of protocol development, 3 patients developed atrial fibrillation [11]. All cases responded to medical intervention. In a series of 102 patients, Wolfsen et al. [14] reported atrial fibrillation in 1 patient who received PDT treatment to a 15-cm length of BE. Cardiac evaluation did not reveal any significant underlying coronary artery disease. The patient responded to oral anticoagulant therapy and converted spontaneously to normal sinus rhythm. Another patient with significant coronary artery disease and a history of heart failure developed recurrent congestive heart failure after a 12-cm segment of BE had been treated. This patient required hospitalization and responded to medical intervention. In a series of 12 patients treated by Overholt et al. [26] evaluation of cardiac enzymes and ECG demonstrated no myocardial abnormalities. It should be noted that treatment parameters in the multicenter study [15] were optimized compared to those patients treated in the initial phases of the study using different light delivery devices, higher light doses, and long treatment segments [11, 14]. We believe atrial fibrillation is related to the depth and extent of esophageal injury and the associated inflammation resulting in some underlying cardiac conduction disturbance. Atrial fibrillation occurs only in cases treated at the level of the left atrium.

Although perforation of the esophagus is another potential complication, no perforation was reported in the multicenter randomized study using the balloon light delivery technique [15]. However, using the diffuser light delivery device, Wolfsen et al. [14] reported perforation in 1 patient who was treated for a 7-cm segment of BE. The patient developed severe chest pain within 2 days of PDT. While contrast esophageal radiography showed no sign of the perforation, CT demonstrated free air in the chest and abdomen indicating a transient perforation of gastroesophageal junction possibly due to vomiting. Patient was admitted for observation, bowel rest, and antibiotics. His symptoms completely resolved within a week without the need of surgery.

Small asymptomatic pleural effusions may develop in some patients. In a group of 14 patients who underwent chest X-ray 48 h after PDT, 6 had bilateral plural effusions, 4 had left pleural effusion, 1 had small right plural effusion, and 3 patients had normal chest X-ray [11]. Overall, pleural effusion was symptomatic in 2% of patients requiring thoracentesis [11]. Patients should be monitored closely for signs and symptoms of dyspnea indicating the possibility of pleural effusion, typically detected 2–4 days after PDT. Pleural effusions typically clear spontaneously over several weeks. Oxygen saturation in the high 80s is typical when patients return for their 48-hour follow-up endoscopy.

Conclusions

Balloon PDT for BE is a scientifically validated outpatient endoscopic treatment that can effectively eliminate Barrett's HGD and reduce the development of cancer. Patient selection should be done carefully to include EUS evaluation of nodular areas. EMR prior to PDT is recommended for nodular areas. High-dose PPI therapy should be administered concurrent with PDT. Long-term follow-up endoscopies should be performed at regular intervals. Chromoendoscopy and adjuvant thermal ablation should be available on follow-up endoscopies for the detection and ablation of residual small islands of Barrett's mucosa. Careful patient education is critical for the management of side effects and to reduce the risk of photosensitivity reactions [27].

References

1 Cameron AJ, Ott BJ, Payne WS: The incidence of adenocarcinoma in columnar-lines (Barrett's) esophagus. N Engl J Med 1985;313:857–859.

2 Miros M, Kerlin P, Walker N: Only patients with dysplasia progress to adenocarcinoma in Barrett's oesophagus. Gut 1991;32:1441–1446.

3 Williamson WA, Ellis FH Jr, Gibbs SP, et al: Barrett's esophagus: prevalence and incidence of adenocarcinoma. Arch Intern Med 1991;151:2212–2216.

4 Birkmeyer JD, Siewers AE, Finlayson EV, et al: Hospital volume and surgical mortality in the United States. N Engl J Med 2002;346:1128–1137.

5 Bonavina L: Early oesophageal cancer: results of a European multicenter survey. Group Européen pour l'Etude des Maladies de l'Oesophage. Br J Surg 1995;82: 98–101.

6 Heitmiller RF, Redmond M, Hamilton SR: Barrett's esophagus with high grade dysplasia. An indication for prophylactic esophagectomy. Ann Surg 1996;224: 66–71.

7 Holsher AH, Bollschweiler E, Schneider PM, Siewert JR: Early adenocarcinoma in Barrett's esophagus. Br J Surg 1997;84:1470–1473.

8 Nigro JJ, Hagen JA, DeMeester TR, et al: Occult esophageal adenocarcinoma: extent of disease and implications for effective therapy. Ann Surg 1999; 230:433–438.

9 Rice TW, Falk GW, Achkar E, Petras RE: Surgical management of high grade dysplasia in Barrett's esophagus. Am J Gastroenterol 1993;88:1832–1836.

10 Thomas P, Doddoli C, Neville P, et al: Esophageal cancer resection in the elderly. Eur J Cardiothor Surg 1996; 10:941–946.

11 Overholt BF, Panjehpour M, Haydek JM: Photodynamic therapy for Barrett's esophagus: follow-up in 100 patients. Gastrointest Endosc 1999;49:1–7.

12 Panjehpour M, Overholt BF, Haydek JM, Lee SG: Results of photodynamic therapy for ablation of dysplasia and early cancer in Barrett's esophagus and effect of oral steroids on stricture formation. Am J Gastroenterol 2000; 95:2177–2184.

13 Wang KK: Current status of photodynamic therapy of Barrett's esophagus. Gastrointest Endosc 1999;49: S20–S23.

14 Wolfsen HC, Hemminger LL, Wallace MB, Devault KR: Clinical experience of patients undergoing photodynamic therapy for Barrett's dysplasia or cancer. Aliment Pharmacol Ther 2004;20:1125–1131.

15 Overholt BF, Lightdale CJ, Wang KK, Canto MI, et al: Photodynamic therapy with porfimer sodium for ablation of high-grade dysplasia in Barrett's esophagus: international, partially blinded, randomized phase III trial. Gastrointest Endosc 2005;62:488–498.

16 Overholt BF, Panjehpour M, Halberg DL: Photodynamic therapy for Barrett's esophagus with dysplasia and/or early stage carcinoma: long-term results. Gastrointest Endosc 2003;58:183–188.

17 Wolfsen HC: Present status of photodynamic therapy for high grade dysplasia in Barrett's esophagus. J Clin Gastroenterol 2005;39:189–202.

18 Wang KK: Combined endoscopic mucosal resection and photodynamic therapy for high grade dysplasia and early cancer in Barrett's esophagus. Tech Gastrointest Endosc 2005;7:69–72.

19 Panjehpour M, Overholt BF, Haydek JM: Light sources and delivery devices for photodynamic therapy in the gastrointestinal tract. Gastrointest Endosc Clin N Am 2000;10:513–532.

20 Overholt BF, Panjehpour M, DeNovo RC, Peterson MG, Jenkins C: Balloon photodynamic therapy of esophageal cancer: effect of increasing balloon size. Lasers Surg Med 1996;18:248–252.

21 Brandt LJ, Blansky RL, Kauvar DR: Repeat laser therapy of recurrent Barrett's epithelium: success with anacidity. Gastrointest Endosc 1995;41:267.
22 Malhi-Chowla N, Wolfsen HC, DeVault KR: Esophageal dysmotility in patients undergoing photodynamic therapy. Mayo Clin Proc 2001;76:987–989.
23 Overholt BF, Panjehpour M: Photodynamic therapy techniques for ablation of Barrett's esophagus. Tech Gastrointest Endosc 2000;2:203–208.
24 Overholt BF, Wang KK, Burdick JS, Lightdale CJ, et al: Five-year efficacy and safety of photodynamic therapy with Photofrin in Barrett's high-grade dysplasia. Gastrointest Endosc 2007;66:460–468.
25 Bronner MP, Overholt BF, Taylor SL, Haggitt RC, et al: Squamous overgrowth is not a safety concern for photodynamic therapy for Barrett's esophagus with high-grade dysplasia. Gastroenterology 2009;136: 56–64.
26 Overholt BF, Panjehpour M, Ayres M: Photodynamic therapy for Barrett's esophagus: cardiac effects. Lasers Surg Med 1997;21:317–320.
27 Phan M, Dyke S, Whittaker MA, Simmerman A, Abrams S, Panjehpour M, Overholt BF: An educational tool for photodynamic therapy of Barrett's esophagus with high-grade dysplasia. Gastroenterol Nurs 2005;28:413–419.

Masoud Panjehpour, PhD
Center of Excellence for Treatment of Barrett's Esophagus, Thomson Cancer Survival Center
1915 White Avenue
Knoxville, TN 37916 (USA)
Tel. +1 865 541 1628, Fax +1 865 541 1585, E-Mail mpanjehp@covhlth.com

Mönkemüller K, Wilcox CM, Muñoz-Navas M (eds): Interventional and Therapeutic Gastrointestinal Endoscopy.
Front Gastrointest Res. Basel, Karger, 2010, vol 27, pp 140–146

Endoscopic Ablation of Barrett's Esophagus Using the HALO® System

David E. Fleischer · Virender K. Sharma

Division of Gastroenterology, Mayo Clinic, Mayo Medical School, Scottsdale, Ariz., USA

Abstract

There is increasing interest in endoscopic treatment for Barrett's esophagus because it is the primary risk factor for adenocarcinoma of the esophagus, and the incidence is increasing. Of the various endoscopic treatments available, radiofrequency ablation is the one that has been studied the most. The principle of radiofrequency technology is to deliver a high power (approx. 300 W) over a short period of time (<300 ms) and to utilize energy density control. Recent studies suggest its utility for patients with low-grade dysplasia and high-grade dysplasia. In most instances, patients with intestinal metaplasia only with no dysplasia are followed with endoscopic surveillance rather than endoscopic treatment. Radiofrequency ablation treatment may be delivered by either a balloon device (HALO^{360}; HALO® system, BÂRRX, Sunnyvale, Calif., USA) or a paddle device attached to the tip of the endoscopy (HALO^{90}). After initial endoscopic treatment a repeat endoscopy is performed in 2–3 months to determine the completeness of the ablation. At the current time, even if there is no residual Barrett's seen at the follow-up examination, surveillance is still advised. This is because the device was first used in 2003 and long-term durability had not been established. It is hoped that when durability has been demonstrated for the removal of both metaplasia and dysplasia, long-term surveillance will not be needed.

There is increasing interest in the endoscopic treatment of Barrett's esophagus (BE). Endoscopic treatment has been utilized for many years [1], but in the past no specific treatment has emerged as an appealing treatment option with appropriate safety, efficacy and ease of treatment for both patients and physicians. Recently there has been a growing amount of literature related to the endoscopic ablation of BE using radiofrequency ablation (RFA) (HALO® system). The indications for RFA are not clearly established. However, there is consensus that this technique is useful for patients with BE and high-grade dysplasia (HGD), BE and intramucosal carcinoma as an adjunct to endoscopic mucosal resection (EMR). The use of RFA for BE with LGD or intestinal metaplasia is not clearly established, and currently considered a relative indication.

Table 1. Endoscopic options for treatment of BE

Multipolar coagulation
Argon plasma coagulation
Photodynamic therapy
Laser therapy
Cryotherapy
RFA (HALO)
Mucosal/submucosal resection
Combination therapy

Table 2. Use of radiofrequency for esophageal diseases

Intestinal metaplasia only
LGD only
HGD only
LGD + HGD
Intramucosal carcinoma
Squamous dysplasia

Procedural Aspects (tables 1, 2)

Patient Preparation

The patient is prepared as for any standard interventional upper endoscopy. Patients with blood dyscrasias or those taking anticoagulant therapy should undergo laboratory tests including a complete blood count and PT-INR.

Technical Aspects

The principle of radiofrequency electrode technology is to deliver high power (approx. 300 W) in a short period of time (<300 ms) and to utilize energy density control. When the HALO^{360} balloon is used, the idea is to have uniform wall tension, which is achievable with a balloon. In addition, tight electrode spacing (<250 μm) leads to more superficial tissue injury. The concept is that this will control the depth of energy penetration to ablate the Barrett epithelium up to the superficial muscularis mucosa without injuring the submucosa. Depths of ablation are generally in the range of 700 μm. The concept is that the Barrett's tissue will not extend into the submucosa. If the submucosa is not injured and there will be less risk of bleeding, fibrosis and stricturing.

The equipment that is utilized for the RFA (HALO® system, BÂRRX, Sunnyvale, Calif., USA) system includes an energy generator, a sizing balloon for HALO^{360} treatments, a treatment delivery balloon (HALO^{360}) for circumferential therapy, and a separate product called the HALO^{90} for focal treatment. The latter is attached to a standard forward-viewing endoscope.

The technique is performed in the following manner [1–4]. After the endoscopic esophageal landmarks are defined, the esophageal wall is sprayed with acetylcysteine 1% and then flushed with water to remove excess mucous for the HALO^{360} ablation procedure. The esophageal diameter is measured with a sizing catheter. It is passed over a stiff guidewire, which is passed endoscopically. After the guidewire passage, the endoscope is removed. An auto-sizing balloon is used to determine the diameter of the esophagus. This is important to allow good contact between the balloon/electrodes and the esophageal wall on the one hand and not to apply excessive pressure on the other. The electrodes on the HALO^{360} treatment catheter are 3 cm in length and treatment is delivered beginning approximately 1 cm above the proximal margin of Barrett's. The location can be achieved by noting the marks on the shaft of the catheter and is usually confirmed with side-by-side endoscopic observation of the ablation procedure. The treatment is delivered using between 10 and 12 J energy settings. Delivery typically lasts 1–3 s. Moving from proximally to distally, the balloon is progressively repositioned allowing for a very small overlap with the previous treatment zone. Ablation is repeated until the entire BE has been treated with radiofrequency energy. In most cases with the HALO^{360}, two treatments are delivered. Generally, the HALO^{360} device is removed after the first series of applications and then cleaned. In addition, the exudative material caused by the burn can be scraped off the esophagus with aggressive washing or using a device similar to the endoscopic cap that is used for mucosal resection. After the initial treatment is delivered, endoscopic observation is made to determine that all the Barrett's has been treated. After that observation is achieved, the procedure for that day is completed. A follow-up endoscopic treatment is usually carried out in 2–3 months.

At the time of the follow-up, a second treatment may be necessary. This can be repeated with the HALO^{360} balloon if there are large areas of Barrett's in the tubular esophagus that have not been eliminated. However, it is far more common that on subsequent treatments after the initial HALO^{360} treatment that the HALO^{90} device will be utilized. The HALO^{90} electrode is fitted on the tip of the endoscope and then the endoscope is advanced into the esophagus. Care must be taken when advancing from the pharynx to the upper esophageal sphincter into the esophagus. In most patients there is little difficulty, but in some patients, particularly those with unusual anatomy, passage may require patience and at times dilation of the upper esophageal sphincter. Prior to assessing the mucosa for further treatment, 1% acetylcysteine is often sprayed to remove mucus and to highlight mucosal features. Narrow band imaging may also be applied. After the residual Barrett's is identified, the HALO^{90} electrode is brought into close contact with the mucosa, the device is deflected for a close apposition of the device with diseased mucosa and then treatment is carried out.

Post-Procedure Care

The procedure is generally well tolerated. However, chest pain occurs in the majority of patients who are treated and generally lasts for a few days. Management with a local solution of viscous Xylocaine® and antacids with non-narcotic analgesics has been effective in most patients. In 1–2% of the patients, the pain has been more severe and longer lasting, and rarely, hospitalization for pain management is required. Follow-up is then carried out in 2–3 months to evaluate the esophagus (see above).

Complications

The RFA using BÂRRX has proven to be a safe procedure, but as with any procedure there are some complications. The most common delayed complication has been the development of esophageal strictures. This is more likely to occur in patients who have had EMRs and in some areas where treatment has been overlapped. The exact incidence is not known, but in published series it has been in the range of 1%. To date, approximately 20,000 patients have been treated and no deaths have been reported. Perforations have occurred, but they are extremely rare and usually happened during insertion or removal of the ablation catheter.

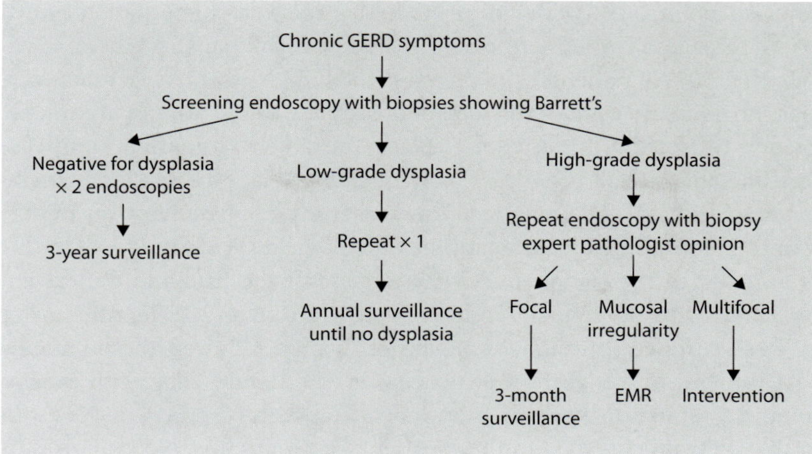

Fig. 1. Surveillance guidelines by the American College of Gastroenterology for BE (2008) [from 3].

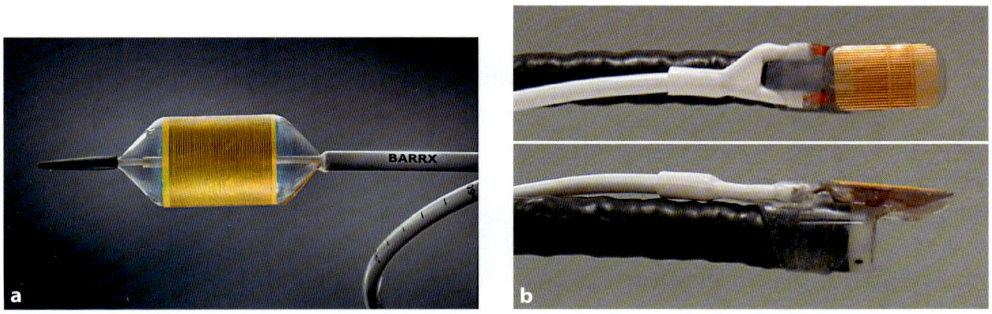

Fig. 2. **a** HALO^{360} balloon with circumferential coils. **b** HALO^{90} with attachment for distal endoscope.

Outcomes

Since the device was released in 2003, there have been an increasing number of abstracts and full publications describing the technology and its clinical use. In 2003 the AIM (ablation of intestinal metaplasia) I Trial began to clarify benefit in patients that had metaplasia without dysplasia [5]. Subsequently, studies in patients with low-grade dysplasia (LGD) and HGD were undertaken. In addition, information has been gathered through patient registries and through cooperative studies.

It can be confusing to 'analyze' the results of RFA treatment for BE without substratifying the analysis. RFA has been used to treat intestinal metaplasia only; to treat LGD only; to treat HGD only; and to treat LGD + HGD +/– intramucosal carcinoma. In addition, RFA has been combined with additional endoscopic modalities and RFA has been studied in patients with squamous dysplasia. Therefore, when one looks at the results, one needs to understand which group of patients is being treated.

Some individuals believe that it is appropriate to use RFA for intestinal metaplasia, while others do not. Those who support its use state that initial studies on its efficacy and safety have been encouraging. They also point out that without predictive markers some patients with a family history or anxiety may desire treatment even if it is not clear that their disease will progress. It is also known that 50% of patients who progress to HGD or esophageal adenocarcinoma have no dysplasia on as many as two previous endoscopies. These are the arguments that are posed in opposition to treating intestinal metaplasia only. They argue that only 10% of patients with intestinal metaplasia will progress. Therefore, why treat 90% of patients who will not have more advanced disease? The longest follow-up study for patients who underwent endoscopic ablation of BE with intestinal metaplasia only is the AIM II Study [6]. In this study, 70 patients were enrolled in the initial effectiveness phase of the trial and underwent circumferential ablation. They had a subsequent endoscopy at 1, 3, 4, 6 and 12 months. After 12 months, 62 patients were enrolled into a study extension, which followed these patients for another 1.5 years. At the end of 2.5 years (30 months), 61 had endoscopy with biopsy. Of those, there was complete remission (CR) of intestinal metaplasia (CR-IM) in 98.4% of patients. There were >1,000 biopsies collected in these patients at 12 months. No strictures or buried glands were seen.

Some have argued that it is unwise to treat patients with intestinal metaplasia only, since most will not go on to more advanced disease. Das et al. [7] performed a study assessing the cost-effectiveness of a combined modality using HALO^{360} followed by HALO^{90} ablation in the management of patients with non-dysplastic BE. The mathematical model compared different strategies in a 50-year-old patient. The assumptions were that the treatment would get rid of Barrett's in 50% of patients and that the costs were 'high'. With this mathematical model, the patient age, cost of ablation and CR rate associated with an ablation are critical determinants of its cost-effectiveness. The authors concluded that ablative therapy is cost-effective over 'surveillance' if the patients are treated at the age less than 55 years, the cost for the procedure is less than USD 7,450 and the CR rate is greater than 66%.

A study by Sharma et al. [8] presented a 2-year follow-up on patients who had been treated for LGD with RFA. Ten patients were initially treated with the HALO^{360} and then HALO^{90}; biopsies were taken at 1, 3, 6, 12 and 24 months. There was CR of dysplasia (CR-D) in 100% of the patients and in all but 1 of the 10 patients there was CR-IM.

A cost-effectiveness study comparing endoscopic surveillance or esophagectomy with RFA for patients with BE and LGD was written by Inadomi et al. [9]. In this study, ablation is the most cost-effective option for patients with LGD if you can achieve CR-IM in 60% of patients and CR of LGD in 70% of patients. For this group of patients, ablation 'dominates' surveillance, which means it is less expensive and more effective.

There are some studies that look at RFA for HGD. The largest series of patients is included in the HGD Registry [10], where 142 patients from 16 centers were included. Eight had previous EMRs. In this collection of patients, results for only 2 patients were treated with circumferential ablation with 12 J/cm^2 because HALO^{90} treatments were unavailable at this time. 92 of the patients were available for follow-up beyond 6 months; the median follow-up was 12 months. The CR for HGD was 90% and the CR for intestinal metaplasia was 53%.

The most important study assessing RFA for dysplasia is the randomized multicenter sham-controlled trial by Shaheen et al. [11], published recently. There were 120 patients with dysplasia, 60 of which had LGD and 60 of which had HGD. In each arm, 2 of 3 patients were randomized to RFA and one third to sham control. The initial treatment was with HALO^{360} and at the follow-up points focal ablation could be instituted if there was residual Barrett's. Follow-up endoscopies with biopsies were carried out at 6, 12, 18 and 24 months in the patients with LGD and at

3, 6, 9, 12, 15, 18, 21, and 24 months in the patients with HGD. The primary endpoints were CR-IM in all patients and CR-D in those with HGD and LGD. The evaluations were done both 'per protocol' and 'intention-to-treat'. Per protocol, 83% of the treated patients had CR-D in the HGD group and none in the sham group. For those patients with LGD, 100% of the treated patients had CR-D and 36% of the patients had CR-D. Regarding CR-IM, it was found in 75% of the patients who were treated with HGD and 87% of the patients with LGD. None of the sham patients had CR-IM. The reason that these results are so impressive is the complete response for a patient is defined as all biopsies negative for either dysplasia or intestinal metaplasia. That is, 1 positive biopsy out of 40 is considered a failure.

For patients with dysplasia and intramucosal carcinoma, many patients are treated with EMR followed by RFA. This is a particularly common strategy if there is an irregularity or nodule seen in the Barrett's segment. The thinking is that the EMR will both remove the pathologic tissue, but also clarify whether or not this management is sufficient for removing the HGD or IMC. After a localized EMR is performed, RFA could then be performed on the flatter and more extensive Barrett's tissue. The leading group in the world for this approach is the group from the Amsterdam Medical Center in the Netherlands led by Bergmann and his colleagues. An example of the efficacy of this strategy is a publication by Gondrie et al. [12, 13], in which 44 patients with dysplasia and intramucosal carcinoma were treated. At 12 months the CR for dysplasia was 98% and the CR for intestinal metaplasia was 98%. Other studies from this group and the European Multicenter Study Group are underway.

Conclusion

RFA with the HALO treatment system is a logical and well-conceived therapy. The device and the technique are still evolving. RFA is effective for eliminating intestinal metaplasia and dysplasia in most patients with BE. Although complications occur, the rate is acceptable. It is the view of the authors that this represents the best endoscopic treatment for flat Barrett's at this time. Combining EMR and RFA has an appeal in certain patients, particularly those who have nodular or elevated foci within the Barrett's. Answers to the questions expressed above will lead to further refinement of this treatment and better definition of the patients for whom this treatment is most appropriate.

References

1 Sharma VK, Fleischer DE: Barrett's esophagus and new therapeutic modalities. Therapy 2007;4:825–840.

2 Sharma P, Falk GW, Weston AP, Reker D, Johnston M, Sampliner RE: Dysplasia and cancer in a large multicenter cohort of patients with Barrett's esophagus. Clin Gastroenterol Hepatol 2006;4:566–572.

3 Wang KK, Sampliner RE: Updated guidelines 2008 for the Diagnosis, surveillance and therapy of Barrett's esophagus. Am J Gastroenterol 2008;103: 788–797.

4 Ganz RA, Utley DS, Stern RA, Jackson J, Batts KP, Termin P: Complete ablation of esophageal epithelium with a balloon-based bipolar electrode: a phased evaluation in the porcine and in the human esophagus. Gastrointest Endosc 2004;60:1002–1010.

5 Sharma VK, Wang KK, Overholt BF, Lightdale CJ, Fennerty MB, Dean PJ, et al: Balloon-based, circumferential, endoscopic radiofrequency ablation of Barrett's esophagus: 1-year follow-up of 100 patients. Gastrointest Endosc 2007;65:185–195.

6 Fleischer DE, Overholt BF, Sharma VK, et al: Endoscopic ablation of Barrett's esophagus: a multicenter study with 2.5-year follow-up. Gastrointest Endosc 2008;68:867–876.
7 Das A, Wells CD, Fleischer DE, Sharma VK, Kim HJ: Determinants of cost-effectiveness of endoscopic ablative therapy for non-dysplastic Barrett's esophagus. Am J Gastroenterol 2006;101:S68(abstr 77).
8 Sharma VK, Kim HJ, Das A, Dean P DePetris G, Fleischer DE: A prospective pilot trial of ablation of Barrett's esophagus with low-grade dysplasia using stepwise circumferential and focal ablation (HALO system). Endoscopy 2008;40:380–387.
9 Inadomi JM, Madanick RD, Somsouk M, Shaheen NJ: Radiofrequency ablation is more cost-effective than endoscopic surveillance or esophagectomy among patients with Barrett's esophagus and low-grade dysplasia. Gastroenterology 2007;132(suppl 1):A53.
10 Ganz RA, Overholt BF, Sharma VK, Fleischer DE, Shaheen NJ, Lightdale CJ, Freeman SR, Pruitt RE, Urayama SM, Gress F, Pavey DA, Branch MS, Savides TJ, Chang KJ, Muthusamy VR, Bohorfoush AG, Pace SC, DeMeester SR, Eysselein VE, Panjehpour M, Triadafilopoulos G: US Multicenter Registry: circumferential ablation of Barrett's esophagus that contains high-grade dysplasia. Gastrointest Endosc 2008;68:35–40.
11 Shaheen NJ, Sharma P, Overholt BF, Wolfsen HC, Sampliner RE, Wang KK, Galanko JA, Bronner MP, Goldblum JR, Bennett AE, Jobe BA, Eisen GM, Fennerty MB, Hunter JG, Fleischer DE, Sharma VK, Hawes RH, Hoffman BJ, Rothstein RI, Gordon SR, Mashimo H, Chang KJ, Muthusamy VR, Edmundowicz SA, Spechler SJ, Siddiqui AA, Souza RF, Infantolino A, Falk GW, Kimmey MB, Madanick RD, Chak A, Lightdale CJ: Radiofrequency ablation in Barrett's esophagus with dysplasia. N Engl J Med 2009;360:2277–2288.
12 Gondrie RE, Pouw CM, Sondermeijer T, et al: Effective treatment of early Barrett's neoplasia with stepwise circumferential and focal ablation using the HALO system. Endoscopy 2008;40:370–379.
13 Gondrie JJ, Rygie AM, Sondermeijer C, et al: Balloon-based circumferential ablation followed by focal ablation of Barrett esophagus containing high-grade dysplasia effectively removes all genetic alterations. Gastroenterology 2007;132(suppl 1):A64.

David Fleischer, MD
Division of Gastroenterology, Mayo Clinic, Mayo Medical School
13400 East Shea Boulevard
Scottsdale, AZ 85259 (USA)
E-Mail Fleischer.David@mayo.edu

Mönkemüller K, Wilcox CM, Muñoz-Navas M (eds): Interventional and Therapeutic Gastrointestinal Endoscopy.
Front Gastrointest Res. Basel, Karger, 2010, vol 27, pp 147–155

Endoscopic Resection for Early Cancers of the Esophagus and Stomach

Hendrik Manner · Oliver Pech · Andrea May · Christian Ell · Jürgen Pohl

Department of Gastroenterology, Dr. Horst Schmidt Klinik Wiesbaden, Medical School of the University of Mainz, Wiesbaden, Germany

Abstract

The advent of endoscopic resection (ER) techniques has enabled gastroenterologists to remove premalignant and early neoplastic lesions throughout the gastrointestinal tract. The indications and techniques of ER are discussed in this article. Before it is performed, accurate evaluation of patients and careful staging of the lesions is mandatory. After ER of the neoplasia, histological assessment of the entire specimen with detailed histological analysis of layer infiltration is crucial. The first long-term follow-up studies of large numbers of patients confirm the excellent effectiveness of ER for well-differentiated mucosal lesions without lymphatic or blood vessel invasion.

Detection of early neoplasias in the gastrointestinal tract has become more frequent as a result of improved endoscopic imaging technology, surveillance programs, and the increasing experience of endoscopists. For many years, radical esophageal resection or gastrectomy was considered to be the treatment of choice for early neoplasias. However, especially in the esophagus surgical resection is associated with significant mortality and morbidity. For these reasons local treatment methods have been introduced and investigated in several studies on cancers that carry a negligible risk of lymph node metastasis. In general, patients are ideal candidates for endoscopic treatment if they are at no risk of lymph node metastasis or lower risk for developing lymph node metastasis compared with the risk of mortality from surgery. This risk of lymph node involvement depends on the location of the neoplasia within the gastrointestinal tract and the depth of tumor invasion. Endoscopic resection (ER) is a promising therapeutic option for removal of superficial gastrointestinal tract carcinomas. Unlike ablative methods such as photodynamic therapy, argon plasma coagulation, or radiofrequency ablation, ER allows complete pathological assessment of the resected specimen including the depth of cancer invasion, degree of cellular differentiation of the cancer, and involvement of lymphatics or vessels. This pathological staging is crucial as it allows the risk of lymph node metastasis to be predicted and refinement of further treatment. There are various ER techniques, of which the most commonly used methods are discussed here.

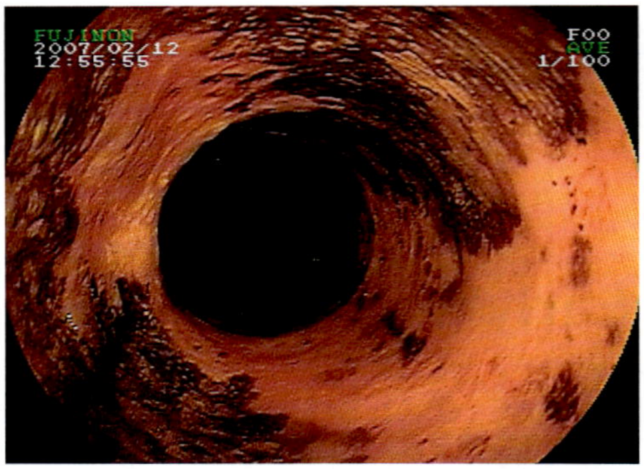

1

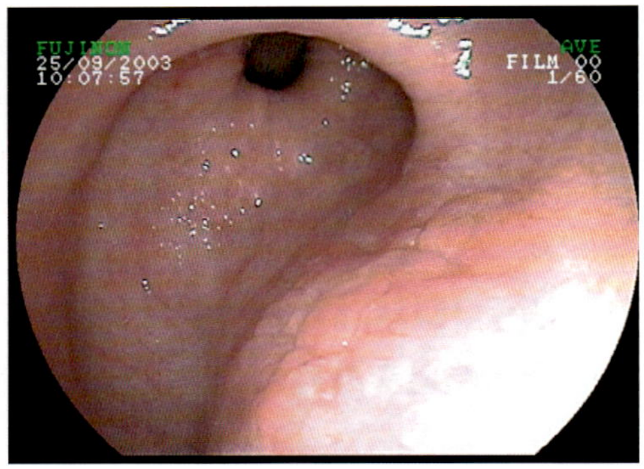

2

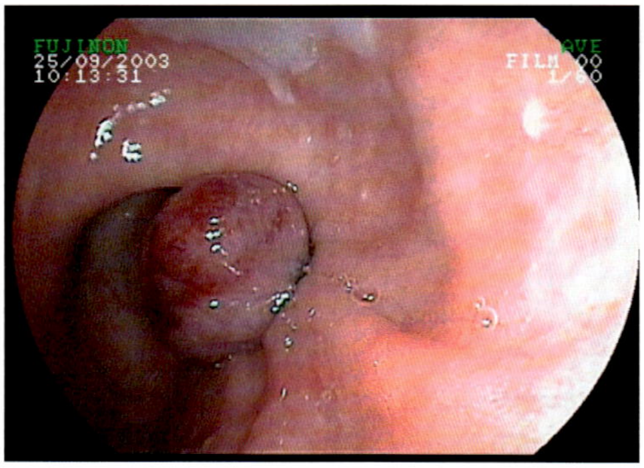

3

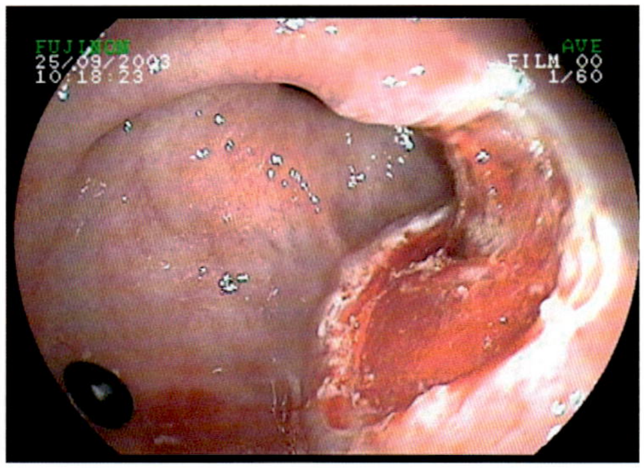

4

Fig. 1. Chromoendoscopy with iodine solution in early squamous cell cancer of the esophagus. **Fig. 2.** Endoscopic finding of early Barrett's cancer. **Fig. 3.** Pseudopolyp created during a ligation procedure for early Barrett's cancer (suck-and-cut ER). **Fig. 4.** Endoscopic finding after suck-and-cut ER of early Barrett's cancer.

Technique and Accessories

Before performing ER, identification of the margins of a lesion is crucial to avoid incomplete resection. For this purpose, conventional chromoendoscopy, e.g. with lugol iodine (squamous cell carcinoma; fig. 1), acetic acid (early Barrett's cancer), or indigo carmine with or without acetic acid (early gastric cancer), are widely used. However, virtual chromoendoscopy techniques like Fujinon intelligent chromoenhancement [1] and narrow-band imaging [2] have also been successfully applied.

There are two different concepts for ER: lesions can either be removed en bloc or piecemeal. Endoscopic resections are commonly performed with the 'suck-and-cut' technique. With this method, mucosa and submucosa are sucked into a cap or tube, and the pseudopolyp created in this way is resected using a diathermy snare (fig. 2–4). The procedure can be performed either with the cap or ligation device. Cap-assisted ER involves the injection of fluid, usually saline or diluted epinephrine, into the submucosa to lift the neoplastic area away from the muscularis propria. The lifted area of mucosa and submucosa is then suctioned into a transparent plastic cap attached to the end of the endoscope, and a cautery snare set inside the plastic cap is closed. Marking the periphery of the lesion with electrocautery before ER helps to determine the lesions margins after submucosal injection for precise direction of ER. Alternatively, the 'suck-and-cut' technique can be applied using a standard ligation device to capture the lesion and make it into a polypoid lesion by deploying the band underneath. However, this technique requires repeated withdrawal and the introduction of the endoscope for band ligation and subsequent resection. A novel multibanding mucosectomy device (Duette®, Cook Ireland Ltd, Limerick, Ireland) has recently been proposed. Since a polypectomy snare can be passed through the ligator handle, ligation and subsequent resection can be performed immediately without removal of the endoscope. A randomized study showed no significant difference between the 'suck-and-ligate' technique and the 'cap-assisted' technique concerning complications and size of the specimen obtained [3].

The major drawback of ER with the suck-and-cut technique appears to be that only small lesions with a diameter of <20 mm can be resected en bloc with tumor-free lateral margins. Larger lesions can usually be resected completely by piecemeal resections, but this method appears to be associated with a higher recurrence rate because of small neoplastic residues resulting from insufficient overlapping of the resection areas [4, 5]. Therefore, a new resection technique called endoscopic submucosal dissection (ESD) was developed to remove large lesions en bloc allowing more accurate histological evaluation of the lateral and basal margins of the lesion [6]. Standard ESD consists of three main steps. First, the lesion margins are marked by electrocautery, and fluids (e.g. hyaluronic acid or glycerol) are injected into the submucosal layer to separate it from the muscular layer. Second, circumferential cuts are made around the lesion. Then, special endoscopic knifes (e.g. insulated tip-knife, hook knife, or flush knife) are used to dissect the submucosal layer underneath the carcinoma in order to obtain a large resection specimen with the neoplasia resected en bloc. The size of the resected specimen obtained with ESD can extend to >10 cm in diameter, but this fascinating new method is associated with several problems and disadvantages. First of all there is a substantial complication rate, including bleedings (8–38%) and perforations (ranging from 4% in non-ulcerated cancers to up to 54% in cases with ulceration) [4–6]. Moreover, ESD requires long procedure times of up to several hours and has a slow learning curve and a high degree of operator dependency. This might be the reason for the fact that even in Japan, the reported en bloc R0 resection rate for gastric neoplasias varies between 55% [7] and more than 95% [8]. At present, ESD has mostly been applied for early gastric carcinoma, and there are only a few reports on cases with early squamous cell cancer or cancer of the esophagogastric junction treated with ESD.

Outcomes

Early Barrett's Adenocarcinoma

Eligibility for ER of Barrett's cancer depends on risk stratification in accordance with known risk factors such as the infiltration depth of the carcinoma (mucosal layer of Barrett's epithelium is divided into four layers, m1–4), grade of differentiation, and lymph vessel or venous infiltration (fig. 5). A large series on patients with Barrett's carcinoma analyzed 350 resected lymph nodes in 41 patients with adenocarcinoma and found that the risk of lymph node involvement was 0% in patients with m1–4 compared to 16% in patients with submucosal infiltration [9]. Limitations for ER of early Barrett's carcinoma should be submucosal infiltration or infiltration of the muscularis mucosae in combination with another risk factor such as poor differentiation or lymph vessel infiltration (table 1).

Surgical series showed that also patients with Barrett's cancer invading the upper third of the submucosa (sm1) have a very low risk of lymph node metastasis [10, 11]. Therefore, the question arises whether also these cancers might be eligible for ER with a curative intent. This question

Table 1. Indications for ER in esophageal neoplasia

	Indication	Expanded indication[1]
Barrett's neoplasia	HGIN, carcinoma, size <20 mm, no risk factors[2], macroscopic types I, IIa, b, c	Carcinoma >20 mm, multifocal cancer, sm1 infiltration without risk factors[2]
Squamous cell neoplasia	HGIN, mucosal cancer, no risk factors[2], macroscopic types I, IIa, b, c	Lesion >20 mm, multifocal cancer

HGIN = High-grade intraepithelial neoplasia.
[1] ER only in highly experienced centers and/or under study conditions.
[2] Risk factors: lymph vessel invasion (L1), venous infiltration (V1), low tumor differentiation (G3).

was answered by a recently published study [12]. ER was associated with favorable outcomes in submucosal Barrett's cancer meeting the following low-risk criteria: invasion not beyond sm1; absence of infiltration into lymph vessels/veins; histological grade G1/2, and macroscopic type I/II. It has to be pointed out that further trials are required before a general recommendation for ER in low-risk sm1 cancers can be given, and ER with a curative intent should only be carried out under study conditions in this group of patients.

While there are only a few cases reports on the successful performance of ESD in patients with Barrett's neoplasia, reports on suck-and-cut ER show very promising results. In several studies, complete remissions of more than 95% have been achieved [13] with no mortality due to Barrett's neoplasia during a 5-year follow-up [14]. However, recurrences or metachronous neoplasia in up to 20–30% [13, 14] represent the major problem with endoscopic therapy in early Barrett's neoplasia, although successful repeat endoscopic treatment is possible in almost all patients. The reasons for the high rate of recurrence appear to be undetected neoplasia in the residual Barrett's segment after treatment and, more importantly, the fact that residual Barrett's metaplasia appears to have an increased risk of malignant transformation in these patients. Ablative therapy, e.g. by argon plasma coagulation or radiofrequency ablation, of the residual Barrett's segment is used in order to reduce recurrence rates.

Although ER is a very safe procedure for resection of esophageal neoplasias, a few complications have been reported. Early complications include perforation (<0.5%) and bleeding (14%) [15]. However, in most cases intra-procedural bleeding is easily controlled by epinephrine injection or metal clip application (or a combination of both). Esophageal stenosis followed ER in 0–30% of cases [13–15] with circumferential resection being a major risk factor.

Squamous Cell Cancer of the Esophagus

Compared to early Barrett's cancer, the risk of lymph node metastasis appears to be higher in patients with squamous cell neoplasia. The mucosal layer of the esophageal squamous epithelium can be divided into three layers (m1–3). Intraepithelial cancers (m1) and cancers invading the lamina propria (m2) are associated with almost no risk of lymph node metastasis [16–18]. The risk appears to be higher with cancers invading the lamina muscularis propria (m3), in the range of 0–10% [16], and with cancers invading the submucosa (50–55%) [17]. Most interestingly, it was shown that even in m3/sm1 tumors, lymph node metastasis was absent if the

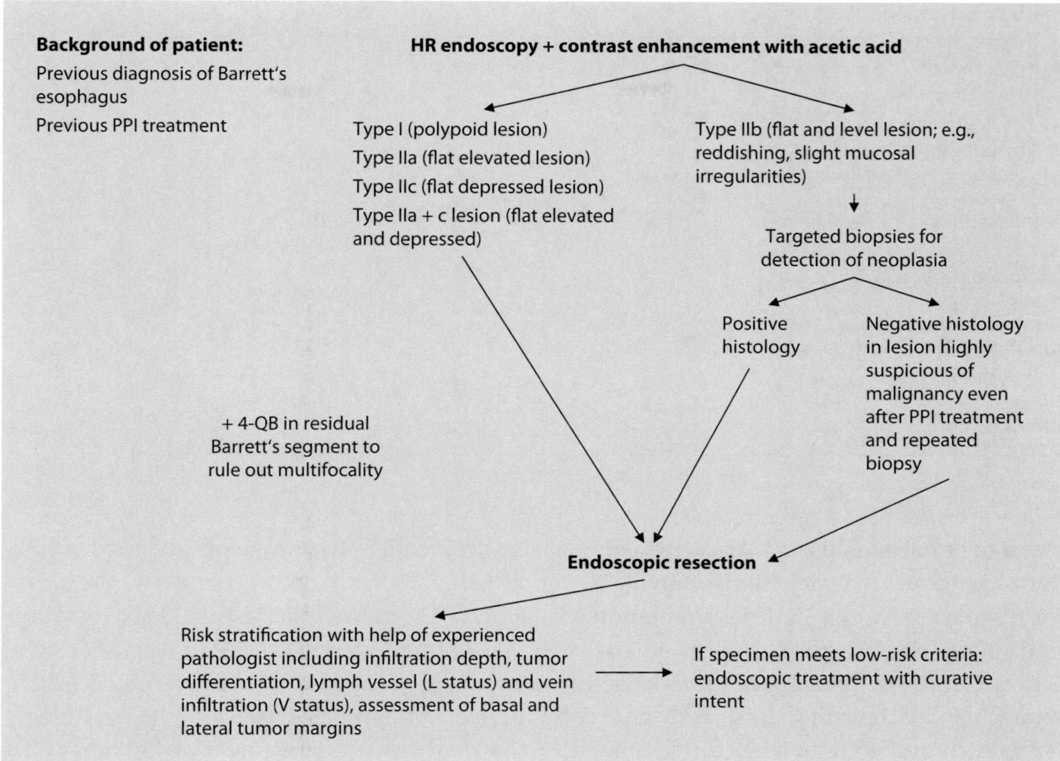

Fig. 5. Algorithm for the detection and endoscopic resection of early Barrett's cancer.

resected specimen did not show lymphatic or blood vessel permeation [16]. Several studies have shown that ER for mucosal squamous cell cancer with low risk of lymph node metastasis is safe and effective. Our group reported a series of 65 patients with high-grade intraepithelial neoplasia and mucosal squamous cell cancer. With ER, complete response was achieved in 95% [19]. However, after successful ER there is a considerable risk of metachronous lesions ranging from 20 to 30% [19, 20]. A recent publication by Fujishiro et al. [21] has reported on ESD in 58 patients with early esophageal squamous cell carcinoma. Complete resection (R0) was possible in 78%. Complications observed in this series included perforations in 7% and strictures in 16% of the cases. In conclusion, ER or ESD of squamous cell carcinoma is indicated for neoplasias with m1 or m2 invasion. Patients with a squamous cell neoplasia invading the muscularis mucosa (m3) should only be treated endoscopically if no further risk factors for lymph node metastasis are present (table 1). In case of submucosal invasion, patients should always be treated using surgery or radiochemotherapy. It remains unclear whether a combination of ER and radiochemotherapy represents an adequate treatment for patients with submucosal invasion or otherwise higher risk of lymph node metastasis, and further studies are needed in order to answer this question.

Gastric Carcinoma

In Japan, ER and ESD are well established alternative treatments to surgery for early gastric carcinoma [22]. Traditionally, indications for endoscopic therapy include well-differentiated

Table 2. Expanded criteria for ER in early gastric cancer

Mucosal cancer Differentiated adenocarcinoma No lymphatic-vascular invasion (L0) If ulcer finding: tumor size <3 cm Without ulcer findings: regardless of tumor size
Undifferentiated mucosal cancer L0 Without ulcer findings Tumor <2 cm
sm1 invasion, < 500 μm Differentiated adenocarcinoma L0 Tumor <3 cm

elevated or flat adenocarcinomas of <20 mm in size, and small (<10 mm) depressed lesions without ulcerations. A large database involving more than 5,000 patients who underwent gastrectomy with meticulous R2 level lymph node dissection [23] showed that the incidence of lymph node metastasis of early gastric cancer was negligible in intramucosal cancers and small (<3 cm) cancers infiltrating the upper third of the submucosa (sm1). Based on these data, extended criteria for endoscopic therapy of early gastric carcinoma were proposed (table 2). Recently, long-term outcomes of ER for small differentiated mucosal early gastric carcinomas of <20 mm in size have been reported in comparison to those of surgical treatment [24]. In the report, the disease-specific 5- and 10-year survival rates were both 99%.

The risk of local recurrence after ER varies between 2 and 35%, and the recurrence rate correlates with the number of resected specimens [22]. However, large studies show that cases of local recurrence could all be cured by repeated endoscopy or surgery [5, 6, 22]. In Western countries, experience with ER for early gastric cancer is still limited, not least due to the fact that the disease is relatively rare. Recently, it was shown that ER can also be effectively used for early gastric cancer in the West, but it is associated with a relevant risk of complications [25]. In this study from our group including 43 patients, the rate of minor complications (not Hb-relevant bleeding) and major complications (Hb-relevant bleeding, perforation) was 18 and 15%, respectively. All complications were managed conservatively. During a mean follow-up of 57 months, recurrent or metachronous lesions were observed in 29% of patients. All lesions were successfully treated by repeated endoscopic treatment. No tumor-related deaths occurred during follow-up.

Staging

Accurate staging is mandatory before ER and ESD of gastric or esophageal cancer. The most important part of the staging procedure is careful evaluation of the neoplasia (table 3) and the borders of the lesion using a high-resolution endoscope and searching for multifocal neoplasia. While for staging of esophageal squamous cell cancer chromoendoscopy with iodine solution is helpful (fig. 1), for adenocarcinoma of the esophagus acetic acid spraying or virtual

Table 3. Japanese classification of gastric carcinoma

Type of lesion	Classification
Polypoid	Type I
Flat and slightly elevated	Type IIa
Flat and level	Type IIb
Flat and depressed	Type IIc
Flat and slightly elevated and depressed	Type IIa + c
Ulcerated	Type III

chromoendoscopy with Fujinon intelligent chromoenhancement or narrow-band imaging have shown promising results.

As mentioned above, the critical importance of accurately determining the depth of invasion of a small esophageal carcinoma is the link between depth of invasion and the likelihood of lymph node metastasis. Endoscopic ultrasound is not only recommended to exclude lymph node metastasis, but also to determine infiltration depth. In the esophagus, it has been shown that the accuracy of EUS for T staging is excellent for differentiating T1 and T2 tumors but poor for distinguishing between the important stages of T1m and T1sm [26, 27]. The only method currently available to accurately determine the depth of invasion is diagnostic ER. Histopathologic workup of the specimen determines if the patient can be safely treated with ER or needs to be referred to surgery for esophageal resection. Concerning T and N staging, EUS is considerably superior to computed tomography in the majority of studies. The major aim of computed tomography is to exclude distant metastases.

Algorithm

An algorithm for the detection and ER of early Barrett's cancer is shown in figure 5. The macroscopic classification of early neoplastic lesions is shown in table 3.

Conclusions

Advanced endoscopic imaging techniques have made early diagnosis of early cancer in the upper gastrointestinal tract easier. This has opened a new chapter in minimal invasive mucosal cancer therapy with fast evolving ER techniques. Especially for early neoplasias of the esophagus, ER and ESD show excellent results and compare very favorably with surgical resection of the organ which carries substantial mortality (5–20%) and morbidity (up to 50%) rates.

It is important to emphasize that after successful ER or ESD a close follow-up program is crucial for surveillance because of the known risk of metachronous or recurrent lesions. En bloc resection with ESD appears to be an attractive new treatment method not only for early gastric, but also for patients with early esophageal malignancy. In terms of complete tumor resection and local cancer recurrence, ESD has proven to be superior to ER. However, only a few experts worldwide have the skills to apply ESD, and the technique is too time-consuming to be implemented to a great extent in daily practice. Therefore, novel techniques and new devices have to be invented to enable safe en bloc resections within certain time limits. In order to minimize complications and optimize the effectiveness of ER, this treatment approach should only be carried out by experienced endoscopists in an appropriate environment (high-volume center).

References

1 Pohl J, May A, Rabenstein T, et al: Comparison of computed virtual chromoendoscopy and conventional chromoendoscopy with acetic acid for detection of neoplasia in Barrett's esophagus. Endoscopy 2007;39: 594–598.

2 Kara MA, Peters FP, Rosmolen WD, et al: High-resolution endoscopy plus chromoendoscopy or narrow-band imaging in Barrett's esophagus: a prospective randomized crossover study. Endoscopy 2005;37:929–936.

3 May A, Gossner L, Behrens A, et al: A prospective randomized trial of two different endoscopic resection techniques for early stage cancer of the esophagus. Gastrointest Endosc 2003;58:167–175.

4 Muto M, Miyamoto S, Hosokawa A, et al: Endoscopic mucosal resection in the stomach using the insulated-tip needle-knife. Endoscopy 2005;37: 178–182.

5 Oka S, Tanaka S, Kaneko I, et al: Advantage of endoscopic submucosal dissection compared with EMR for early gastric cancer. Gastrointest Endosc 2006;64: 877–883.

6 Ono H, Kondo H, Gotoda T, et al: Endoscopic mucosal resection for treatment of early gastric cancer. Gut 2001; 48:225–229.

7 Miyamoto S, Muto M, Hamamoto Y, et al: A new technique for endoscopic mucosal resection with an insulated-tip electrosurgical knife improves the completeness of resection of intramucosal gastric neoplasms. Gastrointest Endosc 2002;55:576–581.

8 Onozato Y, Ishihara H, Iizuka H, et al: Endoscopic submucosal dissection for early gastric cancers and large flat adenomas. Endoscopy 2006;38:980–986.

9 Holscher AH, Bollschweiler E, Schneider PM, et al: Early adenocarcinoma in Barrett's esophagus. Br J Surg 1997;84:1470–1473.

10 Stein HJ, Feith M, Bruecher BL, et al: Early esophageal cancer: pattern of lymphatic spread and prognostic factors for long term survival after surgical resection. Ann Surg 2005;242:566–573.

11 Buskens CJ, Westerterp M, Lagarde SM, et al: Prediction of appropriatness of local endoscopic treatment for high-grade dysplasia and early adenocarcinoma by EUS and histopathologic features. Gastrointest Endosc 2004;60:703–710.

12 Manner H, May A, Pech O, et al: Early Barrett's carcinoma with 'low-risk' submucosal invasion: long-term results of endoscopic resection with a curative intent. Am J Gastroenterol 2008;103:2589–2597.

13 May A, Gossner L, Pech O, et al: Local endoscopic therapy for intraepithelial high-grade neoplasia and early adenocarcinoma in Barrett's esophagus: acute-phase and intermediate results of a new treatment approach. Eur J Gastroenterol Hepatol 2002;14: 1085–1091.

14 Pech O, Behrens A, May A, et al: Long-term results and risk factor analysis for recurrence after curative endoscopic therapy in 349 patients with high-grade intraepithelial neoplasia and mucosal adenocarcinoma in Barrett's esophagus. Gut 2008;57:1200–1206.

15 Seewald S, Akaraviputh T, Seitz U, et al: Circumferential EMR and complete removal of Barrett's epithelium: a new approach to management of Barrett's esophagus containing high-grade intraepithelial neoplasia and intramucosal carcinoma. Gastrointest Endosc 2003, 57:854–859.

16 Tajima Y, Nakanishi Y, Ochiai A, et al: Histopathologic findings predicting lymph node metastasis and prognosis of patients with superficial esophageal carcinoma: analysis of 240 surgically resected tumors. Cancer 2000; 88:1285–1293.

17 Eguchi T, Nakanishi Y, Shimoda T, et al: Histopathological criteria for additional treatment after endoscopic mucosal resection for esophageal cancer: analysis of 464 surgically resected cases. Mod Pathol 2006;19:475–480.

18 Araki K, Ohno S, Egashira A, et al: Pathological features of superficial esophageal squamous cell carcinoma with lymph node and distal metastasis. Cancer 2002;94:570–575.

19 Pech O, May A, Gossner L, et al: Curative endoscopic therapy in patients with early esophageal squamous-cell carcinoma or high-grade intraepithelial neoplasias. Endoscopy 2007;39:30–35.

20 Narahara H, Iishi H, Tatsuta M, et al: Effectiveness of endoscopic mucosal resection with submucosal saline injection technique for superficial squamous carcinomas of the esophagus. Gastrointest Endosc 2000;52:730–734.

21 Fujishiro M, Yahagi N, Kakushima N, et al: Endoscopic submucosal dissection of esophageal squamous cell neoplasms. Clin Gastroenterol Hepatol 2006;4:688–694.

22 Ono H: Early gastric cancer: diagnosis, pathology, treatment techniques and treatment outcomes. Eur J Gastroenterol Hepatol 2006;18:863–866.

23 Gotoda T, Yanagisawa A, Sasako M, et al: Incidence of lymph node metastasis from early gastric cancer: estimation with a large number of cases at two large centers. Gastric Cancer 2000;3:219–225.
24 Uedo N, Ishii H, Tatsuta M, et al: Long-term outcomes after endoscopic mucosal resection for early gastric cancer. Gastric Cancer 2006;8:88–92.
25 Manner H, Rabenstein T, May A, et al: Long-term results of endoscopic resection in early gastric cancer: the Western experience. Am J Gastroenterol 2009;104:566–573.
26 Zuccaro G Jr, Rice TW, Vargo JJ, et al: Endoscopic ultrasound errors in esophageal cancer. Am J Gastroenterol 2005;100:601–606.
27 May A, Guenther E, Roth F, et al: Accuracy of staging in early esophageal cancer using high resolution endoscopy and high resolution endosonography: a comparative, prospective, and blinded trial. Gut 2004;53:634–640.

Dr. Hendrik Manner
HSK Wiesbaden
Ludwig-Erhard-Strasse 100
DE–65199 Wiesbaden (Germany)
Tel. +49 611 432420, Fax +49 611 432418, E-Mail HSManner@gmx.de

Mönkemüller K, Wilcox CM, Muñoz-Navas M (eds): Interventional and Therapeutic Gastrointestinal Endoscopy.
Front Gastrointest Res. Basel, Karger, 2010, vol 27, pp 156–168

Endoscopic Submucosal Dissection of Early Gastric Cancer and Gastric Tumors

Yasumasa Niwa · Ryoji Miyahara · Hidemi Goto

Department of Gastroenterology, Nagoya University Graduate School of Medicine, Nagoya, Japan

Abstract

Endoscopic submucosal dissection (ESD) is a new endoscopic resection technique introduced after endoscopic mucosal resection (EMR) by which the endoscopist can remove a superficial gastrointestinal neoplasm. The endoscopist can determine the incision line preoperatively and can resect even relatively large mucosal tumors en bloc using the ESD technique. ESD has four steps: marking around the lesion, submucosal injection, circumferential incision of the mucosa, and finally dissection of the submucosal layer. ESD requires specific endosurgical knives that are divided into two basic types, the tip-covered type and the tip-noncovered type. The drawbacks of ESD are that it is more time consuming and has a higher rate of complications (bleeding and perforation) compared with EMR. These problems are being overcome gradually with advances in devices and endoscopist skill. The indication for ESD has been extended to not only gastric neoplasia but also esophageal and colonorectal neoplasia.

In 1984, Tada et al. [1] developed endoscopic mucosal resection (EMR), by which the endoscopist could remove a superficial gastrointestinal neoplasm using a two-channel scope with grasper forceps and a snare after local injection of solution into the submucosa, and which can be used to treat flat or even depressed lesions. About 15 years later, a new endoscopic resection technique, endoscopic submucosal dissection (ESD), was invented in Japan. ESD evolved from one of the EMR techniques, ERHSE (endoscopic resection after local injection of a solution of hypertonic saline-epinephrine invented by Hirao et al. [2]). In the late 1990s, Hosokawa and Yoshida [3] and Ono et al. [4] started the development of the IT knife (insulation-tipped diathermic knife) at the National Cancer Center. This is an epoch-making device in the field of endoscopic resection. EMR is a very convenient method for the resection of gastrointestinal tract mucosal tumors in a short operating time. However, it has two drawbacks, namely limited size of resectable tumor and inability of the endoscopist to decide the incision line preoperatively. These have led to a slightly high recurrence rate of resected tumors. With the advent of ESD, the endoscopist can choose the incision line preoperatively and can resect even relatively large mucosal tumors en bloc. In this chapter we will introduce the technique of ESD.

Technique

Figure 1 shows the ESD procedure. The lesion is a IIc type early gastric cancer on the lesser curvature of the antrum. First is marking and injection of solution into the submucosa, followed by circumferential mucosal incision, submucosal dissection, resection, and comparison between pretreatment findings and the resected specimen.

Figure 2 shows the ESD knives. These endosurgical knives are divided into two basic types, the tip-covered type and the tip-noncovered type [5]. These originated from the conventional needle knife. The IT knife (KD-610L, Olympus) is a tip-covered knife. In the tip-noncovered group of endosurgical knives, the hook knife (KD-620 LR, Olympus) was developed by Oyama and Kikuchi [6], the flex knife (KD-630L, Olympus) by Yahagi et al. [7], the triangle-tipped knife by Inoue and Kudo [8], and the FlushKnife (DK2618JN10-30, Fujinon) by Toyonaga et al. [9]. In 2003, the new name *endoscopic submucosal dissection*, ESD, was proposed for this technique that is able to resect completely the superficial neoplasm that was impossible to resect en bloc by EMR. In general, the IT knife is most applicable to gastric tumors and tip-noncovered types for the esophagus or colorectum. In difficult cases, even for gastric neoplasms, a combination of two or three ESD knives is recommended.

ESD is supported by several advances in endoscopic equipment and medical support devices. In addition to endosurgical knives, ESD requires a specific endoscope with water jet and high-frequency generators. The endoscope for ESD is required to have a water jet system because the operator always encounters bleeding during the ESD procedure and needs to stop it immediately. In Japan, the GIF Q260-J (Olympus) high-frequency generator is most commonly used; the ICC 200 or VIO 300 D (ERBE GmbH, Tübingen, Germany) is also essential for ESD because they provide an endo-cut mode, a dry-cut mode, and multiple coagulation modes that are useful for ESD. These high-frequency generators can control the bleeding of a mucosal incision or submucosal dissection easily. Against bleeding of larger vessels in the submucosal layer, we should use hot biopsy or a Coagrasper (FD-410LR, Olympus) with soft coagulation mode.

Indications

The most important point for application of ESD is to detect an early gastric cancer. The endoscopist should obtain a good visual filed while doing esophagoduodenoscopy. Usually the patient is administered 20,000 units of pronase and 1g of sodium hydrogen carbonate as oral premedication to decrease gastric juice and reduce bubbles before examination. If the endoscopist finds bubbles or mucus that disturb the endoscopic view even after such premedications, s/he should wash the unclear area with water containing bubble-reducing agents. To detect early gastric cancer, s/he should take into careful consideration minute changes in the color or surface appearance of the gastric mucosa. Sometimes spraying of indigo carmine can help the endoscopist detect early gastric cancer.

Before ESD, it is important to investigate the histology, the depth, and the lateral margin of the tumor. The indications for conventional EMR are mucosal cancer, differentiated adenocarcinoma, with no ulcer or ulcer scar and <2 cm in diameter. Recently, extended indications for endoscopic resection of early gastric cancer would be necessary because the above criteria are very strict and ESD is able to remove larger tumors compared with conventional EMR. Table 1 shows the indications for conventional EMR and for ESD for early gastric cancer [10, 11]. Since

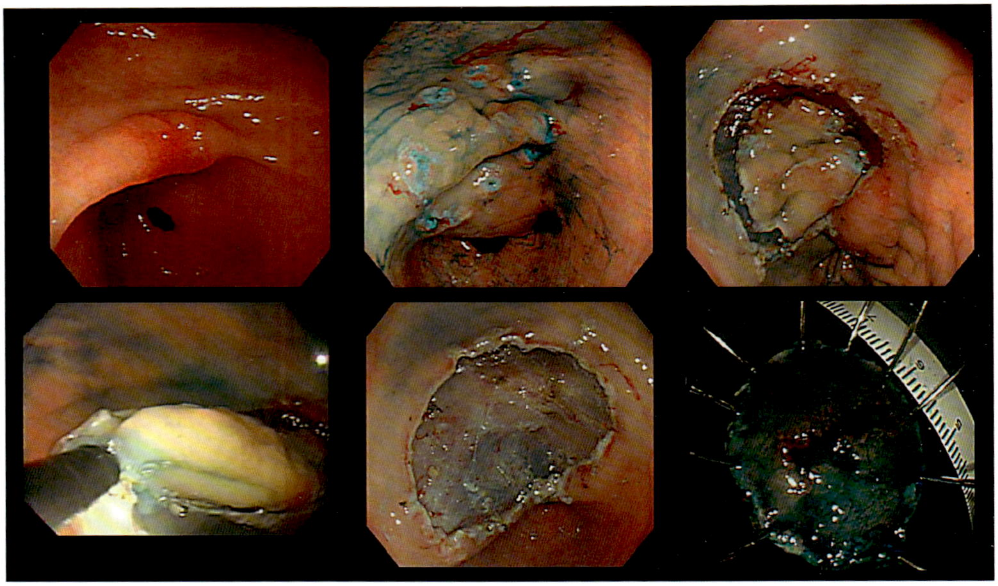

Fig. 1. The ESD procedure. The lesion is a IIc type early gastric cancer on the lesser curvature of the antrum. First is marking and injection of solution into the submucosa, followed by circumferential mucosal incision, submucosal dissection, resection, and comparison between pretreatment findings and the resected specimen.

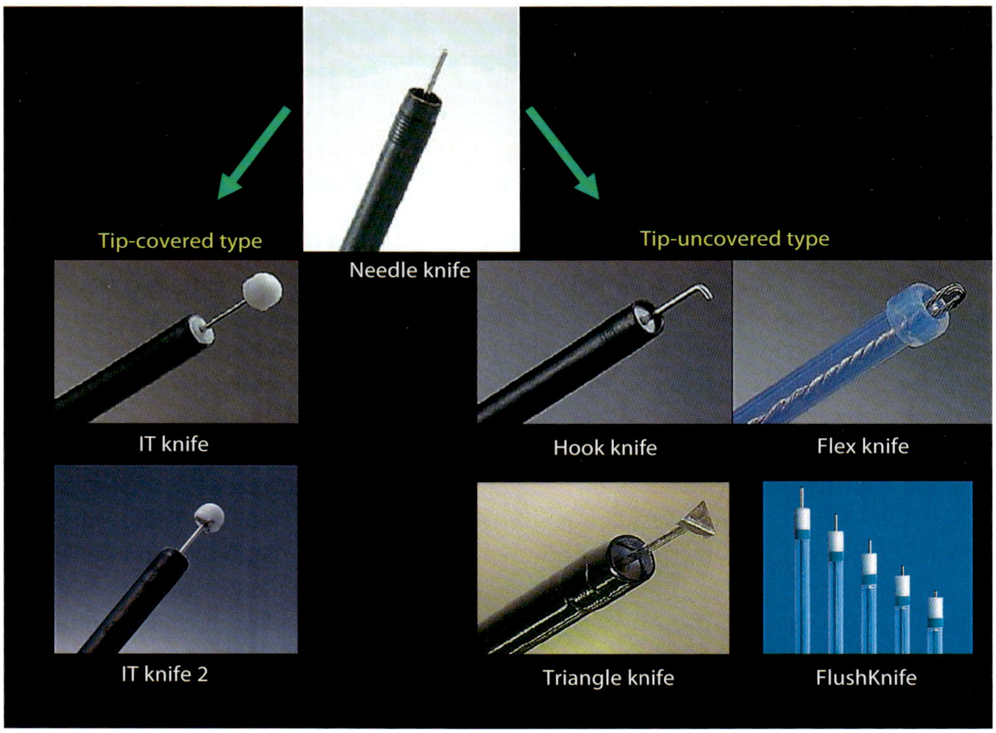

Fig. 2. The ESD knives. These endosurgical knives are divided into two basic types, the tip-covered type and the tip-noncovered type.

Table 1. Indications of EMR or ESD for early gastric cancer

Depth and histology	Mucosal cancer				Submucosal cancer	
	UL(–)		UL(+)		SM1	SM2
	≦20	<20	≦30	<30	≦30	any size
Differentiated	A	B	B	D	B	D
Undifferentiated	C	D	D	D	D	D

A = Guideline criteria for EMR, B = expanded criteria for ESD, C = consider surgery, D = surgery.

ESD enables en bloc resection of larger tumor compared with conventional EMR, we need the new criteria for the indications of early gastric cancer. Gotoda et al. [10, 11] reported that the criterion of lymph node-negative gastric cancer has been defined from a large database of over 5,000 patients with early gastric cancer who underwent gastrectomy with D2 lymph node dissection. According to their papers, differentiated type intramucosal carcinoma without ulcer findings and <3 cm in diameter differentiated type intramucosal carcinoma with ulcer findings do not show lymph node metastasis. Undifferentiated type intramucosal carcinoma is controversial for ESD because the margin of the tumor is not so clear due to its invasive behavior. We recommend endosonography before ESD in addition to abdominal CT. Endosonography shows the layer of the gastric wall so clearly that the submucosal invasion or ulcerated change is recognized objectively.

General Procedure of ESD

Patient position for ESD is the same as for diagnostic esophagoduodenoscopy, the left lateral position. Usually the patient is given a venous infusion and administered a sedative and analgesic. When the operation time is expected to be over several hours, general anesthesia may be recommended.

In general, ESD has four processes: marking around the lesion, submucosal injection, circumferential incision of the mucosa, and finally dissection of the submucosal layer. When we perform ESD, after insertion of the endoscope, we insert an overtube for endoscopic variceal ligation (Sumitomo Bakelite Co. Ltd, Tokyo, Japan) to insert or extract the endoscope smoothly. During ESD in the submucosal layer, since the lens is sometimes clouded with gastric juice, blood, and fat, we have to clean the lens of the endoscope. When we insert a scope with attachment or change endoscopes, the overtube is useful and results in less damage to the patient (fig. 3).

Step 1: Marking

When making marks around the lesion, we use a needle knife. To avoid perforation, we keep in mind the length of the protruded needle. If an endoscopist feels unsettled about needle movement, s/he should put a transparent attachment on the distal tip of the endoscope from the first marking session. This attachment helps the endoscopist keep a constant and stable

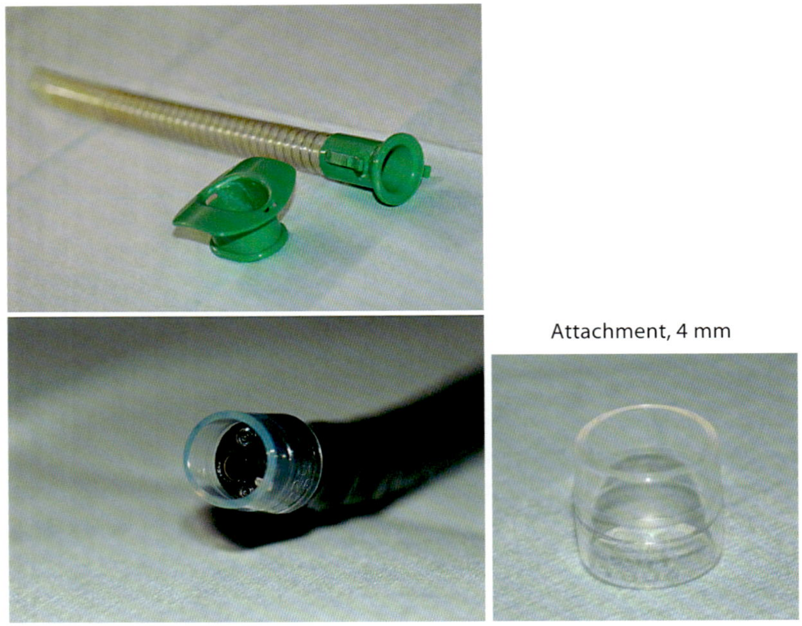

Fig. 3. Upper: An overtube for endoscopic variceal ligation (Sumitomo Bakelite Co. Ltd, Tokyo, Japan). Bottom: An attachment (Olympus, D-201-11804).

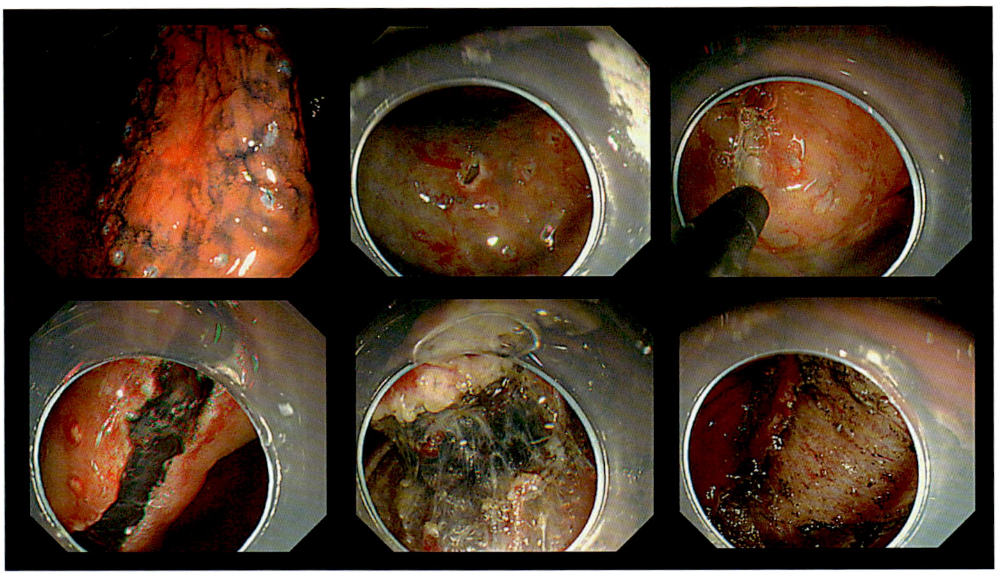

Fig. 4. When the endoscopist injects solution into the submucosa, s/he should keep in mind the position of the first mucosal incision. The endoscopist makes a small hole with a conventional needle knife or tip-non-covered type. Then the operator puts the IT knife into the hole. The IT knife should be used in a drawing manner, from the distal point to the proximal point; visually from the standard point of the angulus, the endoscopist makes the first incision at a point distal from. After the circumferential mucosal incision, the operator should start the submucosal dissection. Following the injection of solution into the submucosa, s/he starts dissecting from the right to the left or in the reverse direction in the submucosa.

distance between the tip of the endoscope and the mucosa. If the patient is prone to easy bleeding, for example, has liver cirrhosis or renal dysfunction, we could choose APC in marking for the gastric body lesions.

Step 2: Submucosal Injection

When the endoscopist injects solution into the submucosa, s/he should keep in mind the position of the first mucosal incision (fig. 4). Usually we add indigo carmine to the injection solution, for example saline, glycerol, or hyaluronic acid. When the endoscopist treats a lesion in the gastric body, hyaluronic acid should be selected because its duration in the submucosal layer is long and helps to avoid perforation [12]. If the operator injects continually, s/he should put the solution into the elevated area. If s/he puts the solution into the flat area, the risk of bleeding might increase.

Step 3: Circumferential Mucosa Incision

Except for the pylorus or cardia, from the standard point of the angulus, the endoscopist makes the first incision at a point distal from the angulus (fig. 5). The endoscopist makes a small hole with a conventional needle knife or tip-noncovered type. The hole should reach below the muscularis mucosa. The appropriate depth will shorten the time needed for mucosal incision. Then the operator puts the IT knife into the hole. The IT knife should be used in a drawing manner from the distal point to the proximal point visually (fig. 4). Usually the line of the mucosal incision should be made outside of the marking line. The operator should always keep in mind the relationship between the direction of the IT knife's advancing line and the marking point. When the operator feels the elevation of mucosa injected with solution flatten, s/he should make additional injections of solution into the submucosa as necessary. In general, with the IT knife it is difficult to cut the mucosa in the transverse direction. If the operator feels difficulty in cutting the mucosa, s/he should change from the IT knife to a needle knife or tip-noncovered type device and the problem may be solved.

Step 4: Dissection of the Submucosal Layer

After the circumferential mucosal incision, the operator should start the submucosal dissection. Following the injection of solution into the submucosa, s/he starts dissecting from the right to the left or in the reverse direction in the submucosa (fig. 4). If the space is narrow, s/he makes space between the mucosa and the proper muscle layer by pushing the distal attachment into the narrow gap. The blade of the IT knife should be moved parallel to the proper muscle layer to avoid perforation. Too high a concentration of indigo carmine in the injection solution might mask the layer of the proper muscle, so it is better to keep the content of indigo carmine in the solution to a minimum. The operator sometimes encounters bleeding in submucosal dissection. If this occurs, s/he should remain calm and stop the bleeding with an endoscopic hemostat, for example, Coagrasper (FD-410LR, Olympus) using the water jet system. If the bleeding point is unclear, s/he might unconsciously continue some dissection near the bleeding point. Even while using the IT knife, s/he should avoid blind maneuvers so as to avoid perforation. When the operator is not able to inspect the lesion closely, s/he should change the position of the scope to retroflexed view, or deflate the air in the stomach to obtain a better view. In case the distance between the tip of endoscope and the dissecting point is large and bleeding or perforation occurs, it is difficult to perform the appropriate endoscopic treatment. If the operator finds large vessels during the dissection, s/he should do precoagulation of the vessels before cutting [13].

When the operator recognizes that the operation time may become too long or the general condition of patient is becoming worse, s/he should finish ESD as soon as possible. If the lesion has been resected except for only central connective tissue in the submucosa, s/he should use a big, stiff snare, such as the Captivator II (Boston Scientific Corp., Natick, Mass., USA) (fig. 6). If the lesion still remains large at this time point, s/he should choose either ending the procedure or removing the lesion using the two-channel EMR technique.

Following Resection of the Tumor
The operator should take care of bleeding or exposed vessels on the artificial ulcer base. Careful observation and diligent treatment of bleeding points or suspected bleeding with a hemostatic device after the resection could prevent late bleeding after ESD.

Generally speaking, the ESD specimen easily corresponds to the endoscopic finding before treatment because of less mucosal damage during the procedure, compared to EMR. The assessment of curative resection of ESD is as follows: EA is equivalent to curative resection; EB is not EA or EC; and EC is vertical margin (+) or lateral margin (+) (table 2) [14]. A patient with EC lesion should be recommended to undergo additional surgical resection with lymph node dissection. Treatment of the patient with EB lesion is controversial. In general, the patient with the lesion of vertical margin (+) or ly (+) or v (+) may be recommended to undergo surgical resection.

New Endosurgical Knives, New Endoscope, and Skillful Technique to Reduce Operation Time

New surgical knives have been developed. The IT knife-2 [15] is typical of the second generation of endosurgical knives (fig. 7a). It has a blade under the tip that enables transverse mucosal incision and submucosal dissection. Some papers have reported that the increased cutting ability of the IT knife-2 has increased the perforation rate but reduced the operation time. The dual knife is a second-generation needle type developed by Yahagi et al. [7] that has a small notch in the tip of the needle (fig. 7b). The FlushKnife BT was developed by Toyonaga et al. [9] (fig. 7c). These new knives have increased the ability to grasp or hook connective tissue in the submucosal layer. When the operator performs submucosal dissection, s/he uses one of the new knives, not tracing the surface of the submucosal layer, but slightly hooking it and turning on the current power.

When it is difficult to detect the lateral margin of the tumor, the use of magnifying observation with narrow band imaging is recommended. Yao et al. [16] reported that minute mucosal differentiated adenocarcinoma of the stomach has irregular microvessels, a demarcation line, and disappearance of regular crypt patterns. Figure 8 shows a lesion that is clearly indicated for ESD after the narrow band imaging illumination.

There are several difficult places that cannot be reached or observed easily during ESD using the GIF Q260-J, for example the incisura angularis or the anterior wall of the gastric body in the long and vertical type of stomach. The GIF Q260-2TM is a new endoscope for difficult ESD cases, and its second bending channel at the proximal part of the endoscope makes it easy to approach difficult locations for ESD using a regular scope. If you do not have new knives available and are not able to approach closely, you should change the GIF Q260-J to the GIF-2T (fig. 9). The latter scope has a much larger angle rate of retroflexion so that the operator is able to observe the lesion more closely.

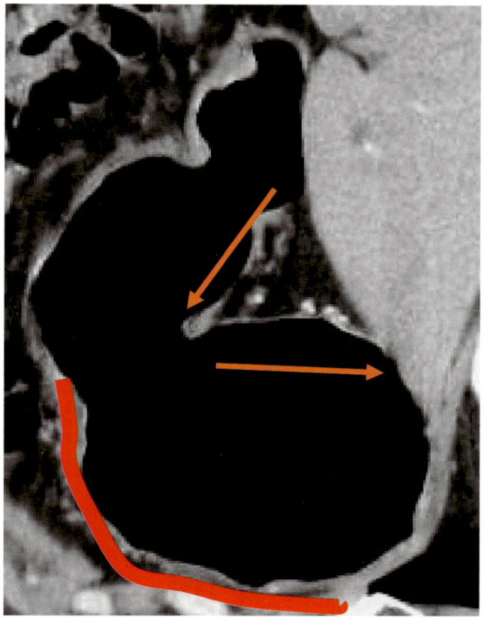

5

Fig. 5. Except for the pylorus and cardia, from the standard point of the angulus, the endoscopist makes the first incision at a point distal from the angulus.

Fig. 6. If the operator recognizes that the operation time may become too long or the general condition of patient is becoming worse, s/he should finish ESD as soon as possible. Operator should use a big, stiff snare, such as the Captivator II (Boston Scientific Corp., Natick, Mass., USA).

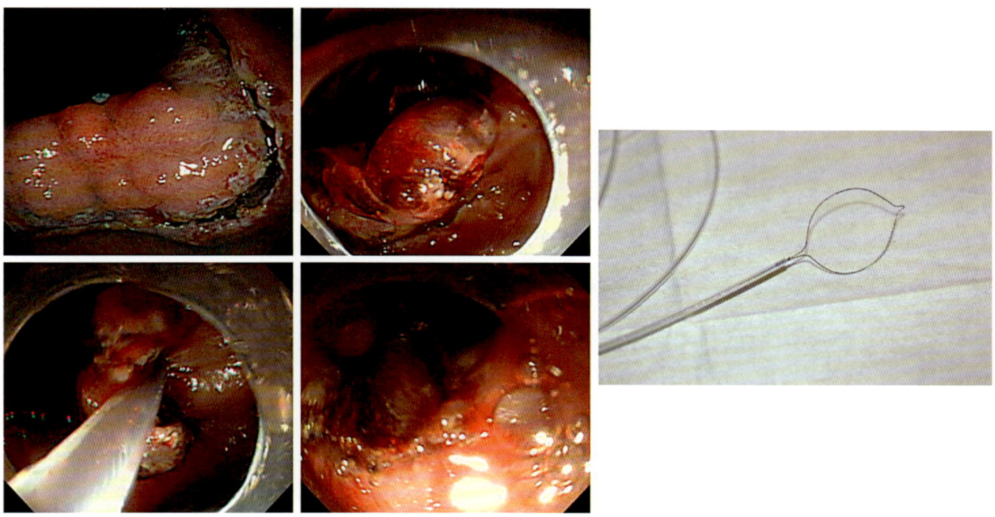

6

Table 2. Assessment of the resected specimen by endoscopic resection

	Depth	Histology	Ulceration	VM(–) LM(–)	LY • V
EA	M	PAP or TUB	(–)	VM(–) LM(–)	LY0 V0
EB	not EA or not EC				
EC	VM(+) or LM(–)				

PAP = Papillary adenocarcinoma, TUB = tubular adenocarcinoma, LY = Lymphatic invasion, V = microvessel invasion, VM = vertical margin, LM = lateral margin.

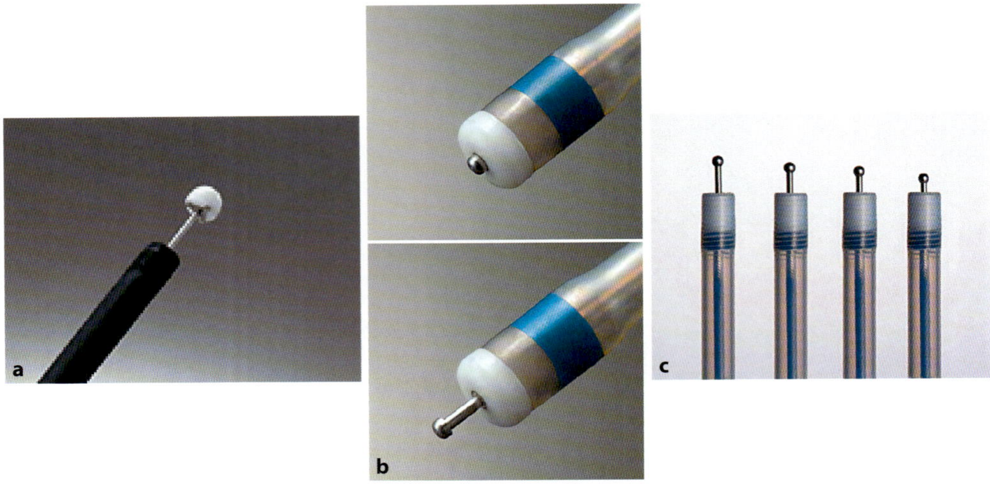

7

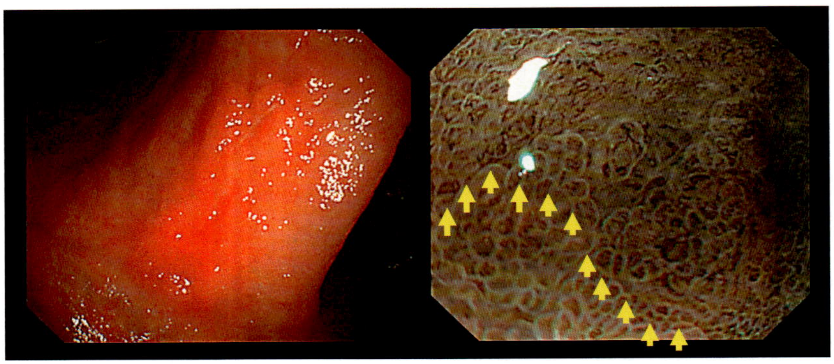

8

Fig. 7. Second generation of ESD knives: the IT knife 2 (**a**), the dual knife (**b**), and the FlushKnife BT (**c**).

Fig. 8. The NBI illumination is able to indicate the margin of tumor clearly.

A shallow mucosal incision sometimes prolongs the ESD time. This figure shows the slightly yellow thin fibrosis band under the surface that is the muscularis mucosa. It disturbs the shrink of the lesion to the central point and is sometimes rich in vascular networks, which leads to bleeding (fig. 10). If the operator recognizes that the incision is shallow, s/he should perform additional trimming at the cut edge or a deeper incision under the muscularis mucosa.

Complications and Limitations

The operator should master how to solve the two major problems during ESD: bleeding and perforation. ESD cannot be performed without some degree of bleeding. We prepare the above-mentioned specific endoscope with a water jet system and the hemostatic devices against bleeding. The latter are the Coagrasper and hot biopsy. The tip of the Coagrasper is so sharp and rotational that the operator is able to grasp the vessel point to point. Coagulation should be selected as soft coagulation (80 W) (fig. 11).

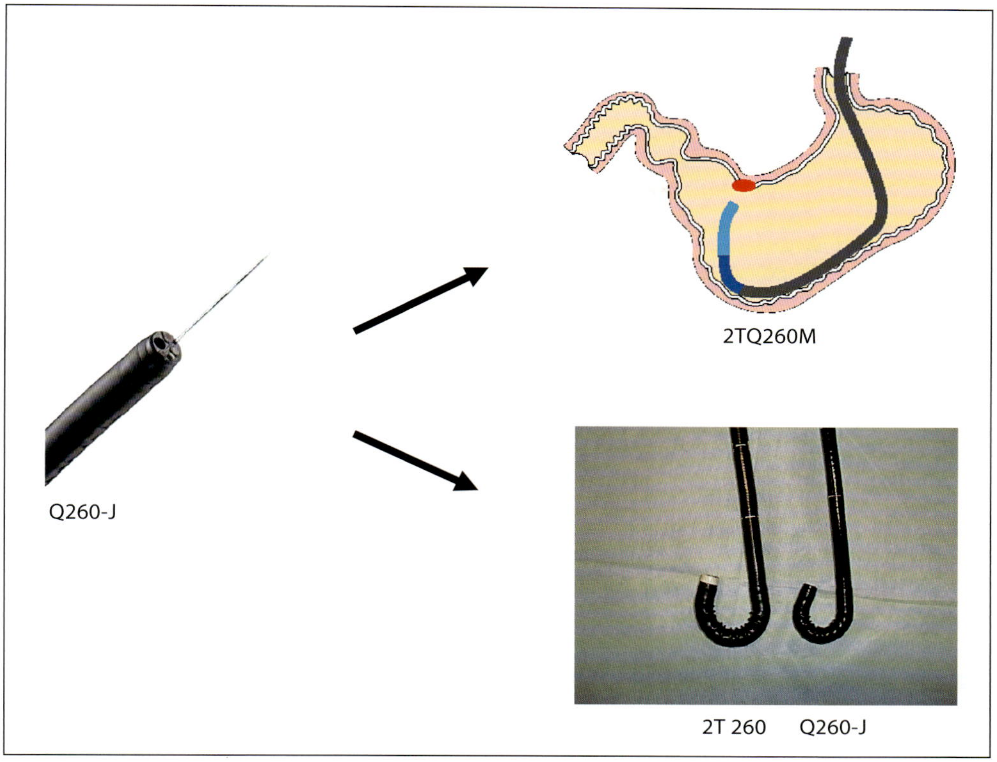

Fig. 9. If you are not able to approach the lesion closely, you should change the GIF Q260-J to the GIF-2T 260 or GIF 2TQ260M.

Perforation is a major complication but not a lethal one if the operator does the appropriate treatment immediately. It sometimes occurs while submucosal dissection is being performed blindly. The risk of perforation depends on the location, with the upper third of the body most prone to perforation, and presence of ulcer adding to the risk [17]. In addition, lesions on the greater curvature of the body are very difficult to inspect obliquely and to resect with IT knife (fig. 5). If the operator recognizes perforation during ESD, s/he should close it from the outside of the perforation using endoclips (HX-600-090; Olympus) or EX-clips (Olympus) (fig. 12). If the operator recognizes late that perforation has occurred and air has leaked from the stomach to the abdomen, s/he should deflate the air in the abdomen. If the general condition of the patient becomes worse, the operator or assistant should deflate air by inserting a catheter from the abdominal surface. From long-term observation, perforation has been reported not to induce the dissemination of gastric cancer [18].

Late bleeding and late perforation sometimes surprise the operator after ESD. Late perforation is believed to originate from too much coagulation at the ulcer bottom during ESD. The rate is unclear, but it occurs suddenly within 1–3 days after ESD. The hole of the perforation is sometimes very large and requires emergent surgical operation.

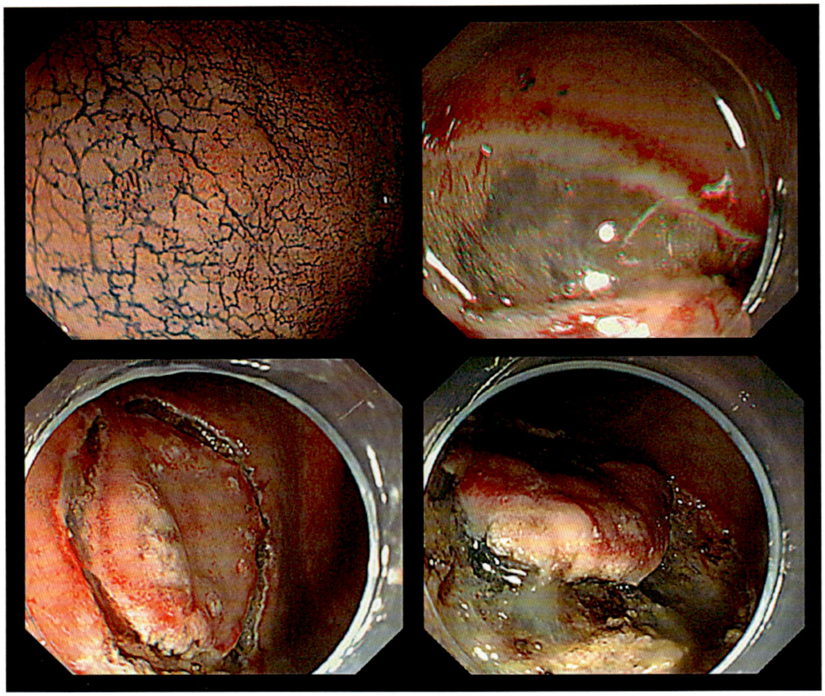

10

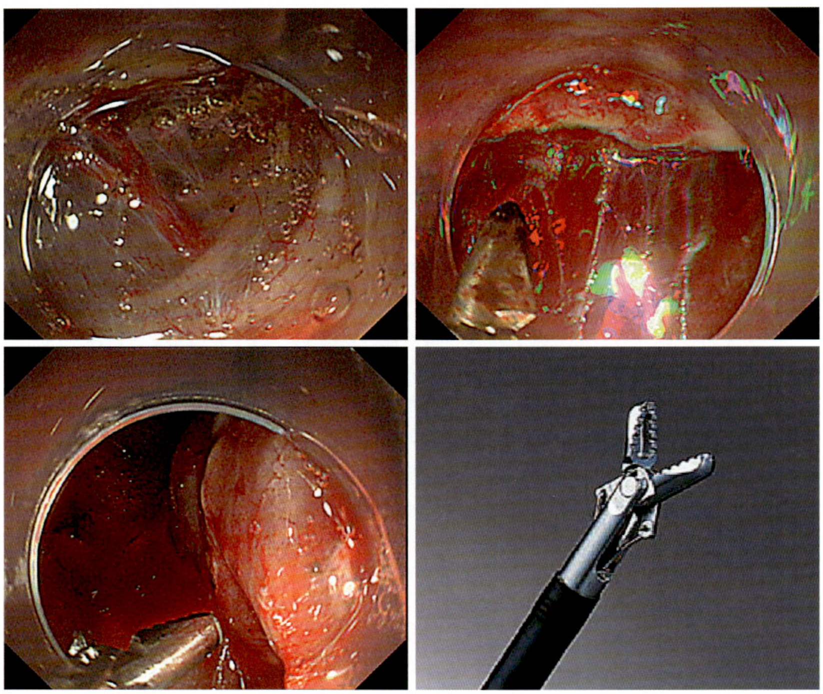

11

Fig. 10. A shallow mucosal incision sometimes prolongs the ESD time. The slightly yellow thin band of fibrosis in the muscularis mucosa disturbs the shrink of the lesion to the central point.

Fig. 11. If a slightly large vessel in the submucosa is found, one should use precoagulation for it with soft coagulation (80 W) using Coagrasper (Olympus).

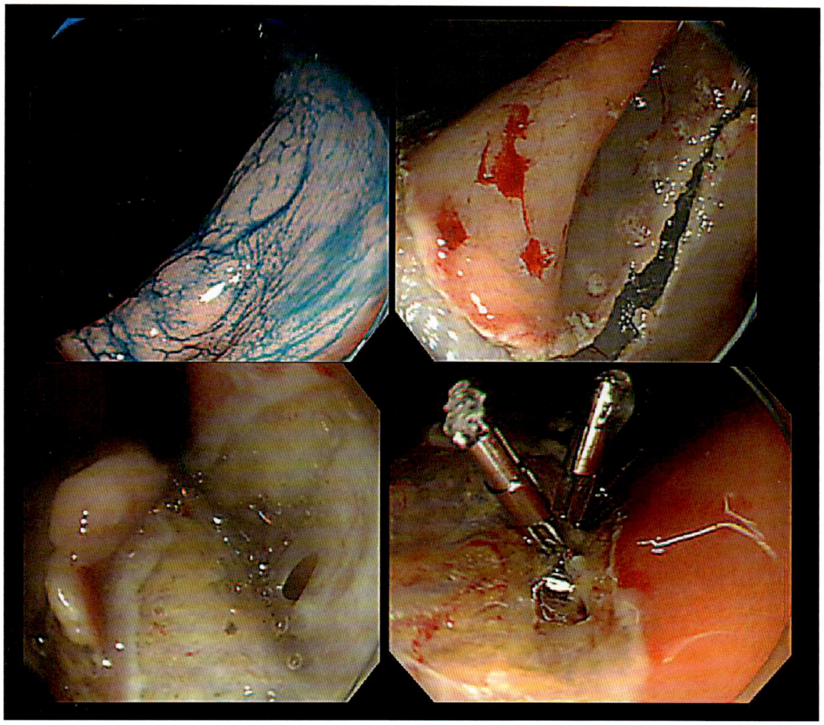

Fig. 12. If the operator recognizes perforation during ESD, s/he should close it from the outside of the perforation using endoclips (HX-600-090; Olympus) or EX-clips (Olympus).

Outcomes

The gastric cancer rate of recurrence in the EMR era was about 15%. This high rate resulted from piecemeal resection of the tumor during EMR. The recurrence rate of gastric cancer treated by ESD is significantly lower than that treated by EMR [4]. Uedo et al. [18] reported that the long-term disease-specific survival rate of EMR for small differentiated mucosal gastric cancer of <20 mm in diameter was 99%.

Conclusion

ESD has replaced EMR for superficial gastric neoplasm treatment in Japan. The drawbacks of ESD, such as a higher rate of complications, requirement for advanced endoscopic technique, and long procedure time, are being overcome with accumulated knowledge, consistently improving technique, and development of new devices and equipment. Even if we are able to remove larger neoplasms in the ESD era than in the EMR era, we need to be mindful of the indications for use of ESD and the histological results of resected specimens. It is necessary for the operator to keep in mind that the result of ESD *must be* equivalent to the result of surgical resection because, although the lesion is being removed without open surgery, it is early gastric cancer.

References

1 Tada M, Shimada M, Murakami F, Mizumachi M, Arima K, Yanai H, et al: Development of strip-off biopsy (in Japanese/English abstract). Gastroenterol Endosc 1984; 26:833–839.

2 Hirao M, Masuda K, Asanuma T, Naka H, Noda K, Matsura K, Yamaguchi O, Ueda N: Endoscopic resection of early gastric cancer and other tumors with local injection of hypertonic saline-epinephrine. Gastrointes Endosc 1988;34:264–269.

3 Hosokawa K, Yoshida S: Recent advances in endoscopic mucosal resection for early gastric cancer (in Japanese/English abstract). Jpn J Cancer Chemother 1998;25:483.

4 Ono H, Kondo H, Gotoda T, Shirao K, Yamaguchi H, Saito D, Hosokawa K, Shimoda T, Yoshida S: Endoscopic mucosal resection for treatment of early gastric cancer. Gut 2001;48:225–229.

5 Tanaka M, Ono H, Hasuike N, Takizawa K: Endoscopic submucosal dissection of early gastric cancer. Digestion 2008;77(suppl 1):23–28.

6 Oyama T, Kikuchi Y: Aggressive endoscopic mucosal resection in the upper GI tract – hook knife EMR method. Min Invas Ther Allied Technol 2002;11:291–295.

7 Yahagi N, Fujishiro M, Kakushima N, Kobayashi K, Hashimoto T, Oka M, et al: Endoscopic submucosal dissection for early gastric cancer using the tip of an electrosurgical snare (thin type). Dig Endosc 2004;16: 34–38.

8 Inoue H, Kudo S: A novel procedure of en bloc EMR using triangle-tipped knife (abstract). Gastrointest Endosc 2003;57:AB86.

9 Toyonaga T, Nishino E, Hirooka T, Dozaiku T, Sujiyama T, Iwata Y, Ono W, Ueda C, Tomita M, Makimoto S, Hayashibe A, Sonomura T: Use of short needle knife for esophageal endoscopic submucosal dissection. Dig Endosc 2005;17:246–252.

10 Gotoda T, Yanagisawa A, Sasako M, Ono H, Nakanishi Y, Shimoda T, Kato Y: Incidence of lymph node metastasis from early gastric cancer: estimation with a large number of cases at two large centers. Gastric Cancer 2000; 3:219–225.

11 Gotoda T, Yamamoto H, Soetikno RM: Review: Endoscopic submucosal dissection of early gastric cancer. J Gastroenterol 2006;41:929–942.

12 Fujishiro M, Yahagi N, Kashimura K, Mizushima Y, Oka M, Enomoto S, Kakushima N, Kobayashi K, Hashimoto T, Iguchi M, Shimizu Y, Ichinose M, Omata M: Comparison of various submucosal injection solutions for maintaining mucosal elevation during endoscopic mucosal resection. Endoscopy 2004;36:579–583.

13 Toyonaga T, Nishino E, Hirooka T, Ueda C, Noda K: Intraoperative bleeding in endoscopic submucosal dissection in the stomach and strategy for prevention and treatment. Dig Endosc 2006;18(suppl 1):S123–S127.

14 Japanese Gastric Cancer Association: Gastric Cancer Treatment Guidelines (in Japanese), ed 2. Tokyo, Kanehara-Shuppan, 2004.

15 Ono H, Hasuike N, Inui T, Takizawa K, Ikehara H, Yamaguchi Y, Otake Y, Matsubayashi H: Usefulness of a novel electrosurgical knife, the insulation-tipped diathermic knife-2, for endoscopic submucosal dissection of early gastric cancer. Gastric Cancer 2008;11:47–52.

16 Yao K, Anagnostopoulos GK, Ragunath K: Magnifying endoscopy for diagnosing and detecting early gastric cancer. Endoscopy 2009;41:462–467.

17 Uedo N, Iishi H, Tatsuta M, Ishihara R, Higashino K, Takeuchi Y, Imanaka K, Yamada T, Yamamoto S, Tsukuma H, Yamamoto S, Tsukuma H, Ishiguro S: Long-term outcomes after endoscopic mucosal resection for early gastric cancer. Gastric Cancer 2006;9:88–92.

18 Ikehara H, Gotoda T, Ono H, Oda I, Saito D: Gastric perforation during endoscopic resection for gastric carcinoma and the risk of peritoneal dissection Br J Surg 2007;94:992–955.

Yasumasa Niwa, MD, PhD
Department of Endoscopy, Aichi Cancer Center Hospital
1-1 Kanokoden, Chikusa-ku, Nagoya 464-8681 (Japan)
Tel. +81 52 762 6111, Fax +81 52 764 2963, E-Mail yniwa@aichi-cc.jp

Mönkemüller K, Wilcox CM, Muñoz-Navas M (eds): Interventional and Therapeutic Gastrointestinal Endoscopy.
Front Gastrointest Res. Basel, Karger, 2010, vol 27, pp 169–173

Pyloric Dilation

C. Carretero · M. Muñoz-Navas

Gastroenterology Department, University Clinic of Navarra, School of Medicine, University of Navarra, Pamplona, Spain

Abstract

Benign pyloric stenosis and gastric outlet obstruction are most commonly caused by peptic ulcer disease. Endoscopic balloon dilation of benign gastric outlet obstruction is a safe, successful, cost-effective, long-lasting alternative to surgery and should be the first-line therapy. Patients with recurrent or intractable symptoms of gastric outlet obstruction, despite multiple attempts at endoscopic dilation, should be considered for surgical intervention.

Peptic ulcer disease is the major cause of benign gastroduodenal obstruction or gastric outlet obstruction in the adult population. Endoscopic therapy of gastrointestinal strictures has become the first line of therapy in the majority of patients thanks to the advances in endoscopic techniques and the introduction of 'through-the-scope' balloon-dilating catheters [1]. Success rates of 80 and 100% have been achieved without complications. Nevertheless, potential complications such as bleeding and perforation should not be ignored [2, 3]. Endoscopic balloon dilation (EBD) has been widely used for peptic ulcer disease; it is also useful for caustic-induced gastric outlet obstruction [4], for postsurgical stenosis [5] and for strictures related to Crohn's disease [6, 7]. These cases usually require more dilations than ulcer-related strictures [4].

Procedural Aspects

The patient is asked to fast for at least 8–12 h prior to the procedure. In case of severe outlet obstruction, the patient's diet should be restricted to liquids at least 24 h before the procedure [1]. Upper endoscopy under conscious sedation is recommended. The stomach and pyloric channel should be carefully examined for the presence of ulcer disease, and biopsy specimens are needed for the study of *Helicobacter pylori* infection. If active ulceration is seen in the pylorus or in the duodenal bulb and always if *H. pylori* is present, we indicate a medical treatment with PPI and antibiotics prior to dilation. The degree of the pyloric stenosis can be assessed by measuring its luminal diameter in reference to the outer diameter of the endoscope and by the ability to advance the endoscope through the stricture into the distal duodenum. This may help to choose the initial size of the dilator to be used. Slim (5.9 mm outer diameter) and super-slim (4.9 mm) endoscopes (Olympus GIF-XP160 and GIF N180 respectively) are extremely useful to go

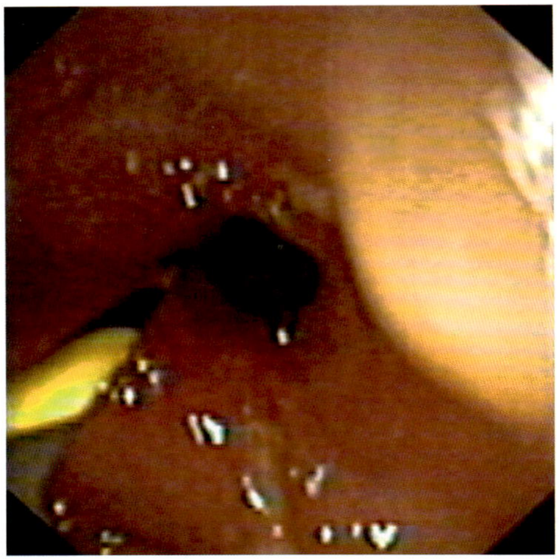

1

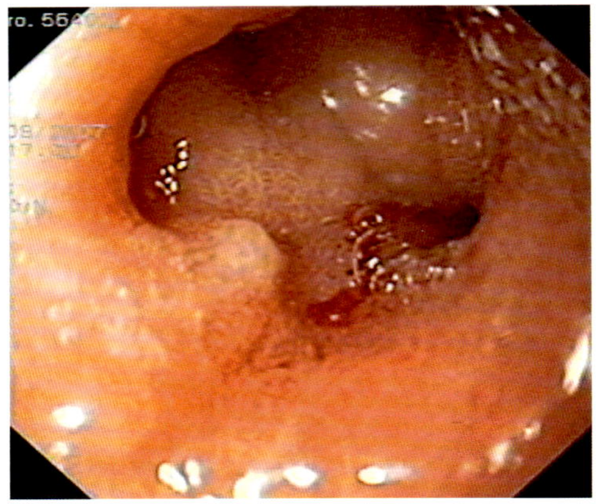

2

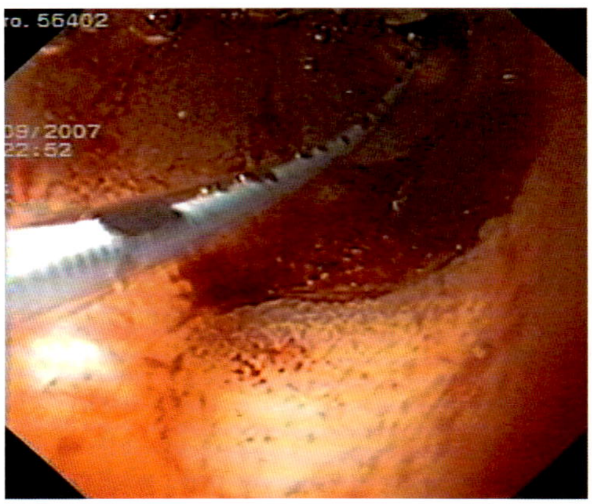

3

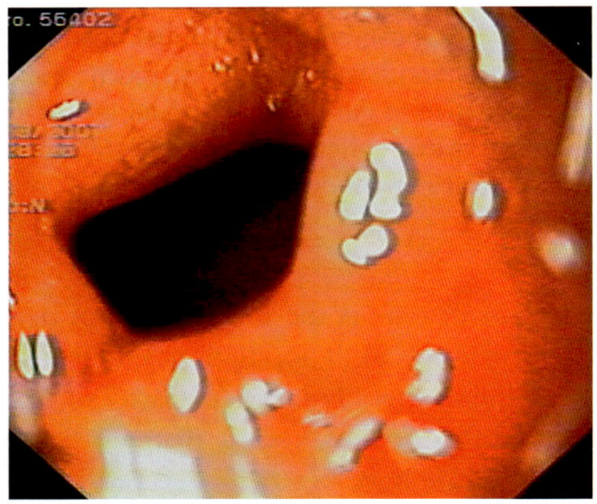

4

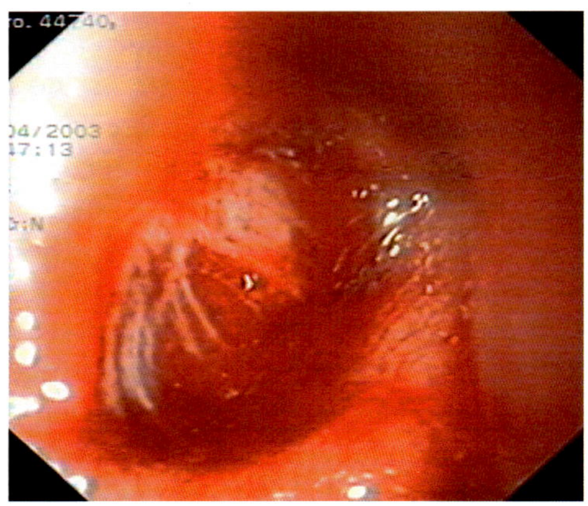

5

Fig. 1. Endoscopic view with a slim endoscope with the guidewire introduced into the distal part of the duodenum.

Fig. 2. Endoscopic view of pyloric stenosis.

Fig. 3. Endoscopic view of an inflated through-the-scope balloon catheter properly positioned in a pyloric stricture.

Fig. 4. Endoscopic view of pyloric stenosis immediately after successful dilation.

Fig. 5. Endoscopic view of a duodenal perforation immediately after pyloric dilation.

through the stricture, allowing the endoscopist to study the length of the stricture, to examine the duodenum and also to introduce easily the guidewire into the distal part of the duodenum (fig. 1). The most commonly balloon dilators used are the controlled radial expansion wire-guided balloon dilators (Boston Scientific Corp., Natick, Mass., USA). These balloons have a flexible tip that minimizes the risk of perforation and they are able to deliver three distinct pressure-controlled diameters with a high degree of radial vector force at any given pressure.

Apply silicone spray to the balloon and gently rub over the entire balloon surface to ensure uniform coverage. Advance the balloon catheter into the scope using short, 2- to 3-cm movements. A guidewire is used to advance the balloon, enhancing its placement. It is possible to use a common guidewire and place it under endoscopic guidance with a slim or super-slim endoscope. Another option is to use a wire-guided balloon dilator. Once the balloon is positioned across the stricture, it is inflated with either sterile water or sterile saline by using a pressure gun, up to the pressure recommended by the manufacturer to achieve the desired diameter. This procedure is usually performed under direct endoscopic visualization (fig. 2–4), although in some cases it can also be performed under fluoroscopic guidance [6]. In this case, sterile saline mixed with a contrast agent is used. The balloon diameter should be selected by the clinical condition of the patient and by the endoscopic appearance of the stricture. The procedure is repeated in 1–2 weeks, until outlet obstruction symptoms disappear.

Studies about gastric outlet obstruction of peptic origin show a response from as low as 16% [8] to as high 88% [9], with disappearance of all the associated lesions, as reflux esophagitis and gastric ulcers [9]. Recent reports suggest that endoscopic therapy combined with *H. pylori* eradication can provide sustained relief in such patients [10–12] and there have been reports of resolution of gastric outlet obstruction after eradication of the infection [1]. In corrosive induced pyloric stenosis, intralesional steroid injections combined with EBD can be an effective treatment [13]. Cost comparisons suggest that the surgical approach to gastric outlet obstruction, with vagotomy and pyloroplasty, is approximately 10-fold higher compared with endoscopic treatment [14].

Limitations and Complications

EBD for benign pyloric stenosis is usually effective and offers symptom relief in the majority of patients, however treatment failure occurs in a small group of patients [1]. Perng et al. [15] prospectively studied 42 patients with benign gastric outlet obstruction who underwent EBD in order to identify factors that predict failure of endoscopic therapy. The only statistically significant prognostic factor was the need for more than two courses of balloon dilation in order to achieve symptom relief [15]. In another study, duration of endoscopic treatment (<1 vs. >1 year) and number of dilatations (<3 vs. >3) were statistically significant prognostic factors that predicted the need for surgery [16]. Complications of EBD include perforation and bleeding. Perforation complicates the procedure in 0–12% of patients [4, 6, 9]. The incidence of perforation seems to be related to the diameter of the balloon used, increasing after 16 mm dilation [6, 12]. 15 mm may be the optimal size for dilation of a strictured gastric outlet [17].

Postprocedure Care

Following dilation, as after every endoscopic dilation of the GI tract, we recommend to explore endoscopically the dilated stenosis in order to see the lesion and diagnose possible complications, such as bleeding or perforation (fig. 5). If bleeding is present, we will try to see clearly the lesion and will treat endoscopically if possible. If perforation is present, its management depends on the size of the hole. If it is small it could be possible to close the hole with hemoclips [18] and in some cases with the combined use of hemoclips and endoloops [19]. If the perforation is too big it is better to go to surgery.

After the procedure the patient is monitored for signs and symptoms of perforation and bleeding. Afterwards the patients are allowed to take clear liquids and the diet is advanced to a regular diet as tolerated. In case of active *H. pylori* infection, appropriate antimicrobial and acid-suppressive therapy should be administered [1]. If dilation fails, symptoms frequently recur, or perforation occurs, surgery can be performed without compromising patient outcomes [17].

Tricks

These include the following: (1) The use a slim endoscope to: (i) see the whole stenosis, (ii) pass to the second part of the duodenum, and (iii) easily pass the guidewire. (2) If *H. pylori* infection is present, previous treatment of the infection is highly recommended. (3) Do not use dilators >16 mm in order to avoid the risk of perforation. (4) Finally, explore endoscopically the treated stenosis immediately after finishing the dilation in order to diagnose without delay possible complications.

References

1 Yusuf TE, Brugge WR: Endoscopic therapy of benign pyloric stenosis and gastric outlet obstruction. Curr Opin Gastroenterol 2006;22:570–573.

2 Griffin SM, Chung SC, Leung JW, Li AK: Peptic pyloric stenosis treated by endoscopic balloon dilatation. Br J Surg 1989;76:1147–1148.

3 Schmudderich W, Harloff M, Riemann JF: Through-the-scope balloon dilatation of benign pyloric stenoses. Endoscopy 1989;21:7–10.

4 Kochhar R, Dutta U, Sethy PK, Singh G, Sinha SK, Nagi B, et al: Endoscopic balloon dilation in caustic-induced chronic gastric outlet obstruction. Gastrointest Endosc 2009;69:800–805.

5 Muñoz-Navas M, García L, Macías E, Val J, Zozaya JM: Through-the-scope balloon dilatation of benign gastric outlet stenosis. Medium and long-term results. Endoscopy 1992;24:629–630.

6 Kim JH, Shin JH, Di ZH, Ko GY, Yoon HK, Sung KB, et al: Benign duodenal strictures: treatment by means of fluroscopically guided balloon dilation. J Vasc Interv Radiol 2005;16:543–548.

7 Matsui T, Hatakeyama K, Ikeda K, Yao T, Takenaka K, Sakurai T: Long-term outcome of endoscopic balloon dilation in obstructive gastroduodenal Crohn's disease. Endoscopy 1997;29:640–645.

8 Kuwada SK, Alexander GL: Long-term outcome of endoscopic dilation of non-malignant pyloric stenosis. Gastrointest Endosc 1995;41:15–17.

9 Muñoz-Navas M, Jimenez J, Subtil JC, Betes M, Macias E, Borda F: Long-term outcome of endoscopic dilation of benign gastric outlet obstruction. Gastrointest Endosc 1997;45:AB97.

10 Kochhar R, Sethy PK, Nagi B, Wig JD: Endoscopic balloon dilatation of benign gastric outlet obstruction. J Gastroenterol Hepatol 2004;19:418–422.

11 Cherian PT, Cherian S, Singh P: Long-term follow-up of patients with gastric outlet obstruction related to peptic ulcer disease treated with endoscopic balloon dilatation and drug therapy. Gastrointest Endosc 2007;66:491–497.

12 Lam YH, Lau JY, Fung TM, Ng EK, Wong SK, Sung JJ, et al: Endoscopic balloon dilation for benign gastric outlet obstruction with or without *Helicobacter pylori* infection. Gastrointest Endosc 2004;60:229–233.

13 Kochard R, Sriram PV, Ray JD, Kumar S, Nagi B, Sing K: Intralesional steroid for corrosive induced pyloric stenosis. Endoscopy 1998;30:734–736.

14 Kozarek RA, Botoman VA, Patterson DJ: Long-term follow-up in patients who have undergone balloon dilation for gastric outlet obstruction. Gastrointest Endosc 1990;36:558–561.

15 Perng CL, Lin HJ, Lo WC, Lai CR, Guo WS, Lee SD: Characteristics of patients with benign gastric outlet obstruction requiring surgery after endoscopic balloon dilation. Am J Gastroenterol 1996;91:987–990.

16 Boylan JJ, Gradzka MI: Long-term results of endoscopic balloon dilatation for gastric outlet obstruction. Dig Dis Sci 1999;44:1883–1886.
17 DiSario JA, Fennerty MB, Tietze CC, Hutson WR, Burt RW: Endoscopic balloon dilation for ulcer-induced gastric outlet obstruction. Am J Gastroenterol 1994;89:868–871.
18 Fujii T, Ono A, Fu KI: A novel endoscopic suturing technique using a specially designed so-called '8-ring' in combination with resolution clips. Gastrointest Endosc 2007;66:1215–1220.
19 Matsuda T, Fujii T, Emura F, Kozu T, Saito Y, Ikematsu H, et al: Complete closure of a large defect after EMR of a lateral spreading colorectal tumor when using a two-channel colonoscope. Gastrointest Endosc 2004;60:836–838.

Muñoz-Navas, MD, PhD
Gastroenterology Department, University Clinic of Navarra
School of Medicine, University of Navarra
ES–31008 Pamplona (Spain)
Tel. +34 948296730, Fax +34 948296500, E-Mail mmunoz@unav.es

Mönkemüller K, Wilcox CM, Muñoz-Navas M (eds): Interventional and Therapeutic Gastrointestinal Endoscopy.
Front Gastrointest Res. Basel, Karger, 2010, vol 27, pp 174–184

Stents for Gastric Outlet Obstruction

Jesús García-Cano

Department of Digestive Diseases, Hospital Virgen de la Luz, Cuenca, Spain

Abstract

The term malignant gastric outlet obstruction (MGOO) refers to cancers located in three areas that prevent proper gastric empting: antropyloric zone, pylorobulbar area and descending duodenum or postbulbar area. Tumoral strictures in these anatomical regions can be rechanneled by means of self-expanding metal stents (SEMS) as a palliative measure. Dedicated enteral SEMS are very similar for colonic obstruction and MGOO and differ from esophageal and biliary endoprosthesis. Endoscopic insertion of SEMS for MGOO relies on crossing the stricture with a guidewire inserted through the working channel of a therapeutic endoscope. Afterwards, the undeployed SEMS is glided over the guidewire inside the working channel and opens up, bridging the entire stricture. Both endoscopic and fluoroscopic monitoring during the procedure are the best methods to achieve success. Insertion of SEMS for MGOO takes part in advanced therapeutic endoscopy. These interventions are not as complex as, for instance, endoscopic retrograde cholangiopancreatography, but special interventional skills are needed for the endoscopic team. An average 94% technical success and 87% clinical success have been reported. However, palliation for these patients should not only focus on food passage but also on other factors that might decrease the quality of life. A complication rate of <30% can occur. The majority of complications are minor in severity but perforation and death have been reported. In general, palliation of MGOO by means of SEMS insertion compares favorably with surgical palliation.

Obstruction is a pathological phenomenon common to all tubular organs of the body. The pathophysiological consequences vary in relation to the anatomical location of the obstruction. Technological advances allow the use of different materials to build self-expanding metal stents (SEMS). SEMS are meshed cylindrical tubes of various lengths and widths that can be inserted in a folded state. This property allows their passage beyond severe strictures, usually without the need of previous dilation. Once inside the obstructed area, SEMS are opened by a release mechanism that provides sufficient diameter to re-canalize the stenosed area. SEMS can be modified according to the anatomic location, and are used to achieve patency in the obstruction of tubular structures such as the coronary arteries, trachea, and most of the digestive tract and bile duct [1].

Nowadays, stents woven from a single length of nickel-titanium alloy (nitinol) are replacing designs made from multiple strands of stainless steel wire, because they have a smoother finish, the risk of trauma to the bowel wall is reduced, and stent failure from entanglement of wire ends is avoided. Furthermore, nitinol stents are softer and more flexible, but retain shape-memory of their original configuration [2].

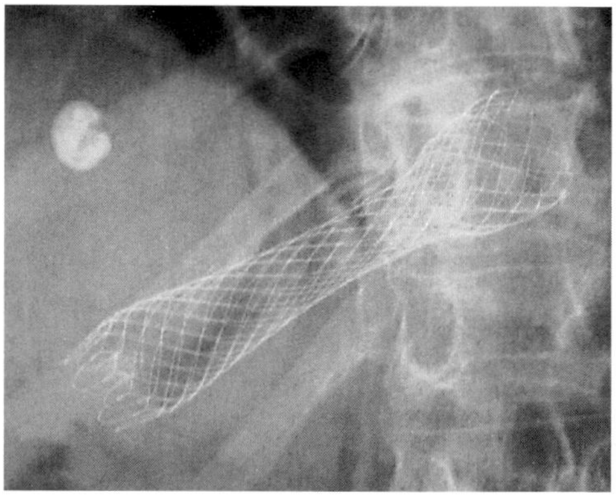

Fig. 1. Enteral Wallflex (made of nitinol) in the stomach. The flared end is located orally in the upper part to prevent migration.

The term enteral SEMS includes endoprostheses for the treatment of malignant gastric outlet obstruction (MGOO) and malignant colorectal obstructions. Usually, the design in both cases is similar, although the endoprosthesis has an end wider than the rest of the stent, which is located orally in relation to the obstruction to help prevent SEMS migration (fig. 1). Since stents for MGOO are inserted by upper endoscopic techniques, and colorectal ones via the anus, this wider portion is already located in the folded endoprosthesis at a different end. Due to technological improvement, stent models can now be specifically designed to re-canalize tumoral obstructions of the gastric outlet (antrum, pylorus, and duodenum). MGOO refers to cancers located in three areas that prevent proper gastric empting (fig. 2). Many reports on the use of SEMS for MGOO have included heterogeneous patient groups with different cancers such as pancreaticobiliary cancer, duodenal cancer, and gastric cancer.

Often, because of advanced disease and poor general condition, surgical intervention in patients with malignant upper intestinal obstruction can be associated with significant morbidity and mortality rates. In addition, it has been reported that delayed gastric emptying after gastrojejunostomy (GJJ) occurs in up to 57% of patients and leads to prolonged hospital stay.

Therefore, patients with MGOO from nonresectable cancer frequently are not surgical candidates but require some form of palliative care. In this way, SEMS are being used to palliate MGOO since the 1990s [3].

SEMS for MGOO as opposed to stents for malignant colorectal obstruction [4] are usually inserted only with a palliative purpose. The concept of using SEMS as a bridge to surgery has not yet been clearly established for stents for MGOO. Unlike acute colonic obstruction, which needs urgent treatment, obstruction of the gastric outlet can be managed with nil per os and fluidotherapy, sometimes with aspiration by a nasogastric tube if surgery is not delayed too much.

Patient Preparation

The simplest way to diagnose MGOO is upper endoscopy plus biopsy in patients with typical clinical symptoms (vomiting, food intolerance, stomach dilatation with retained food). An image technique for the TNM assessment would be advisable.

As in all other digestive procedures, written informed consent must be obtained from each patient before the endoscopic intervention. The procedure, outcomes and possible complications

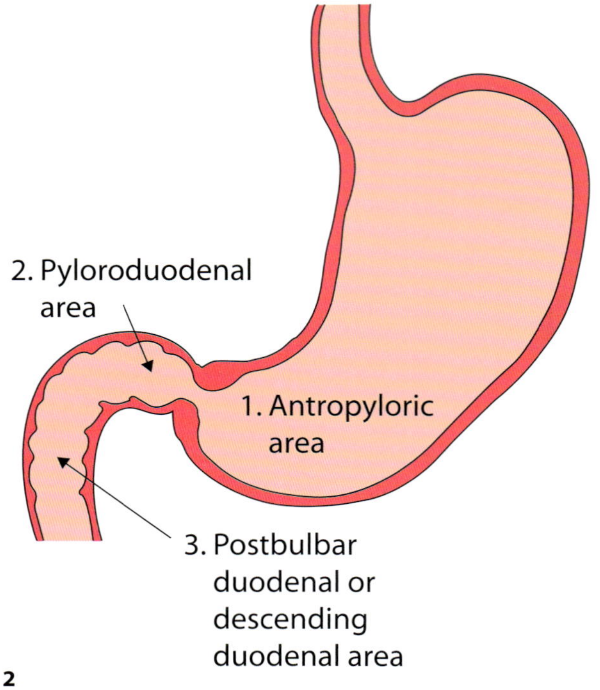

2

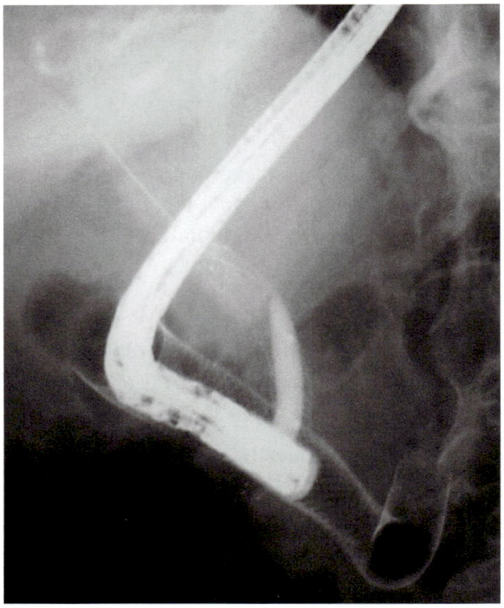

3

Fig. 2. The term malignant gastric outlet obstruction (MGOO) refers to cancers located in three areas that prevent adequate gastric emptying. **Fig. 3.** After a duodenal stent has been inserted covering the papillary area, cannulation of the bile duct by ERCP is very difficult and time-consuming. Sometimes it succeeds, as in this case. Balloon dilation was performed to solve an obstruction of a previously inserted biliary stent.

should also be explained to some close relatives, unless the patient is unwilling. Potentially curable disease has to be excluded. However, the patient can undergo curative surgery after stenting, sometimes with no special surgical complications because of the stent. The only disadvantage can be the previous unnecessary costs of the stenting procedure.

Barium studies of the upper gastrointestinal tract and cross-sectional images like those obtained by CT are not completely necessary to perform the procedure. However, as much information as possible should be obtained to overcome any technical difficulties that can appear during the stenting procedure.

In the same way, dysphagia scores or quality-of-life questionnaires are not completely necessary on exclusively clinical grounds, but often they can offer appropriate information about the patient's clinical status. Food intake can be assessed using the standardized Gastric Outlet Obstruction Scoring System (GOOSS): 0 = no oral intake; 1 = liquids only; 2 = soft foods, and 3 = solid food/full diet [5].

The gastric cavity must be cleaned of retained food as much as possible to facilitate the endoscopic procedure and avoid aspiration. Sometimes, patients have to have a nasogastric tube to ensure proper cleaning, apart from being on nil per os for at least 8 h before the procedure.

Biliary patency must be evaluated, especially in patients with tumors located in the descending duodenum (fig. 2). Patients with suspected biliary obstruction (cholestatic liver biochemistry) should undergo biliary drainage by insertion of an expandable metal stent, either endoscopically or radiologically. In patients already with a plastic biliary stent in place, it might be better to replace it with an expandable metal biliary stent. One must keep in mind that, after a duodenal stent has been inserted covering the papillary area, cannulation of the bile duct by endoscopic retrograde cholangiopancreatography (ERCP) is very difficult, time consuming (fig. 3) and sometimes, almost impossible. However, Mutignani et al. [6] published a study in which they were successful placed a biliary stent through the meshes of duodenal stents. After achieving biliary cannulation they either widened the meshes of the enteral stent with a pneumatic balloon or removed those covering the papilla with a rat-tooth foreign body forceps or argon plasma coagulation. They even treated patients with concurrent biliary and duodenal obstruction by initially placing a duodenal stent followed by a biliary stent, which was successful in 13 of 14 patients (95%). These results provide evidence that enteral balloon dilation of the duodenal stricture to reach the papilla for placement of a biliary stent before enteral SEMS placement is not a prerequisite. In this way, the risk of perforation for malignant stricture dilation is avoided. But these results come from a single expert center, and it remains to be established whether the same results could be achieved in the community.

Choosing the Appropriate Stent

Most published data relate to patients treated with enteral stents that can be inserted through the working channel of the scope (also called TTS). Until recently, the duodenal Wallstent (Boston Scientific, Natick, Mass., USA) was the most used SEMS [7]. This is a stainless steel woven stent that is preloaded on a delivery system that can be introduced through the working channel of a therapeutic endoscope with subsequent deployment controlled by both fluoroscopic and endoscopic views. The limited flexibility of the metal wire mesh of the Wallstent might contribute to stent migration. Also, the sharp ends of the metal meshes of the Wallstent may injure the intestinal wall, could lead to ulceration with the associated risk of bleeding and perforation. Recently, the same manufacturer launched a new enteral stent, Wallflex, which is made of nitinol instead of stainless steel. This new stent was constructed to provide improved flexibility while maintaining lumen integrity; it has looped ends to reduce the risk of mucosal injury and has a proximal flared end (fig. 1) to minimize the risk of stent migration [8]. The duodenal Wallflex stent is available with a diameter of 27 mm at the flared end and 22 mm at the body. The usual lengths are 6, 9, and 12 cm. The stent is already preloaded on a 10-french delivery system. This SEMS is uncovered (bare) over the mesh, and this allows the tumor to penetrate the metal cells, thus decreasing migration. However, the tumor can grow into the stent and obstruct it over time.

Other enteral stents made of nitinol are the Niti-S Duodenal [9] and Colonic Stent D-type (Taewoong Medical, Seoul, Korea). According to the manufacturer, the D-weaved feature contributes to the flexibility for proper adjustment with the curved anatomy of the duodenum. It also has blunt ends to avoid mucosal damage. The Hanaro stent (M.I. Tech Co. Ltd., Seoul, Korea) also has flare-shaped ends [10]. Niti-S and Hanaro stents are available as uncovered or covered types with different lengths. Covered stents have polyurethane in the body and in the distal flare portion, whilst the proximal end is uncoated to prevent migration. Covered stents have some risk of biliary outflow blockage when the papilla of Vater is covered by the SEMS.

In addition, endoscopists can also use non-TTS stents [11] such as the Ultraflex esophageal stent (Boston Scientific, Natick, Mass., USA).

It is important to place stents that are long enough to extend around flexures; 9 cm is usually the minimum length required to cover a bend, and shorter stents often require extension with a second one. All stents shorten during deployment and this must be taken into account. Fortunately, most delivery systems allow re-sheathing of a partially deployed stent if things go wrong.

As a general rule, endoscopists mostly choose TTS duodenal stents. Selection of the manufacturer often relates to availability, ease of use, and the previous experience of the whole endoscopic team (physicians and endoscopy assistants).

Technique

Stent placement is usually done with the patient under conscious sedation (midazolam and/or fentanyl). A therapeutic endoscope (working channel ≥3.7 mm), either forward (gastroscope, colonoscope) or side viewing (duodenoscope as for ERCP), is used for placement of the TTS enteral stent. Experience with instruments used for ERCP such as catheters and guidewires is very useful for successful insertion of duodenal and other digestive stents.

If the patient is in the prone position (as sometimes in ERCP) the 'C' of the descending duodenum is better delineated and anatomical orientation is improved (fig. 4). But the placement procedure can also be done with the patient in the usual position for upper endoscopy (left lateral decubitus).

The most critical step for SEMS insertion is the passage of a guidewire through the tumoral stricture to place it beyond the tumor, in healthy tissue (fig. 5). The undeployed stent is then glided over this guidewire and may be opened inside the tumor, thus solving the obstruction. Fluoroscopy guidance is the best method to ensure that the guidewire has been properly positioned. Besides, events beyond the stricture, such as stent opening, can be appropriately monitored by fluoroscopy. Malignant stricture dilation should be avoided for the possible risk or perforation.

Procedure Description

The endoscope with a therapeutic working channel is located in the proximal part of the tumor. A guidewire of 0.875 mm (0.035 inch) in diameter, fitted with an atraumatic hydrophilic tip, is passed through the working channel and the whole stenosed segment. This passage is confirmed by fluoroscopy. A biliary catheter used for ERCP is then introduced over the guidewire and the obstruction is delineated by contrast injection. The length of the stricture is also assessed. The catheter is then withdrawn and the undeployed stent is inserted over the guidewire. Ideally, the length of the stent has to exceed the stricture length by at least 2 cm. If one single stent does not cover the entire stricture, two stents can be overlapped (fig. 5). Once the SEMS is inside the stricture, it is gradually opened up to place it correctly with the proximal and distal ends located in healthy areas. During stent release the distal end, which is seen in the endoscopic view, shortens towards the stricture, therefore continuous adjustment is necessary. It is not advisable to advance a partially deployed stent, but it may be pulled back if it has been placed too distally. Care must be taken not to release the stent by accident. It is safer to re-sheath the stent and start again.

Preferably the flared proximal end of the stent should be placed proximal to the pylorus in the prepyloric distal antrum, which is called the transpyloric position (fig. 6), except when the

Fig. 4. If the patient is in the prone position for SEMS insertion, as sometimes in ERCP, the 'C' of the descending duodenum is better delineated and anatomical orientation is improved, as can be seen by this Wallstent inserted for a malignant duodenal stricture in the second part of the duodenum.

Fig. 5. Insertion technique of a self-expanding metal stent to palliate a duodenal obstruction secondary to pancreatic cancer. **a**. Endoscopic view of the stricture in the bulbar apex crossed by a guidewire. **b**. Radiological view. The guidewire located at the angle of Treitz passes the tumor. **c**. To open the whole stricture, two overlapped Wallstents were used from the pylorus up to the third portion of the duodenum. Previously, a Zilver stent had been placed in the common bile duct to palliate the patient's obstructive jaundice. Reproduced from García-Cano et al. [12] with permission.

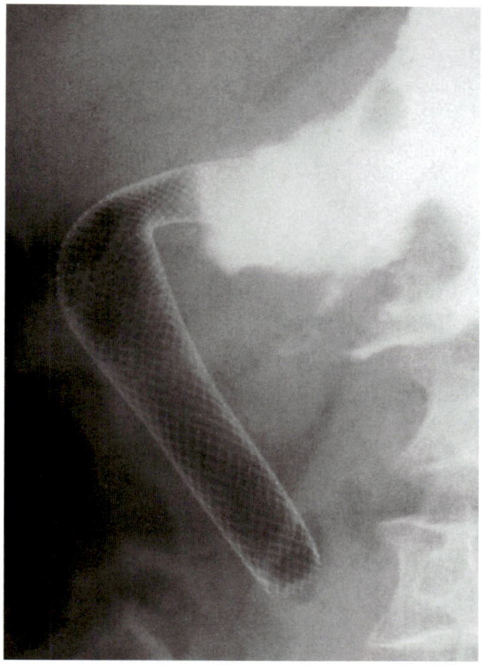

4

5

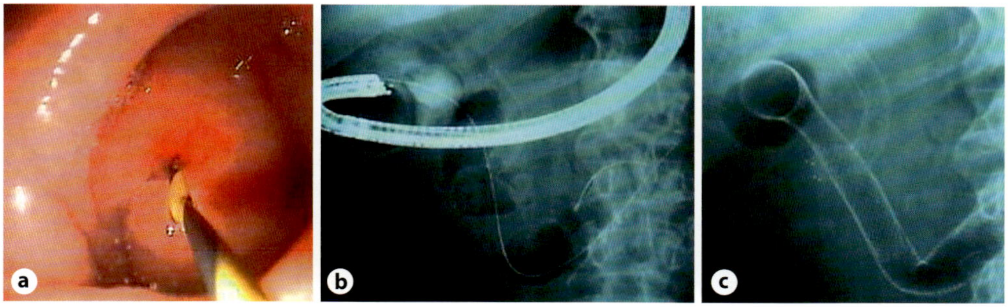

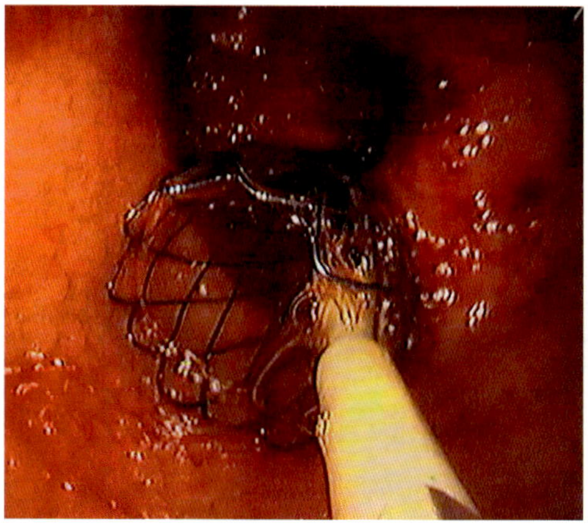

Fig. 6. A Wallflex stent immediately after release. The yellow rod in which it was mounted and folded may be seen. The end is in the gastric antrum outside the pylorus. This is called the transpyloric position for stents. Reproduced from García-Cano et al. [12] with permission.

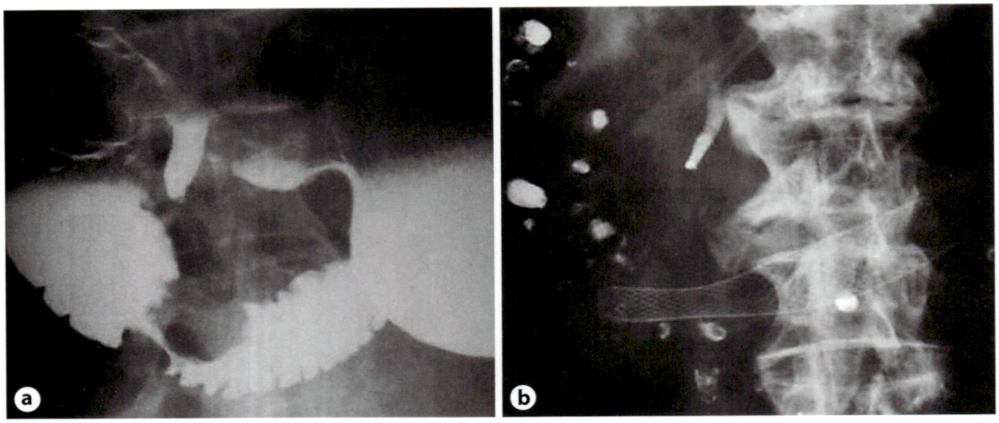

Fig. 7. **a** A 90-year-old patient with a tumoral stricture in the inferior duodenal angle. The barium contrast also reveals the common bile duct. **b** A Wallstent immediately after placement between the second and third duodenal portions. Reproduced from García-Cano et al. [12] with permission.

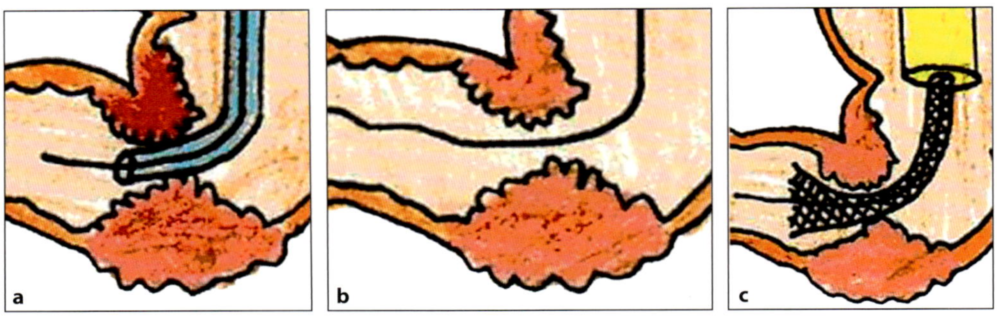

Fig. 8. Drawings showing a method for stent insertion by means of an ultrathin endoscope [13]. **a** An ultrathin gastroscope is employed to pass the severe tumoral strictures causing gastric outlet obstruction. A guidewire is placed beyond the stricture. **b** The ultrathin endoscope is removed leaving the guidewire in place. During withdrawal, the characteristics of the stricture (length, shape) are assessed. **c** The guidewire is then backloaded into a therapeutic endoscope. Insertion of a through-the-scope (TTS) stent is then performed. If a non-TTS SEMS is chosen, insertion and deployment can be monitored with the endoscope side-to-side. Courtesy of Dr. Elisa Bermejo-Saiz.

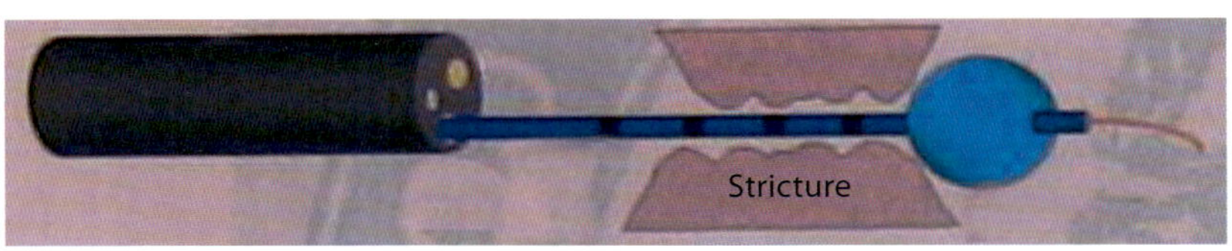

Fig. 9. A balloon with visible endoscopic marks can be useful to measure the length of the stricture, according to Kwon et al. [14].

obstruction is in the more distal duodenum (fig. 7). This is not based on any literature but on the general belief of the endoscopists that the anti-migration end of the stent works better if placed prepylorically.

If fluoroscopy facilities are not available, other techniques can be used. Nowadays, several models of very small-caliber endoscopes (ultrathin endoscopes, UTEs) are available. They are able to pass through many strictures in the digestive tract. According to our previously described technique [13], once the tumor is traversed by a 6-mm diameter endoscope (for instance Pentax EG-1870 K), a guidewire is left in place through the UTE working channel (fig. 8). Subsequently the UTE is removed, leaving the guidewire in place beyond the stenosis. This guidewire is then inserted in a retrograde manner in the therapeutic endoscope working channel, and an SEMS is placed over it. This technique is riskier because only upstream events (in the endoscopic view) are properly monitored, whilst downstream maneuvers are done blindly.

The small caliber endoscope can also be used together with fluoroscopy to negotiate difficult strictures. Usually, there is no need for dilation before insertion. After stent deployment hydrostatic balloon dilatation is rarely performed when the extent of SEMS expansion is considered inadequate.

Kwon et al. [14] described another method for insertion of SEMS without fluoroscopy. A balloon catheter is inserted as far as possible past the stenosis; an air-inflated balloon catheter was then slowly retrieved; the length of stenosis is measured with marking, and an adequate length of SEMS is inserted in that order. This method is even riskier than the UTE, because the duodenum beyond the stricture is not seen at all. However, the balloon catheter with marks can be useful to properly measure the stricture length when using fluoroscopy (fig. 9). At the end of the procedure the position of the stent must be confirmed endoscopically and fluoroscopically (or with radiographs).

Enteral SEMS insertion can be performed on an outpatient basis. However, it is recommended to keep patients in hospital for 24 h, and try tolerance to liquids the next day.

Outcomes

Evaluation of results achieved with endoscopic SEMS insertion to palliate MGOO must focus on several issues: (1) technical success (adequate placement of the stent bridging the entire stricture); (2) clinical success (improving symptoms related to delayed gastric emptying, i.e., vomiting, and the subjective perception of the patient of adequate food passage); (3) occurrence of complications, early or late, related to stent insertion; (4) comparison with the standard surgical care for MGOO, which is GJJ, and (5) improving the global quality of life of patients.

Holt et al. [15] reported a review of published series from 1996 to 2004. There were in total 433 patients. Technical success was 94%, and clinical success 87%. Stent migration was seen in 16% of covered stents and 2.7% of uncovered ones. Stent patency was 105 days. There were no intervention-related deaths, patients had a short procedure-related hospital stay, and they were able of resuming oral intake usually within 4 days after stent placement.

Early major complications (in the 7 days after the procedure) have been reported on average in 1% (0–10%). The most severe is perforation. If a gastroduodenal perforation occurs during insertion, an urgent procedure will probably be needed under difficult conditions. Recently, the closure of a perforation due to a gastroduodenal SEMS by means of another covered SEMS has been reported [16]. Other types of major early complications are bleeding, migration, aspiration

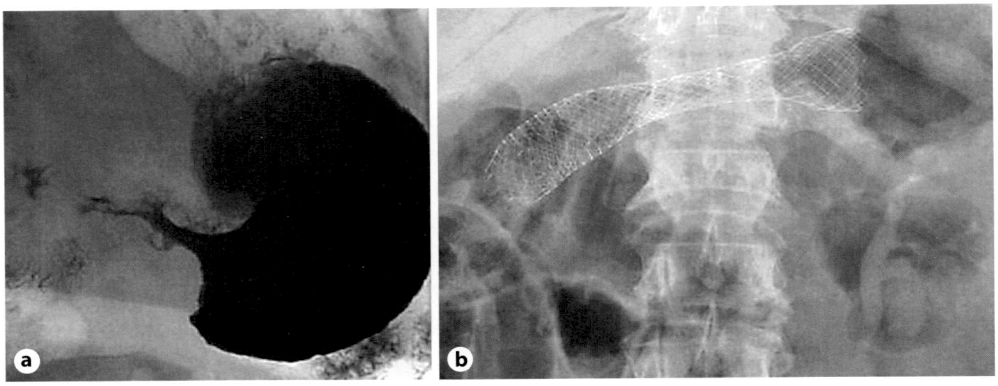

10

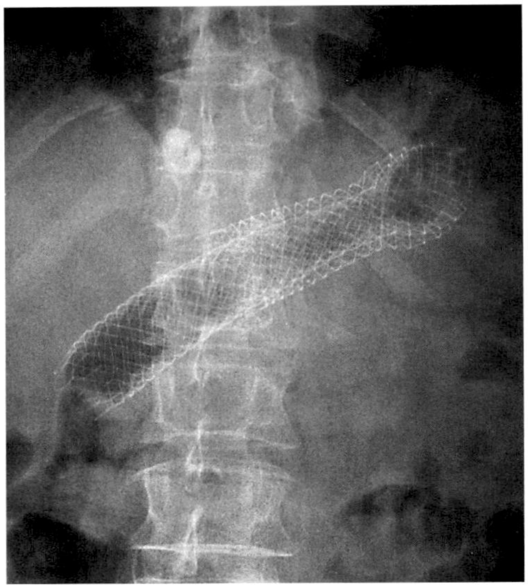

11

Fig. 10. **a** Tumoral gastric obstruction located in the antropyloric area. **b** A Wallflex stent was inserted from the beginning of the descending duodenum until the non-affected antrum. Both stent ends are open demonstrating that the stricture has been properly re-canalized. Nevertheless, the patient's obstructive symptoms did not improve and he had to undergone surgery. Sometimes dysfunction occurs in stents which are apparently in the correct position.

Fig. 11. Wallflex stent obstruction solved by insertion of a longer SEMS in the same patient as in figure 1.

pneumonia, cholangitis and dysfunction. The term dysfunction refers to a delayed gastric emptying through a SEMS which is apparently in the correct position (fig. 10). Carcinomatosis or multiple small bowel obstructions have to be ruled out if the GOOSS does not improve. Some migrated stents can pass via the anus without the patient's knowledge. Patients receiving chemotherapy have more frequent migration specially with covered SEMS.

Minor early complications have been reported in 26% (0–30%); mainly mild pain. The most frequent late complication is obstruction by tumor growth into mesh cells that can be easily solved endoscopically by the insertion of new stents (fig. 11). It is important to know that the biological activity and response to chemotherapy or radiotherapy can differ according to the type of cancer, which might affect the stent patency and clinical outcome.

As treatment of MGOO with SEMS exspands from specialized centers to the community, figures for success and complications are less good, but remain highly acceptable. In this way, in a retrospective study performed in 15 Spanish centers, Pérez-Miranda et al. [17] found that a good clinical outcome was achieved in 58/71 (81.7%) patients, with 3 severe complications (perforation, aspiration pneumonia and mesenteric ischemia), all resulting in death (3/71 or 4.2%).

They conclude that SEMS offer good palliation to most patients with MGOO, but perhaps prior reports seem to underestimate complications.

A particular situation is obstruction at the anastomosis site after surgery. Song et al. [18] found that simultaneous double stent placement (covered and uncovered) is technically feasible and effective for palliative treatment of recurrent malignant obstruction after gastric surgery. Double stent placement was found to be important to prevent tumor ingrowth, especially very early restenosis, and to have a more prolonged stent patency. They suggest that this procedure should be considered rather than an uncovered stent alone as the primary choice for palliation of obstruction in such patients.

In a systematic review by Jeurnink et al. [19] on stents versus GJJ for the palliation of MGOO, they found better results in initial clinical success (89% stents vs. 72% GJJ) and minor complications in the patient series (9% stents vs. 33% GJJ). Hospital stay was prolonged after GJJ compared to stent placement (13 vs. 7 days). On the other hand, recurrent obstructive symptoms were more common after stent placement (18% stents vs. 1% GJJ). The mean survival was 105 days after stent placement and 164 days after GJJ. Mean costs reported by Mittal et al. [20] in 2004 were USD 8,680 for stent placement, USD 20,060 for open GJJ, and USD 16,552 for laparoscopic GJJ.

Therefore, stent placement may be associated with more favorable results in patients with a relatively short life expectancy, while GJJ could be preferable in patients with a more prolonged prognosis. However, the paucity of evidence from large randomized trials may have influenced the results, and consequently trials of sufficient size are needed to determine which palliative treatment modality is optimal in certain subgroups of patients with MGOO.

Finally, whilst the GOOSS improves in the majority of patients after SEMS placement, some studies fail to achieve a significant improvement in the global quality of life during the remainder of patients' lives. It appears feasible that palliative treatment for these patients should definitely not only be focused on food passage but also on other factors that might potentially decrease the quality of life, such as pain, deterioration of the patient's physical condition and mental support [21].

Conclusions

Endoscopic placement of an enteral SEMS offers effective palliation by means of a minimally invasive procedure for patients with nonresectable MGOO. Stent insertion has a faster relief of symptoms compared to open or laparoscopic GJJ. As a consequence, hospital stay is usually shorter in the majority of patients. Many of them are able to eat soft solids after 1–4 days. Technical and clinical success rates are high and mortality related to the procedure is rare after stent placement. In addition, costs are lower than surgical palliative GJJ. However, the longer the patient survives, the higher the risk of stent re-obstruction from tumor overgrowth or ingrowth, although SEMS can be reopened by inserting a new stent.

After SEMS placement obstructive symptoms can improve until death. However, to achieve progress in global quality of life, efforts have not only to be focused on food passage but on other physical and mental conditions.

References

1 Baron TH: Expandable metal stents for the treatment of cancerous obstructions of the gastrointestinal tract. N Engl J Med 2001;344:1681–1687.
2 Laasch HU, Martin DF, Maetani I: Enteral stents in the gastric outlet and duodenum. Endoscopy 2005;37:74–81.
3 Kozarek RA, Ball TJ, Patterson DJ: Metallic self-expanding stent application in the upper gastrointestinal tract: caveats and concerns. Gastrointest Endosc 1992;38:1–6.
4 García-Cano J, González-Huix F, Juzgado D, et al: Use of self-expanding metal stents to treat malignant colorectal obstruction in general endoscopic practice (with videos). Gastrointest Endosc 2006;64: 914–920.
5 Adler DG, Baron TH: Endoscopic palliation of malignant gastric outlet obstruction using self-expanding metal stents: experience in 36 patients. Am J Gastroenterol 2002;97:72–78.
6 Mutignani M, Tringali A, Shah SG, et al: Combined endoscopic stent insertion in malignant biliary and duodenal obstruction. Endoscopy 2007;39:440–447.
7 Dormann A, Meisner S, Verin N, et al: Self-expanding metal stents for gastroduodenal malignancies: systematic review of their clinical effectiveness. Endoscopy 2004;36:543–550.
8 van Hooft J, Mutignani M, Repici A, et al: First data on the palliative treatment of patients with malignant gastric outlet obstruction using the WallFlex enteral stent: a retrospective multicenter study. Endoscopy 2007;39:434–439.
9 Maetani I, Isayama H, Mizumoto Y: Palliation in patients with malignant gastric outlet obstruction with a newly designed enteral stent: a multicenter study. Gastrointest Endosc 2007;66:355–360.
10 Nassif T, Prat F, Meduri B, et al: Endoscopic palliation of malignant gastric outlet obstruction using self-expandable metallic stents: results of a multicenter study. Endoscopy 2003;35:483–489.
11 Maetani I, Ukita T, Tada T, et al: Metallic stents for gastric outlet obstruction: reintervention rate is lower with uncovered versus covered stents, despite similar outcomes. Gastrointest Endosc 2009 ;69:806–812.
12 García-Cano J, Sánchez-Manjavacas N, Viñuelas-Chicano M, et al: Palliative management of malignant gastric outlet obstruction with endoscopically inserted self-expanding metal stents (in Spanish and English). Rev Esp Enferm Dig 2008;100:320–326.
13 García-Cano J: Use of an ultrathin gastroscope to allow endoscopic insertion of enteral wallstents without fluoroscopic monitoring. Dig Dis Sci 2006 ;51:1231–1235.
14 Kwon C-I, Ko KH, Han C, et al: A new method of endoscopic stent insertion for gastrointestinal luminal stenosis without fluoroscopic assistance. Gastrointest Endosc 2007;65:AB280.
15 Holt AP, Patel M, Ahmed MM: Palliation of patients with malignant gastroduodenal obstruction with self-expanding metallic stents: the treatment of choice? Gastrointest Endosc 2004;60:1010–1017.
16 Small AJ, Petersen BT, Baron TH: Closure of a duodenal stent-induced perforation by endoscopic stent removal and covered self-expandable metal stent placement (with video). Gastrointest Endosc 2007; 66:1063–1065.
17 Pérez-Miranda M, Espinós J, Juzgado D, et al: Palliation of malignant gastric outlet obstruction (GOO) with through-the-scope (TTS) expandable metal stents (EMS): a multicenter descriptive study. Gastrointest Endosc 2005; 61:AB178.
18 Song GA, Kang DH, Kim TO, et al: Endoscopic stenting in patients with recurrent malignant obstruction after gastric surgery: uncovered versus simultaneously deployed uncovered and covered (double) self-expandable metal stents. Gastrointest Endosc 2007;65:782–787.
19 Jeurnink SM, van Eijck CH, Steyerberg EW, et al: Stent versus gastrojejunostomy for the palliation of gastric outlet obstruction: a systematic review. BMC Gastroenterol 2007;7:18.
20 Mittal A, Windsor J, Woodfield J, et al: Matched study of three methods for palliation of malignant pyloroduodenal obstruction. Br J Surg 2004;91: 205–209.
21 van Hooft JE, Uitdehaag MJ, Bruno MJ: Efficacy and safety of the new WallFlex enteral stent in palliative treatment of malignant gastric outlet obstruction (DUOFLEX study): a prospective multicenter study. Gastrointest Endosc 2009;69:1059–1066.

J. García-Cano
Hospital Virgen de la Luz
ES–16002 Cuenca (Spain)
Tel. +34 660 010621, Fax +34 969 230407, E-Mail j.garcia-cano@terra.es

Mönkemüller K, Wilcox CM, Muñoz-Navas M (eds): Interventional and Therapeutic Gastrointestinal Endoscopy.
Front Gastrointest Res. Basel, Karger, 2010, vol 27, pp 185–197

Stents for Postoperative Upper Gastrointestinal Leaks

Daniel Schubert

Department of Surgery, Otto von Guericke University, Magdeburg, Germany

Abstract

Anastomotic leaks are the most severe complication after upper gastrointestinal surgery and a major source for mortality and morbidity. Meanwhile, endoscopic procedures, especially the placement of self-expanding stents, are an attractive treatment option to close the leak and to promote the healing process under these conditions. Endoscopic stent placement should be the treatment of choice in patients with symptomatic (septic), non-ischemic and sufficiently drained anastomotic leaks up to 60% of the anastomotic circumference after gastroesophageal surgery. Complete anastomotic healing of postsurgical leaks after stent placement, without the need of further surgical procedures, was reported in 67–100% with an acceptable mortality of 0–33%. The most frequent complications after stent placement seem to be the migration of the graft and strictures after stent removal, which can be treated in the majority of cases sufficiently by an endoscopic reintervention. Surgical reexploration must be considered if clinical improvement of the patient is not achieved with endoscopic treatment.

Anastomotic leaks after gastroesophageal resection continue to be a major source of mortality and morbidity, especially when leakage follows an intrathoracic anastomosis [1–4]. The incidence of this complication has been reported to be between 4 and 17% and it is responsible for approximately 40% of postoperative deaths [2–4]. The spectrum of manifestations of anastomotic leakage ranges from clinically silent to early fulminant leaks. A key issue is that there are no uniform methods for treating patients with symptomatic anastomotic leakage. Appropriate treatment must therefore be matched to the individual patient. Traditionally, some authors suggest surgical reexploration and repair (e.g. resection and diversion procedures), whereas others recommend a more conservative approach using parenteral nutrition, nasogastric decompression, perianastomotic drainage in the form of intercostal drains, or CT-guided percutaneous drainage and broad-spectrum antibiotics. However, aggressive surgical treatment is often associated with poor results and considerable mortality and morbidity, especially after delayed diagnosis of the leakage [1, 3]. A conservative approach is indicated only in selected patients with asymptomatic, non-septic and small anastomotic leaks, and it is associated with long hospitalization and long time enteral or parenteral nutrition support. Conservative treatment of clinically significant leaks was associated with mortality up to 30–45% and with a high rate of persistent leaks [5, 6].

However, during the past decade, the principles of management of postoperative anastomotic leaks after upper gastrointestinal surgery have shifted increasingly toward a more less surgically invasive but, nevertheless, endoscopically interventional approach, including endoscopic application of fibrin glue injections, use of clips and covered self-expanding stents to seal leakages [7]. Especially the use of stent seems to be a promising treatment option for many patients [7].

Clinical Presentation of Anastomotic Leaks

A postoperative leakage of the anastomotic suture is the most frequent and severe surgical complication following upper gastrointestinal surgery and the major source for surgical mortality [8]. For that reason, not only obvious clinical and laboratory signs suggestive of an anastomotic complication, such as body temperature >38°C, significant leukocytosis and increasing levels of C-reactive protein and procalcitonin and/or purulent exudation from the local drain, postoperative psychosyndrome, but also every disturbance of a normal postoperative course should lead to the suspicion of the presence of an anastomotic leak, which will require immediate diagnostic interventions. Endoscopy should be the first diagnostic step to detect a suspected postoperative leakage. The detection rate of postoperative anastomotic leaks and the sensitivity of endoscopy in experienced hands are superior to conventional radiological contrast studies in this context [9, 10]. For that reason, routine contrast studies after upper gastrointestinal surgery are not currently recommended [9, 10]. Endoscopy should clarify the following therapeutically relevant points: (1) size of the leakage (percent of the anastomotic circumference); (2) vitality and perfusion of the anastomotic line and interponate; (3) distance of the anastomosis from the mouth; (4) approximate luminal diameter, and (5) degree of contamination of the perianastomotic region, e.g. perianastomotic abscess formation, putrid fluid retention.

Non-ischemic anastomotic leaks up to 60% (two thirds) of the anastomotic circumference are suitable for endoscopic stent placement (fig. 1). Endoscopic treatment cannot be recommended for dehiscences of more than 60–70% of the anastomotic suture, complete dehiscences and anastomoses with an ischemic and devitalized anastomotic line (or interponate). A reoperation in these cases is mandatory. Furthermore, an early leakage occurring within the first 48–72 h postoperatively is mostly the result of relevant technical or surgical defaults (problems with the stapling device, difficulties with the suture line). An immediate surgical reexploration and revision of such early leaking and well-drained anastomosis can be effective and helpful, prior to a relevant perianastomotic inflammation.

In selected patients with non-symptomatic minor leaks (up to 10% of the anastomotic circumference, without septic signs), fibrin glue injection or endoscopic clipping could be an alternative and inexpensive treatment option for rapidly leak closure.

In many cases of larger dehiscences (more than 30% of the anastomotic suture), and especially after delayed leak diagnosis, an advanced putrid pleural or mediastinal inflammation of the perianastomotic region is seen (fig. 2). If possible, large dehiscences should be passed with an endoscope in order to explore the perianastomotic pleural or mediastinal cavity with regard to the degree of contamination. In those cases an endoscopic lavage and debridement of the perianastomotic region, prior to endoscopic leak closure, is useful, whenever significant putrid pleural inflammation is endoscopically detectable [11, 12]. This procedure, which equates traditional surgical cleansing of infected wounds, results in elimination of bacteria,

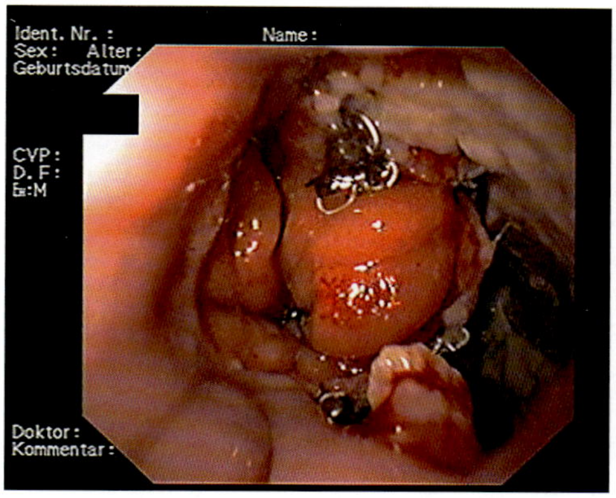

1

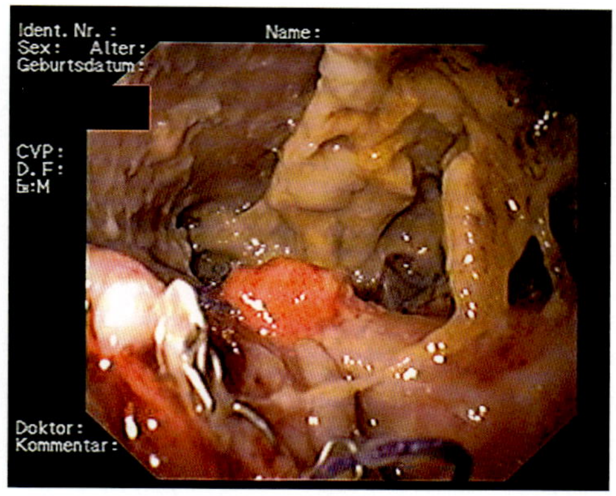

2

Fig. 1. Anastomotic leakage 5 days after an extended gastrectomy. Note that nearly 50% of the circumference is dehisced, without ischemia and tension. This is a good scenario for an endoscopic management.

Fig. 2. Anastomotic leakage 5 days after extended gastrectomy (same patient as in figure 1). Endoscopic view into the perianastomotic mediastinum with purulent surface and necrotic tissue. As is mandatory, endoscopic debridement was performed prior to stent placement in this patient.

noxious necrotic tissue and remains of gastrointestinal fluids from the fistula and the perianastomotic mediastinum and should thus lead to an improvement of the clinical situation and of local as well as systemic inflammation [11–14]. Endoscopic lavage and debridement should be performed daily or at 2-day intervals until the anastomotic fistula is sufficiently cleaned and incipient granulation and no more putrid tissue are seen. If these criteria are fulfilled, the anastomotic leak can be closed by stent placement [11, 12].

Radiological diagnostics, i.e. CT scans (mostly repetitive CT scans) and, if necessary, conventional contrast studies should resolve the following points in addition to endoscopy: (1) sufficient external drainage of the leak; (2) non-drained mediastinal/pleural or abdominal effusions, and (3) advanced pleural or abdominal infection, i.e. empyema or abscesses.

Appropriate external drainage of an anastomotic leak to minimize contamination of the perianastomotic region is a crucial precondition for endoscopic leak closure via stent placement. Endoscopic leak closure of non-drained leaks cannot be recommended. The stent would prevent the transit of internal effluent of toxic and infectious material from the contaminated perianastomotic region into the intestinal tract, resulting in perianastomotic fluid retention, abscess formation, pleura empyema, and in the worst case, mediastinitis.

In cases of non-drained or insufficiently drained leaks, the additional placement of drains or catheters (pigtails or chest drains) under CT guidance should be pursued in order to eliminate infectious fluid retentions prior to or in addition to endoscopic stent placement. However, there are some exceptions for such minimally invasive and interventional leak management, where surgery is still needed, in addition to endoscopic stent placement. Interventional external drain placement is mostly not suitable and sufficient in septic patients with pleural abscesses or empyema, due to intrathoracic leakages. In this scenario a radical surgical approach, i.e. evacuation of empyema and pleural decortication, for septic focus clearance should be considered (fig. 3). Relaparotomy, lavage and drainage of the abdominal cavity is inevitable in undrained intraabdominal esophageal leaks (e.g. after gastrectomy), which often lead to a diffuse contamination of the peritoneal cavity or when peritonitic signs are seen.

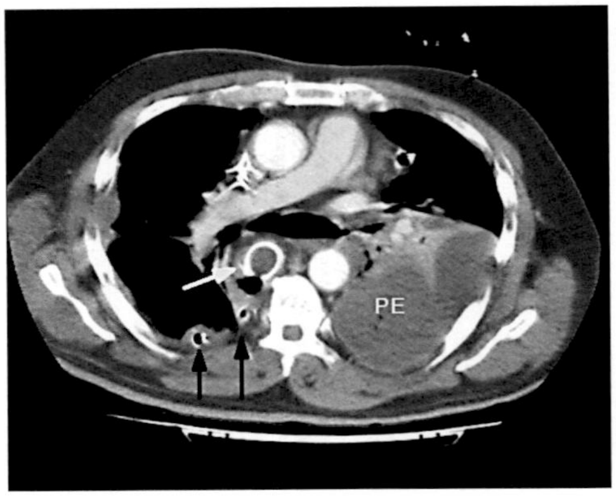

3

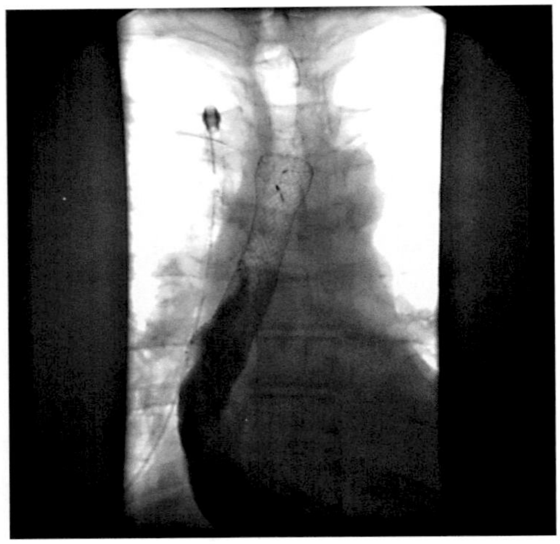

4

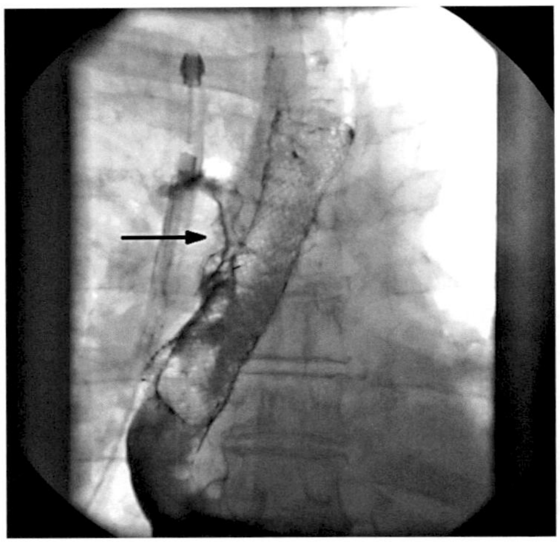

5

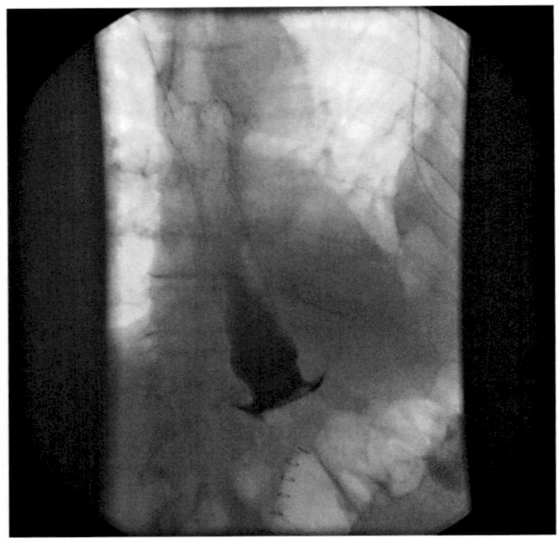

6

Fig. 3. CT scan of a septic patient with an anastomotic leakage after esophageal resection, with left-sided pleural empyema (PE) communicating with the leakage. The leak was covered by stent placement (white arrow). The right pleural cavity and mediastinum is sufficiently drained by intraoperatively placed chest drains (black arrows). The patient required an additional surgical evacuation (thoracoscopy) of the PE and placement of additional drainage of the left-sided pleura.

Fig. 4. First contrast swallow after stent placement for an anastomotic leak following esophageal resection. The swallow suggests a complete leak closure (see also figure 5).

Fig. 5. After 3 contrast swallows (same patient as in figure 4), with progressive filling of the gastric pull-up, retrograde regurgitation of the contrast medium from distal, alongside the stent into the pleura is seen (arrow), demonstrating persistent leakage in this patient.

Fig. 6. A specially designed, fully covered SEMS (ECO Cardia Umbrella®, Leufen Medical, Aachen, Germany) was placed for best anchorage and for leak closure and to decrease the reflux of gastric fluids from distally. This patient had undergone resection of the esophagogastric junction and developed an incongruent, leaking esophagogastric anastomosis. This specially designed stent allows for complete leak closure and prevents persistent leaks due to stent influx and reflux.

Technique of Endoscopic Stent Placement

The patient is placed in a supine position and endoscopy is performed under analgosedation. In cases where additional surgical procedures are contemplated (e.g. evacuation of pleural empyema, peritoneal lavage and drainage), the stent placement should be performed simultaneously under general anesthesia. Use of fluoroscopy (i.e. C-arm) is strongly recommended. However, in emergency settings, stent placement is feasible too, without fluoroscopic guidance, alongside the endoscope under direct visualization [15].

A standard guidewire is placed endoscopically crossing the anastomotic line. The anastomotic leak should be identified with radiopaque markers. All stents used for closing anastomotic leaks should be partially or fully covered (please refer to the Results section for an overview of different types of stents used for the closure of gastrointestinal anastomosis leaks). The unreleased stent is advanced over the guidewire and placed with its proximal and distal radiopaque markers above and below the leaking anastomosis. Now, the stent is delivered under fluoroscopic guidance or under direct visual control with the endoscope according to the instructions for use of the manufacturer. The stent should be deployed with at least 3–4 cm overlap proximal and distal to the leak with its covered part. Stents with a *proximal* release mechanism are recommended for this approach. After stent deployment, endoscopy is performed once again, to confirm correct stent placement and adequate leak closure. Additional nasojejunal tubes are not mandatory in cooperative patients, but very useful in ventilated patients: the nasojejunal tube helps for decompression and enteral feeding. However, oral fluid nutrition is feasible 4 h after stenting.

Technical Notes

Some differences and aspects regarding to esophageal anatomy and configuration of leaking upper gastrointestinal anastomoses need to be addressed. Complete leak closure is not seen in every leaking anastomosis in spite of technically perfect stent placement. This fact may be explainable due to esophageal anatomy and physiology, which may result in stent migration due to the contraction waves occurring during deglutition. In contrast to the bile duct, the esophagus is a non-rigid, motile tube, and it is technically demanding to seal a very contractile leaking tube with a less flexible stent graft completely. Nevertheless, in those cases the implanted stents reduce contamination of the perianastomotic region to a considerable extent, which is an essential precondition for the healing process of leaking anastomoses. Presumably, another advantage of stents is their pressure on the esophageal wall, which induces rapidly granulations and promotes accelerated physiological tissue repair for the definitive leak closure. Dehiscent esophagojejunal end-to-end or end-to-side anastomoses (e.g. after gastrectomy) are optimally suitable for stent placement. The inner diameter of the esophagus is approximately identically to the jejunal lumen. This fact allows mostly direct and complete leak closure for esophagojejunal inflow as well as for jejunoesophageal reflux, due to optimal stent adaption at the inner esophageal and jejunal walls with a minimal risk for stent dislocation. Stent placement is much more difficult in incongruent esophageal anastomoses with a gastric or colonic interponate or a jejunal pouch. The wider inner diameter of the interponate decreases stent anchoring ability distally and leak closure from the interponate site. Complete leak closure for regular influx but not for reflux from the interponate back into the stented esophagus is often seen in those cases (fig. 4, 5). Additionally, the migration rate is higher. It is important to use a large covered stent with its maximal diameter configuration under these conditions. For best anchorage, the stent should be placed as far as possible at the esophageal site. Partially covered stents, to minimize migration, or custom-made grafts with larger diameters or stents with specifically designed distal ends (tulip ends, mushroom shape, umbrella design) (fig. 6–8) are very useful in this situation.

Adjunctive Therapy
For an interventional-endoscopic approach to be successful, close cooperation between surgeon, ICU specialist, endoscopist and radiologist is required. Most patients with anastomotic leaks following upper gastrointestinal surgery require intensive care treatment due to septic and multiorgan failure. The early initiation of supportive systemic strategies to decrease the dared consequences of sepsis and mediastinitis is mandatory. The use of broad-spectrum antibiotics is essential under these conditions. An intensive monitoring of systemic inflammation and immunologic competence, i.e. leukocyte counts, C-reactive protein level, interleukin and procalcitonin, is required. If the clinical situation and systemic inflammation is not improving under endoscopic treatment, immediate reevaluation, i.e. endoscopy and radiologic diagnostics (repetitive CT scans), or surgery is required.

Endoscopic Stent Removal

Because of their long-term complications, like stent ingrowth or overgrowth with resultant secondary strictures, fistulization and upper gastrointestinal hemorrhage, stents should be removed when definitive anastomotic healing is expected. Nevertheless, general recommendations for the optimal duration of stenting for an anastomotic leak do not exist and are not easy to define due to various factors influencing patient recovery and definitive anastomotic healing. The reported time for stent retrieval after placement for anastomotic upper gastrointestinal leaks ranges from 2 up to 20 weeks [15–20]. Leak closure will generally be heralded by an absent inflammatory response. We believe that anastomotic healing can be expected at the earliest 2 weeks after stent placement in smaller leaks and should be completed at the latest after 10 weeks in most of the larger or complicated leaks, depending on initial leak size, patients course and stent type (fully or partially covered) etc., so that stent removal should be conducted within this period in the majority of cases [11, 12]. Infrequently, a second stent therapy is needed in the presence of a persistent leak.

Stent removal (or replacement) can be accomplished in a safe and easy way preferably within 6 weeks (partially covered SEMS) [21] or 3 months (fully covered SEMS or plastic stents) [18, 19, 22] after placement. Stent retrieval becomes more and more difficult after this period, when the ends of the stent (mainly partially covered stents) become embedded in the esophageal mucosa. Further alterations of the anastomoses and esophageal wall, like secondary fistulization, can be expected after delayed stent removal. In cases of persistent leaks after stent removal, the defect can be sealed by fibrin glue, endoscopic clipping or by placement of a new stent (larger diameter and length or different design) [12].

Technique
Stent removal is performed using a standard gastroscope and a rat-toothed forceps under analgosedation and direct visualization. To pull out the stent, the proximal stent end or the retrievable thread is grasped with the forceps. However, in our opinion, it is easier and safer to grasp the distal end of the stent (or the distally located retrievable thread) and to invaginate the stent up into itself to extract it from the esophagus. The invagination technique is particularly safe and

7 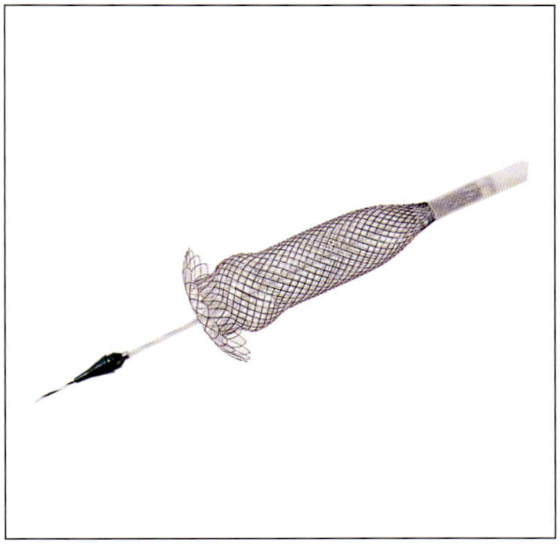

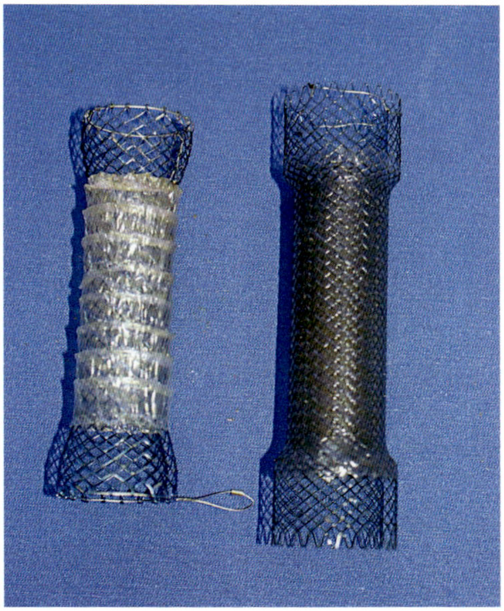 8

Fig. 7. ECO Cardia Umbrella Stent® (Leufen Medical, Aachen, Germany) with specially designed distal stent end (umbrella design) for optimal leak closure from distal in incongruent anastomoses.

Fig. 8. Two partially covered SEMS.

effective for the retrieval of proximal ingrown stents. Sometimes, in cases of stent ingrowth or overgrowth, it is useful to reduce granulation tissue at the proximal stent end using argon plasma coagulation. Endoscopy should be always performed after stent removal to rule out complications such as bleeding or persistent fistulization. A contrast swallow using water-soluble contrast should be performed to confirm complete leak closure.

Procedure-Associated Complications

Stent Migration

Stent migration is the most frequent procedure-associated complication after stent placement for leaking anastomoses. It should be pointed out that stents were originally designed for (malignant) strictures, and stent adhesion in a non-stenotic, contractile esophagus is not always possible. Distal migration is the commonest problem after stenting, especially in incongruent esophageal anastomoses with a wider gastric or colonic interponate or jejunal pouch. After incomplete distal migration (the stent migrates distally underneath the anastomotic dehiscence, but not completely into the interponate) the proximal stent end can be grasped firmly with a forceps, in order to pull up the graft and to correct its position. This maneuver is usually successful. In cases of repeated distal migrations, the stent should be replaced by a stent with a larger diameter and length, or a fully covered stent should be replaced by a partially covered one for better anchorage. Complete distal stent migration into the interponate requires mostly stent retrieval and placement of a new stent, but endoscopic stent removal can be difficult under these conditions. The fully expanded stent ends are not easy to pull through a relatively narrower

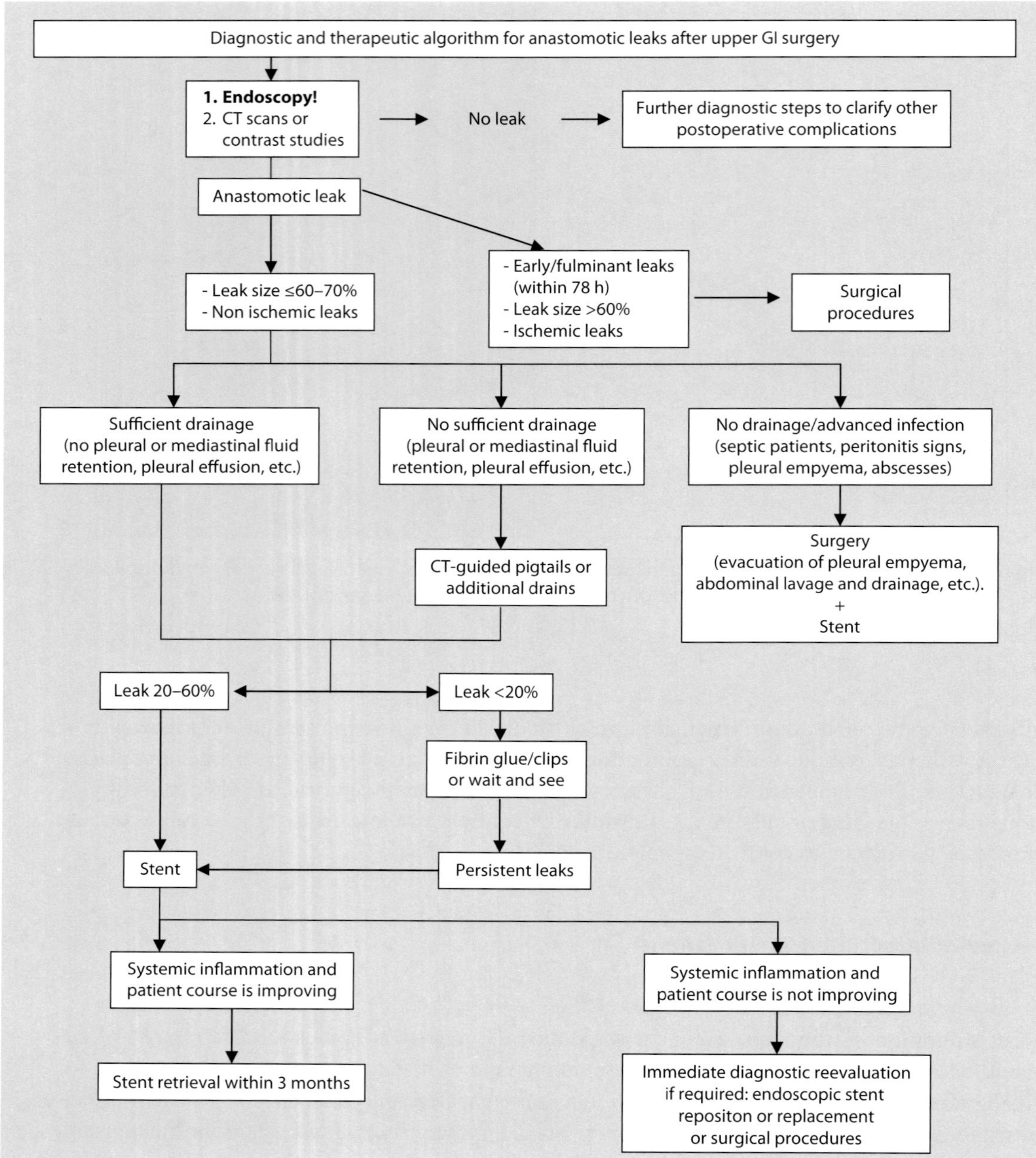

Fig. 9. Diagnostic and therapeutic algorithm for anastomotic leaks after upper gastrointestinal surgery.

anastomosis. In those cases it is easier to pass the migrated stent completely with the endoscope and to grasp the distal end with a forceps, in order to invaginate the stent up into itself for removal. Sometimes it is useful to place at first a new larger diameter stent. Subsequently, the complete migrated stent can be removed by pulling it through the previously placed stent using the invagination technique.

In contrast, proximal migration is infrequent. Endoscopic reposition, by pulling down the stent, often fails. Removal of the migrated graft and placement of a larger stent are frequently needed to cover the leakage.

Gastrointestinal Bleeding

Gastrointestinal bleeding after stent placement or stent retrieval is a rare complication which requires usual endoscopic treatment options for hemostasis. An extremely rare and fatal complication is gastrointestinal bleeding resulting from an esophagoaortic fistula, with a mortality rate of nearly 100%. Merely, additional vascular stenting of the thoracic aorta may be a treatment option in individual cases.

Anastomotic Strictures

Anastomotic strictures after stent placement are less frequent than stenoses following conventional treatment or fibrin glue injections for anastomotic leaks. This fact is another argument for the use of stents for the treatment of anastomotic leaks. Anastomotic strictures can be treated endoscopically with good results. Usually, surgery is not required.

Results

The use of stents to seal non-malignant esophageal leaks has been increasingly described during the last years [11, 16–28]. Up to now, there are various series about the successful placement of covered stents to close anastomotic leaks after esophageal or gastric, and more recently, bariatric surgery [11, 16–29]. Complete anastomotic healing of postsurgical leaks after stent placement, without the need of further surgical procedures, has been reported in 67–100% of selected cases with an acceptable mortality of 0–33% (table 1). Hereby, stent placement was technically correct in nearly 100% of the patients without difficulties (table 1). The commonest problem after stenting seems to be the migration of the graft, with a recurrence of a symptomatic leakage, which can be treated in the majority of cases sufficiently by endoscopic reposition of the stent or by stent replacement.

Both fully and partially covered metallic stents and covered plastic stents have been found suitable to seal anastomotic leakages in various studies [11, 16–29]. But the crucial question, what stent type should be preferred, cannot been answered yet and further technical innovations of current stents are needed. However, it is clear that all stents should be partially or completely covered, and have an adequate diameter, preferably with larger distal expansion. The cover will decrease leakage into the fistula and the dilated proximal end will help anchor the stent proximally, and thus decrease the chances of distal migration. Currently available stents show different features and have both advantages and disadvantages. The commonly used Polyflex® stent is completely covered by a soft silicon layer, which may result in less proliferation and inflammatory tissue. In contrast, metal stents (partially covered) mostly become strongly embedded in the esophageal mucosa, and stent retrieval is often more tricky. Another advantage of the Polyflex® stent is that it narrows under pressure, this is in contrast to, for example, metal stents, and can thus be removed more easily. But an important disadvantage of those stents, in this context, is an increased risk for migration (up to 37%) [24] in contrast to metal stents. In addition, the diameter of the delivery device is larger than that of the most commonly used metal stents, i.e. 12–14 mm, and the Polyflex® stent needs to be loaded into the delivery device before placement.

Table 1. Outcome after stent placement for anastomotic leaks and non malignant esophageal perforations

Reference (first author)	n	Stent	Correct stent placement, %	Complete leak healing, %	Mortality %	Migration %	Retrieval %
Doniec [16]	21	SEMS partially covered	90	80.1	23.8	5	56.5
Freeman [23]	21	Polyflex	100	95	5	24	100
Gelbman [18]	9	Polyflex	100	67	33	30	100
Han [22]	8	SEMS fully covered	100	100	0	0	100
Hunerbein [19]	9	Polyflex	100	88.9	0	22	100
Kauer [20]	10	SEMS fully covered	100	70	20	40	62.5
Leers [21]	31	SEMS partially covered	100	92	6.5	3	100
Ott [30]	12	Polyflex	100	42	n.a.	33	100
Radecke [15, 26]	15	Polyflex	100	73	n.a.	20	n.a.
Langer [24]	24	Polyflex	92	89	25	37.5	50
Evrad [17]	4	Polyflex	100	100	0	0	100
Roy-Choudhury [27]	14	SEMS partially covered	100	93	7	0	0
Tueberger [27]	32	SEMS fully covered	100	78	15.6	n.a.	70
Own patients	17	Polyflex	100	82	12	35	100
Own patients	21	SEMS fully covered	100	86	14	10	95

n.a. = No data available.

Table 2. Characteristics of recently used stent types for sealing of anastomotic leaks and non-malignant esophageal perforations (– low, + high)

	SEMS (partially covered)	SEMS (fully covered)	Polyflex
Delivery device, diameter in mm	5–10	5–10	12/14
Costs	+(++)	+(++)	–
Effectiveness in leak sealing	+(++)	+(++)	+(++)
Induction of stenoses	++	+	+
Risk for migration	–	+	++
Easy to removal	–	+	++

Initially, we used the Polyflex® stent for treating anastomotic leaks. Recently, we changed our initially endoscopic approach, due to frequent migrations of these plastic stents and repetitive incomplete leak closure, by using the new generation of fully covered metallic stents, which are also easy to remove within 3–4 months. The pros and cons of current available stent types are summarized in table 2.

Evidence-based guidelines for endoscopic treatment of anastomotic upper gastrointestinal leaks do not exist up to now, because of lacking prospective studies comparing different stent types, i.e. plastic versus metallic stents and partially covered versus fully covered stents, and different treatment strategies, i.e. endoscopic versus surgical or conservative treatment under defined conditions.

Conclusion

Anastomotic leaks are the most severe and feared complication after gastroesophageal surgery and a major source of mortality and morbidity. Successful management of an anastomotic leak after upper gastrointestinal surgery requires sufficient drainage of the leakage to eliminate the contamination of the perianastomotic region and to control ongoing sepsis. It is also important to secure the intestinal passage and enteral feeding during the healing process. The optimal therapeutic strategy depends on a variety of influencing factors, such as size of the leakage, perfusion of the interponate, patient's condition, degree of sepsis and drainage of the leak, and ranges from a strict conservative approach in selected patients with small, well-drained and asymptomatic leaks to aggressive surgery (resection and diversion procedures) in septic patients with early and fulminant undrained leaks.

Despite the lack of prospective, randomized studies, the temporary placement of self-expanding and covered stents seems to be a very effective and safe, minimally invasive modality to treat these leaks, and it can reduce morbidity and mortality of this life-threatening complication after upper gastrointestinal surgery. With regard to published studies and our own experience, endoscopic stent placement should be the treatment of choice in patients with symptomatic (septic), non-ischemic and sufficiently drained anastomotic leaks involving up to 60% of the anastomotic circumference. Adequate drainage of the leakage must be established prior to sealing the leak with a stent, because once covered by a stent, the leak no longer allows internal drainage of infectious fluid into the intestinal tract and septic complications of the perianastomotic region are to be expected. In addition, endoscopic lavage and debridement, prior to stent placement, can be helpful to reduce pleural and mediastinal contamination in selected patients. To prevent mechanical and other stent-related complications, the stent should be removed or replaced preferably within 6 weeks (partially covered SEMS) or 3 months (fully covered SEMS and plastic stents). An interventional-endoscopic management of anastomotic leaks should be based on a multidisciplinary approach involving the surgeon, endoscopist, radiologist and ICU specialist. Surgical reexploration must be immediately considered if clinical improvement of the patient is not achieved with endoscopic treatment.

References

1 Alanezi K, Urschel JD: Mortality secondary to esophageal anastomotic leak. Ann Thorac Cardiovasc Surg 2004; 10:71–75.

2 Blewett CJ, Miller JD, Young JE, Bennett WF, Urschel JD: Anastomotic leaks after esophagectomy for esophageal cancer: a comparison of thoracic and cervical anastomoses. Ann Thorac Cardiovasc Surg 2001;7:75–78.

3 Griffin SM, Lamb PJ, Dresner SM, Richardson DL, Hayes N: Diagnosis and management of a mediastinal leak following radical oesophagectomy. Br J Surg 2001; 88:1346–1351.

4 Hofstetter W, Swisher SG, Correa AM, Hess K, Putnam JB Jr, Ajani JA, Dolormente M, Francisco R, Komaki RR, Lara A, et al: Treatment outcomes of resected esophageal cancer. Ann Surg 2002;236:376–384.

5 Sauvanet A, Baltar J, Le MJ, Belghiti J: Diagnosis and conservative management of intrathoracic leakage after oesophagectomy. Br J Surg 1998;85:1446–1449.

6 Turkyilmaz A, Eroglu A, Aydin Y, Tekinbas C, Muharrem EM, Karaoglanoglu N: The management of esophagogastric anastomotic leak after esophagectomy for esophageal carcinoma. Dis Esophagus 2009;22:119–126.

7 Siersema PD: Treatment of esophageal perforations and anastomotic leaks: the endoscopist is stepping into the arena. Gastrointest Endosc 2005;61:897–900.

8 Bartels H, Siewert JR: Therapy of mediastinitis in patients with esophageal cancer (in German). Chirurg 2008;79:30–37.

9 Lamb PJ, Griffin SM, Chandrashekar MV, Richardson DL, Karat D, Hayes N: Prospective study of routine contrast radiology after total gastrectomy. Br J Surg 2004; 91:1015–1019.

10 Tirnaksiz MB, Deschamps C, Allen MS, Johnson DC, Pairolero PC: Effectiveness of screening aqueous contrast swallow in detecting clinically significant anastomotic leaks after esophagectomy. Eur Surg Res 2005;37: 123–128.

11 Schubert D, Scheidbach H, Kuhn R, Wex C, Weiss G, Eder F, Lippert H, Pross M: Endoscopic treatment of thoracic esophageal anastomotic leaks by using silicone-covered, self-expanding polyester stents. Gastrointest Endosc 2005;61:891–8916.

12 Schubert D, Pross M, Nestler G, Ptok H, Scheidbach H, Fahlke J, Lippert H: Endoscopic treatment of mediastinal anastomotic leaks (in German). Zentralbl Chir 2006; 131:369–375.

13 Nguyen NT, Mailey BA, Hinojosa MW, Chang K: Natural orifice management of anastomotic leaks after minimally invasive esophagogastrectomy. Surg Innov 2008; 15:249–252.

14 Wehrmann T, Stergiou N, Vogel B, Riphaus A, Kockerling F, Frenz MB: Endoscopic debridement of paraesophageal, mediastinal abscesses: a prospective case series. Gastrointest Endosc 2005;62:344–349.

15 Radecke K, Lang H, Frilling A, Gerken G, Treichel U: Successful sealing of benign esophageal leaks after temporary placement of a self-expanding plastic stent without fluoroscopic guidance. Z Gastroenterol 2006;44: 1031–1038.

16 Doniec JM, Schniewind B, Kahlke V, Kremer B, Grimm H: Therapy of anastomotic leaks by means of covered self-expanding metallic stents after esophagogastrectomy. Endoscopy 2003;35:652–658.

17 Evrard S, Le Moine O, Lazaraki G, Dormann A, El N, I, Deviere J: Self-expanding plastic stents for benign esophageal lesions. Gastrointest Endosc 2004; 60:894–900.

18 Gelbmann CM, Ratiu NL, Rath HC, Rogler G, Lock G, Scholmerich J, Kullmann F: Use of self-expandable plastic stents for the treatment of esophageal perforations and symptomatic anastomotic leaks. Endoscopy 2004; 36:695–699.

19 Hunerbein M, Stroszczynski C, Moesta KT, Schlag PM: Treatment of thoracic anastomotic leaks after esophagectomy with self-expanding plastic stents. Ann Surg 2004; 240:801–807:

20 Kauer WK, Stein HJ, Dittler HJ, Siewert JR: Stent implantation as a treatment option in patients with thoracic anastomotic leaks after esophagectomy. Surg Endosc 2008;22:50–53.

21 Leers JM, Vivaldi C, Schafer H, Bludau M, Brabender J, Lurje G, Herbold T, Holscher AH, Metzger R: Endoscopic therapy for esophageal perforation or anastomotic leak with a self-expandable metallic stent. Surg Endosc 2009; [Epub ahead of print].

22 Han XW, Li YD, Wu G, Li MH, Ma XX: New covered mushroom-shaped metallic stent for managing anastomotic leak after esophagogastrostomy with a wide gastric tube. Ann Thorac Surg 2006;82:702–706.

23 Freeman RK, Ascioti AJ, Wozniak TC: Postoperative esophageal leak management with the Polyflex esophageal stent. J Thorac Cardiovasc Surg 2007; 133:333–338.

24 Langer FB, Wenzl E, Prager G, Salat A, Miholic J, Mang T, Zacherl J: Management of postoperative esophageal leaks with the Polyflex self-expanding covered plastic stent. Ann Thorac Surg 2005;79:398–403.

25 Pennathur A, Chang AC, McGrath KM, Steiner G, Velo-Rivera M, Awais O, Gooding WE, Christie NA, Gilbert S, Landreneau RJ, et al: Polyflex expandable stents in the treatment of esophageal disease: initial experience. Ann Thorac Surg 2008;85:1968–1972.

26 Radecke K, Gerken G, Treichel U: Impact of a self-expanding, plastic esophageal stent on various esophageal stenoses, fistulas, and leakages: a single-center experience in 39 patients. Gastrointest Endosc 2005;61: 812–818.

27 Roy-Choudhury SH, Nicholson AA, Wedgwood KR, Mannion RA, Sedman PC, Royston CM, Breen DJ: Symptomatic malignant gastroesophageal anastomotic leak: management with covered metallic esophageal stents. AJR Am J Roentgenol 2001;176:161–165.
28 Tuebergen D, Rijcken E, Mennigen R, Hopkins AM, Senninger N, Bruewer M: Treatment of thoracic esophageal anastomotic leaks and esophageal perforations with endoluminal stents: efficacy and current limitations. J Gastrointest Surg 2008;12:1168–1176.
29 Eubanks S, Edwards CA, Fearing NM, Ramaswamy A, de la Torre RA, Thaler KJ, Miedema BW, Scott JS: Use of endoscopic stents to treat anastomotic complications after bariatric surgery. J Am Coll Surg 2008;206:935–938.
30 Ott C, Ratiu N, Endlicher E, Rath HC, Gelbmann CM, Schölmerich J, Kullmann F: Self-expanding Polyflex plastic stents in esophageal disease: various indications, complications, and outcomes. Surg Endosc 2007;21:889–896.

Daniel Schubert, MD
Klinik für Allgemein-, Viszeral- und Gefässchirurgie, Otto von Guericke Universität Magdeburg
Leipziger Strasse 44, DE–39120 Magdeburg (Germany)
Tel. +49 391 67 15500, Fax +49 391 67 15570, E-Mail daniel.schubert@med.ovgu.de

Mönkemüller K, Wilcox CM, Muñoz-Navas M (eds): Interventional and Therapeutic Gastrointestinal Endoscopy.
Front Gastrointest Res. Basel, Karger, 2010, vol 27, pp 198–208

Percutaneous Endoscopic Gastrostomy

L. López Rosés · E. Castro Ortiz

Gastroenterology Department, Xeral-Calde Hospital, Lugo, Spain

Abstract

Percutaneous endoscopic gastrostomy (PEG) has become one of the most frequently used procedures to administer nutrition and also as an alternative to the surgical approach or nasogastric tubes. The technique is simple, safe and cheap; it can be performed by any moderately experienced endoscopist and so, since the original description in 1980, has become a popular method around the world. The main PEG indication is the nutrition of patients that cannot swallow, although there are other utilities. Contraindications and complications are very unusual in clinical practice. There are three technical modalities for the placement of the gastrostomy tube, with no one being better than the other. This chapter tries to explain in a very practical way the main aspects of the procedure and it especially focuses on technical points, incorporating some useful tricks that can help solve some eventually embarrassing situations.

Percutaneous endoscopic gastrostomy (PEG) was first described by Ponsky and Gauderer in the year 1980 and was quickly accepted as a useful alternative to surgical gastrostomy and nasogastric tubes [1]. The endoscopic technique requires less instrumentation, reduces the stay in hospital and as a result, the economic cost compared to the surgical technique [2], and secondly, it avoids annoying and unsightly nasogastric tubes.

The standardization of this technique, the marketing of the kits and the simplicity in the replacement of the probe has made the PEG the procedure of choice in patients requiring long-term enteral nutrition. This chapter will review the indications, the contraindications, the different techniques of implantation and the possible complications of the placement of PEG tubes.

Indications

As a general rule, the implant of a PEG is indicated for those patients that, having a functioning gastrointestinal tract, suffer from dysphagia or any other problem that precludes nutrition by mouth for at least 4 weeks and for which there is no contraindication or inability to the introduction of an endoscope down to the stomach. In practice, the most common cause is represented by the neuromuscular diseases that occur with pharyngoesophagic motor impairment [3]. However, it can also be used in patients with obstructive dysphagia,

Table 1. Indications for PEG

Neurological disorders
Stroke
Anoxic encephalopathy
Alzheimer's disease
Multiple sclerosis
Parkinson's disease
Amyotrophic lateral sclerosis
Brain tumors
Huntington's chorea
Polio
Obstructive neoplasia
Head and neck tumors
Carcinoma of the esophagus
Carcinoma of cardia
Muscle diseases
Myotonic dystrophy
Dermatomyositis/polymyositis
Oculopharyngeal muscular dystrophy
Amyloidosis
Gastric decompression
Abdominal carcinomatosis
Hyperemesis gravidarum
Miscellaneous
Nutritional complement
Tracheoesophageal fistula
Chronic gastric volvulus
Macroglossia
Badly tasting drugs (pediatric use)
Recurring bronchial aspirations

especially secondary to head and neck tumors [4]. On the other hand, other utilities apart from nutrition have been described; for example, it can be used as a method for gastrointestinal decompression [5], prevention of recurrent gastric volvulus [6] or for the administration of badly tasting medicine to children [7]. Table 1 summarizes the main indications.

Contraindications

Different situations may contraindicate the implantation of a PEG, or by promoting the complications or by technically preventing it (table 2). The impossibility to pass the endoscope down to the stomach, severe disorders of coagulation, massive ascites, severe infections of the wall or the abdominal cavity, pyloric or intestinal obstruction, neoplastic infiltration of the abdominal wall or limited life expectancy are considered absolute contraindications. The presence of ascites, morbid obesity, portal hypertension, subtotal gastrectomy or peritoneal dialysis are relative contraindications. At present, recent myocardial stroke [8], the presence of a ventricular peritoneal shunt [9] or extensive burns of the abdominal wall are not considered contraindications [10].

Table 2. Contraindications for PEG

Absolute contraindications
Inability to pass the endoscope into the stomach
Severe disorders of coagulation and incorrigible
Massive ascites
Infection of the abdominal wall
Peritonitis
Neoplastic infiltration of abdominal wall
Pyloric or intestinal obstruction
Short life expectancy
Nervous anorexia
Relative contraindications
Morbid obesity
Ascites
Portal hypertension data
Peritoneal dialysis
Subtotal gastrectomy

Patient Preparation

The patient should fast for at least 6 h and his/her coagulation tests should be within the hemostatic levels. To reduce the risk of septic complications it is important to administer a dose of a broad-spectrum antibiotic 30 min before the process (e.g., 1 g of intravenous cefazolin) and perform a thorough cleansing and disinfection of the oropharyngeal cavity [11, 12]. Informed consent must be properly completed.

Material Needed

To implant a PEG, the material normally used for an upper gastrointestinal endoscopy is necessary. The technique is performed under analgesic sedation, therefore all the necessary material should be available for its administration and monitoring. An additional aspirator should also be prepared. Everything must also be prepared to create a sterile field in the anterior abdominal wall, local anesthetic, scalpels, a small trocar, a guidewire, a polypectomy snare and the gastrostomy tube, of which there are many models on the market and come in kits with all the necessary materials for its implantation (fig. 1). The material which the tubes are made of is silicone or polyurethane. The use of either one is indifferent [13].

Implant Technique

The procedure is performed with the patient in supine decubitus position. For this reason there must be an additional aspirator to collect oropharyngeal secretions throughout the whole process. Before proceeding to place the probe, an endoscopic exploration of the esophagus, stomach and duodenum is performed in order to rule out any circumstance that contraindicates the implant. As regards the placement of the probe itself, the basic principle consists in insufflating the stomach considerably, so that its anterior wall is in intimate contact with the anterior abdominal wall, thereby achieving a secure area in which to create a gastrocutaneous fistula without interposition of other organs.

There are three different methods for the placement of the probe. Some variations on them have also been described.

Pull Method or the Ponsky-Gauderer Method [1]
The technique is performed with the patient in the supine decubitus position, although to introduce the endoscope he/she may be placed in left lateral decubitus. Having explored the upper digestive tract, the site where the probe will be inserted should be chosen. For this, with the distal end of the endoscope placed in the stomach, insufflation is applied, and after darkening the room, the patient's abdominal wall is inspected to try to visualize the point of maximum transillumination, that it is usually located in the epigastrium slightly to the left. Then pressure with a finger is applied on this point, verifying endoscopically that this action causes a clear imprint in the gastric lumen (fig. 2, 3). This maneuver is the most important part of the procedure, as we ensure a secure puncture area in which to introduce the probe. To avoid that the probe once attached causes pain to the patient, we must be careful not to choose the insertion point at <2 cm below the costal ridge [14].

The skin is then disinfected, a sterile field is prepared and the selected point is infiltrated with local anesthesia, making the needle penetrate the abdominal wall and its tip be seen in the stomach. Then, with a scalpel, a skin incision of about 1 cm is made. The next step is to introduce the trocar with its stylet from the outside and through the incision to the gastric cavity, all of this under endoscopic control. Once this is done, the endoscopist will get the trocar using a polypectomy snare. Now the stylet will be withdrawn and the guidewire will be inserted through the trocar until the tip penetrates several centimeters into the stomach. At that time, and manipulating the handle of the snare, the endoscopist will release his hold on the trocar and catch the guide (fig. 4, 5). Immediately thereafter, the endoscope will be withdrawn, which will drag behind it the guide to make it come out of the mouth of the patient. In this way we will have the guidewire entering through the abdominal wall and coming out through the patient's mouth. After this, the pointed end of the gastrostomy tube is knocked to the end of the wire that comes out of the mouth, then the wire is tractioned from the opposite end, so that the probe penetrates through the mouth, sliding along the esophagus and stomach and finally, penetrates the gastric wall and the abdominal wall and appears on the exterior through the incision previously performed (fig. 6). The endoscope is then reintroduced and the tube pulled until the retainer cap of the probe presses against the gastric wall (fig. 7). Having done this, the outside retainer is placed avoiding excessive tension, for which we must verify that the probe can rotate on its axis (fig. 8).

Push or Sacks-Vine Method [15, 16]
Basically it is similar to the previous one. It differs in the type of probe that is used, which is linked to a long, semirigid and pointed tube, so keeping the guide thread taut, the catheter is inserted by pushing it from the mouth of the patient until it comes out through the abdominal wall (fig. 9). The rest of the process is identical to the pull method.

The Introducer Method or the Russell Method [17]
Using this technique, the endoscope is inserted only once, and also prevents the gastrostomy tube passing through the mouth, which may be desirable in certain situations. The steps are identical

1

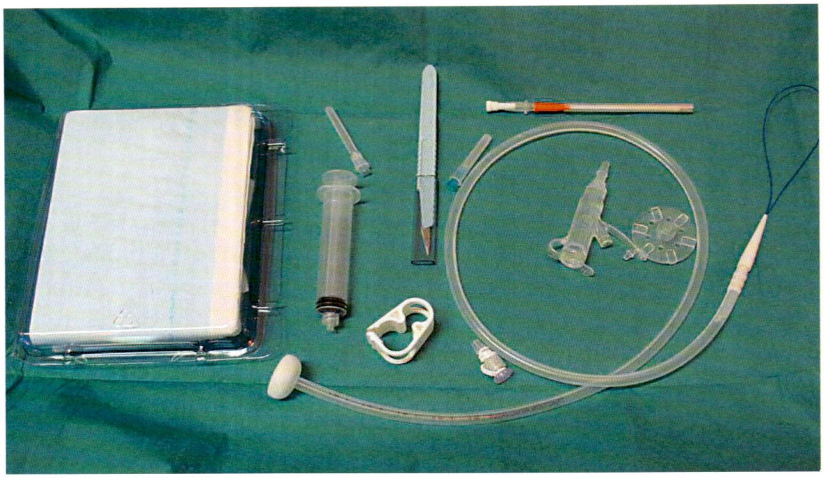

2

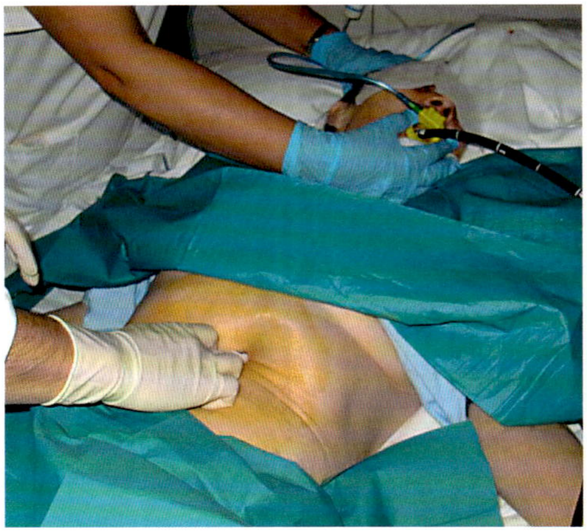

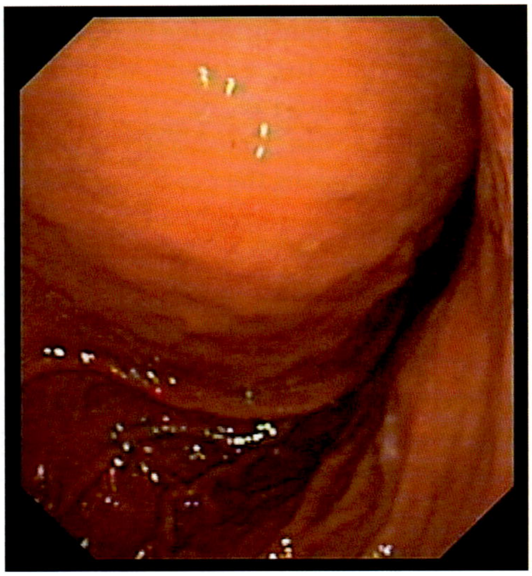

3

Fig. 1. Material needed for the PEG, included in a commercial kit.

Fig. 2, 3. External and endoscopic image of the digital imprint in the gastric cavity.

to those of previous techniques until the trocar is inserted. From then the guide is introduced, the trocar is removed and several plug-shaped dilators are introduced. Finally a thicker sheath trocar is introduced, through which the gastrostomy tube which is a Foley type passes. Then the balloon is inflated, the sheath is removed, the probe is pulled until it stops and finally is fixed externally with a retainer, as in the other techniques.

Postprocedual Care

During the early days, wound care will be undertaken. Later, cleansing with soapy water once a day will be sufficient, keeping the area without covering up with bandages or dressings. It is

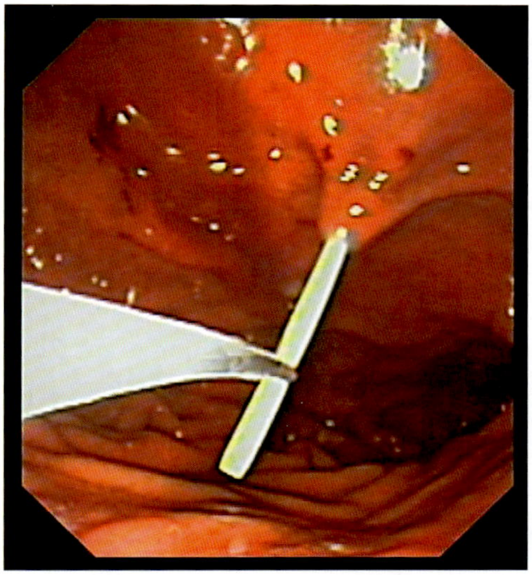

4

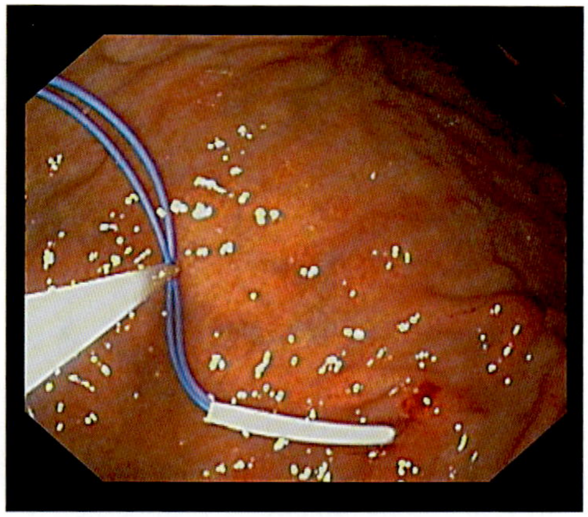

5

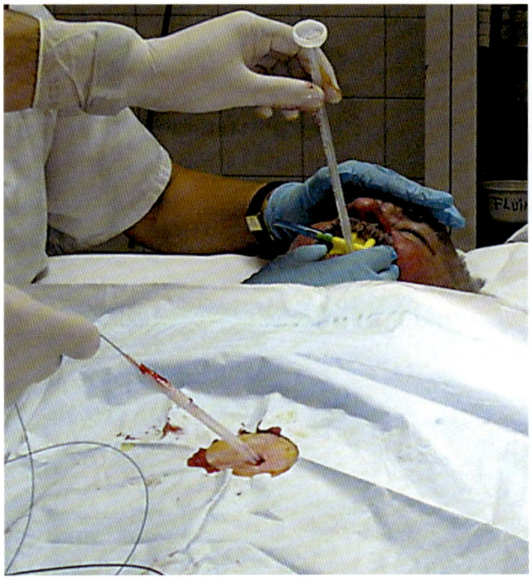

6

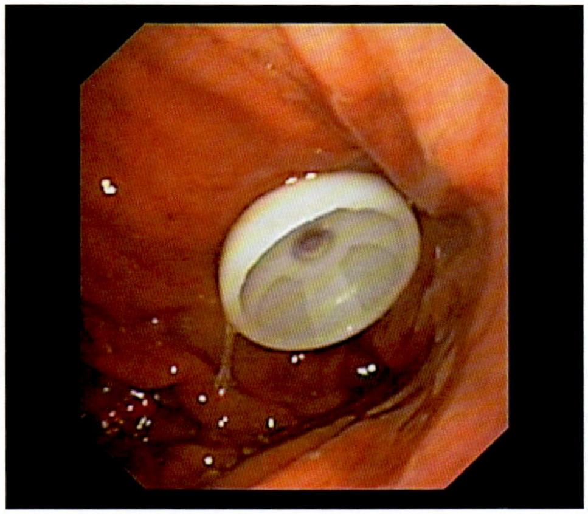

7

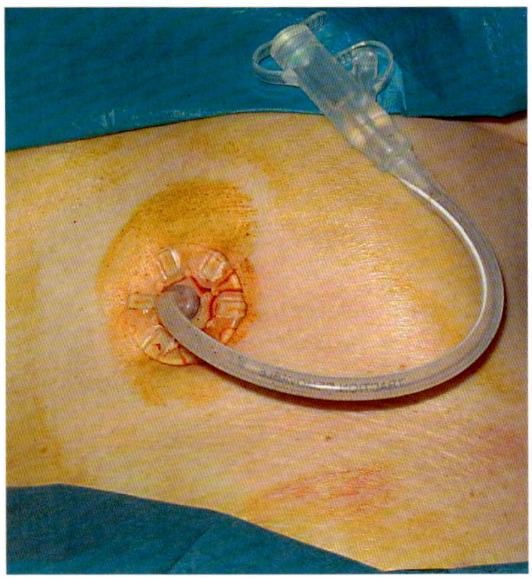

8

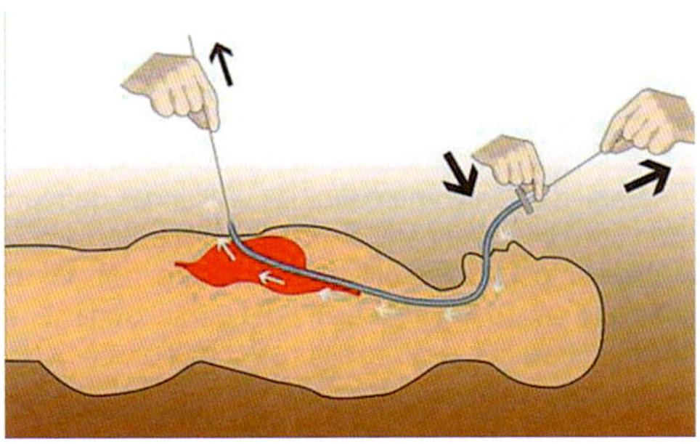

9

Fig. 4, 5. Pull method. The snare grabs the catheter first and then the guidewire. **Fig. 6.** Pull method. Pulling the wire, the probe penetrates through the mouth and exits through de abdominal wall. **Fig. 7.** Gastric internal bumper. **Fig. 8.** Final aspect of the PEG with the external retainer. **Fig. 9.** Schematic representation of the push technique.

possible that the patient will complain of pain where the puncture took place, the days after the implantation. In this case, and once discarded complications, the necessary analgesia will be administered. The intake of food can be started immediately after placing the probe but in many hospitals 24 h is waited. To prevent the internal bumper from migrating and getting stuck to the wall of the stomach, it is highly desirable, several weeks after the implant, to loosen the tension of the outer retainer, sliding it along the tube towards the proximal end 2–3 cm, and also regularly checking that the probe can be rotated on its axis.

Removal and Replacement of the Probe

If the dysphagia or any other indication that would have led to the implantation of the PEG has disappeared, the tube can be withdrawn. However, 2–3 weeks must have passed after the placement, as this is the time required for the gastrocutaneous fistula to mature, to become fibrous and prevent the passage of gastric contents into the peritoneal cavity after the removal of the probe; the fistulous hole will close spontaneously within a few days. If the internal bumper of the gastrostomy tube is soft, one can simply remove the tube by pulling it up from the outside until one overcomes its resistance. If the retainer is rigid, it will be necessary to cut the tube where it meets the skin and insert the endoscope to remove the retainer through the mouth.

On the other hand, and as a consequence of the action of the acid, the probes deteriorate in some time and must be replaced. In this case, after the removal of the probe of the first implant, a substitution probe of the same caliber will be put in its place. There are two types of these probes on the market: with a balloon retainer or with a circular retainer which includes a rectifier. They are both placed from the outside without the need for endoscopic control, and can be both put in place by nurses. It is important to ensure that the probe glides smoothly through the fistula and its tip reaches the stomach light. In case of doubt, its correct position should be checked by endoscopy or radiology. Replacement button-type probes, with a flat profile, can also be found on the market and they are especially useful in patients with an active life or in children. However, its use should be individualized, as some serious complications associated with them have been described [18, 19].

Useful Tricks

As in other endoscopic procedures, it is useful to know a number of tricks that will help us avoid some complications and which will help us resolve issues that may arise during the implantation or replacement of the PEG.

Reduction of the Risk of Stoma Infection

Stoma infection by germs carried from the oropharynx during the implantation of the probe is the most frequent complication. Cleansing and disinfection of the mouth and pharynx together with antibiotic prophylaxis decreases the risk. One can also use two tricks to avoid this complication: (1) Leave an overtube placed in the first pass of the endoscope, so during the implant maneuvers, when the probe is pulled, contact with the oropharynx is avoided [20]. (2) The use of the Russell method.

Difficulty to Introduce the Endoscope

At times and for different reasons, it is very difficult to pass the endoscope through the mouth or the pharyngoesophageal junction. If the push or pull methods are used, it is necessary to reintroduce the endoscope to check the correct position of the probe, with which the problem repeats itself. We can avoid this problem in several ways: (1) Placing the probe without reintroducing the endoscope, that is to say without endoscopic control, sensing by touch the moment the retainer cap presses against the internal gastric wall and adjusting the external retainer to approximately 4 cm of the marks indicated in centimeters on the outer tube [14]. (2) Reinserting the gastroscope guided by the probe itself, by knotting its distal end to a polypectomy handle, so that the endoscope and the probe form a single body [21]. (3) Using the Russell method. (4) Performing the gastrostomy through the nose. The procedure for placement of the probe may be conducted wholly through the nose, using ultrathin or pediatric endoscopes and conventional probes, with the sole condition that the internal retainer is soft and can be folded for insertion through the nostrils [22].

Avoiding the Puncture of Adjacent Organs (Especially Liver and Transverse Colon)
To prevent viscera from being placed between the abdominal wall and the stomach, we can use various tricks: (1) Insufflating the stomach sufficiently, so that there is extensive contact between the anterior gastric and abdominal wall. (2) Placing the patient in an anti-Trendelenburg position. In this way the transverse colon caudally tends to fall not standing between the stomach and the abdominal wall. (3) Introducing the trocar connected to a syringe with serum, gently pulling on the plunger while punctioning and advancing towards the stomach light. The sight of bubbles before viewing the tip of the trocar in the stomach will announce that a hollow organ has been penetrated [21]. (4) Selecting the puncture site assisted by ultrasonographic endoscopy.

Patients without Adequate Transillumination in the Abdominal Wall
In certain occasions a failure of correct transillumination may occur. However, it is possible to select a safe insertion point in several ways: (1) Checking that the external digital compression produces a very clear imprint on the gastric light. (2) Locating the insertion point guided by fluoroscopy, CT or ultrasonographic endoscopy [23].

Results

There are comparative studies between the three techniques for the placement of the PEG but none has shown significant differences in terms of treatment success or complications [24, 25]. The success rate of the technique is greater than 95% [26]. In a large meta-analysis a morbidity and mortality of 9.4 and 0.53% was respectively estimated [27]. In other series the morbidity rate ranged from 9 to 17%, but major complications occur in only 1–3% of cases [28, 29].

Complications

Major Complications
(1) *Hemorrhage:* Produced by accidental puncture of a vessel. If bleeding occurs in the stomach it can be seen as an upper gastrointestinal bleeding, and if it is produced by peritoneal puncture of a vessel as hemoperitoneum. This complication is more common in patients with portal hypertension.

(2) *Acute peritonitis:* It is produced by the passage of gastric contents into the peritoneal cavity. It has been described in patients whose probe was tried to be changed within 2–3 weeks. In these cases, the fistulous tract may not yet be ripe and the end of the replacement tube instead of entering the stomach is located in the peritoneal cavity [30]. What can also occur if the probe

is placed with excessive tension is an ischemic necrosis of the gastric wall and a migration of the probe towards the peritoneal cavity.

(3) *Bronchial aspiration:* It is the most common major complication. It can occur during the procedure of the placement of the probe. It is therefore important to aspirate the oropharyngeal secretions throughout the procedure. It can also occur following the administration of nutrition. To prevent it, the patient should be incorporated 30° while he/she is fed, and shall be kept in this position for the following 2 h.

(4) *Necrotizing fasciitis:* It is the most serious complication but also the less common and is associated with high mortality. It is an infection and subsequent necrosis of the soft tissues of the abdominal wall. It is accompanied by fever, cellulitis and edema, and subcutaneous emphysema can be observed. It requires treatment with broad-spectrum antibiotics and surgical debridement.

(5) *Gastrocolic fistula:* It occurs when the transverse colon is placed between the gastric wall and the abdominal wall by placing the PEG. It can cause acute symptoms of intestinal obstruction or peritonitis, or evolve in a hidden way, with chronic subocclusive symptoms. Sometimes this complication is found when the first replacement of the probe takes place and the end of the replacement tube is placed at the level of the light of the colon, causing diarrhea when nutrition is administered. To solve this, it may be enough to remove the tube to close the fistula spontaneously, but occasionally surgical treatment will be required.

(6) *Metastatic tumor implantation at the stoma:* Cases of metastasis of oropharyngeal and esophageal tumors in the stoma due to the dragging of malignant cells during the placement of the probe have been described [31]. With the Russell technique or the placement of an overtube, we can avoid this complication.

Minor Complications

(1) *Infection of the stoma:* It is the most frequent complication. It is managed with antibiotics and local treatment. It is sometimes necessary to withdraw the probe.

(2) *Extrusion of the probe (buried bumper):* It consists of the migration of the internal retainer towards the gastric wall, leaving an impact on it and sometimes being completely covered by gastric mucosa, hindering or preventing both nutrition and the replacement of the tube. To avoid this we must avoid excessive tension on the external retainer by loosening the outside retainer and by regularly rotating the probe on its axis.

(3) *Overflowing:* It consists on the oozing of gastric contents around the tube, causing skin irritation and interfering with the patient's care and hygiene.

(4) *Miscellaneous:* Complications that can usually be resolved without major difficulties are: hematoma of the abdominal wall or stomach, fever, subcutaneous emphysema, asymptomatic pneumoperitoneum, granuloma of ostomy, catheter obstruction, rupture of the tube and others.

Some Tricks to Resolve Some Complications

Burial of the Retainer in the Gastric Wall (Buried Bumper Syndrome)

There are several ways to resolve this complication: (1) Introduce a dilatation balloon [32] or a Savary dilator with a diameter slightly greater than that of the probe [33] through the lumen of it and push to the gastric cavity until the retainer is unstuck. For this maneuver, we can help ourselves by pulling the dilator with a polypectomy snare introduced through the working channel of the endoscope. (2) Putting a new probe by the pull method, inserting the guidewire through the lumen of the buried probe; in this way, when we pull the wire the new probe will drag the old and it will become unstuck [34]. (3) Make incisions with a needle knife sphincterotome or with argon plasma coagulation, on the lining that covers the internal retainer to release and remove it.

Stenosis of the Stoma

Very often if the probe is removed and the substitution probe is not placed promptly, the fistulous tract narrows, preventing the entry of the substitution probe. To solve this complication we can: (1) Dilate the fistula with Savary plugs or balloon dilators. (2) Introduce the replacement tube over a biopsy forceps used as a guide which are introduced by the stoma to the stomach [35]. (3) Introduce a guidewire by the fistulous tract and then perform the complete first implant procedure.

Peritube Leakage of Gastric Contents

It can be solved: (1) Removing the probe for several hours for the fistulous tract narrow and then placing the replacement probe. (2) Replacing the probe with another one with a larger caliber. (3) Removing the PEG and finally placing a new tube in another location.

Conclusion

The PEG procedure is technically simple and accessible to any endoscopist, providing quick, inexpensive enteral access with few complications. In this chapter we have reviewed in a concise way the technical aspects, indications, contraindications and complications of the technique. However, we must take into account that the endoscopist should not merely be a technician who only places the probe, but who must be involved in the process advising the clinicians responsible for the patient, the patient himself/herself and his/her family, describing the advantages, disadvantages risks of the technique and its alternatives. The decision to place probes for artificial feeding, especially in the final stages of life, must be based on the expectations of the progression of the disease, the chances of obtaining benefits and the desires of the patient and his family.

References

1 Gauderer NW, Ponsky JL, Izan RJ Jr: Gastrostomy without laparotomy: a percutaneous endoscopic technique. J Pediatr Surg 1980;15:872–875.

2 Steigmann GV, Goff JS, Silas D, Pearlman N, Sun J, Norton L: Endoscopic versus operative gastrostomy: final results of a prospective randomized trial. Gastrointest Endosc 1990;36:1–5.

3 Ponsky JL, Gauderer MWL: Percutaneous endoscopic gastrostomy: indications, limitations, techniques and results. World J Surg 1989;13:165–172.

4 Stellata TA: Expanded applications of percutaneous endoscopic gastrostomy. Gastrointest Endosc Clin N Am 1992;2:249–257.

5 Cannizzaro R, Bortoluzzi R, Valentini M, Scarabelli C, Campagnutta E, Sozzi M, et al: Percutaneous endoscopic gastrostomy as a decompressive technique in bowel obstruction due to abdominal carcinomatosis. Endoscopy 1995;27:317–320.

6 Eckhauser ML, Ferron JP: The use of dual percutaneous endoscopic gastrostomy in the management of chronic intermittent gastric volvulus. Gastrointest Endosc 1985; 31:140–142.

7 Gauderer MWL: An updated experience with percutaneous endoscopic gastrostomy in children. Gastrointest Endosc Clin Am 1992;2:195–205.

8 Cappel MS, Iocovone FM Jr: The safety and efficacy of percutaneous endoscopic gastrostomy after recent myocardial infarction: a study of 28 patients and 40 controls at four university teaching hospitals. Ann Gastroentrol J 1996;91:1599–1604.

9 Graham SM, Flowers JL, Scott TR, Lin F, Rigamonti D: Safety of percutaneous endoscopic gastrostomy in patients with a ventriculoperitoneal shunt. Neurosurgery 1993;32:932–934.

10 Patton ML, Haith LR, Germain TJ, Goldman WT, Raymond JT: Use of percutaneous endoscopic gastrostomy in burn patients. Surg Endosc 1994;8:1067–1071.

11 Sharma VK, Howden CW: Meta-analysis of randomized controlled trials of antibiotic prophylaxis before percutaneous endoscopic gastrostomy. Am J Gastroenterol 2000;95:3133–3136.
12 Saadeddin A, Freshwater DA, Fisher NC, Jones BJ: Antibiotic prophylaxis for percutaneous endoscopic gastrostomy for non-malignant conditions: a double-blind prospective randomized controlled trial. Aliment Pharmacol Ther 2005;22:565–570.
13 Santori S, Trevisani L, Nielsen I: Longevity of silicone and polyurethane catheters in long-term enteral feeding via percutaneous endoscopic gastrostomy. Aliment Pharmacol Ther 2003;17:853–856.
14 DeLegge MH: Percutaneous endoscopic gastrostomy. Am J Gastroenterol 2007;102:2620–2623.
15 Sacks BA, Vine HS, AM speakers, HP Ellison, D Shropshire, R Lowe A non-operative technique for establishment of a gastrostomy in the dog. Invest Radiol 1983; 18:485–487.
16 Foutch PG, Woods CA, Talbert GA, Sanowski RA: Critical analysis of the Sacks-Vine gastrostomy tube: a review of 120 consecutive procedures. Am J Gastroenterol 1988;83:812–815.
17 Russell TR, Brotman M, Forbes N: Percutaneous gastrostomy: a new simplified and cost-effective technique. Am J Surg 1984;148:132–137.
18 Gauderer MWL, Picha GL, Izant RJ Jr: The gastrostomy button. A simple, skin level non-refluxing device for long-term enteral feedings. J Pediatr Surg 1984;19:803–805.
19 Kozarek RA, Payne M, Barkin J, Goff J, Gostout C: Prospective multicenter evaluation of a initially placed button gastrostomy. Gastrointest Endosc 1995;41:105–108.
20 Maetani I, Yasuda M, Seiko M, Ikeda M, Tada T, Ukita T, et al: Efficacy of an overtube for reducing the risk of peristomal infection after PEG placement: a prospective, randomized comparison group. Gastrointest Endosc 2005;61:522–527.
21 Ponsky JL: Percutaneous endoscopic gastrostomy. J Gastrointest Surg 2004;8:901–904.
22 Vitale MA, Villoti G, D'Alba L, De Cesare M, Frontespezi S, Lacopini G: Unsedated transnasal PEG placement in selected patients. Endoscopy 2005;37:48–51.
23 Chaves DM, Kumar A, Lera ME, et al: EUS-guided percutaneous endoscopic gastrostomy for enteral feeding tube placement. Gastrointest Endosc 2008;68:1168–1172.
24 Hogan RB, DeMarco DC, Hamilton JK, Walker CO, Polter CE: Percutaneous endoscopic gastrostomy: to push or to pull. Gastrointest Endosc 1986;32:253–258.
25 Kozarek RA, Ball TJ, Ryan JA: When push comes to shove: a comparison between two methods of percutaneous endoscopic gastrostomy. Am J Gastroenterol 1986; 81:642–646.
26 Larson DE, Burton DD, Schroeder KW, et al: Percutaneous endoscopic gastrostomy Indications, success, complications and mortality in 314 consecutive patients. Gastroenterology 1987;93:48–52.
27 Wollman B, D'Agostino HB, Walus-Wigle JR, et al: Radiologic, endoscopic and surgical gastrostomy, an institutional evaluation and meta-analysis of the literature. Radiology 1995;197:699–704.
28 Disario J: Endoscopic approaches to enteral nutritional support. Best Pract Res Clin Gastroenterol 2006;20:605–630.
29 Lin HS, Ibrahim HZ, Kheng JW, et al: Percutaneous endoscopic gastrostomy: strategies for prevention and management of complications. Laryngoscope 2001;111: 1847–1852.
30 Bender JS, Levison MA: Complications after percutaneous endoscopic gastrostomy removal. Surg Laparosc Endosc 1991;1:101–103.
31 Khurama V, Singh T: Percutaneous endoscopic gastrostomy site metastasis in esophageal cancer. Gastrointest Endosc 2005;62:612.
32 Strock P, Weber J: Buried bumper syndrome: endoscopic management using a balloon dilator. Endoscopy 2005; 37:279.
33 Klein S, Hear BR, Soloway RD: The 'buried bumper syndrome: a complication of percutaneous gastrostomy. Am J Gastroenterol 1990;85:448–51.
34 Venu RP, Brown RD, Pastika BJ, et al: The buried bumper symdrome: a simple management approach in two patients. Gastrointest Endosc 2002;56:582–584.
35 Kumer S, Dreyer JS: Stylet reinforcement method for replacement of a percutaneous gastrostomy tubes: a useful technique using endoscopic biopsy forceps. Endoscopy 2004,36:466.

L. López Rosés, MD
Gastroenterology Department, Xeral-Calde Hospital
ES–27004 Lugo (Spain)
E-Mail leolopezroses@hotmail.com

Mönkemüller K, Wilcox CM, Muñoz-Navas M (eds): Interventional and Therapeutic Gastrointestinal Endoscopy.
Front Gastrointest Res. Basel, Karger, 2010, vol 27, pp 209–214

Direct Percutaneous Endoscopic Jejunostomy

Todd H. Baron

Department of Medicine, Division of Gastroenterology and Hepatology, Mayo Clinic, Rochester, Minn., USA

Abstract

Direct percutaneous endoscopic jejunostomy is a method of placing a jejunal feeding tube directly into the small bowel in a manner similar to placement of a percutaneous endoscopic gastrostomy tube. The advantages over other endoscopic methods of jejunal feeding include anchoring of the tube into the small bowel and large luminal diameter. Successful placement is achieved in approximately 85% of patients and the procedure is more technically challenging to perform than for percutaneous endoscopic gastrostomy. This chapter reviews the method of direct percutaneous endoscopic jejunostomy tube placement and outcome following attempted placement.

Direct percutaneous endoscopic jejunostomy (DPEJ) was described more than 20 years ago. The technique for DPEJ placement has been described [1, 2] though is not standardized. The alternative to DPEJ placement is percutaneous endoscopic gastrostomy (PEG) placement with jejunal extension (PEG-J). The advantages of DPEJ over PEG-J are the ability to place a larger diameter feeding tube (decreased clogging) and the anchoring of the tube into the jejunum since the J-extension tube of a PEG-J often migrates back into the stomach. In fact, DPEJ has been shown to provide better long-term placement than PEG-J [3].

Indications for and Contraindications of DPEJ Placement

Long-term jejunal feeding is necessary in a variety of clinical situations (table 1). These include patients considered at high risk for or have been documented to have aspiration of gastric feedings, those with non-functional stomachs (diabetic gastroparesis), patients with esophageal obstruction, and patients needing tube placement for feeding or venting and whose stomachs are not accessible or amenable for PEG placement (subtotal gastrectomy, distal esophagectomy with gastric pull-up).

Preprocedural Evaluation

Prior to the DPEJ, laboratory evaluation as for PEG should be undertaken including CBC, platelets, and coagulation parameters. The type of endoscope used is based on whether the patient has native gastrointestinal anatomy or surgically altered anatomy. In patients with native anatomy, colonoscopes or enteroscopes are required to pass beyond the ligament of Treitz. Surgeries in which a standard upper endoscope is long enough to reach the jejunum are seen in table 2. Preprocedural antibiotics should be administered as in PEG placement.

Required Accessories

A standard PEG tray is needed. A colonic length polypectomy snare is needed when a longer endoscope is used, since the standard PEG tray snare has a length for passage through a standard upper endoscope. Glucagon or another antiperistaltic agent should be readily available to administer in order to reduce motility.

Position

The patient is kept in the supine position. If possible the head of bed can be raised to reduce the risk of aspiration if retained food (e.g. in the setting gastroparesis) is present. Alternatively, the patient can be placed in the left lateral decubitus position until the small bowel is entered.

DPEJ Insertion

After the endoscope has been passed into the duodenum, an antiperistaltic agent can be administered. Immediately after the endoscope has been passed into the jejunum the endoscopist and assistant should look for an area of transillumination, since on occasion, an ideal location will be found upon insertion and not withdrawal of the endoscope. In most cases, the light transillumination will be located in the left upper quadrant, though one should be aware that the light may be seen virtually anywhere in the abdomen and may be found in the left flank or in the pelvis. Abdominal scars do not necessarily need to be avoided since a loop of small bowel may be adhered and fixed at this point. Although transillumination and indention are required to safely perform DPEJ, the transillumination is frequently not as bright as for PEG placement. Thus, the transillumination button on the processor should be used liberally and all room lights and extraneous display monitors should be turned off.

Once an area of transillumination and indentation has been identified, the person performing the non-endoscopic portion of the procedure needs to act quickly, since the transillumination location may change during the course of the procedure. The abdomen is quickly prepped and draped and lidocaine is used for local anesthesia. At this point, the middle-length needle in the PEG tray is used as a 'finder needle'. Once this needle has been passed transabdominally and is identified endoscopically, it should be grasped as firmly as possible with the snare to fix the small bowel close to the abdominal wall. The trocar is then passed percutaneously alongside the finder needle in the same trajectory (fig. 1). When the trocar is visible endoscopically, the finder needle is released from the snare and the trocar is endoscopically grasped with the snare (fig. 2). Care must be taken to grasp the trocar tightly enough that it is not released, but not so tight that it kinks the catheter once the stylet has been removed. The remainder of the examination proceeds as with PEG placement as the loop is passed through the trocar and grasped (fig. 3) and the endoscope is

Table 1. Indications and contraindications for DPEJ placement

Indications	
1.	Patients whose stomach is obstructed or non-functional (diabetic gastroparesis)
2.	Patients at high-risk or with documented aspiration of gastric feedings
3.	Patients with previous gastric resection or gastric bypass in whom PEG placement (for feeding or venting) is not feasible
4.	Intrathoracic stomach in those patients requiring enteral access
5.	Patients with complications of acute and chronic pancreatitis
6.	Patients with distal esophageal carcinoma - preoperative nutritional support to avoid PEG which may interfere with gastric pull-up
Contraindications	
1.	Large volume ascites
2.	Uncorrected coagulopathy
3.	Inability to obtain informed consent
4.	Intra-abdominal perforation
5.	Pregnancy

Table 2. Postsurgical anatomy in which an upper endoscope may be used for DPEJ placement

Prior subtotal gastrectomy with inability to transilluminate or indent
Prior total gastrectomy
Ivor-Lewis (distal esophagus and proximal gastric resection)
Billroth II
Gastric bypass with Roux-en-Y gastrojejunostomy
Pancreaticoduodenectomy with antrectomy (Whipple procedure) with inability to transilluminate and indent

withdrawn. The endoscope does not need to be reinserted to confirm proper location (fig. 4) after it has been pulled into position unless excessive resistance is encountered (which occasionally occurs at the pylorus), or if the tube feels like it is in place under the skin but the length of external tube is excessive (the tube should be at the 2- to 3-cm mark externally when in correct position).

Fluoroscopy has been described as being helpful during DPEJ placement, although it may allow one to identify the tip of the endoscope in relation to the surface of the abdomen. Its use, however, is not a substitute for adequate transillumination and indentation.

Special Considerations

Altered Anatomy. In patients with Billroth II or Whipple anatomy where there is an afferent and efferent jejunal limb, the tube should be placed into the efferent limb or the location where the limbs meet. For example, in patients with Billroth II anatomy, one can locate the papilla or proximal stump of the afferent limb endoscopically, then withdraw the endoscope and pass the endoscope into the other limb. On occasion, in patients with Billroth II anatomy the best transillumination is found at the branch point between the two limbs. Assuming that the patient did well

1 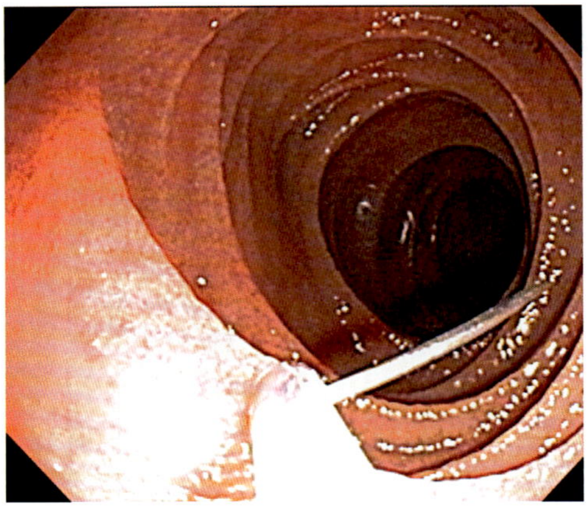

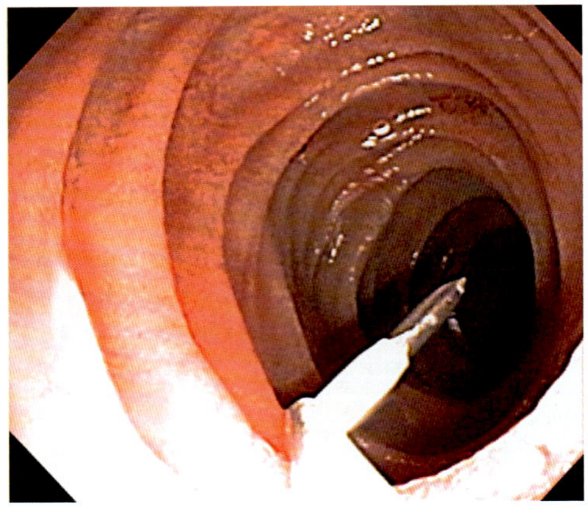 2

3 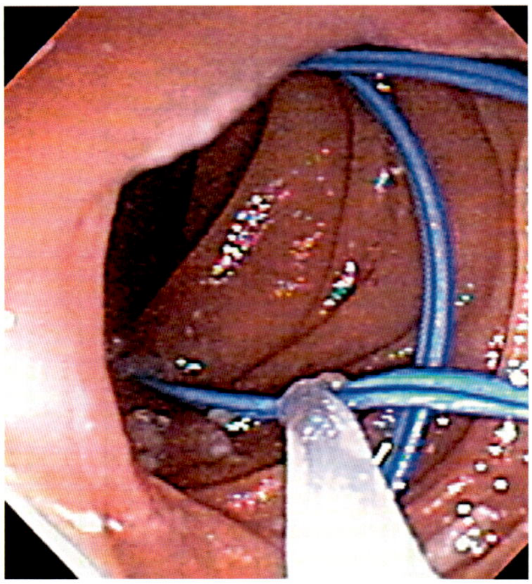

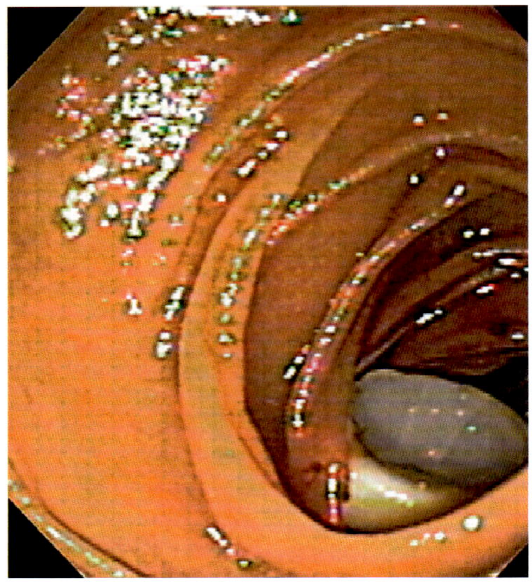 4

Fig. 1. Endoscopic view taken during DPEJ placement. The middle-length needle is grasped with the snare to maintain adherence to the anterior abdominal wall. **Fig. 2.** The trocar has been passed into the jejunal limb and grasped. **Fig. 3.** The loop has been passed through the trocar and grasped with the snare. **Fig. 4.** Endoscopic view showing position of the 20-french tube in the jejunum.

with per oral intake prior to PEG (neurologic dysphagia), this location should be adequate for jejunal feeding. In patients with Roux-en-Y gastrojejunostomy, the jejunal limb is the only efferent limb leading away from the stomach and usually easily reached with an upper endoscope.

Gastric Decompression. Some patients with severe gastroparesis require both gastric decompression and jejunal feeding.

Transgastric DPEJ. In some instances, a patient with an existing PEG needs DPEJ feeding. It is technically feasible to pass a small caliber endoscope transgastrically through a mature PEG tract beyond the ligament of Treitz and perform DPEJ. The feeding tube is pulled through the PEG tract [4, 5].

Timing of Postprocedural Feeding

In the absence of complications, the tube may be used for fluid and medications 4 h after placement. Tube feeding is usually initiated 12 h after placement.

DPEJ Removal and Replacement

There is almost no published information concerning removal of DPEJ tubes. It is unknown what duration of time is required for maturation of the PEJ tract and safety of traction removal. Based upon PEG data, the tract should be mature at 4 weeks. At that time, conversion to skin level devices may be undertaken in the usual fashion. One should consider fluoroscopic confirmation of correct tube positioning after traction removal and replacement. If balloon replacement tubes are used, we inflate with less than the recommended volume of water (half the recommended volume) to keep the balloon volume small enough to prevent obstruction of the jejunal lumen.

Complications have been noted with traction removal of DPEJ tubes including bleeding and tract disruption with intraabdominal leakage. Therefore, some endoscopists prefer endoscopic removal by passing the endoscope into the jejunum, grasping the bumper with a snare, and cutting the tube externally. The endoscope is then withdrawn with the tube. In each individual patient the risk of traction removal of the tube must be weighed against the risk of endoscopic removal (which carries risks of sedation and perforation).

Outcomes

In the largest series to date, of over 300 patients undergoing DPEJ placement the success rate was approximately 70%. Adverse events from DPEJ placement or removal occurred in 22.5% of cases including bowel perforation, jejunal volvulus, bleeding, abdominal wall infection and aspiration. Persistent enterocutaneous fistula after removal occurs at a higher rate than with PEG removal and up to 15% [6]. Obesity appears defined as a body mass index of at least 30, decreases DPEJ tube placement success rates and increased complication rates. The success rate was 96% for underweight patients, 81% for patients with a normal body mass index, 73% for overweight patients, and 60% for obese patients [7]. Thus, DPEJ placement, though a viable alternative for long-term enteral feeding, has a lower success rate and higher complication rate than PEG in adults. Limited data suggest DPEJ placement is safe and effective [8].

References

1 Shike M, Latkany L: Direct percutaneous endoscopic jejunostomy. Gastrointest Endosc Clin N Am 1998;8:569–580.

2 Baron TH: Direct percutaneous endoscopic jejunostomy. Am J Gastroenterol 2006;101:1407–1409.

3 Fan AC, Baron TH, Rumalla A, Harewood GC: Comparison of direct percutaneous endoscopic jejunostomy and PEG with jejunal extension. Gastrointest Endosc 2002;56:890–894.

4 Baron TH: Direct percutaneous endoscopic jejunostomy through a mature gastrostomy tract. Gastrointest Endosc 2002;56:946–947.

5 Nishiwaki S, Araki H, Shirakami Y, Kawaguchi J, Asano T, Iwashita M, Tagami A, Hatakeyama H, Hayashi T, Maeda T, Naganawa S, Saitoh K: Direct percutaneous endoscopic jejunostomy using a transgastrostomic endoscope in patients with previous endoscopic gastrostomy. Endoscopy 2009;41(suppl 2):E36–E37.
6 Maple JT, Petersen BT, Baron TH, Gostout CJ, Wong Kee Song LM, Buttar NS: Direct percutaneous endoscopic jejunostomy: outcomes in 307 consecutive attempts. Am J Gastroenterol 2005;100:2681–2688.
7 Mackenzie SH, Haslem D, Hilden K, Thomas KL, Fang JC: Success rate of direct percutaneous endoscopic jejunostomy in patients who are obese. Gastrointest Endosc 2008;67:265–269.
8 Virnig DJ, Frech EJ, Delegge MH, Fang JC: Direct percutaneous endoscopic jejunostomy: a case series in pediatric patients. Gastrointest Endosc 2008;67: 984–987.

Todd H. Baron, MD
200 First Street SW, Charlton 8
Rochester, MN 55905
Tel. +1 507 266 6931, Fax +1 507 266 3939, E-Mail baron.todd@mayo.edu

Mönkemüller K, Wilcox CM, Muñoz-Navas M (eds): Interventional and Therapeutic Gastrointestinal Endoscopy.
Front Gastrointest Res. Basel, Karger, 2010, vol 27, pp 215–220

Therapeutic Small Bowel Endoscopy

Peter B.F. Mensink · Huseyin Aktas

Department of Gastroenterology and Hepatology, Erasmus MC, University Medical Center, Rotterdam, The Netherlands

Abstract

Double-balloon enteroscopy was first introduced in 2001, followed by single-balloon enteroscopy in 2007, allowing endoscopic evaluation and therapy of the small bowel. Since the introduction of both balloon-assisted enteroscopy techniques, endoscopic therapeutic options have evolved rapidly. Argon plasma coagulation, polypectomy, dilation therapy of strictures, and therapy of the pancreatico-biliary system in patients with surgically altered proximal intestinal anatomy: have all been successfully introduced to treat pathological findings in all segments of the small bowel. The clinical impact of treatment of vascular malformations, polypectomy and strictures caused by chronic inflammation therapy seems evident. The overall complication rate of therapeutic balloon-assisted enteroscopy seems acceptable, but is higher compared to therapeutic colonoscopy which needs further attention in future.

Double-balloon enteroscopy (DBE) was introduced in 2001 by Yamamoto et al. [1] as a new endoscopic modality for visualization of the entire small bowel. In 2007 the single-balloon enteroscopy (SBE) technique was introduced [2]. Recently, the term balloon-assisted enteroscopy (BAE) was introduced as a unifying terminology referring to both techniques [3]. In the current chapter, this new term will be used referring to DBE and/or SBE. BAE is now considered the standard endoscopic technique for visualization and endoscopic therapy of the small bowel. Complete small bowel evaluation is achieved in up to 25 and 86% of procedures in respectively SBE and DBE, mostly using the combined oral and rectal approach with tattoo or hemoclip marking [2, 4]. The main advantages of BAE are controlled visualization, targeted biopsy sampling for pathologic evaluation and the ability to perform therapeutic interventions under direct endoscopic visualization. Currently, injection therapy, tattooing, argon plasma coagulation (APC), polypectomy, placement of (hemo)clips, and dilation of strictures are considered standard interventions during a BAE procedure. In selected cases, pancreaticobiliary procedures can be performed using BAE, after surgical reconstructions that impede standard duodenoscopy. The introduction of larger diameter working channels in the latest versions of the enteroscopes, and the development of especially designed materials, have both led to easier access and advanced therapeutic opportunities in the small bowel. In this chapter we will give an overview concerning the current possible therapeutic endoscopic interventions with BAE (table 1).

Table 1. Therapeutic options using balloon enteroscopy

Hemostasis for small bowel bleeding	
	Argon plasma coagulation
	Injection of epinephrine, fibrin glue or Histoacryl
	Placement of clips
Crohn's disease	
	Stricture dilation using through-the-scope balloon
Small bowel polyps and tumors	
	Polypectomy
	Endoscopic mucosal resection
	Lesion marking with submucosal injection with India ink
	Small bowel stent placement for malignant strictures
Removal of foreign body (e.g. capsule endoscope)	
PEG placement in altered bowel anatomy (gastric bypass, Roux-en-Y)	
ERCP in altered bowel anatomy (gastric bypass, Roux-en-Y)	

Technique and Accessories

Both the SBE and DBE technique use longer 'enteroscope' in combination with an additional fixation of the endoscope and/or the overtube by using inflatable balloon(s). The DBE system uses a two-balloon system, while the SBE system uses angulation of the tip the endoscope to fixate the tip of the endoscope. In theory, both systems can be used to visualize the entire small bowel. Currently, the DBE system consists of two commercially available enteroscopes: the EN-450P5/20, 'pediatric type' or the EN-450T5, 'therapeutic type' (Fujinon Inc., Saitama, Japan). Both enteroscopes are 200 cm in length, but differ in outer diameter of the enteroscope and working channel: 8.5 and 9.4, and 2.2 and 2.8 mm, respectively. The majority of therapeutic accessories like injectors, APC catheters, polypectomy snares, endoloops and baskets can be used and are available for both types of enteroscopes. CRE-dilation balloons and hemoclips can only be used by the therapeutic type enteroscope because of the wider working channel provided by this enteroscope. The SBE enteroscope, SIF-Q180 (Olympus Optical Co., Ltd, Tokyo, Japan) is also 200 cm in working length, has an outer diameter of 9.2 mm and a working channel of 2.8 mm. Both the DBE and SBE systems use an overtube of 145 and 140 cm length, respectively. The overtube of the DBE system is polyethylene-based, while the SBE system uses silicone-based overtubes. Also, both systems use a remotely controlled pump system to in- and deflate the balloon(s).

Therapy and Outcome

Argon Plasma Coagulation. APC is a method of non-contact electrocoagulation in which current is applied to tissues by means of ionized argon gas (argon plasma) (table 2). BAE is widely used in evaluating the causes of obscure gastrointestinal bleeding (OGIB). Angiodysplasia, or arteriovascular malformations (AVMs), and tumors are the most important causes of OGIB [4–7]. APC of AVMs can lead to cessation of the gastrointestinal bleeding resulting in decrease or stop

Table 2. Outcomes and complication rates of therapeutic BAE

Indication/therapy	Clinical impact	Complication rate
Angiodysplasia/APC	59–89%	0.9–1.6%
Polyps*/polypectomy	unknown, seems positive	3.3–10.8%
Dilation/strictures (mainly CD)	71–74%	0–2.9%
Altered anatomy/ERCP BAE	85–94%	0–5%

BAE = Balloon-assisted enteroscopy; APC = argon plasma coagulation; CD = Crohn's disease; * = FAP (familial adenomatous polyposis); PJS (Peutz-Jegher syndrome).

of transfusion requirements [5]. The real clinical impact of treatment of angiodysplasia or AVMs is currently a point of discussion: primary data concerning this issue showed promising results, but a recent study with longer follow-up has reported more disappointing results [8]. May et al. [9] showed that APC is also effective in hemostasis of Dieulafoy lesions in the small bowel. APC during BAE is also an applicable treatment of small and flat adenomas and can be used if these adenomas are endoscopically difficult to remove because of challenging position [10].

The energy levels used in APC treatment is of significant importance, in combination with the diameter of the APC probe for prevention of possible complications (i.e. perforation). A standard catheter diameter of 1.5 mm (4.5 Fr) in combination with energy levels of 30–40 W (APC 300/Erbotom ICC 200) or 15–25 W and pulse 2 mode (Vio APC 2, both Erbe Elektromedizin, Tübingen, Germany) seems safe [9, 10].

Polypectomy. Small bowel polyps and tumors are a common finding in patients undergoing BAE [11]. Small bowel polyps include hyperplastic polyps, adenomas mostly in relation with familial adenomatous polyposis and hamartomatous polyps associated with the Peutz-Jeghers syndrome (PJS). Before the introduction of BAE, patients with PJS underwent, mostly repeated, polypectomy or enterectomy during urgent or planned laparotomies. BAE is an effective approach to screen the whole small bowel for polyps and if indicated to remove these polyps. An additional indication for repeated polyp surveillance with BAE in these patients might be the malignancy rate of 2–3% for polyps 11 cm [10, 11]. 18 polypectomies (varying in polyp size of 10–60 mm in diameter) during DBE were successfully performed in 2 patients with PJS, reported by Ohmiya et al. [12]. They concluded that PJS-associated complications (intussusception, bleeding and tumorigenesis) can be reduced by enteroscopic polypectomies [12]. May et al. [9] performed successfully 44 polypectomies for polyps ranging in diameter from 10 to 50 mm. In PJS patients with endoscopic unresectable polyps or acute small bowel obstruction due to intussusception, laparotomy remains the first-choice treatment.

Polypectomies can be carried out with a polypectomy snare after submucosal injection of the stalk of the polyp with a diluted epinephrine-saline solution (1:100,000). After resection, polyps can be captured with the polypectomy snare or a polyp retriever with a nitinol basket. Using a large-diameter overtube, the endoscope can be pulled back through the overtube outside the patient, with the overtube staying in position. After removal of the resected polyp, the endoscope can be reinserted via the overtube, resuming the enteroscopy. Adequate sedation by propofol or general anesthesia is preferred for these patients, in which the procedures are more time-consuming and possibly more difficult by agitation of the patients [6]. So far, the experience of enteroscopic resection of flat adenomas or (early) cancers in the small bowel by BAE is limited. Only a few (case) reports have been published, describing resection of an early carcinoma in the afferent loop of a Roux-en-Y anastomosis and resection of a flat adenoma, both clinically successful [6, 13].

Dilation Therapy. Many chronic inflammatory diseases can cause strictures in the small bowel. Crohn's disease is one of the most common inflammatory diseases, often causing strictures in the small bowel. These strictures are mostly located in jejuno-ileal and ileal region (respectively 36 and 32%), but can also be located more proximal in the small bowel [9, 14]. BAE dilation therapy seems a safe and clinical useful alternative for, repeated, surgical therapy in these patients. Especially in patients with the need for repeated small bowel surgery, endoscopic dilation therapy might prevent short bowel problems in the future. Endoscopic dilation therapy can be performed using the 'through-the-endoscope' balloon dilation technique in enteroscopes with a large-diameter working channel. An alternative technique is placement of a guidewire through the stenosis, consequently removal of the endoscope (leaving the overtube in position) and insertion of a dilation balloon over the guidewire. After the dilation, the enteroscope can be reintroduced via the overtube, and the effect of treatment can be visualized. In general, all enteroscopic dilation procedures are performed using fluoroscopy guidance. Fukumoto et al. [14] showed in a large series of small bowel strictures that in 87% of patients the lesions could be identified with DBE. They showed a success rate of 71% after dilation therapy (74% in the Crohn's stricture patients), after a mean follow-up of almost 12 months. The overall mean number of dilations was 1.6 per patient (1.5 in the Crohn's patients). Of the Crohn's disease stricture patients who had initial endoscopic dilation therapy, 17% had repeated dilation therapy and almost 9% eventually needed surgical therapy.

ERCP Procedures. Conventional endoscopic retrograde cholangiopancreaticography (ERCP) in patients after gastric or biliodigestive surgery can be challenging and is, depending on the type of surgery, often unsuccessful. Using BAE, deep insertion of these endoscopically difficult-to-reach bowel loops seems feasible, and diagnostic and therapeutic interventions of the pancreatico-biliary system can be performed [15–22]. Haruta et al. [15] reported the first treatment of a stricture in a hepaticojejunal anastomosis after liver transplantation in a child, using BAE. Repeated enteroscopic balloon dilations were necessary for a long-term success. More recently, Aabakken et al. [16] showed a success rate of 94% (17 out of 18) in reaching the end of the afferent limb of the Roux-en-Y anastomosis using BAE. They performed the majority of procedures (10 out of 13) in patients after liver transplantation for primary sclerosing cholangitis. A diagnosis was established in up to 85% of patients and therapy was successful in the majority of cases [17].

Enteral Stent Placement. Ross et al. [23] reported on the technique of enteral stent placement using BAE. In their case series, self-expanding metal stents were placed as a palliative measure in patients with stenosing small bowel tumors.

Foreign Body Extraction. DBE also enables the removal of foreign bodies from the small intestine making surgical intervention unnecessary. Numerous cases of successful retrieval of retained capsule endoscopes using the oral or anal approach are described in the current literature [24].

Complications

Recently, two large multicenter studies have presented data concerning complications and DBE [25, 26]. The complication rate after diagnostic DBE procedures was 0.8% and comparable in both studies. The complication rate of therapeutic DBE procedures was 4.3%, this rate being higher compared to therapeutic colonoscopy [25]. A single-center study by May et al. [9], focusing especially on complications after therapeutic DBE, reported an overall complication rate of 3.4%. In the latter study a rather high complication rate of 10.8% was reported after polypectomy. In the international multicenter study, one acute pancreatitis was reported after a pancreatico-biliary intervention in a patient with a Roux-en-Y biliodigestive anastomosis. Several other case reports document the risk of complications after therapeutic interventions using DBE [27, 28]. The first two published series concerning SBE procedures reported both one complication, accounting for a complication rate of 1.2 and 2.7%, respectively [2, 29].

Conclusions

The introduction of BAE has given the endoscopist the opportunity to perform therapeutic endoscopic interventions in all regions of the small bowel. In a short time, therapeutic BAE has evolved to a wide range of different endoscopic therapies. In the past few years a lot of experience has been gathered, especially concerning APC treatment (AVMs and angiodysplasia), polypectomy (PJS), dilation therapy (Crohn's disease) and ERCP procedures in patients with surgically altered proximal intestinal anatomy. These BAE therapeutic interventions seem of clinical benefit in selected patients, although currently controversy exists about the long-term outcome following endoscopic therapy in OGIB patients. Hopefully in the coming years prospective studies will give answers concerning this interesting clinical problem. The clinical impact of dilation of small bowel Crohn's disease strictures and polypectomies in the PJS appears to be evident, but larger and longer follow-up studies after therapy have to be conducted. The concomitant introduction of anti-TNF medication in Crohn's disease patients treated with dilation therapy for small bowel strictures can possibly improve the outcome in these patients. The overall complication rate of therapeutic BAE seems acceptable, but is slightly higher compared to therapeutic colonoscopy. Further improvement of enteroscopy techniques, endoscopic materials and patient sedation methods will hopefully lead to a higher clinical impact and lower complication rate of therapeutic BAE in future.

References

1 Yamamoto H, Sekine Y, Sato Y, Higashizawa T, Miyata T, Iino S, et al: Total enteroscopy with a nonsurgical steerable double-balloon method. Gastrointest Endosc 2001;53:216–220.

2 Tsujikawa T, Saitoh Y, Andoh A, Imaeda H, Hata K, Minematsu H, et al: Novel single-balloon enteroscopy for diagnosis and treatment of the small intestine: preliminary experiences. Endoscopy 2008;40: 11–15.

3 Mönkemüller K, Fry LC, Bellutti M, Malfertheiner P: Balloon-assisted enteroscopy: unifying double-balloon and single-balloon enteroscopy. Endoscopy 2008;40:537.

4 Zhong J, Ma T, Zhang C, et al: A retrospective study of the application on double-balloon enteroscopy in 378 patients with suspected small-bowel diseases. Endoscopy 2007;39:208–215.

5 Kwan V, Bourke MJ, Williams SJ, Gillespie PE, Murray MA, Kaffes AJ, et al: Argon plasma coagulation in the management of symptomatic gastrointestinal vascular lesions: experience in 100 consecutive patients with long-term follow-up. Am J Gastroenterol 2006;101:58–63.

6 Kaffes AJ, Siah C, Koo JH: Clinical outcomes after double-balloon enteroscopy in patients with obscure gastrointestinal bleeding and a positive capsule endoscopy. Gastrointest Endosc 2007;66:304–309.

7 Sun B, Rajan E, Cheng S, Shen R, Zhang C, Zhang S, et al: Diagnostic yield and therapeutic impact of double-balloon enteroscopy in a large cohort of patients with obscure gastrointestinal bleeding. Am J Gastroenterol 2006;101:2011–2015.

8 Madisch A, Schmolders J, Brückner S, Aust D, Miehlke S: Less favorable clinical outcome after diagnostic and interventional double-balloon enteroscopy in patients with suspected small-bowel bleeding? Endoscopy 2008; 40:731–734.
9 May A, Nachbar L, Pohl J, Ell C: Endoscopic interventions in the small bowel using double-balloon enteroscopy: feasibility and limitations. Am J Gastroenterol 2007;102:527–535.
10 Mönkemüller K, Fry LC, Ebert M, et al: Feasibility of double-balloon enteroscopy-assisted chromoendoscopy of the small bowel in patients with familial adenomatous polyposis. Endoscopy 2007;39:52–57.
11 Fry LC, Neumann H, Kuester D, Kuhn R, Bellutti M, Malfertheiner P, Mönkemüller K: Small bowel polyps and tumours: endoscopic detection and treatment by double-balloon enteroscopy. Aliment Pharmacol Ther 2008;29:135–142.
12 Ohmiya N, Taguchi A, Shirai K, Mabuchi N, Arakawa D, Kanazawa H, et al: Endoscopic resection of Peutz-Jeghers polyps throughout the small intestine at double-balloon enteroscopy without laparotomy. Gastrointest Endosc 2005;61:140–147.
13 Kuno A, Yamamoto H, Kita H, Sunada K, Yano T, Hayashi Y, et al: Double-balloon enteroscopy through a Roux-en-Y anastomosis for EMR of an early carcinoma in the afferent duodenal limb. Gastrointest Endosc 2004; 60:1032–1034.
14 Fukumoto A, Tanaka S, Yamamoto H, Yao T, Matsui T, Iida M, et al: Diagnosis and treatment of small-bowel stricture by double-balloon endoscopy. Gastrointest Endosc 2007;66:S108–S112.
15 Haruta H, Yamamoto H, Mizuta K, Kita Y, Uno T, Egami S, et al: A case of successful enteroscopic balloon dilation for late anastomotic stricture of choledochojejunostomy after living donor liver transplantation. Liver Transpl 2005;11:1608–1610.
16 Aabakken L, Bretthauer M, Line PD: Double-balloon enteroscopy for endoscopic retrograde cholangiography in patients with a Roux-en-Y anastomosis. Endoscopy 2007;39:1068–1071.
17 Maaser C, Lenze F, Bokemeyer M, Ullerich H, Domagk D, Bruewer M, et al: Double-balloon enteroscopy: a useful tool for diagnostic and therapeutic procedures in the pancreaticobiliary system. Am J Gastroenterol 2008; 103:894–900.
18 Chu YC, Yang CC, Yeh YH, Chen CH, Yueh SK: Double-balloon enteroscopy application in biliary tract disease – its therapeutic and diagnostic functions. Gastrointest Endosc 2008;68:585–591.
19 Moreels TG, Roth B, Vandervliet EJ, Parizel PM, Dutré J, Pelckmans PA: The use of the double-balloon enteroscope for endoscopic retrograde cholangiopancreatography and biliary stent placement after Roux-en-Y hepaticojejunostomy. Endoscopy 2007;39 (suppl 1): E196–E197.
20 Koornstra JJ: Double-balloon enteroscopy for endoscopic retrograde cholangiopancreaticography after Roux-en-Y reconstruction: case series and review of the literature. Neth J Med 2008;66:275–279.
21 Fähndrich M, Sandmann M, Heike M: A facilitated method for endoscopic interventions at the bile duct after Roux-en-Y reconstruction using double-balloon enteroscopy. Z Gastroenterol 2008;46:335–338.
22 Mönkemüller K, Fry LC, Bellutti M, Neumann H, Malfertheiner P: ERCP using single-balloon instead of double-balloon enteroscopy in patients with Roux-en-Y anastomosis. Endoscopy 2008;40:E19–E20.
23 Ross AS, Semrad C, Waxman I, Dye C: Enteral stent placement by double-balloon enteroscopy for palliation of malignant small bowel obstruction. Gastrointest Endosc 2006;64:835–837.
24 Rejchrt S, Kopacova M, Tacheci I, Bures J: Interventional DBE for Crohn's, gastrointestinal bleeding and foreign body extraction. Tech Gastrointest Endosc 2008;10:101–106.
25 Mensink PB, Haringsma J, Kucharzik T, Cellier C, Pérez-Cuadrado E, Mönkemüller K, et al: Complications of double-balloon enteroscopy: a multicenter study. Endoscopy 2007;39:613–615.
26 Möschler O, May AD, Müller MK, Ell C; DBE-Studiengruppe Deutschland: Complications in double-balloon enteroscopy: results of the German DBE register. Z Gastroenterol 2008;46:266–270.
27 Spahn TW, Kampmann W, Eilers M, et al: Small-bowel perforation after endoscopic resection of a Peutz-Jeghers polyp in an infant using double-balloon enteroscopy. Endoscopy 2007;39:E217.
28 Matsushita M, Shimatani M, Uchida K, et al: Mechanism of acute pancreatitis after peroral double-balloon enteroscopy. Endoscopy 2007;39:480–481.
29 Kawamura T, Yasuda K, Tanaka K, Uno K, Ueda M, Sanada K, Nakajima M: Clinical evaluation of a newly developed single-balloon enteroscope. Gastrointest Endosc 2008;68: 1112–1116.

Peter Mensink, MD, PhD
Department of Gastroenterology and Hepatology, Erasmas MC University Medical Center
PO Box 2040, NL–3000 CA Rotterdam (The Netherlands)
Fax +31 10 4634680, E-Mail p.mensink@erasmusmc.nl

Mönkemüller K, Wilcox CM, Muñoz-Navas M (eds): Interventional and Therapeutic Gastrointestinal Endoscopy.
Front Gastrointest Res. Basel, Karger, 2010, vol 27, pp 221–239

Middle Gastrointestinal Bleeding

Klaus Mönkemüller[a,b] · Helmut Neumann[b] · Lucía C. Fry[a,b]

[a]Department of Internal Medicine, Gastroenterology, Hepatology and Infectious Diseases, Marienhospital, Bottrop, and [b]Department of Gastroenterology, Hepatology and Infectious Diseases, Otto-von-Guericke University, Magdeburg, Germany

Abstract

Middle gastrointestinal (GI) bleeding (MGIB) refers to small bowel bleeding originating distal to the ampulla of Vater and proximal to the ileocecal valve. The differential diagnosis of small bowel bleeding is broad and includes among many others: angioectasias, ulcers, erosions, tumors, jejunitis, ischemic and portal enteropathy. The preferred endoscopic methods to investigate small bowel bleeding include capsule endoscopy and balloon-assisted enteroscopy. Push enteroscopy remains an important option for lesions suspected to be located in the proximal 60–70 cm of jejunum. Spiral enteroscopy is emerging as another useful enteroscopic method to investigate the small bowel. Other important tests in the evaluation of MGIB include angiography, red blood cell scans, computed tomography (CT), small bowel enteroclysis, magnetic resonance imaging (MRI) and CT or MRI enterography/enteroclysis. In this article we will focus on the approach and management of MGIB.

Traditionally gastrointestinal (GI) bleeding (GIB) has been classified as upper and lower [1]. Upper GIB (UGIB) is defined as hemorrhage originating from the oropharynx to the ligament of Treitz, and lower GIB (LGIB) is defined as bleeding distal to the ligament of Treitz [1]. However, this classification is inexact as we currently know that the small bowel represents significant sources for occult and overt GIB [2–7]. Given the small bowel's importance as a source of bleeding, the new term 'mid-gastrointestinal bleeding' (MGIB) was proposed [8]. However, the exact anatomical landmarks to define MGIB remain to be defined. Although some authors propose the area of the small bowel distal to the ligament of Treitz to the ileocecal valve, we prefer to use the ampulla of Vater as the proximal landmark. First, the ligament of Treitz is an anatomical landmark that only rarely can be localized endoscopically. Second, we always recommend utilizing the duodenoscope in cases of obscure overt GIB to rule out hemobilia, hemosuccus pancreaticus or hemorrhage around the papilla of Vater.

Before discussing the approach to MGIB we want to emphasize that MGIB is not the same as obscure GIB (OGIB). OGIB is defined as bleeding of unknown origin that persists or recurs after a negative initial esophagogastroduodenography (EGD) and colonoscopy [1]. Per definition one would assume that if an EGD and colonoscopy were negative the source of GIB should be in the small bowel, and OGIB has been equated with MGIB. However, studies during the push enteroscopy (PE) era and recent studies using double-balloon enteroscopy clearly show that up to 30% of OGIB can be found within reach of conventional endoscopes (i.e. EGD and/or colonoscopy) [9–12]. When evaluating patients with OGIB it is important to repeat both EGD and colonoscopy because a significant number of these patients will have bleeding lesions in the esophagus, stomach or colon that were overlooked during the initial workup [1, 11, 12]. Commonly overlooked lesions include Cameron's erosions, fundic varices, peptic ulcer disease, angiectasias, Dieulafoy's lesion and gastric antral vascular ectasias in the upper GI tract, and angiectasias and neoplasms in the lower GI tract [1].

Differential Diagnosis of Middle Gastrointestinal Bleeding

OGIB accounts for about 5% of episodes of GIB [1]. Thus, it is estimated that 3–4% of cases of bleeding originate from the small bowel. However, this number may be an underestimation as it is becoming clear that previously unknown or recognized lesions such as portal enteropathy, Non-steroidal anti-inflammatory drug (NSAID) enteropathy and tumors are an important source of OGIB [2–8, 13, 14]. Table 1 lists reported causes of MGIB. Figures 1–18 exemplify causes of MGIB.

Approach to MGIB

Most patients being evaluated for MGIB have already undergone a clinical, laboratory and endoscopic investigation. However, as with any GI hemorrhage the most important aspect is to obtain a thorough history and to perform a thorough physical examination. It will never harm to have a repeat detailed history and physical examination. In addition, a thorough review of the medical records and transfer documentation is essential.

History and Physical Examination

Despite every technological advance, a thorough investigation of the patient's history and physical examination is still necessary to assess the etiology of bleeding. Severe bleeding is usually manifested as melena or hematochezia, which usually results in hemodynamic alterations reflected by resting tachycardia (pulse ≥100 beats/min) and hypotension (systolic blood pressure <100 mm Hg). Clues such as dry mucous membranes, non-distensible neck veins, and decreased urinary output also point towards significant intravascular volume depletion. Patients with slow bleeding may only have hemoccult-positive stools. On physical examination look for clues such as stigmata of chronic liver disease, emaciation, cachexia, heart failure and subtle signs such as angioectasias of the lips and tongue.

Internal risk factors for GIB include a positive family history of celiac disease, hereditary hemorrhagic diseases (e.g. Rendu-Osler-Weber syndrome, von Willebrand disease), aortic stenosis (Heyde's syndrome) or even polyposis syndromes (hamartomatous familial polyposis syndromes including Peutz-Jeghers syndrome, juvenile polyposis syndrome, Cowden disease, and Ruvalcaba-Myhre-Smith syndrome and adenomatous polyposis syndromes including the classic familial adenomatous polyposis, Gardner syndrome and Turcot syndrome) [1]. External risk factors contain medication use (e.g. coumarins, NSAIDs, aspirin) and prior surgeries (e.g. abdominal aortic aneurysm repair, liver transplantation, bowel resection) [1]. Physical examination, especially

Table 1. Reported causes of small bowel bleeding

Vascular diseases	
	Angiodysplasias
	Dieulafoy's lesions
	Ischemic enteritis
	Varices
	Arteriovenous malformations
	Portal enteropathy
Inflammatory and autoimmune diseases	
	Behcet's disease
	Non-steroidal anti-inflammatory drug (NSAID)-induced
	Antihypertensive drug-induced
	Intestinal tuberculosis
	Crohn's disease
	Duodenal ulcers
	Amyloidosis
	Radiation injury
	Ulcers of unknown origin
	Eosinophilic enteritis
	Anastomotic ulcers
Polyps and tumors	
	Inflammatory polyps
	Gastrointestinal stromal tumor
	Adenoma
	Adenocarcinoma
	MALT lymphoma
	Follicular lymphoma
	Lipoma
	Hamartoma
	Metastasis
	Hemangioma
	Carcinoids
	Adenomyoma
	Lymphangioma
	Leiomyosarcoma
	Cronkhite-Canada syndrome
	T-cell lymphoma
	Gardner's syndrome
Diverticulosis	
	Meckel's diverticula
	Diverticula retracted by tumors
	Diverticula retracted by adhesions
Infections	
	Whipple's disease
	Strongyloidiasis
	Cytomegalovirus
	Mycobacterium avium complex
	M. tuberculosis
	Blastomycosis

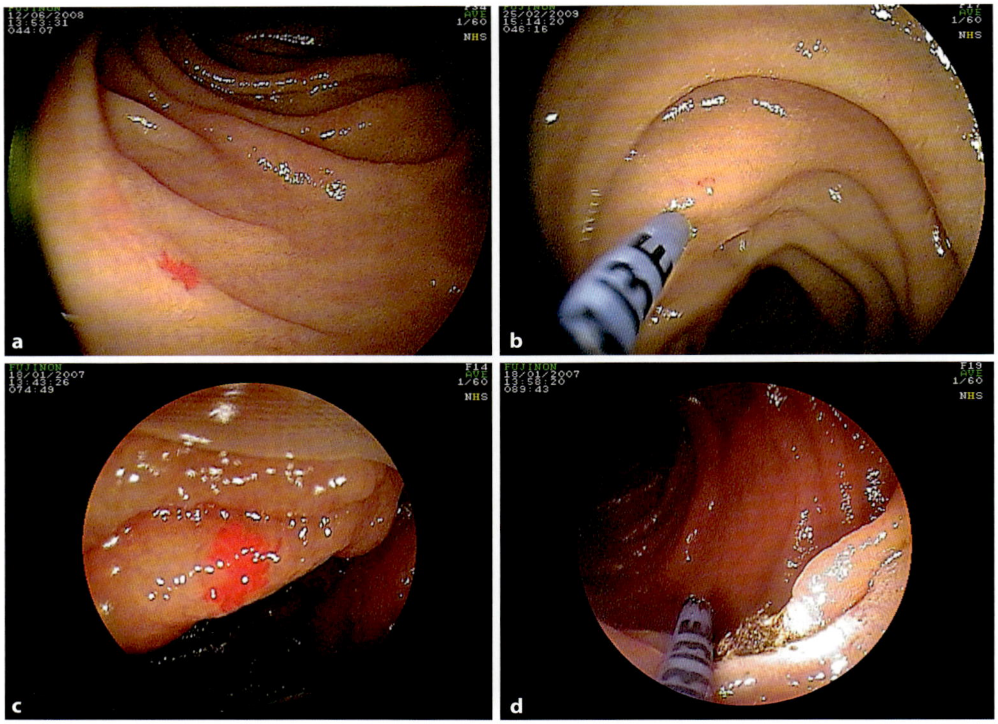

Fig. 1. The most common cause of small bowel bleeding is angioectasias. A jejunal angoectasia (**a**) which is being cauterized with argon plasma coagulation (APC; **b**). A larger ileal angiectasia (**c**) was ablated with APC (**d**). When applying APC to the small bowel, we use 20–30 W, as higher power settings can result in perforation due to the thin small bowel wall.

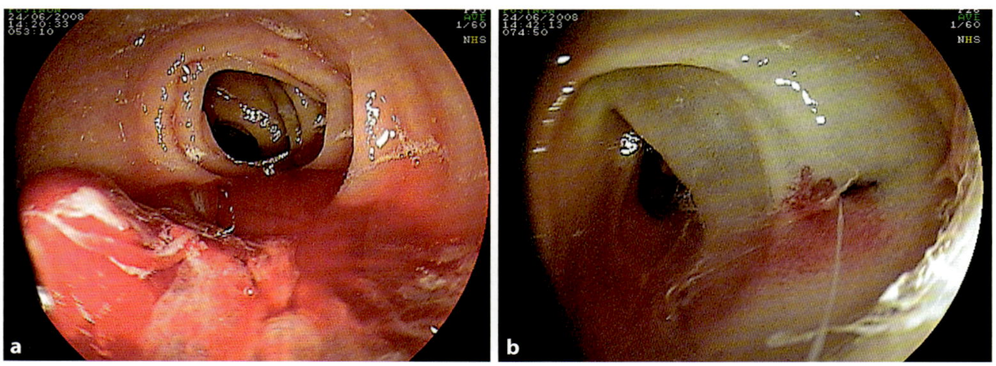

Fig. 2. An advantage of double balloon enteroscopy in patients with overt GI bleeding is the ability to inspect the bleeding lesion in a to-and-fro manner, to wash the bleeding lesion with water, to remove the clot, to apply endoscopic therapy and to mark the lesion with india ink, should endoscopic therapy fail. **a** A large clot on top of a Dieulafy lesion. **b** A bleeding angioectasia. By using the immersion technique active bleeding can be better appreciated.

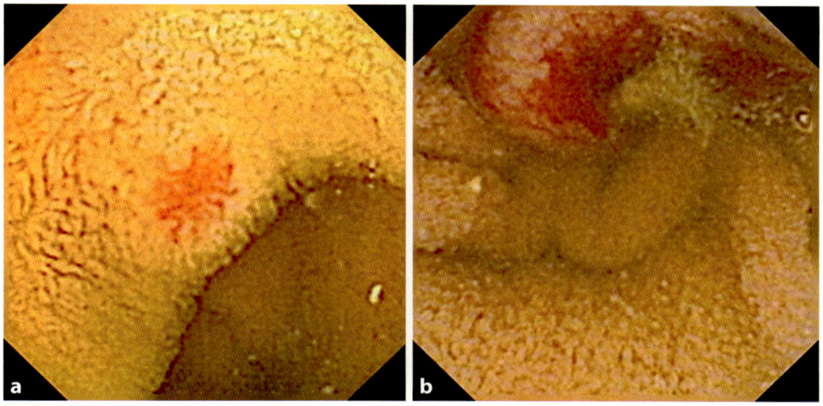

Fig. 3. Capsule endoscopy is also very useful to characterize angioectasias. **a** Classic angiectasias. **b** Bleeding angioectasia.

4

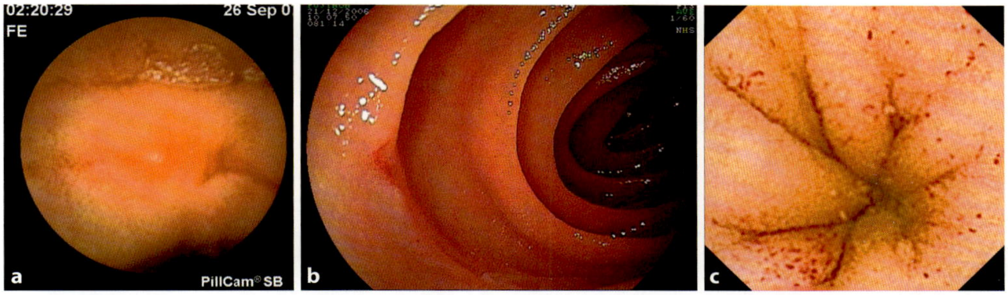

5

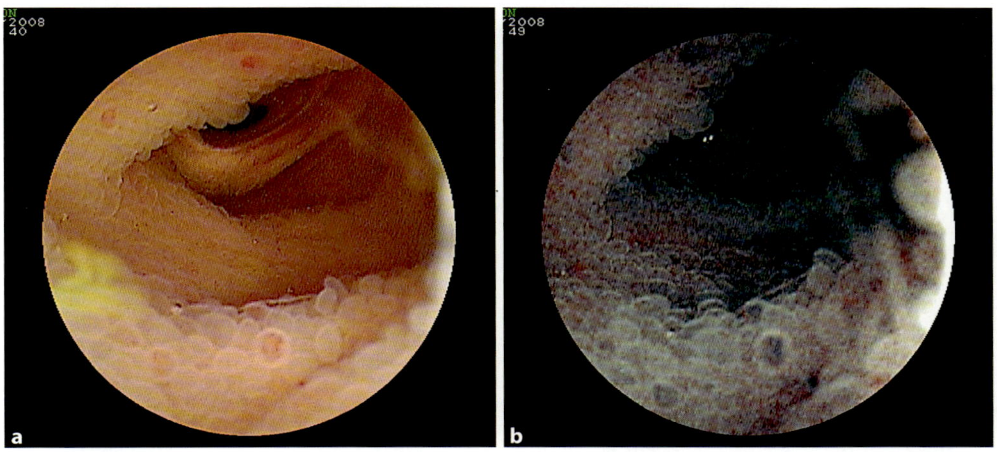

Fig. 4. These pictures are from patients that presented with obscure occult GI bleeding. **a** A capsule, endoscopic view of an NSAID-induced ulcer. **b** A 'punched-out' linear ulcer on top of a fold in a patient taking NSAIDs. **c** Multiple submucosal hemorrhages ('petechiae') in another patient taking NSAIDs.

Fig. 5. The double balloon system form Fujinon enables the use of magnification and virtual chromoendoscopy (Fujinon intelligent chromoendoscopy). By combining a magnification of ×1.5 and the underwater view ('immersion technique') the villi can be seen in clear detail. Note the edematous appearance of these villi in a patient taking NSAIDs (**a, b**). Blood (submucosal hemorrhage) or mini-angioectasias can be seen inside of some villi (**a**). This becomes more apparent when using FICE.

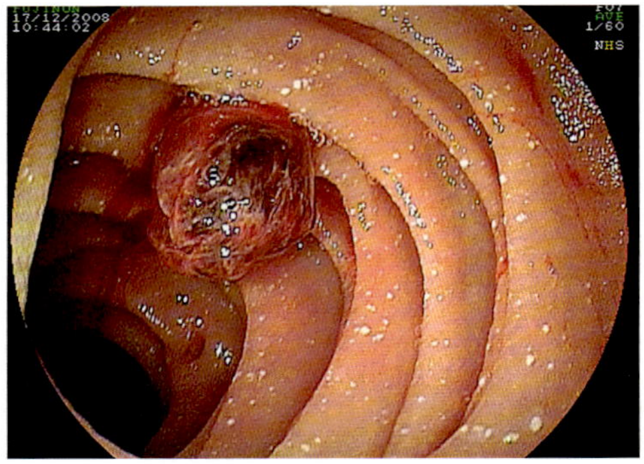

Fig. 6. Note the large adherent clot on top of a Dieulafoy lesion.

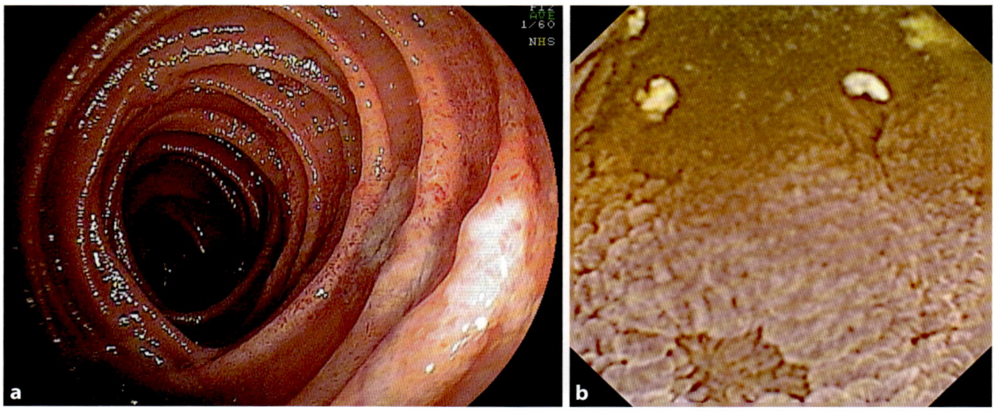

Fig. 7. Various form of enteritis can also result in obscure GI bleeding. This patient had ischemic jejunopathy. The finding is more impressive when seen with double balloon enteroscopy (**a**) than when seen using capsule endoscopy (**b**).

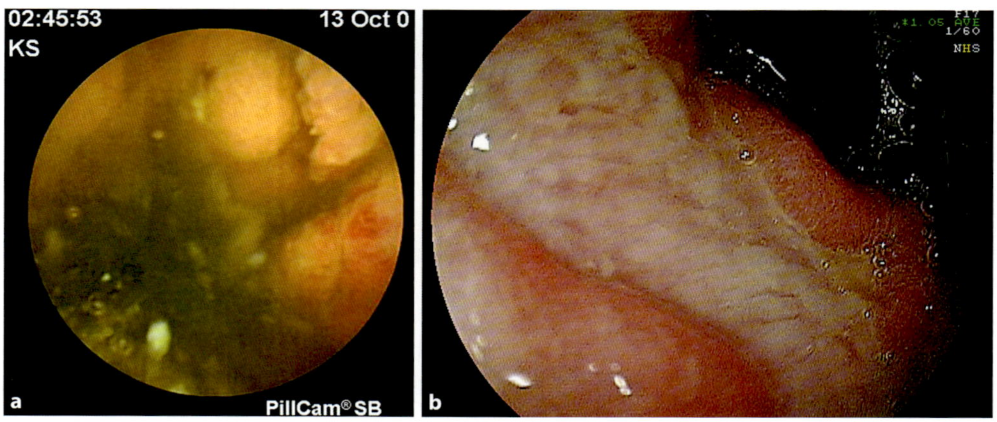

Fig. 8. This patient presented with obscure occult GI bleeding. Capsule endoscopy revealed nonspecific swelling and reddening of the mucosa (**a**). Double balloon enteroscopy revealed a large, ulcerated gastrointestinal stromal tumor (**b**).

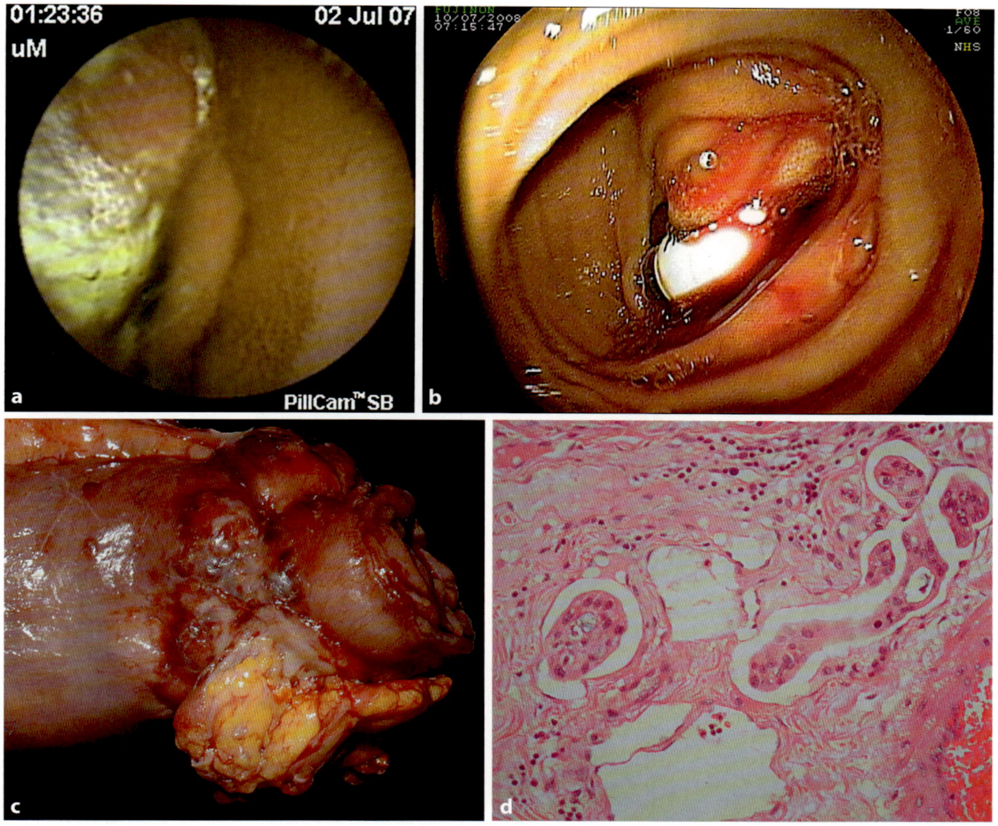

9

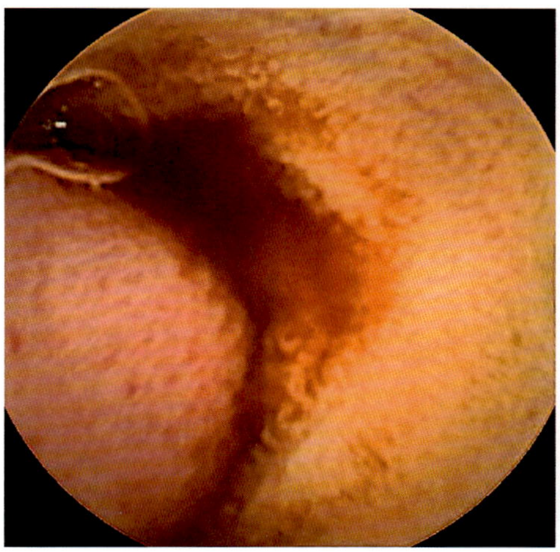

10

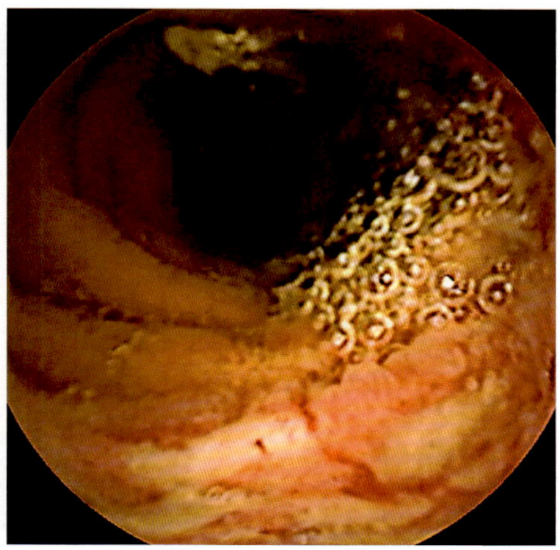

11

Fig. 9. Adenocarcinoma of the small bowel. Capsule endoscopy revealed a tumor in the jejunum, approximately 2 h after passing the pylorus (**a**). The capsule sent permanent images of this structure until its battery expired, suggesting capsule impaction. This was confirmed at double balloon enteroscopy (**b**). The surgical resection specimen shows a stenosing jejunal adenocarcinoma (**c**, **d**). **Fig. 10.** Although capsule endoscopy does not permit the retrieval of tissue, it can be helpful to infer the presence of a tumor. **Fig. 11.** NSAID use is not only associated with small bowel erosions but also with large round ulcers such as this case.

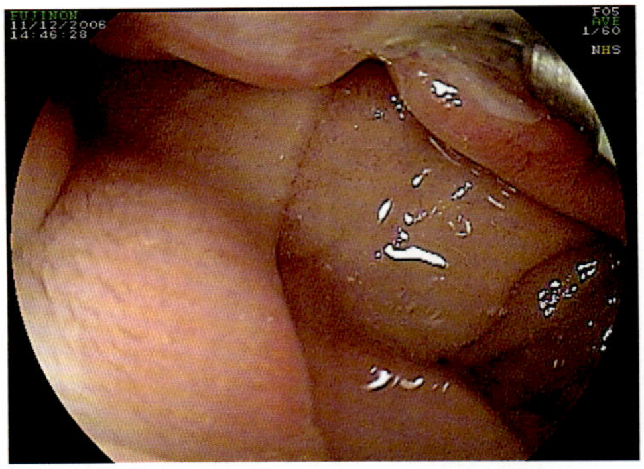

12

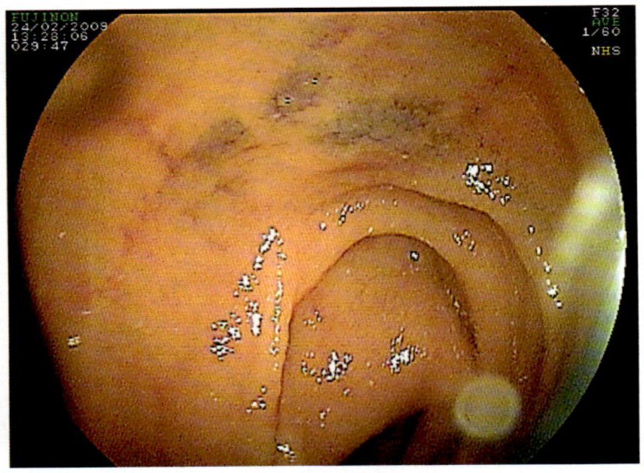

13

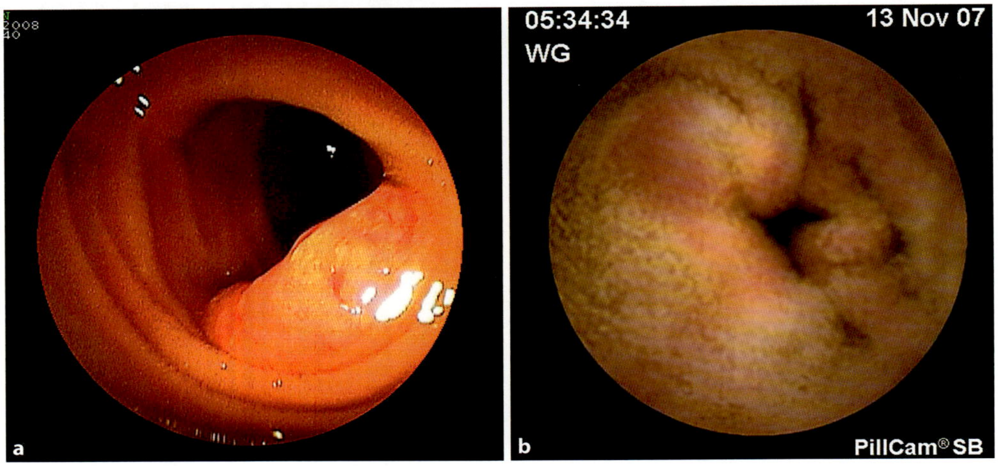

14 a b

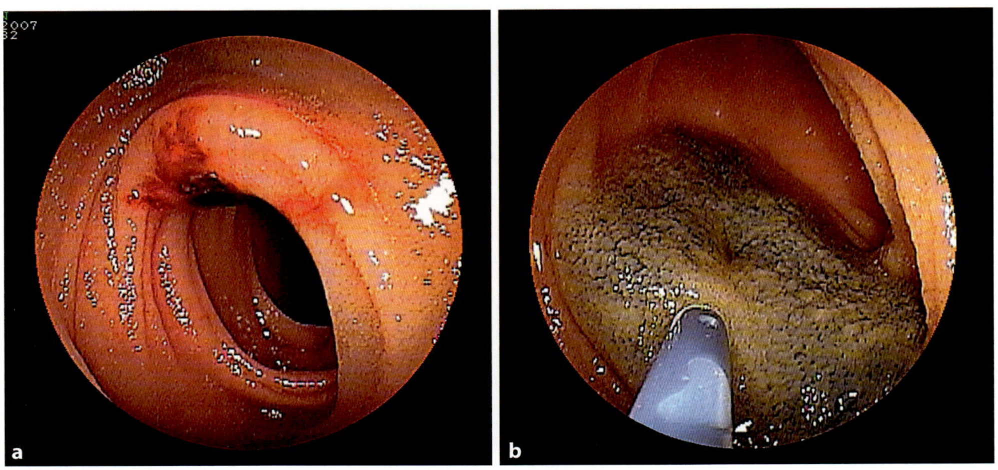

15 a b

Fig. 12. One of the major advantages of double-balloon enteroscopy is the retrieval of tissue for diagnosis, such as this neuroendocrine tumor. **Fig. 13.** Whether small bowel venectasias are a cause of bleeding is a matter of debate. However, in patients with blue rubber bleb syndrome or patients with ectopic varices, there is no question that these veins can bleed. **Fig. 14.** This patient with obscure occult GI bleeding had a Non-Hodgkin's lymphoma involving the ileum (**a**). Capsule endoscopy performed 6 months prior revealed edema and erythema of some mucosal folds (**b**). **Fig. 15.** Bleeding small bowel tumor (neuroendocrine tumor; **a**). The location was marked with submucosal ink, in order to facilitate the location of the lesion (**b**).

Fig. 16. Angioectasias are the most common cause of obscure GI bleeding.

Fig. 17. In the presence of melena or active bleeding, the diagnostic accuracy of capsule endoscopy is low. The only diagnosis that can be made is that there is some sort of active bleeding. If a patient presents with obscure overt GI bleeding on Friday afternoon, would it be worth performing capsule endoscopy? Or should the clinician wait until Monday to perform an elective capsule endoscopy or enteroscopy? Or should an angiography be performed? Or would it be worthwhile to perform an 'emergent balloon enteroscopy'.

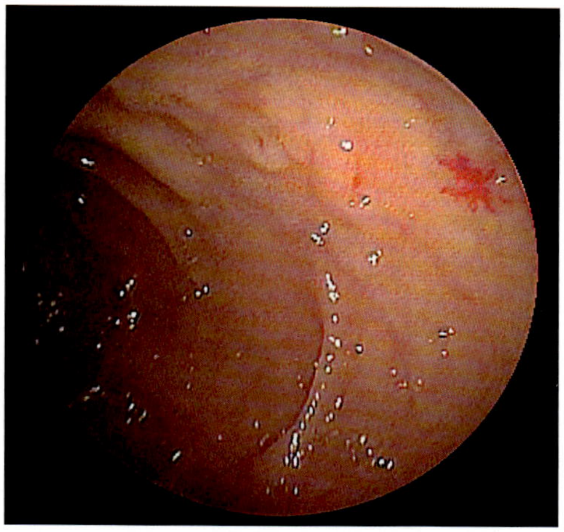

16

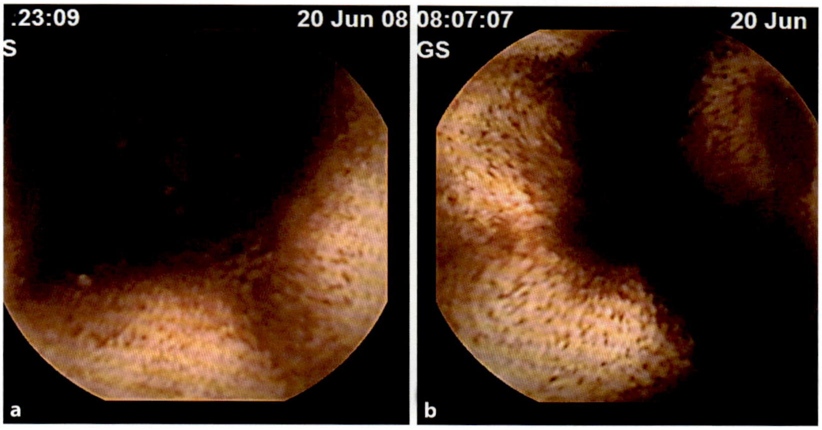

17

regarding a detailed dermatological evaluation, may also be useful to make a differential diagnosis of the etiology for obscure GI bleeding [15]. For example, Rendu-Osler-Weber syndrome (synonym hereditary hemorrhagic telangiectasia) is an autosomal dominant disorder characterized by the appearance of multiple punctate telangiectasias on skin and mucous membranes. The number and size of lesions increases with increasing age and the overall incidence of GI bleeding, about 33%, appears to develop in the fourth or fifth decade of life [16]. A rare disorder, characterized by the development of cavernous hemangiomas in the skin and gastrointestinal tract, is the so-called blue rubber bleb nevus syndrome. Patients usually present with iron deficiency anemia from occult GI bleeding. Characteristically, the skin lesions occur in childhood (but even in the adult) and are usually blue in color and easily compressible which results in an empty, slowly refilling sac [15]. Klippel-Trénaunay-Weber syndrome, another disease leading to obscure GI bleeding, is characterized by a triad of port-wine stains, varicose veins, and bony and soft tissue hypertrophy involving just one extremity (hemihypertrophy) [17].

Laboratory investigation will help to estimate the severity of blood loss and in the evaluation of the coagulation status, including the liver reserve. While the laboratory data are being processed, resuscitation of the patient should proceed. The next step is to stabilize the patient, securing airways, providing oxygen supply if the anemia is severe. Large bore intravenous access,

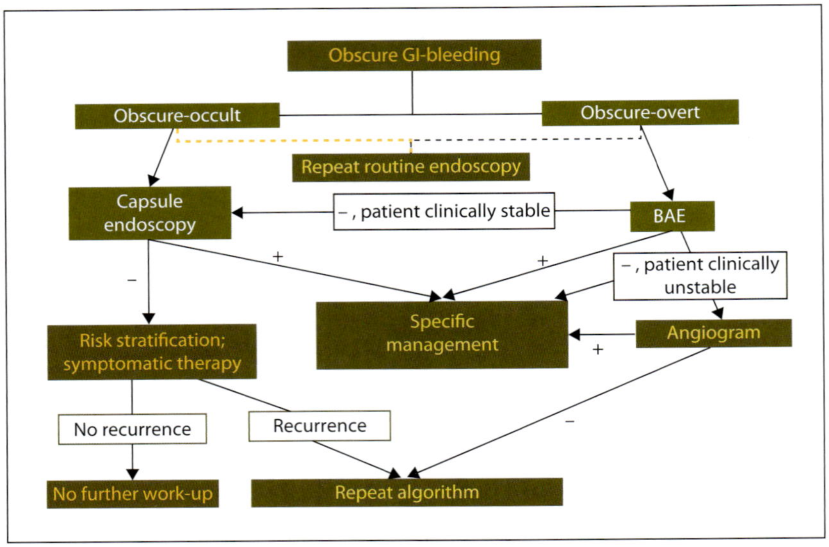

Fig. 18. Proposed algorithm for the approach to obscure GI bleeding. BAE = Balloon-assisted enteroscopy.

judicial use of crystalloids, plasma expanders or packed red cells can be dictated by the clinical setting.

Methods to Investigate MGIB

The preferred approach to investigate MGIB is endoscopic, mainly capsule endoscopy (CE) and balloon-assisted enteroscopy (BAE). PE remains an important option for lesions suspected to be located in the proximal 60–70 cm of the jejunum. Spiral enteroscopy was recently introduced as another useful enteroscopic method to investigate the small bowel. Other important tests in the evaluation of MGIB include angiography, red blood cell scans, computed tomography (CT), small bowel enteroclysis, magnetic resonance imaging (MRI) and CT or MRI enterography/enteroclysis as described below. Table 2 lists all the currently used methods to investigate MGIB.

Endoscopic Evaluation

Until the end of the last century the traditional method to endoscopically investigate the small bowel was PE [3]. However, both BAE techniques, double-balloon enteroscopy (DBE) and single-balloon enteroscopy (SBE), have replaced PE as the methods of choice to perform deep small bowel investigation and to perform endoscopic interventions within the small intestine [18]. Because both SBE and DBE depend on 1 or 2 balloons to advance the scope we propose to name these methods BAE [19]. Very recently, spiral enteroscopy was introduced for deep small bowel intubation that uses a special overtube (DSB, discovery small bowel) to pleat the small bowel [20]. Preliminary data suggest that DSB represents a rapid, safe and effective new technique for small bowel intubation compared to BAE techniques [20].

Table 2. Methods currently used to investigate MGIB and suggested utility

Method	Suggested utility
Capsule endoscopy	3
Double-balloon enteroscopy	3
Single-balloon enteroscopy	3
Spiral enteroscopy	2–3
Push enteroscopy	1
Technetium 99m-labeled red blood cell nuclear scan	2
Technetium 99m pertechnetate scintigraphy (Meckel scan)	2
Angiography	2
Small bowel series	1
Barium enteroclysis	1
CT enterography	2–3
CT enteroclysis	2–3
MRI enterography	2–3
MRI enteroclysis	2–3
CT angiography	2

CT = Computed tomography; MRI = magnetic resonance imaging. 1 = Low utility, 2 = average utility, 3 = high utility.

Capsule Endoscopy

The diagnostic yield for CE in MGIB varies from 38 to 91%, which was confirmed by large meta-analyses [6, 21, 22]. The most common diagnosis found on CE include among others: angioectasias, active bleeding lesions, erosions, tumors, and ulcers [6, 21, 22]. One important issue when using CE is the significant miss rate reported for small bowel tumors and other lesions [23–25]. This is a paradoxical issue, as one would expect the capsule endoscope to get stuck at tumorous areas. However, several studies indicate this significant failure rate [23–25]. Thus, in patients with persistent anemia and occult GIB it is wise to use other methods to search for a potential tumor.

In the setting of OGIB CE can be utilized to 'screen' the small bowel. If a lesion is found, then an invasive endoscopy, surgery or other testing method can be used [26, 27].

The main advantages of CE are its noninvasiveness and no need for sedation. At the moment, the major disadvantages are the inability to wash a bleeding lesion and the inability to perform any therapeutic intervention. Of note, currently new wireless capsule devices are under investigation, allowing both diagnostic and therapeutic tasks [28].

Balloon-Assisted Enteroscopy

The diagnostic yield for BAE in MGIB varies from 38 to 91% [29–31]. Data from independent studies have been confirmed by systematic reviews and meta-analyses [29–31]. Pasha et al. [29] performed a systematic review of the literature to determine the diagnostic and therapeutic yield of DBE in patients with OGIB. Thirteen studies including 906 patients were analyzed. DBE detected a potential bleeding source in 66% of patients, which included angioectasias (25.6%), inflammatory lesions (16.1%) and small bowel neoplasms (13.9%). Interestingly, small-bowel ulcers and tumors are the most common diagnostic findings in series originating from Far Eastern countries, whereas in European and North/South American studies the commonest diagnostic finding is angioectasias.

BAE directly influences management in 44–80% patients resulting in a new diagnosis, change in management or improved outcomes in 60–70% of patients with OGIB [29].

It is not quite clear why the diagnostic rates are so variable. It is likely that the difference in diagnostic yield depends on a combination of factors, including indication (obscure overt versus obscure occult), quality and completeness of pre-BAE investigations, timing of BAE, as well as performance of a pre-BAE CE. Studies with the highest yield included a large number of patients with previous CE, whereas lower yields were achieved in patients investigated without previous CE [6, 22, 29, 30]. Also, higher yields are generally achieved when the indication was obscure overt bleeding as compared to obscure occult GIB [31–33].

Compared to CE BAE has the following advantages: ability to clean a lesion, inspect the lesion back and forth, and application of therapy. The major disadvantages are its invasiveness, the need for sedatives as well as endoscopy and sedative-associated complications [34].

Determination of the Primary Route of Insertion of BAE (Oral or Antegrade versus Anal or Retrograde)

The choice for either the oral or the anal route depends on the suspected location of the lesion within the small bowel based on the clinical manifestations, results of laboratory, radiological and CE examinations [4, 35–37]. In the case of spiral enteroscopy, no studies using the anal route have been published yet. For OGIB CE is currently the main instrument used to indicate the preferential endoscope insertion route for BAE [38]. Nevertheless, it would be hard to justify performing a CE in a patient with clinical significant bleeding, as this approach will only delay the diagnosis. Therefore, we need to remember that CE mainly serves as a topographical indicator of where the bleeding comes from. As mentioned before, CE, at the moment, cannot be moved to and from the lesion, no water can be applied to clean the lesion, and in cases of active bleeding the CE may only see blood whereas an intervention is not possible. For this reason we prefer to perform an endoscopy (i.e. BAE) in patients with active bleeding, as the yield and chances of performing an intervention are much higher. In cases of OGIB the stool color can also help to direct the BAE route: the oral route in the case of melena and the anal route in the case of hematochezia. However, this approach has not been validated yet. In general, total enteroscopy by BAE is not required in the majority of patients with OGIB, as the potential bleeding source can generally be identified without entire small bowel visualization [11]. Nonetheless, about one third of patients will require 2 separate BAEs to make an adequate diagnosis [39].

Unfortunately, total enteroscopy is not always achievable. Success rates of total small bowel investigation (oral insertion and reaching the cecum) using the antegrade approach range from 0 to 5%, and total enteroscopy using the oral and anal approach range from 0 to 86% [4, 35, 36, 40]. Reasons for failing to achieve total enteroscopy include marked intestinal adhesion caused by previous abdominal or pelvic surgery, type of enteroscope used (thin diagnostic BAE versus therapeutic BAE) and the endoscopist's level of experience [41].

Comparison of DBE with CE

Several studies have compared BAE to CE in patients with OGIB [42–44]. Most studies report concordant findings, just 1 prospective study report higher yields for CE than for DBE (80 vs. 60%) [42].

In a large multicenter US study, the diagnostic yield of DBE and CE were retrospectively evaluated in a group of 115 patients with OGIB [45]. CE found a potential bleeding source in 55% of patients. In these patients DBE confirmed a potential bleeding source in 41 (65%). These results are hypothesized to depend on an overestimation of CE findings. In the 52 patients with negative CE, DBE was positive in 16 (30%). Of note, DBE detected 4 large adenocarcinomas that were missed by CE [45]. This is a very important finding and a clinician should not be reassured by a negative finding in a patient with persistent anemia.

Radiologic Evaluation

Technetium 99m-Labeled Red Blood Cell Nuclear Scan

This technique has the ability to detect GIB at a rate of 0.1–0.4 cm^3 of blood loss/min and allows scanning for up to 24 h [46]. An early positive bleeding scan is predictive of patients who may benefit from angiography or endovascular therapeutic interventions [47, 48]. Furthermore, it seemed that these scans may be useful to direct the timing of angiography [48]. Nevertheless, its role in patients with OGIB is still controversial. It seemed that particularly in delayed images (obtained 3–4 h after injection of the radioactive material) the nuclear scan may be beneficial to detect active bleeding [49]. Nevertheless, it has been demonstrated that the ability to localize the bleeding source is weak [49]. Probably, this depends on misinterpretation of the bleeding location because of a higher likelihood of radiotracer movement through the bowel away from the bleeding source in delayed images [50].

Technetium 99m Pertechnetate Scintigraphy (Meckel Scan)

Although Meckel's diverticulum is the most prevalent congenital abnormality of the GI tract (present in approximately 2% of the population), it is often difficult to diagnose [51]. The Meckel scan is the investigation of choice to detect these diverticula with a sensitivity of 64–100% [52, 53]. In approximately 50% of cases ectopic tissue is found, consisting gastric tissue in 60–85% [54]. The test relies on uptake of pertechnetate anions by ectopic gastric mucosa, therefore visualizing the malformation. Of note, the sensitivity is better in children than in adults and can be improved by pretreatment with ranitidine [55–57].

Small Bowel Series and Barium Enteroclysis

The role of both techniques in the diagnosis of GIB has declined with the introduction of new endoscopic methods (e.g. CE and BAE) but also with the introduction of more sensitive radiologic testing's as described below. Small bowel series and barium enteroclysis with methylcellulose have poor sensitivities of l <5 and 10–20%, respectively, in the case of OGIB [58, 59]. Different studies compared small bowel radiographs and CE for suspected small bowel diseases [22, 60]. According to these studies, the diagnostic yield of CE is considerably higher (67 vs. 8%; $p < 0.00001$). Furthermore, radiographic testing was not able to demonstrate angiectasias, suggested as the most common cause of small bowel bleeding [22, 60]. In a retrospective review of enteroclysis in patients with OGIB and chronic abdominal pain of undetermined etiology by Malik et al. [61], enteroclysis only changed management in 10% of patients. Therefore, unless the clinical findings suggest small bowel obstruction (e.g. in the course of tumors, Crohn's disease or NSAID intake) neither small bowel series nor enteroclysis play a role in the evaluation of MGIB.

Computed Tomography and Magnetic Resonance Enterography and Enteroclysis

Computed tomography (CT)/magnetic resonance imaging (MRI) enterography and CT/MRI enteroclysis are both hybrid techniques that combine the methods of fluoroscopic intubation-infusion small bowel examinations with that of abdominal CT or MRI [58]. The techniques can be performed using either neutral enteral contrast material with intravenous contrast material or positive enteral contrast material without intravenous contrast material via a peroral (enterography) or nasojejunal approach (enteroclysis). Conscious sedation is used in most patients to adequately perform the examination [58]. Preliminary data suggest the utility of helical CT in identifying OGIB including angiodysplasias reporting a diagnostic yield of 45% [62–64]. Very recently, Huprich et al. [64] described their initial experience with a 64-section CT system using neutral enteric contrast material and a 3-phase acquisition in 22 patients with OGIB. They compared the findings with capsule and traditional endoscopic, surgical, and angiographic results. CT enterographic findings were positive for a bleeding source in 46% of patients, compared to 36% in the CE group. Furthermore, CT enterography helped to identify 3 lesions which were not detected by CE, suggesting a possible role of multiphase, multiplanar CT enterography in the evaluation of OGIB [64]. In a small retrospective case series MRI enterography detected a 37-mm polyp in the proximal ileum that was not seen by CE, even after careful retrospective review of the capsule video [24]. In another case report MRI enterography was able to detect a gastrointestinal stromal tumor in the distal jejunum, which was not seen by CE [65]. At least, Gölder et al. [66] compared the diagnostic yield of CE and MRI enteroclysis in 14 patients with OGIB. CE revealed the bleeding site in 36% of patients whereas MRI enteroclysis did not reveal any intestinal abnormalities [66]. Therefore, at the moment, the main advantage of CT/MRI enterography or enteroclysis is the identification of small bowel strictures prior to CE and the possibility of providing detailed information on mural and extramural findings, which cannot be detected by endoscopic approaches [67, 68].

Angiography

The main advantage in the setting of angiography is the possibility for both diagnosis and therapy (with embolization). Angiography has the ability to detect GIB at a rate of 0.5–1 cm^3 of blood loss/min (equivalent to about 2–3 units of blood loss/day), therefore being less sensitive for GIB compared to technetium 99m-labeled red blood cell nuclear scans [46]. Although angiography has the ability to also diagnose non-bleeding lesions like angiectasias, which represent the main bleeding cause of OGIB (<40%) in patients older than 40 years, the overall yield of this technique is poor [1, 46]. Overall yields have been reported at 27–77% with improved yields of 61–72% in patients with active bleeding [46]. Provocative angiography has been reported in several small series [69, 70]. Bloomfeld et al. [70] investigated provocative angiography (with the use of tolazoline – a vasodilator, heparin and/or urokinase) in patients with gastrointestinal hemorrhage of unknown origin. While no complications attributed to the provocative bleeding occurred, an angiographically identifiable lesion was only identified in 29% of cases, suggesting that provocative angiography in the setting of obscure occult GIB seemed to be safe but effective only in very selected patients [70]. Data regarding the use of angiography in the setting of MGIB are still pending.

CT Angiography

CT angiography uses less oral contrast agent compared to CT enterography or CT enteroclysis, therefore luminal distension is distinctive less. A helical CT is performed after catheterization of the abdominal aorta before and after intra-arterial contrast injection. The bleeding site is then recognized as a hyper-dense area due to the extravasation in the intestinal lumen [1, 71]. Previously, Ettore et al. [71] analyzed the usefulness of CT angiography in 18 consecutive patients with OGIB and reported a diagnostic yield of 72% [71]. Junquera et al. [72] studied the accuracy of CT angiography for the diagnosis of colonic angiodysplasias in 18 patients and described sensitivity, specificity and positive predictive values of 70, 100 and 100%, respectively, when compared with colonoscopy and mesenteric angiography [72].

Current Algorithm for MGIB

The diagnostic and treatment algorithm for MGIB is based on the principles of investigating OGIB. However, in MGIB specific small bowel lesions are diagnosed and treated. The diagnostic work-up of patients with MGIB should be individualized on the basis of their clinical presentation. In cases of obscure occult GIB it appears best to start with a CE, and perform BAE only if a potential source is identified [1, 73, 74]. In patients with suspicious findings, BAE can be used to either confirm the lesion through visualization and retrieval of tissue or to provide endoscopic therapy. However, as shown in various reports, relevant lesions can be missed by CE [23–25]. Thus, BAE should be strongly considered in patients at a higher risk of a small bowel lesion despite negative CE. These include patients with iron deficiency anemia, weight loss and diarrhea.

In patients with obscure overt GIB it appears that BAE should be the initial test because of the high likelihood of finding a potentially treatable lesion [39, 73]. Nevertheless, there are no prospective studies comparing the diagnostic yield of CE and BAE in this setting. Definite indications for starting with a BAE in this setting are suspicion of small bowel stricture (clinically or by other imaging techniques) and in patients with surgically modified anatomy (especially those with an afferent intestinal loop) [37].

Furthermore, the timing of BAE in obscure overt GIB has not been defined, and it is commonly considered 'emergent' when performed within the first 48 h of presentation. In our opinion, a true emergent BAE should be performed within 24 h and preferably 12 h after patient presentation.

The remaining tests such as angiography, technetium scans and others should be utilized based on an individual basis. If the bleeding is massive, then an angiography should be strongly considered. If there is a suspicion of Meckel's diverticulum, then a technetium 99m Meckel scan should be performed. CT and MRI are useful when tumors such as gastrointestinal stromal tumors, neuroendocrine tumors or adenocarcinoma are suspected. If the patient has inflammatory signs then searching for Crohn's disease, Becquet's or other vasculopathies is warranted. In these scenarios the use of CT and MRI enterography/enteroclysis is warranted.

Conclusions

For the first time we have presented the approach to MGIB in a book. The time has come to rewrite the books and reclassify GIB. Now GIB is divided into upper (originating in the upper GI tract, above the papilla of Vater, or for some other experts, the ligament of Treitz), middle (from the papilla of Vater to the ileocecal valve) and lower (from the terminal ileum to the anus).

The preferred endoscopic methods to investigate small bowel bleeding include CE and BAE. PE remains an important option for lesions suspected to be located in the proximal 60–70 cm of jejunum. Newly developed radiologic methods like CT or MRI enterography seemed to be promising in the setting of MGIB, especially when combined with CE. One of the major weaknesses of BAE is that it is a time-consuming procedure, requiring special training and more staff than for standard endoscopies. But reaching a diagnosis and establishing a therapeutic plan in patients with previously negative upper and lower endoscopies and radiologic studies is certainly rewarding and worth the time spend pushing and pulling the BAE. Although some experts propose the routine use of CE before BAE in MGIB, we believe that BAE should be the first method of investigation in situations when a diagnostic biopsy or therapeutic interventions are anticipated. In patients without anticipated intervention (biopsy or endoscopic therapy), it appears that the optimal evaluation of the small intestine should start with a noninvasive CE and a targeted BAE could be performed afterwards if a suspicious lesion is found.

Radiological tests should be utilized on an individual basis. In case of massive bleeding an angiography should be strongly considered. When Meckel's diverticulum is suspected, a Meckel scan should be performed. CT and MRI are useful when tumors are suspected.

References

1 Raju GS, Gerson L, Das A, Lewis B; American Gastroenterological Association: American Gastroenterological Association (AGA) Institute technical review on obscure gastrointestinal bleeding. Gastroenterology 2007;133:1697–1717.

2 Yamamoto H, Sekine Y, Sato Y, Higashizawa T, Miyata T, Iino S, Ido K, Sugano K: Total enteroscopy with a nonsurgical steerable double-balloon method. Gastrointest Endosc 2001;53:216–220.

3 Mönkemüller K, Weigt J, Treiber G, Kolfenbach S, Kahl S, Röcken C, Ebert M, Fry LC, Malfertheiner P: Diagnostic and therapeutic impact of double-balloon enteroscopy. Endoscopy 2006;38:67–72.

4 Heine GD, Hadithi M, Groenen MJ, Kuipers EJ, Jacobs MA, Mulder CJ: Double-balloon enteroscopy: indications, diagnostic yield, and complications in a series of 275 patients with suspected small-bowel disease. Endoscopy 2006;38:42–48.

5 Zhong J, Ma T, Zhang C, Sun B, Chen S, Cao Y, Wu Y: A retrospective study of the application on double-balloon enteroscopy in 378 patients with suspected small-bowel diseases. Endoscopy 2007;39: 208–215.

6 Leighton JA, Triester SL, Sharma VK: Capsule endoscopy: a meta-analysis for use with obscure gastrointestinal bleeding and Crohn's disease. Gastrointest Endosc Clin N Am 2006;16:229–250.

7 Tsujikawa T, Saitoh Y, Andoh A, Imaeda H, Hata K, Minematsu H, Senoh K, Hayafuji K, Ogawa A, Nakahara T, Sasaki M, Fujiyama Y: Novel single-balloon enteroscopy for diagnosis and treatment of the small intestine: preliminary experiences. Endoscopy 2008;40:11–15.
8 Ell C, May A: Mid-gastrointestinal bleeding: capsule endoscopy and push-and-pull enteroscopy give rise to a new medical term. Endoscopy 2006;38:673–675.
9 Zaman A, Hapke R, Flora K, Rosen H, Benner K: Prevalence of upper and lower gastrointestinal tract findings in liver transplant candidates undergoing screening endoscopic evaluation. Am J Gastroenterol 1999;94:895–899.
10 Chak A, Koehler MK, Sundaram SN, Cooper GS, Canto MI, Sivak MV Jr: Diagnostic and therapeutic impact of push enteroscopy: analysis of factors associated with positive findings. Gastrointest Endosc 1998;47:18–22.
11 Fry LC, Bellutti M, Neumann H, Malfertheiner P, Mönkemüller K: Incidence of bleeding lesions within reach of conventional upper and lower endoscopes in patients undergoing double-balloon enteroscopy for obscure gastrointestinal bleeding. Aliment Pharmacol Ther 2009;29:342–349.
12 Manes G, Bianchi Porro G: Missed lesions with conventional endoscopy discovered by double-balloon enteroscopy: endoscopist or instrument? Aliment Pharmacol Ther 2009;29:918–919.
13 Matsumoto T, Kudo T, Esaki M, Yano T, Yamamoto H, Sakamoto C, Goto H, Nakase H, Tanaka S, Matsui T, Sugano K, Iida M: Prevalence of non-steroidal anti-inflammatory drug-induced enteropathy determined by double-balloon endoscopy: a Japanese multicenter study. Scand J Gastroenterol: 2008;43: 490–496.
14 Fry LC, Neumann H, Kuester D, Kuhn R, Bellutti M, Malfertheiner P, Monkemuller K: Small bowel polyps and tumours: endoscopic detection and treatment by double-balloon enteroscopy. Aliment Pharmacol Ther 2008 [Epub ahead of print].
15 Braverman IM: Skin signs of gastrointestinal disease. Gastroenterology 2003;124:1595–1614.
16 Kjeldsen AD, Kjeldsen J: Gastrointestinal bleeding in patients with hereditary hemorrhagic telangiectasia. Am J Gastroenterol 2000;95:415–418.
17 Sato T, Ohta K, Ohyama S, Suenaga M, Ueno M, Oya M, Yamamoto J, Yamaguchi T, Muto T, Kato Y: Klippel-Trenaunay-Weber syndrome and duodenal hemorrhage. Gastrointest Endosc 2003;58:756–757.
18 Matsumoto T, Moriyama T, Esaki M, Nakamura S, Iida M: Performance of antegrade double-balloon enteroscopy: comparison with push enteroscopy. Gastrointest Endosc 2005;62:392–398.
19 Mönkemüller K, Fry LC, Bellutti M, Malfertheiner P: Balloon-assisted enteroscopy: unifying double-balloon and single-balloon enteroscopy. Endoscopy 2008;40: 537.
20 Akerman PA, Agrawal D, Cantero D, Pangtay J: Spiral enteroscopy with the new DSB overtube: a novel technique for deep peroral small-bowel intubation. Endoscopy 2008;40:974–978.
21 Jones BH, Fleischer DE, Sharma VK, Heigh RI, Shiff AD, Hernandez JL, Leighton JA: Yield of repeat wireless video capsule endoscopy in patients with obscure gastrointestinal bleeding. Am J Gastroenterol 2005;100:1058–1064.
22 Triester SL, Leighton JA, Leontiadis GI, Fleischer DE, Hara AK, Heigh RI, Shiff AD, Sharma VK: A meta-analysis of the yield of capsule endoscopy compared to other diagnostic modalities in patients with obscure gastrointestinal bleeding. Am J Gastroenterol 2005;100:2407–2418.
23 Ross A, Mehdizadeh S, Tokar J, Leighton JA, Kamal A, Chen A, Schembre D, Chen G, Binmoeller K, Kozarek R, Waxman I, Dye C, Gerson L, Harrison ME, Haluszka O, Lo S, Semrad C: Double balloon enteroscopy detects small bowel mass lesions missed by capsule endoscopy. Dig Dis Sci 2008;53:2140–2143.
24 Postgate A, Despott E, Burling D, Gupta A, Phillips R, O'Beirne J, Patch D, Fraser C: Significant small-bowel lesions detected by alternative diagnostic modalities after negative capsule endoscopy. Gastrointest Endosc 2008;68:1209–1214.
25 Chong AK, Chin BW, Meredith CG: Clinically significant small-bowel pathology identified by double-balloon enteroscopy but missed by capsule endoscopy. Gastrointest Endosc 2006;64:445–449.
26 Somsouk M, Gralnek IM, Inadomi JM: Management of obscure occult gastrointestinal bleeding: a cost-minimization analysis. Clin Gastroenterol Hepatol 2008;6:661–670.
27 Gerson L, Kamal A: Cost-effectiveness analysis of management strategies for obscure GI bleeding. Gastrointest Endosc 2008;68:920–936.
28 Valdastri P, Quaglia C, Susilo E, Menciassi A, Dario P, Ho CN, Anhoeck G, Schurr MO: Wireless therapeutic endoscopic capsule: in vivo experiment. Endoscopy 2008;40:979–982.
29 Pasha SF, Leighton JA, Das A, Harrison ME, Decker GA, Fleischer DE, Sharma VK: Double-balloon enteroscopy and capsule endoscopy have comparable diagnostic yield in small-bowel disease: a meta-analysis. Clin Gastroenterol Hepatol 2008;6:671–676.
30 Chen X, Ran ZH, Tong JL: A meta-analysis of the yield of capsule endoscopy compared to double-balloon enteroscopy in patients with small bowel diseases. World J Gastroenterol 2007;13:4372–4378.
31 Mönkemüller K, Fry LC, Neumann H, Rickes S, Malfertheiner P: Diagnostic and therapeutic utility of double balloon endoscopy: experience with 225 procedures. Acta Gastroenterol Latinoam 2007;37: 216–223.
32 Kaffes AJ, Siah C, Koo JH: Clinical outcomes after double-balloon enteroscopy in patients with obscure GI bleeding and a positive capsule endoscopy. Gastrointest Endosc 2007;66:304–309.

33 Sun B, Rajan E, Cheng S, Shen R, Zhang C, Zhang S, Wu Y, Zhong J: Diagnostic yield and therapeutic impact of double-balloon enteroscopy in a large cohort of patients with obscure gastrointestinal bleeding. Am J Gastroenterol 2006;101:2011–2015.
34 Mensink PB, Haringsma J, Kucharzik T, Cellier C, Pérez-Cuadrado E, Mönkemüller K, Gasbarrini A, Kaffes AJ, Nakamura K, Yen HH, Yamamoto H: Complications of double balloon enteroscopy: a multicenter survey. Endoscopy 2007;39:613–615.
35 May A, Nachbar L, Ell C: Double-balloon enteroscopy (push-and-pull enteroscopy) of the small bowel: feasibility and diagnostic and therapeutic yield in patients with suspected small bowel disease. Gastrointest Endosc 2005;62:62–70.
36 Di Caro S, May A, Heine DG, Fini L, Landi B, Petruzziello L, Cellier C, Mulder CJ, Costamagna G, Ell C, Gasbarrini A; DBE-European Study Group: The European experience with double-balloon enteroscopy: indications, methodology, safety, and clinical impact. Gastrointest Endosc 2005;62:545–550.
37 Neumann H, Mönkemüller K, Malfertheiner P: Obscure overt GI bleeding secondary to angiodysplasias at the hepaticojejunostomy diagnosed and successfully treated with double-balloon enteroscopy. Gastrointest Endosc 2008;67:563–565.
38 Gay G, Delvaux M, Fassler I: Outcome of capsule endoscopy in determining indication and route for push-and-pull enteroscopy. Endoscopy 2006;38:49–58.
39 Mönkemüller K, Bellutti M, Fry LC, Malfertheiner P: Enteroscopy. Best Pract Res Clin Gastroenterol 2008;22: 789–811.
40 May A, Nachbar L, Schneider M, Ell C: Prospective comparison of push enteroscopy and push-and-pull enteroscopy in patients with suspected small-bowel bleeding. Am J Gastroenterol 2006;101:2016–2024.
41 Mehdizadeh S, Han NJ, Cheng DW, Chen GC, Lo SK: Success rate of retrograde double-balloon enteroscopy. Gastrointest Endosc 2007;65:633–639.
42 Hadithi M, Heine GD, Jacobs MA, van Bodegraven AA, Mulder CJ: A prospective study comparing video capsule endoscopy with double-balloon enteroscopy in patients with obscure gastrointestinal bleeding. Am J Gastroenterol 2006;101:52–57.
43 Nakamura M, Niwa Y, Ohmiya N, Miyahara R, Ohashi A, Itoh A, Hirooka Y, Goto H: Preliminary comparison of capsule endoscopy and double-balloon enteroscopy in patients with suspected small-bowel bleeding. Endoscopy 2006;38:59–66.
44 Matsumoto T, Esaki M, Moriyama T, Nakamura S, Iida M: Comparison of capsule endoscopy and enteroscopy with the double-balloon method in patients with obscure bleeding and polyposis. Endoscopy 2005;37:827–832.
45 Mehdizadeh S, Ross A, Gerson L, Leighton J, Chen A, Schembre D, Chen G, Semrad C, Kamal A, Harrison EM, Binmoeller K, Waxman I, Kozarek R, Lo SK: What is the learning curve associated with double-balloon enteroscopy? Technical details and early experience in 6 US tertiary care centers. Gastrointest Endosc 2006;64:740–750.
46 Singh V, Alexander JA: The evaluation and management of obscure and occult gastrointestinal bleeding. Abdom Imaging 2009;34:311–319.
47 Hammond KL, Beck DE, Hicks TC, Timmcke AE, Whitlow CW, Margolin DA.:Implications of negative technetium 99m-labeled red blood cell scintigraphy in patients presenting with lower gastrointestinal bleeding. Am J Surg 2007;193:404–407.
48 Ng DA, Opelka FG, Beck DE, Milburn JM, Witherspoon LR, Hicks TC, Timmcke AE, Gathright JB Jr: Predictive value of technetium Tc 99m-labeled red blood cell scintigraphy for positive angiogram in massive lower gastrointestinal hemorrhage. Dis Colon Rectum 1997;40: 471–477.
49 Howarth DM, Tang K, Lees W: The clinical utility of nuclear medicine imaging for the detection of occult gastrointestinal haemorrhage. Nucl Med Commun 2002; 23:591–594.
50 Howarth DM: The role of nuclear medicine in the detection of acute gastrointestinal bleeding. Semin Nucl Med 2006;36:133–146.
51 Elsayes KM, Menias CO, Harvin HJ, Francis IR: Imaging manifestations of Meckel's diverticulum. AJR Am J Roentgenol 2007;189:81–88.
52 Schwartz MJ, Lewis JH: Meckel's diverticulum: pitfalls in scintigraphic detection in the adult. Am J Gastroenterol 1984;79:611–618.
53 Sfakianakis GN, Conway JJ: Detection of ectopic gastric mucosa in Meckel's diverticulum and in other aberrations by scintigraphy: I. Pathophysiology and 10-year clinical experience. J Nucl Med 1981;22:647–654.
54 Martin JP, Connor PD, Charles K: Meckel's diverticulum. Am Fam Physician 2000;61:1037–1042.
55 Zuckerman GR, Prakash C, Askin MP, Lewis BS: AGA technical review on the evaluation and management of occult and obscure gastrointestinal bleeding. Gastroenterology 2000;118:201–221.
56 Swaniker F, Soldes O, Hirschl RB: The utility of technetium 99m pertechnetate scintigraphy in the evaluation of patients with Meckel's diverticulum. J Pediatr Surg 1999;34:760–764.
57 Rerksuppaphol S, Hutson JM, Oliver MR: Ranitidine-enhanced 99mtechnetium pertechnetate imaging in children improves the sensitivity of identifying heterotopic gastric mucosa in Meckel's diverticulum. Pediatr Surg Int 2004;20:323–325.
58 Maglinte DD, Sandrasegaran K, Lappas JC, Chiorean M: CT Enteroclysis. Radiology 2007;245:661–671.

59 Moch A, Herlinger H, Kochman ML, Levine MS, Rubesin SE, Laufer I: Enteroclysis in the evaluation of obscure gastrointestinal bleeding. AJR Am J Roentgenol 1994;163:1381–1384.
60 Costamagna G, Shah SK, Riccioni ME, Foschia F, Mutignani M, Perri V, Vecchioli A, Brizi MG, Picciocchi A, Marano P: A prospective trial comparing small bowel radiographs and video capsule endoscopy for suspected small bowel disease. Gastroenterology 2002;123:999–1005.
61 Malik A, Lukaszewski K, Caroline D, Parkman H, DeSipio J, Banson F, Bazir K, Reddy L, Srinivasan R, Fisher R, Miller L: A retrospective review of enteroclysis in patients with obscure gastrointestinal bleeding and chronic abdominal pain of undetermined etiology. Dig Dis Sci 2005;50:649–655.
62 Grassi R, di Mizio R, Romano S, Cappabianca S, del Vecchio W, Severini S: Multiple jejunal angiodysplasia detected by enema-helical CT. Clin Imaging 2000;24:61–63.
63 Miller FH, Hwang CM: An initial experience: using helical CT imaging to detect obscure gastrointestinal bleeding. Clin Imaging 2004;28:245–251.
64 Huprich JE, Fletcher JG, Alexander JA, Fidler JL, Burton SS, McCullough CH: Obscure gastrointestinal bleeding: evaluation with 64-section multiphase CT enterography – initial experience. Radiology 2008;246:562–571.
65 Moawad FJ, LaRock TR, Biondi MC, Cash BD, Kurland JE: A case of obscure gastrointestinal bleeding secondary to a small bowel gastrointestinal stromal tumor detected by magnetic resonance enterography. Medscape J Med 2008;10:263.
66 Gölder SK, Schreyer AG, Endlicher E, Feuerbach S, Schölmerich J, Kullmann F, Seitz J, Rogler G, Herfarth H: Comparison of capsule endoscopy and magnetic resonance (MR) enteroclysis in suspected small bowel disease. Int J Colorectal Dis 2006;21:97–104.
67 Filippone A, Cianci R, Milano A, Valeriano S, Di Mizio V, Storto ML: Obscure gastrointestinal bleeding and small bowel pathology: comparison between wireless capsule endoscopy and multidetector-row CT enteroclysis. Abdom Imaging 2008;33:398–406.
68 Crook DW, Knuesel PR, Froehlich JM, Eigenmann F, Unterweger M, Beer HJ, Kubik-Huch RA: Comparison of magnetic resonance enterography and video capsule endoscopy in evaluating small bowel disease. Eur J Gastroenterol Hepatol 2009;21: 54–65.
69 Shetzline MA, Suhocki P, Dash R, Rockey DC: Provocative angiography in obscure gastrointestinal bleeding. South Med J 2000;93:1205–1208.
70 Bloomfeld RS, Smith TP, Schneider AM, Rockey DC: Provocative angiography in patients with gastrointestinal hemorrhage of obscure origin. Am J Gastroenterol 2000;95:2807–2812.
71 Ettorre GC, Francioso G, Garribba AP, Fracella MR, Greco A, Farchi G: Helical CT angiography in gastrointestinal bleeding of obscure origin. AJR Am J Roentgenol 1997;168:727–731.
72 Junquera F, Quiroga S, Saperas E, Pérez-Lafuente M, Videla S, Alvarez-Castells A, Miró JR, Malagelada JR: Accuracy of helical computed tomographic angiography for the diagnosis of colonic angiodysplasia. Gastroenterology 2000;119:293–299.
73 Pennazio M: Bleeding update. Gastrointest Endosc Clin N Am 2006;16;251–266.
74 Pennazio M, Santucci R, Rondonotti E, Abbiati C, Beccari G, Rossini FP, De Franchis: Outcome of patients with obscure gastrointestinal bleeding after capsule endoscopy: report of 100 consecutive cases. Gastroenterology 2004;126:643–653.

Klaus Mönkemüller, MD, PhD, FASGE
Department of Gastroenterology, Hepatology and Infectious Diseases, Marienhospital
Josef-Albers-Strasse 70
DE–46236 Bottrop (Germany)
Tel. +49 2041 106 1000, Fax +49 2041 106 1009, E-Mail klaus.moenkemueller@mhb-bottrop.de

Mönkemüller K, Wilcox CM, Muñoz-Navas M (eds): Interventional and Therapeutic Gastrointestinal Endoscopy.
Front Gastrointest Res. Basel, Karger, 2010, vol 27, pp 240–253

Endoscopic Therapy for Lower Gastrointestinal Bleeding

Ivan Jovanović · Tomica Milosavljević

Clinic for Gastroenterology and Hepatology, Clinical Center of Serbia, Belgrade, Serbia

Abstract

Lower gastrointestinal bleeding (LGIB) refers to blood loss of recent onset originating from a site distal to terminal ileum. It is less common than upper GI bleeding, but if it is massive, it can be a serious clinical condition. Management of GI bleeding includes initial assessment, resuscitation and triage, history and physical examination, laboratory evaluation and upper endoscopy, if necessary followed by colonoscopy. Total colonoscopy is a procedure of choice for evaluation of patients with LGIB but in some cases can be complemented with angiography and/or nuclear medicine scintigraphy and surgery. Data show that careful early colonoscopy is highly effective for both diagnosis and therapeutic intervention of patients with severe LGIB. The localization of the bleeding source has priority over any therapeutic actions and early colonoscopy facilitates identification of bleeding site or bleeding stigmata which enables successful endoscopic therapy and prevents rebleeding. Injection therapy, together with thermal and mechanical modalities, can be used for treatment of most acutely bleeding lesions.

Lower gastrointestinal bleeding (LGIB) refers to blood loss of recent onset originating from a site distal to terminal ileum. It is less common than upper GI bleeding, but if it is massive, it can be a serious clinical condition. Approximately 20% of acute hemorrhage presents as massive LGIB. A recent US population-based study estimated an annual incidence rate of lower GI bleeding at 20.5/100,000 [1]. The most common diagnoses were diverticulosis, colorectal cancer and ischemic colitis [1]. The mean age of presentation ranged from 63 to 77 years and there was a 200-fold increase in the frequency of lower GI bleeding from the third to ninth decade of life [2–7]. The severity of LGIB is variable but overall mortality is low (2.4–4%) among patients admitted with lower GI bleeding compared with 23.1% in patients who developed lower GI bleeding while hospitalized for another reason. Mortality is more common in older adults, those with intestinal ischemia and comorbid illnesses [1, 2, 7].

The causes of LGIB may be arbitrarily grouped into several categories: anatomic (diverticulosis), vascular (angiodysplasia, ischemic, radiation-induced), inflammatory (infectious, IBD), and neoplastic. In addition, LGIB can occur after therapeutic interventions such as following polypectomy. LGIB can also be grouped by its intensity – occult, acute mild, acute massive. Acute LIGB is arbitrarily defined as bleeding of less than 3 days in duration that may result in instability of vital signs, anemia, and/or the need for blood transfusion. Chronic LGIB is a passage of blood per rectum over a period of several days or longer and usually implies intermittent or slow loss of blood. The patient with chronic bleeding can have occult fecal blood, occasional episodes of melena or maroon stools, and small quantities of visible blood per rectum.

Management of Gastrointestinal Bleeding

Initial Assessment, Resuscitation and Triage

The patient who presents with acute lower GI bleeding may complain of passing bright red blood per rectum, dark blood with clots, or, less commonly, melena. In fact, clinical manifestation can range from hematochezia with hemodynamic instability, to melena or rectal bleeding without hemodynamic compromise. The color can suggest the source as the darker blood denotes more proximal source of bleeding, except for cases of massive bleeding from the upper GI. Blood originating from the left colon typically is bright red. In comparison, bleeding from the right side of the colon usually appears dark or maroon-colored and may be mixed with stool. However, rapid transit of blood from the right side of the colon or massive upper GI bleeding can present as bright red blood per rectum. Melena suggests upper gastrointestinal bleeding (UGIB), although bleeding from the cecum may present in this manner. Thus, although helpful, the distinctions based upon stool color are not absolute. Patients may have chronic GI bleeding with asymptomatic iron-deficiency anemia, or hemoccult-positive stool on screening for colorectal cancer. In most cases of lower GI bleeding there are no symptoms of abdominal pain, except if there is ischemia and IBD.

The triage and initial assessment of patients presenting with presumed acute lower GI bleeding is based on the dynamics and severity of hemorrhage. Large volume hemorrhage can have major cardiovascular effect and symptoms associated with blood loss may be present even before any blood appears per rectum. Hypotension (systolic blood pressure <100 mm Hg), tachycardia (>100 beats/min), sweating, thirst, postural hypotension (blood pressure fall of 15 mm Hg when the patient sits up from recumbent position or pulse increase of 15 beats/min) even collapse indicates a significant blood loss of at least 20–30% of blood volume.

Patients presenting to the emergency room with hemodynamic instability require rapid clinical assessment, intravenous access with at least two large-diameter IV lines and laboratory evaluation (see below). Initial volume replacement should be with crystalloids and then with blood. Admission to hospital is required for most patients presenting with acute, massive lower GI bleeding. Those who present with mild bleeding without evidence of continued bleeding, but have had a significant drop from baseline hemoglobin (>2.0 g/l) and have a need for transfusion should also be hospitalized. In general, young patients with self-limited GI bleeding who present without hemodynamic instability and who have no significant comorbid conditions may be managed as outpatients.

History and Physical Examination

After the patient is stabilized, one should take detailed history, particularly noting GI symptoms, previous episodes of bleeding, drug intake particularly regarding anticoagulants or inhibitors of

1
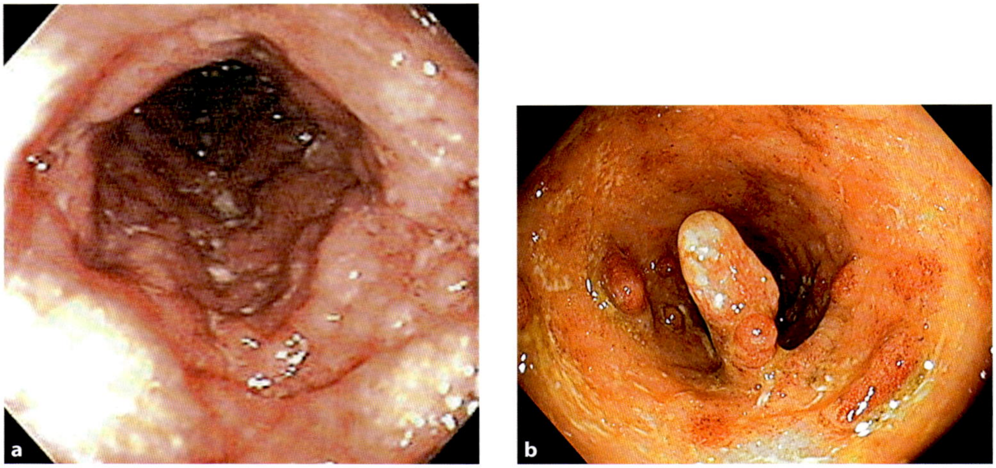

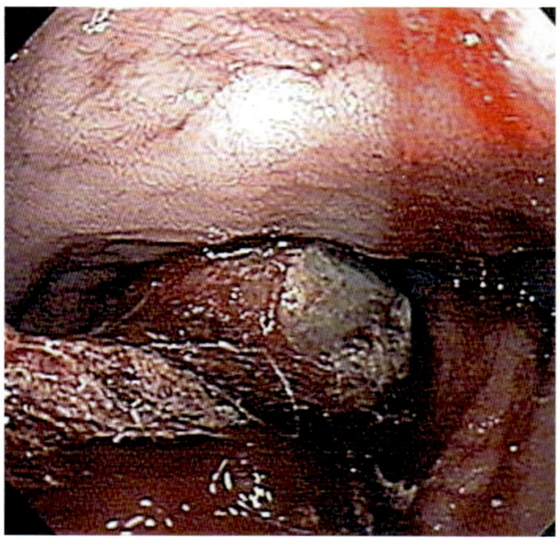

2

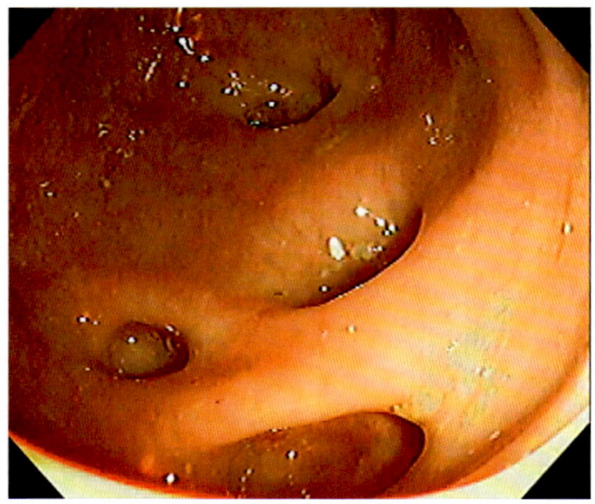

3

Fig. 1. **a** Diffuse mucosal edema and bleeding in a patient with ulcerative colitis. **b** Large pseudopolyp and multiple subepithelial hemorrhages in ulcerative colitis. **Fig. 2.** Elderly male with rectal bleeding. Colonoscopy revealed a large mass (prostate cancer) penetrating into the rectosigmoid lumen.

Fig. 3. The most common causes of lower GI bleeding are diverticula. However, in the absence of a bleeding diverticulum, other sources should be considered and searched for.

platelet aggregation (clopidrogel, salicylates and NSAIDs). Patients with suspected lower GI bleeding should also be asked about hemorrhoids, associated diarrhea, change in bowel habits, recent polypectomy, family history of GI disorders, history of inflammatory bowel disease, prior abdominal aneurysm repair, pelvic radiation therapy (for prostatic or gynecologic malignancies), bleeding disorders, other diseases and treatments that could cause clotting defects (fig. 1a, b). Patient age is also relevant. Bleeding is more common among younger patients due to IBD, from Meckel's diverticulum, or juvenile polyps, while middle-aged patients tend to bleed from diverticular disease and neoplasms (fig. 3, 4). Colonic diverticula and arteriovenous malformations (angiodysplasias) are more common source of bleeding in elderly patients [1, 2, 6, 7]. Infectious causes of LGIB include common bacterial pathogens such as *Salmonella*, *Shigella* and *Campylobacter*. *Clostridium difficile* and *Cytomegalovirus* can also result in colonic bleeding (fig. 5, 6).

Thorough physical examination should be undertaken as it can provide helpful clues (i.e. abdominal masses, tenderness and bruits, mucosal teleangiectasias in case of collagen vascular disorders and Osler-Weber-Rendu disease, etc.). A digital rectal examination is conditio sine qua non to exclude anorectal pathology as well as confirming the patient's description of the appearance of the stool.

Laboratory Evaluation

This should include a complete blood count (CBC) with platelet count, prothrombin time/partial thromboplastin time (PT/PTT), international normalized ratio (INR) and creatinine/blood urea nitrogen (BUN) in order to assess renal function in case of resuscitation purposes and also in case of need for angiography. Blood type and cross-matches should also be obtained. Usually, otherwise healthy patients with a hemoglobin level >80 g/l do not require transfusion, but in elderly cases (>65 years) and comorbid patients, Hgb should be maintained at >100 g/l as it allows safe and diagnostic and therapeutic endoscopy. Clotting defects that precipitate bleeding should promptly be corrected with fresh-frozen plasma and in some cases with platelet transfusion when needed (platelet count <50,000).

Upper Endoscopy (Esophagogastroduodenoscopy, EGD)

Distinguishing between an upper and lower source of bleeding is usually relatively straightforward. However, 10–15% of patients presenting as 'lower GI bleeding' actually bleed from the upper GI tract [2, 7]. These patients are usually unstable hemodynamically. Nasogastric tube aspirate may fail to identify bleeding from the upper GI tract [8]. Thus, an EGD is mandatory in patients with LGIB and hemodynamic changes.

Techniques (fig. 6–10)

General. Patients with bright red hematochezia and minimal blood loss can initially be evaluated with anoscopy and flexible sigmoidoscopy. Otherwise, a total colonoscopy is a procedure of choice for evaluation [9]. The diagnostic accuracy of colonoscopy ranges from 48 to 86% in the setting of LGIB, and cecal intubation is achieved in greater than 95% of attempts [10–13]. However, as the localization of the site and source of bleeding requires ongoing bleeding, these figures are likely to be overestimated in terms of the utility of colonoscopy as most bleedings stop spontaneously. Still, even if the source of bleeding is not found, it can be of benefit to document the finding in colon. Furthermore, if total colonoscopy is feasible and no source of bleeding is found, then the ileal intubation is a prerequisite to exclude bleeding from the small bowel. Although retrograde passage from colon can occur, ileal blood in most cases indicates a small-bowel origin. Richter et al. [5] also demonstrated that the yield from colonoscopy is greater when done earlier in the hospital stay, and patients who undergo colonoscopy for LGIB have a shorter length of stay compared with those who did not [14, 15].

Angiography. Angiography should be reserved for those patients with active bleeding and continued hemodynamic instability in whom endoscopy is not feasible [16, 17]. Selective

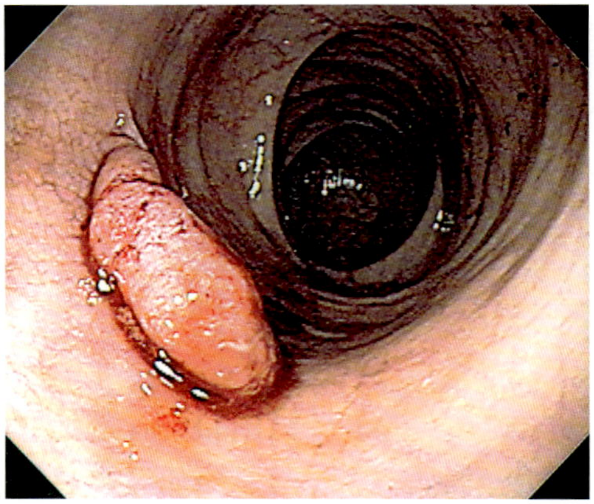

4

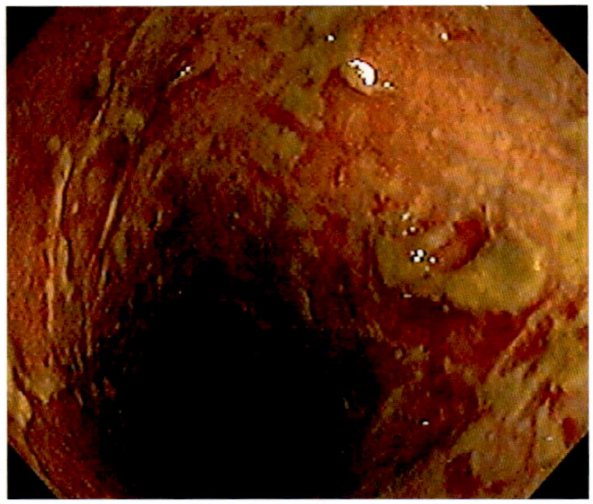

5

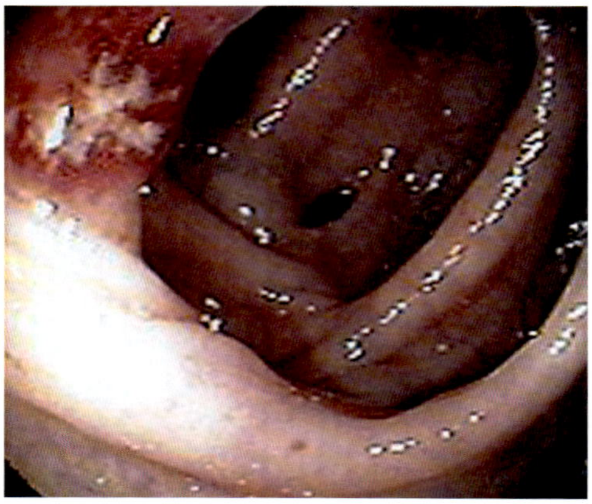

6

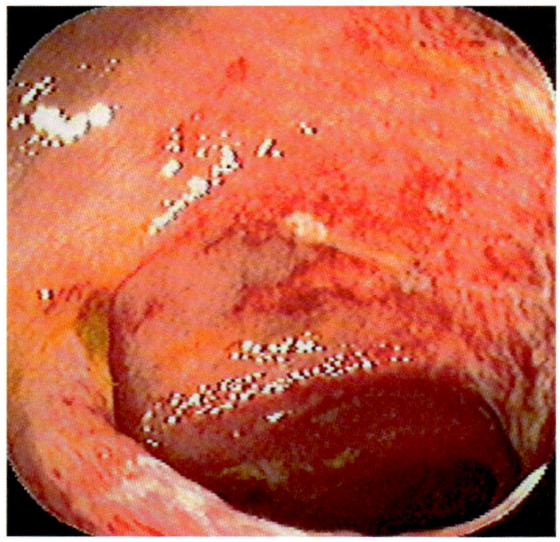

7

Fig. 4. Colon cancers generally result in anemia (right-sided colon cancer) or obstruction (left colon cancer). However, overt bleeding is not uncommon, specially in patients who take anticoagulant therapy. **Fig. 5.** *Clostridium difficile* colitis can occasionally result in frank rectal bleeding.
Fig. 6. Cytomegalovirus colitis should always be considered in the differential diagnosis of lower GI bleeding in any immunosuppressed patient (e.g. HIV, status post-transplant). Endoscopically, CMV results in ulcers or stellate erosions such as this case.
Fig. 7. Most of the patients with ischemic colitis do not require any intervention to control bleeding, since it usually stops spontaneously and lesions are diffuse in character. **Fig. 8.** SRUS bleeding vessel.

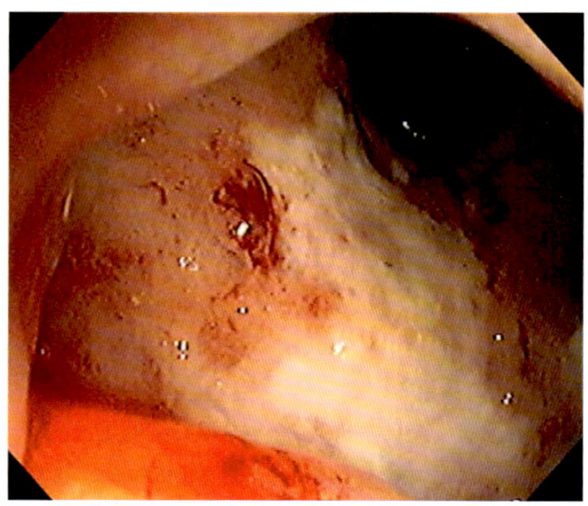

8

angiography has diagnostic yield ranging from 27 to 67% with a complication rate of 2–4% (contrast-induced renal failure, arterial injury and mesenteric ischemia), but it requires bleeding rate of at least 1.0–1.5 ml/min. Angiographic location allows vasopressin infusion and/or embolization. Provocative angiography with short-acting agents such as heparin, tolazoline or

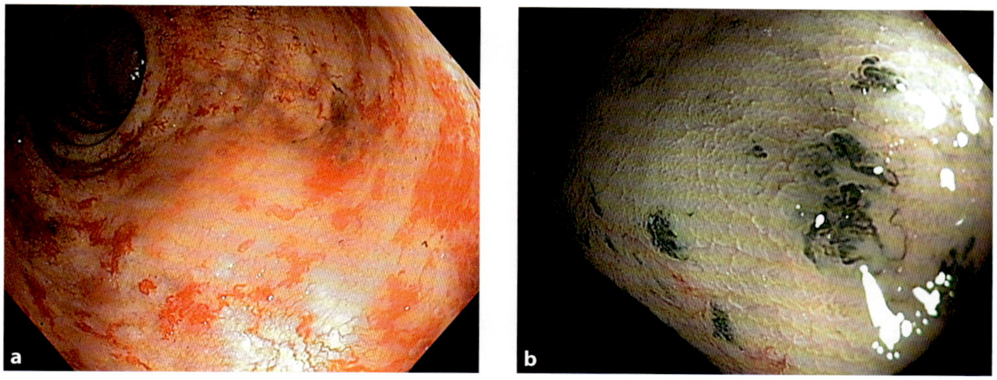

Fig. 9. **a** Radiation treatment of pelvic malignancies frequently causes acute and chronic changes which can take the form of teleangiectasias and hemorrhagic changes of rectal mucosa as a spectrum of radiation proctitis (cf. fig. 4). **b** Narrowband imaging of radiation proctitis.

urokinase has unclear success and it is not generally recommended unless patient is not immediately referred to surgery.

Nuclear Medicine Scintigraphy. Nuclear scans have poor accuracy in localizing the bleeding site and are difficult to interpret. The threshold rate of GI bleeding for localization with radioisotope scanning is about 0.1 ml/min or more. Nuclear scans are either technetium sulfur colloid (short half-life) or technetium-labeled red blood cells. A colonic resection should not be only based on the results of a nuclear scan.

Surgery. Surgery is generally reserved for patients whose bleeding site is identified by angiography but who are inappropriate for, or fail, angiographic therapy. Besides, surgical intervention is required when hemodynamic instability persists despite resuscitation or severe bleeding recurs. Guidelines for the evaluation of patients with LGIB are provided in the algorithm shown in figure 10 [17].

Endoscopic Treatment. Hemodynamic and respiratory stability of the patient is a prerequisite for the safe and complete emergency endoscopy. Intravenous sedation should be avoided in hemodynamically unstable patients. The experience and skill of the endoscopist is of critical value for the successful completion of the procedure. Another factor determining the outcome of hemostatic procedure is knowledge of the limitations of hemostatic techniques and timing. A delayed decision to refer a patient to surgery and irrational repeated attempts to achieve hemostasis can be just as devastating as bleeding by itself.

Colon Preparation. In a case of active LGIB, the colon must be cleansed prior to the procedure. Examining unprepared colon gives a very little yield to the diagnosis of the source of bleeding. Therefore, most experts suggest quick purge of the colon with 4–6 liters of PEG (polyethylene glycol) either per os or through the nasogastric tube together with some prokinetics (metoclopramid i.v.) in order to speed up peristalsis. The only exception from this generally accepted policy is when there is a high suspicion of rectal bleeding, when rectosigmoidoscopy can be performed on an unprepared colon.

Timing of Examination. Several studies have shown that colonoscopy is safe and effective when performed within 12 h of admission although two recent studies challenged the utility of early colonoscopy [20, 21]. In their settings, urgent colonoscopy had no advantage over expectant

Table 1. Most common causes of massive LGIB

Children and adolescents
Meckel's diverticulum
Juvenile polyps
Inflammatory bowel diseases
Adults
Diverticulosis
Inflammatory bowel diseases
Colorectal neoplasia
Infectious colitis
Adults >60 years of age
Angiodysplasia
Diverticulosis
Colorectal neoplasia
Ischemic colitis

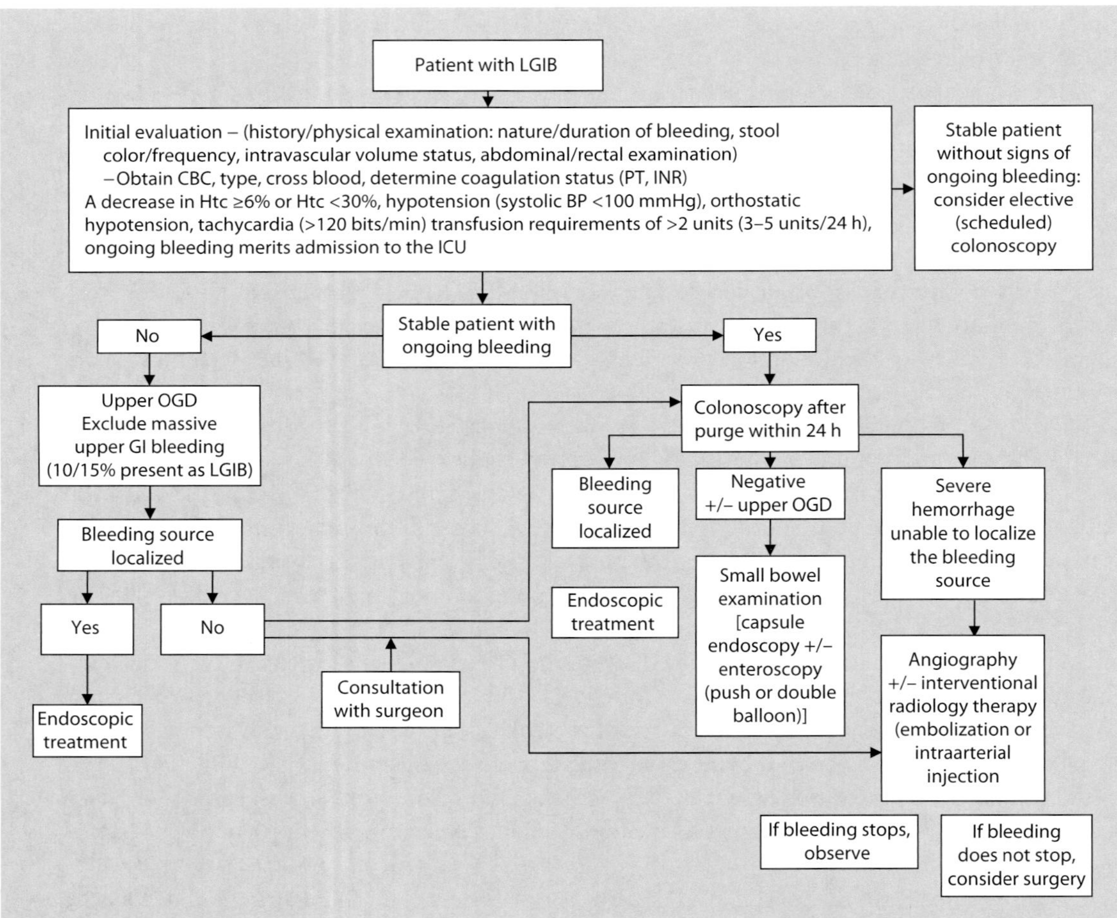

Fig. 10. Guidelines for the evaluation of patients with LGIB.

colonoscopy in terms of diagnostic yield, subsequent therapy, hospital stay and overall clinical outcome. Thus, decisions concerning care for patients with acute LGIB and timing of colonoscopy should be based on individual experience and local expertise. It is our practice to perform colonoscopy the following morning and after the patient is stabilized in the ICU (within 12–24 h of admission). If the patient stops bleeding, colonoscopy is usually deferred until 48–72 h.

Equipment. Endoscopic hemostasis should be attempted with a 3.7- to 4.2-mm large-channel colonoscope to allow blood and colon content to be suctioned through the working channel alongside an accessory. Alternatively, a double-channel colonoscope can be used when available, which enables accessories manipulation independently from aspiration.

Accessories (also see Accessories Used for Hemostasis in Gastrointestinal Bleeding, pp. 18–36)

Outcomes

Data show that careful early colonoscopy is highly effective for both diagnosis (sensitivity of proximally 86% ranging from 48 to 90%) and therapeutic intervention of patients with severe LGIB [22, 23]. Early colonoscopy is also associated with a shorter hospital stay and it is more cost-effective (cost saving of approximately USD 10,000 per patient) than other strategies for diagnosis and treatment of severe hematochezia [14, 15]. Early colonoscopy facilitates identification of bleeding site or bleeding stigmata which enables successful endoscopic therapy and prevents rebleeding. Some experts therefore strongly advocate early colonoscopy to prevent rebleeding through endoscopic therapy. The UCLA/Center for Ulcer Research and Education (CURE) group found a 53% rebleeding rate among non-treated patients with recent diverticular bleeding, but no rebleeds over a period of 3 years among endoscopically treated patients [24]. The implications of these studies are that a shorter hospital stay, along with elimination of further diagnostic tests and procedures, can lower hospitalization costs. Other uncontrolled studies have not demonstrated a convincing improvement in rebleeding rates [20, 21, 25, 26]. A case series from the Mayo Clinic [30], two non-randomized studies [20, 26] as well as a randomized controlled trial form Duke University [21] failed to document a benefit (mortality, hospital stay, ICU stay, transfusion requirements, early rebleeding, or late rebleeding) from an early colonoscopy.

Regardless of the approach (urgent vs. expectant colonoscopy), mortality rates for LGIB remain low and under 5% [2, 27], unless bleeding starts after hospital admission (23%) for another reason [2]. Urgent colonoscopy is not essential for initial evaluation of acute LGIB but it has a major advantage over the other hemostatic techniques as it can become therapeutic at the same time. Spontaneous resolution of bleeding is also common without further medical intervention besides initial resuscitation. Patients presenting with lower GI bleeding should nonetheless undergo colonoscopy within a reasonable period of time from admission to rule out other significant pathology, including neoplasm. Thus, the approach algorithm should be developed according to the available resources and expertise.

Therapeutic Intervention in Specific Lesions

Hemorrhoids. Hemorrhoidal bleeding is the most common cause of mild and intermittent lower GI bleeding. Bleeding is typically with bright red blood on the surface of the stool, on the toilet paper and/or in the toilet bowl. It may occur from any grade of hemorrhoids, but it is more severe from the advanced stadium. The majority of patients require treatment. Treatment of

Table 2. Diagnosis in elderly patients with lower GI bleeding

Diverticular bleeding	43%
Vascular ectasias	20%
Colonic cancer or polyp	9%
Radiation proctitis	6%
Ischemic colitis	4%
Miscellaneous causes	11%
Source not determined	11%

hemorrhoids in our settings is usually carried out by coloproctology surgeons and it is beyond the interest of this chapter (book). The diagnosis can be confirmed on anoscopy and/or flexible sigmoidoscopy and for those patients >50 years of age, colonoscopy is recommended.

Diverticular Bleeding. The prevalence of diverticulosis is estimated as 30–50% in asymptomatic individuals ≥50 years [2, 6, 7]. Bleeding will occur in 15–17% of patients with diverticulosis, being massive in approximately one-third. Affected patients have an appreciable risk of rebleeding (14–38%). The UCLA/CURE group found that among 17 patients with stigmata of recent diverticular hemorrhage there was a very high rebleed rate of 53% and an emergency surgery rate of 35% [3, 4, 24].

Many patients are elderly, with comorbid conditions that contribute to morbidity and mortality rates which together approximate 10–20% [1, 2, 6].

It is very rare for bleeding to coexist with diverticulitis which reflects non-inflammatory pathogenesis of the bleeding. Bleeding usually occurs in the neck or in the base of the diverticulum and in 75–80% stops spontaneously. Therefore, the diagnosis is often made by finding diverticula on colonoscopy in the absence of another identifiable cause of lower GI bleeding (50%) [28]. A clot is rarely seen in the diverticulum that has bled (20%) [28, 29]. Patients with a single self-limited episode of diverticular hemorrhage can be managed conservatively. The remaining 15% with stigmata of significant bleeding seen on colonoscopy such as adherent clots, a non-bleeding visible vessel, or active bleeding are more likely to require transfusion and specific hemostasis intervention which can now be successfully delivered by colonoscopy [24, 26, 28, 30]. Endoscopic treatment of bleeding secondary to diverticulosis includes epinephrine injection, contact thermal modalities, hemoclip application, band ligation and combination of the above.

In theory, early endoscopy would facilitate identification of bleeding site, but endoscopic treatment of diverticular bleeding is not always preferred for at least two reasons: first, most often, bleeding stops spontaneously, and second, it is often difficult to localize the bleeding diverticulum in case of the active bleeding as non-bleeding diverticuli can contain blood (especially in a case of extensive left colon diverticular disease). Last but not the least, thermal treatment of the bleeding diverticulum has been associated with a perforation of the colon.

Our experience with endoscopic treatment of patients found to be bleeding from colonic diverticuli is similar to the treatment of bleeding ulcer disease. Endoscopic treatment of diverticula with active bleeding, non-bleeding visible vessel or an adherent clot is treated with paradiverticular injection of a 1:10,000 dilution of epinephrine in 0.5 aliquots using a standard Teflon sheath injection catheter with a 4-mm needle extension. A submucosal injection of 1–2 ml in 2–4 sites around the diverticulum is often sufficient [28–31]. After a period of observation, the site is lavaged with water and observed for hemostasis. Subsequently, the bleeding vessel is cauterized with multipolar probe (10–15 W, 1-s pulses with light tamponade pressure). The perforation

Table 3. Aetiology of lower gastrointestinal bleeding

Reference (first author)	Diverti-culosis %	Angio-dysplasia %	Colitis %	Neoplasm %	Anorectal %	Miscella-neous %	Small intestine %	Unknown %
Longstreth 1997 [2]	3	41	16	9	5	14	NA	NA
Jensen 1997 [4]	40	23	12	15	5	4	NA	NA
Richter 1995 [5]	12	48	6	11	3	6	NA	NA
Chaudhry 1998 [12]	20	11.8	33	11	14	7	12.1	3.5
Ohyama 2000 [13]	5.2	1.2	27	2.9	3.2	14.5	4.9	11
Strate 2003 [15]	3	30	21	6	14	28	NA	NA
Boley 1979 [54]	11	40	12	14	NA	NA	NA	NA
Jansen 1988 [55]	17	30	9	11	4	7	9	6
Leitman 1989 [56]	24	27	10	15	NA	NA	NA	NA

risk is substantially higher when the vessel is located at the base of the diverticulum. In this circumstance, clipping of the visible vessel or entire diverticulum might be a safer alternative [32]. Adherent clot is usually washed and suctioned or, if resistant, removed with a basket or snare with prior injection of epinephrine at the base of the clot. The exposed vessel is then coagulated with a multipolar probe or clipped [30–32].

More recently, the treatment of bleeding diverticuli with band ligation has been demonstrated, with inversion of the diverticulum by suction and its banding. Farrell et al. [34] and Tucker [35], based on the previous work of Witte [33], have reported cases of diverticular bleeding treated by elastic band ligation and suggested that this might be a promising method not only for the hemostasis, but for diverticular reversion as well.

Bleeding is rarely massive on presentation, requiring emergent diagnostic angiography followed by intraarterial infusion of vasopressin or segmental resection.

Vascular Anomalies. Angiodysplasia accounts for another 20–30% of cases of hematochezia. Colonic angiodysplasia occurs in approximately 1% of the adult population and is one of the most common causes of massive LGIB in patients over the age of 65 years [2, 6, 7]. It is also one of the major causes of GI bleeding, particularly recurrent bleeding, in patients with end-stage renal disease. They are usually a few millimeters in size but may be as big as 1 cm or larger [36]. They are most commonly seen in the right colon and can be single or multiple [36]. While angiodysplasia can be found anywhere along the colon, significant bleeding occurs most frequently from those lesions located in the cecum [36]. Patients who bleed typically present with occult blood loss. However, marked acute bleeding, causing orthostatic or hypotension, can occur.

Endoscopic hemostasis has been successfully reported using thermal modalities (bipolar probe, heater probe, and APC) as well as injection therapy [37–40]. The recommended power setting for multipolar probe is 10–12 W with 1- to 2-s pulses. Applications are repeated until the lesion is completely obliterated and hemostasis achieved. Often a prominent feeding or draining vascular structure is identified and more cautery may be required to completely coagulate this site. The cauterized areas should be flashed with water and observed for repeated applications if necessary. Transmural injury resulting in perforation has been reported but is uncommon. Alternatively, hemostasis can be achieved with a heater probe using a setting of 10–15 J. Both modalities are equally efficient in long-term follow-up in terms of number of bleeding episodes, blood transfusions and hematocrits when compared to prior to endoscopic treatment. Coagulation complications can be expected in 5% of the treated patients and they include recurrent delayed hemorrhage due to postcoagulation ulceration and postcoagulation syndrome.

Among all available techniques and accessories, APC appears to be the simplest and safest modality. Argon gas offers superficial coagulation that can be easily applied to multiple and widespread locations. However, care must be taken in the right colon, as perforations after APC have been reported.

For treatment of vascular ectasias in the colon, a meticulous preparation is necessary and endoscopic trauma and suction of the mucosa should be avoided. Treatment is easier in en-face view and when the lesion is not actively bleeding, although, in a case of side-firing APC probe, truly, it does not make a difference if you approach the lesion in a tangential manner. Before the start of the procedure, the position of all lesions needs to be carefully observed. The most dependent ones should be treated first. Also, smaller lesions should be treated first as the treatment of larger lesions often provokes bleeding and which can obscure the view. Large lesions should be treated from the periphery to the center while smaller ones can be targeted directly.

The ascending colon and cecum are the thinnest part of the colon, and too much insufflation further thins the wall. Therefore, it is wise to aspirate excess air in between attacks. Effective ablation can also be achieved with contact devices such as a multipolar cautery device or the heater probe. There is evidence that vascular malformations tend to recur, therefore endoscopic surveillance is necessary, particularly in patients with multiple lesions.

Colorectal Neoplasm. Although colorectal cancer is most commonly associated with occult blood loss rather than acute bleeding, patients with rectosigmoid lesions may present with hematochezia (fig. 4). Colonoscopy in this setting is primarily diagnostic.

Ischemic Colitis. Most of the patients with ischemic colitis do not require any intervention to control bleeding, since it usually stops spontaneously and lesions are diffuse in character (fig. 7). Endoscopy is usually diagnostic and it is indicated in the setting of possible inflammatory or ischemic colitis, unless there is clinical evidence for perforation. In some cases, focal bleeding ulcers or stigmata of hemorrhage can be treated endoscopically. Otherwise, endoscopic findings as well as mucosal biopsies are diagnostic.

Solitary Rectal Ulcer Syndrome. Endoscopic treatment consists of injection of diluted epinephrine (1:10,000) circumferentially around the bleeding point. In addition, visible vessel can be further cauterized with a bipolar probe using a power setting of 12–16 W or with a heater probe at 10–15 J. A cold polypectomy snare should be used to remove the clot after an injection of diluted epinephrine around the pedicle. After the vessel is exposed, it can be further cauterized as described. Ever since the introduction of endoclips, we increasingly use a combination of injection therapy and hemoclips for hemostasis of bleeding rectal ulcers.

Treatment of Radiation Proctitis. Radiation treatment of pelvic malignancies frequently causes acute and chronic changes which can take the form of teleangiectasias and hemorrhagic changes of rectal mucosa as a spectrum of radiation proctitis (fig. 4). Endoscopy therapy includes coagulation with bipolar [37], heater probe [37, 38], APC [39–42] and Nd:YAG lasers [43, 44], which all have been used successfully to treat bleeding from radiation-induced angiectasias. Recently, APC has become the treatment of choice which provides controlled, superficial, non-contact coagulation. It is very important to apply coagulation carefully in order to avoid the creation of deeper ulceration in a fragile ischemic mucosa. Multiple sessions are usually required [41, 42]. The use of APC to treat radiation proctitis is effective as it can lead to an improvement of symptoms and bleeding episodes after an average of two sessions carried out at an interval of 4 weeks.

Postpolypectomy Bleeding. Bleeding is the most common complication of polypectomy. Reported risk factors for postpolypectomy bleeding during colonoscopy include older age (≥65 years), large polyps (>2 cm), thick stalks, sessile polyps, right colon polyps and use of pure cut electrosurgical current [45–47]. Delayed postpolypectomy bleeding may be associated with hypertension [47], aspirin [48, 49], NSAIDs [49], or resuming anticoagulants [49, 50]. Endoscopic management techniques include re-snaring the stalk (without cautery), epinephrine injection, thermal coagulation, hemoclips, and endoloops [51].

Other Causes. Dieulafoy lesions rarely lead to bleeding from the small bowel and colon. Hemostasis of Dieulafoy lesions can be achieved by epinephrine injection, thermal coagulation, band ligation, and clipping; nevertheless, no single modality has been proven superior to the others [52, 53].

Conclusion

To conclude, localization of the bleeding source has priority over any therapeutic actions. In this respect, colonoscopy is superior to other diagnostic methods and is recommended in the early evaluation of acute LGIB. The diagnostic yield of urgent colonoscopy in acute LGIB is high. Injection therapy, together with thermal and mechanical modalities, can be used for treatment of most acutely bleeding lesions. Still, if there is a profuse bleeding that cannot be controlled endoscopically, angiography is the means of choice. Subtotal colectomy has proven advantageous over segmental resection if the bleeding site is unclear, but preoperative localization of bleeding should be attempted by all available diagnostic means. In approaching patients with LGIB, also consider the patient's age, general condition, bleeding source, and availability of technology at the treating hospital (endoscopy, interventional angiography, nuclear medicine, surgeons) and skills of all treating personal. Nevertheless, it is important to take into account an ability to transfer patients to the tertiary center. Therefore, a diagnostic and therapeutic approach is more dependent on local expertise and availability than on an algorithmic approach.

References

1 Farrell JJ, Friedman LS: Gastrointestinal bleeding in the elderly. Gastroenterol Clin North Am 2001;30: 377–407.

2 Longstreth GF: Epidemiology and outcome of patients hospitalized with acute lower gastrointestinal hemorrhage: a population-based study. Am J Gastroenterol 1997;92:419–424.

3 Wong Kee Song LM, Baron T: Endoscopic management of acute lower gastrointestinal bleeding. Am J Gastroenterol 2008;103:1881–1887.

4 Jensen DM, Machicado GA: Colonoscopy for diagnosis and treatment of severe lower gastrointestinal bleeding. Routine outcomes and cost analysis. Gastrointest Endosc Clin N Am 1997;7:477–498.

5 Richter JM, Christensen MR, Kaplan LM, Nishioka NS: Effectiveness of current technology in the diagnosis and management of lower gastrointestinal hemorrhage. Gastrointest Endosc 1995;41:93–98.

6 Rios A, Montoya MJ, Rodrigez JM, et al: Acute lower gastrointestinal hemorrhages in geriatric patients. Dig Dis Sci 2005;50:898–904.

7 Wilcox CM, Clark WS: Causes and outcome of upper and lower gastrointestinal bleeding: The Grady Hospital experience. South Med J 1999;92:44–50.

8 Cuellar RE, Gavaler JS, Aleksander JA, et al: Gastrointestinal tract haemorrhage. The value of nasogastric aspirate. Arch Intern Med 1990;150:1381–384.

9 Davila RE, Rajan E, Adler DG, Egan J, Hirota WK, Leighton JA, Qureshi W, Zuckerman MJ, Fanelli R, Wheeler-Harbaugh J, Baron TH, Faigel DO: ASGE Guideline: The role of endoscopy in the patient with lower-GI bleeding. Gastrointest Endosc 2005;62:656–660.

10 Peura DA, Lanza FL, Gostout CJ, Foutch PG: The American College of Gastroenterology Bleeding Registry: Preliminary findings. Am J Gastroenterol 1997;92:924–928.

11 ASGE Guideline: The role of endoscopy in the patient with lower-GI bleeding. Gastrointest Endosc 2005:62: 656–660.

12 Chaudhry V, Hyser MJ, Gracias VH, Gau FC: Colonoscopy: the initial test for acute lower gastrointestinal bleeding. Am Surg 1998;64:723–728.

13 Ohyama T, Sakurai Y, Ito M, et al: Analysis of urgent colonoscopy for lower gastrointestinal tract bleeding. Digestion 2000;61:189–192.

14 Schmulewitz N, Fisher DA, Rockey DC: Early colonoscopy for acute lower GI bleeding predicts shorter hospital stay: a retrospective study of experience in a single center. Gastrointest Endosc 2003; 58:841–846.

15 Strate LL, Syngal S: Timing of colonoscopy: impact of length of hospital stay in patients with acute lower intestinal bleeding. Am J Gastroenterol 2003;98:317–722.

16 Zuccaro G: Management of adult patients with lower gastrointestinal bleed. ACG Guidelines. Am J Gastroenterol 1998;93:1202–1208.

17 Faigel DO, Dominitz JA, Eisen GM and members of ASGE Standards of Practice Committee: An annotated algorithmic approach to acute lower gastrointestinal bleeding. Gastrointest Endosc 2001;53: 859–863.

18 Hunter JM, Pezim ME: Limited value of technetium-99m-labeled red cell scintigraphy in localization of lower gastrointestinal bleeding Am J Surg 1990;159:504–506.

19 Levy R, Barto W, Gani J: Retrospective study of the utility of nuclear scintigraphic-labelled red cell scanning for lower gastrointestinal bleeding. ANZ J Surg 2003;73:205–209.

20 Angtuaco TL, Reddy SK, Drapkin S, et al: The utility of urgent colonoscopy in the evaluation of acute lower gastrointestinal tract bleeding: a 2-year experience from a single center. Am J Gastroenterol 2001;96:1782–1785.

21 Green BT, Rockey DC, Portwood G, et al: Urgent colonoscopy for evaluation and management of acute lower gastrointestinal hemorrhage: a randomized controlled trial. Am J Gastroenterol 2005;100:2395–2402.

22 Zuckerman GR, Prakash C: Acute lower gastrointestinal bleeding. Part I. Clinical presentation and diagnosis. Gastrointest Endosc 1998;48:606–616.

23 Zuckerman GR, Prakash C: Acute lower gastrointestinal bleed. Part II. Etiology, therapy, and outcomes. Gastrointest Endosc 1999;49:228–238.

24 Jensen DM, Machicado GA, Jutabha R, Kovacs TO: Urgent colonoscopy for the diagnosis and treatment of severe diverticular haemorrhage. N Engl J Med 2000; 342:78–82.

25 Smooth RL, Gostout CJ, Rajan E, et al: Is early colonoscopy after admission for acute bleeding needed? Am J Gastroenterol 2003;98:1996–1999.

26 Bloomfeld R, Shetzline M, Rockey DC: Urgent colonoscopy for the diagnosis and treatment of severe diverticular haemorrhage. N Engl J Med 2000;342:1608–1609.

27 Rios A, Montoya MJ, Rodriguez JM, et al: Severe acute lower gastrointestinal bleeding: risk factors for morbidity and mortality. Langenbecks Arch Surg 2007;392:165–171.

28 Prakash C, Chokshi H, Walden DT, Aliperti G: Endoscopic hemostasis in acute diverticular bleeding. Endoscopy 1999;31:460–463.

29 Foutch PG, Zimmerman K: Diverticular bleeding and the pigmented protuberance (sentinel clot): clinical implications, histopathological correlation, and results of endoscopic intervention. Am J Gastroenterol 1996;91: 2589–2593.

30 Bloomfeld RS, Rockey DC, Shetzline MA: Endoscopic therapy of acute diverticular haemorrhage. Am J Gastroenterol 2001;96:2367–2372.

31 Ramirez FC, Johnson DA, Zierer ST, Walker GJ, Sanowski RA: Successful endoscopic hemostasis of bleeding colonic diverticula with epinephrine injection. Gastrointest Endosc 1996;43:167–170.

32 Simpson PW, Nguyen MH, Lim JK, Soetikno RM: Use of endoclips in the treatment of massive colonic diverticular bleeding. Gastrointest Endosc 2004;59:433–437.
33 Witte JT: Band ligation for colonic bleeding: modification of multiband ligating devices for use with a colonoscope. Gastrointest Endosc 2000;52:762–765.
34 Farrell JJ, Graeme-Cook F, Kelsey PB: Treatment of bleeding colonic diverticula by endoscopic band ligation: an in-vivo and ex-vivo pilot study. Endoscopy 2003;35:823–829.
35 Tucker LE: Diverticular bleeding: novel treatment with band ligation. Mo Med 2004;101:61–63.
36 Hochter W, Weingart J, Kuhner W, Frimberger E, Ottenjann R: Angiodysplasia in the colon and rectum. Endoscopic morphology, localisation and frequency. Endoscopy 1985;17:182–185.
37 Jensen DM, Machicado GA, Cheng S, Jensen ME, Jutabha R: A randomized prospective study of endoscopic bipolar electrocoagulation and heater probe treatment of chronic rectal bleeding from radiation teleangiectasia. Gastrointest Endosc 1997;45:20–25.
38 Fuentes D, Monserat R, Isern AM, et al: Colitis due to radiation: endoscopic management with heat probe. GEN 1993;47:165–167.
39 Silva RA, Correia AJ, Dias LM, Viana HL, Viana RL: Argon plasma coagulation therapy for hemorrhagic radiation proctosigmoiditis. Gastrointest Endosc 1999; 50:221–224.
40 Fantin AC, Binek J, Suter WR, Meyenberger C: Argon beam coagulation for treatment of symptomatic radiation-induced proctitis. Gastrointest Endosc 1999;49:515–518.
41 Tam W, Moore J, Schoeman M: Treatment of radiation proctitis with argon plasma coagulation. Endoscopy 2000;32:667–672.
42 Olmos JA, Marcolongo M, Pogorelsky V, Varela E, Davolos JR: Argon plasma coagulation for prevention of recurrent bleeding from GI angiodysplasias. Gastrointest Endosc 2004;60:881–886.
43 Buchi KN, Dixon JA: Argon laser treatment of hemorrhagic radiation proctitis. Gastroint Endosc 1987; 33:27–30.
44 Gostout CJ, Bowyer BA, Ahlqnist DA, et al: Mucosal vascular malformations of the gastrointestinal tract: clinical observations and results of endoscopic neodymium: yttrium-aluminum garnet laser therapy. Mayo Clin Proc 1988;63:993–1003.
45 Van Gossum A, Cozzoli A, Adler M, Taton G, Cremer M: Colonoscopic snare polypectomy: analysis of 1,485 resections comparing two types of current. Gastrointest Endosc 1992;38:472–475.
46 Kim HS, Kim TI, Kim WH, et al: Risk factors for immediate postpolypectomy bleeding of the colon: a multicenter study. Am J Gastroenterol 2006;101:1333–1341.
47 Watabe H, Yamaji Y, Okamoto M, et al: Risk assessment for delayed hemorrhagic complication of colonic polypectomy: polyp-related factors and patient-related factors. Gastrointest Endosc 2006;64:73–78.
48 Nakajima H, Takami H, Yamagata K, et al: Aspirin effects on colonic mucosal bleeding: implication for colonic biopsy and polypectomy. Dig Colon Rectum 1997;40:1484–1488.
49 Hui AJ, Wong RM, Ching JY, et al: Risk of colonoscopic polypectomy bleeding with anticoagulants and antiplatlet agents: analysis of 1,657 cases. Gastrointest Endosc 2004;59:44–48.
50 Sawhney MS, Salfiti N, Nelson DB, Lederle FA, Bond JH: Risk factors for severe delayed postpolypectomy bleeding. Endoscopy 2008;40:115–119.
51 Waye JD: Management of complications of colonoscopic polypectomy. Gastroenterologist 1993;1:158–164.
52 Lee YT, Walmsley RS, Leong RW, et al: Dieulafoy's lesion. Gastrointest Endosc 2003;58:236–243.
53 Fukumori D, Sasaki T, Sato M, Sakai K, Ohmori H, Yamamoto F: Massive rectal bleeding from a Dieulafoy's ulcer of the rectum. Int Surg 2004;89:63–66.
54 Boley SJ, DiBase A, Brandt LJ, Sammartano RJ: Lower intestinal bleeding in the elderly. Am J Surg 1979;137:57–64.
55 Jensen DM, Machicado GA: Diagnosis and treatment of severe haematochezia. The role of urgent colonoscopy after purge. Gastroenterology 1988;95:1569–1574.
56 Leitman IM, Paull DE, Shires GT III: Evaluation and management of massive lower gastrointestinal haemorrhage. Ann Surg 1989;209:175–180.

Ivan Jovanović, MD, PhD
Clinic for Gastroenterology and Hepatology
Clinical Center of Serbia
CS–11000 Belgrade (Serbia)
Tel./Fax +381 11 361 5587, E-Mail ivangastro@beotel.rs

Mönkemüller K, Wilcox CM, Muñoz-Navas M (eds): Interventional and Therapeutic Gastrointestinal Endoscopy.
Front Gastrointest Res. Basel, Karger, 2010, vol 27, pp 254–268

Principles and Technique of Colon Polypectomy

Klaus Mönkemüller[a,b] · Helmut Neumann[b] · Lucia C. Fry[a,b]

[a]Department of Internal Medicine, Gastroenterology, Hepatology and Infectious Diseases, Marienhospital, Bottrop, and [b]Department of Gastroenterology, Hepatology and Infectious Diseases, Otto-von-Guericke University, Magdeburg, Germany

Abstract

Colorectal cancer (CRC) is one of the leading causes of death from cancer worldwide. It is accepted that CRC originates from colon adenomas. Removal of colon adenomas is associated with a reduction in the incidence of CRC. Thus, CRC could theoretically be prevented by the detection and removal of adenomatous polyps. Standard polyp removal methods include the use of biopsy forceps and various types of electrocautery snares. Advanced endoscopic and imaging techniques such as cap-assisted colonoscopy, chromoendoscopy, and virtual chromoendoscopy may be helpful in the detection and characterization of polyps. A basic prerequisite for colonoscopic polypectomy is adequate training in colonoscopy and polypectomy. Minor and major complications such as bleeding and perforation occur in roughly 10% of advanced polypectomies. Therefore, the colonoscopist should be capable of managing most of these complications. The objective of this paper is to present the principles, theory and technique of basic colon polypectomy.

Definition of Colon Polyp

Colon polyps are classified based on endoscopic and histologic criteria. The name 'polyp' derives from Greek, means 'many-footed', and is used to characterize the protrusions of an octopus [1]. Colon polyps are classified based on endoscopic and histologic criteria [1–4]. There is an ongoing debate on how to best define a colon 'polyp' endoscopically [4–6]. Polyps with a stalk, stem, pedicle or peduncle are referred to as 'pedunculated' polyps and those without a pedicle are categorized as 'sessile' polyps [1, 2] (fig. 1, 2). The third type of colon polyp is the 'flat lesion' [2, 4] (table 1; fig. 1, 3). Most flat polyps are adenomas, and thus are also called 'flat adenomas' [2–6]. Flat adenomas have special biologic and genetic characteristics that make them more aggressive [4–6]. Even if small, these lesions can harbor advanced neoplasia or even carcinoma [4–7]. Thus, removal of these lesions should be performed using mucosectomy techniques. Some flat and sessile polyps tend to spread across a larger surface of mucosa and are called 'carpet-shaped' or laterally spreading lesions or polyps [2–6] (fig. 4).

The appearance of the mucosa is also used to categorize polyps. The surface can be smooth, normal, granular, nodular or villous [2]. Breaks in the mucosa are more common in the presence of cancer. Mucosal breaks can be categorized into erosions and ulcerations [2]. When ulcers

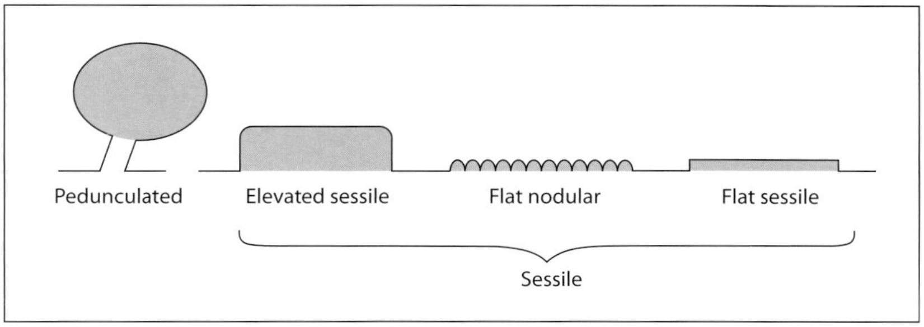

Fig. 1. Diagram showing the most common polyp shapes: pedunculated, sessile and flat.

involve large parts of an exophytic lesion then the polyp or tumor is categorized as exulcerated, whereas when the ulcer reaches into the deeper layers it is called excavated. Large polyps can also have the appearance of a 'cauliflower' and are called vegetant(ing) or fungating [2]. The use of advanced imaging techniques such as magnification and chromoendoscopy have helped to characterize colon polyps [8–12]. In addition to allowing a detailed appreciation of the mucosal surface ('pit pattern'), these techniques also enable the investigation of the capillary pattern ('submucosal capillary loops') and the polyp margins [12] (fig. 5, 6). In neoplasia there is increased angiogenesis. Thus, investigation of the vessel pattern may help predict the stage of neoplasia [8–11]. However, currently no data exist supporting the routine use of these techniques to classify polyps. Furthermore, the ability to predict invasive carcinoma using these techniques is not much higher than using standard video endoscopic imaging methods [13]. Ultimately, the diagnosis of the type of lesion and depth of invasion of neoplasia will be done by the pathologist.

The endoscopist has to carefully document the location, morphology, size and appearance of each polyp seen.

Patient Preparation

The patient should undergo a detailed preoperative history and physical examination and be informed by the physician about the benefits, alternatives and risks of colonoscopic polypectomy. Informed consent should not only include information about the endoscopic risks, but also those risks associated with sedation and potentially missing a lesion. Although every effort is paid to thoroughly investigate the colon, colon polyps can be missed, even in expert hands [14]. Routine preoperative laboratory blood testing is not indicated before polypectomy, unless there is clinical evidence or suspicion of a blood dyscrasia or patients are being treated with coumarin oral anticoagulants or heparin and its derivatives. Even though colon polypectomy is considered a high risk endoscopic procedure, the limited data available do not demonstrate any increased risk of bleeding after polypectomy in patients taking non-steroidal anti-inflammatory drugs, aspirin or clopidrogel [15, 16]. Thus, we do not routinely stop these medications before polypectomy. However, if an endoscopic mucosal resection or removal of a large polyp is planned electively, we ask the patient to stop aspirin or clopidrogel (not both) 1 week before the procedure. Both, the British Society of Gastroenterology and the American Society of Gastrointestinal Endoscopy guidelines are very useful to guide the endoscopist in the management of anticoagulants such as warfarin or heparin and its derivatives in the peri-endoscopic period [15, 16].

Table 1. Comparison of standard and new polyp classifications

Polyp morphology	Standard	Paris-Japanese[1]
Pedunculated	Pedunculated	Protruding polypoid, pedunculated, type I
Sessile	Sessile-LST	Protruding polypoid, sessile, type I
	Flat-LST	Superficial, polypoid lesion Pedunculated (0-Ip) Sessile (0-Is) Mixed (0-Isp)
		Superficial, non-polypoid lesion Slightly elevated (0-IIa) Completely flat (0-IIb) Slightly depressed (0-IIc)
		Superficial, mixed types Elevated and depressed (0-IIa + IIc) Depressed and elevated (0-IIc + IIa) Sessile and depressed (0-Is + IIc)

LST = Laterally spreading tumor or 'carpet-shaped' polyp; p = pedunculated; s = sessile; a = elevated; b = flat; c = depressed.
Reproduced with permission from Mönkemüller et al. [1].
[1] The Paris-Japanese classification defines a protruding polypoid lesion as a lesion that is elevated >2.5 mm above the surrounding mucosa, superficial or non-polypoid lesions should be elevated <2.5 mm or be depressed <2.5 mm. A type 0 lesion is defined as a superficial, sessile, polypoid, flat/depressed, or excavated lesion. A type I lesion is defined as a protruding polypoid lesion.
Adapted from both the Kyoto and Paris workshops [4, 6].

The two most important determinants of an adequate colon examination are: (1) colonoscopist's expertise, which encompasses having had adequate training, and (2) adequate colon preparation, which is essential for adequate mucosal visualization and removal of polyps. If the colon inadequately prepared we recommend repeating colonoscopy on another occasion. Although currently the rate of colon perforation after polypectomy is negligible, the presence of stool will certainly make any peritonitis worse.

Tips and Tricks for Polypectomy

There is a large variety of snares available for polypectomy (table 2). Broadly, snares are made of monofilament or braided steel wire. Whereas the depth of cut may be less with the monofilament snare, the rapidity of the cutting effect is somewhat less with braided snares. Thus, monofilament snares may be preferred for polyps located in the cecum, where the wall thickness is less. Braided snares also provide better stability for ensnaring maneuvers. However, there is no set rule for what type of snare to use. We have found that the standard braided snares are useful for performing polypectomy in any part of the colon. Before catching and snaring a polyp it is important to place the polyp in an adequate position.

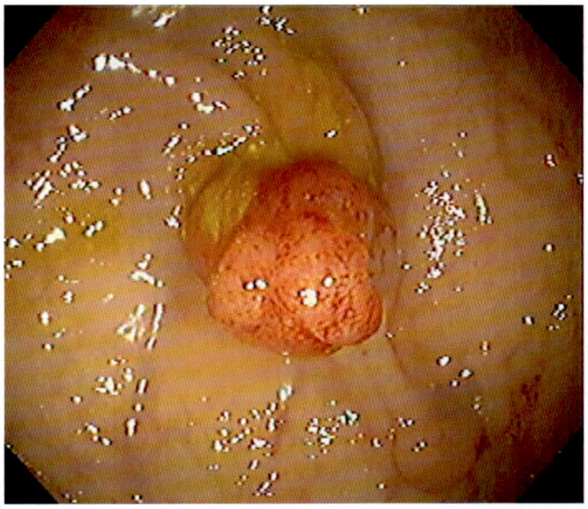

2

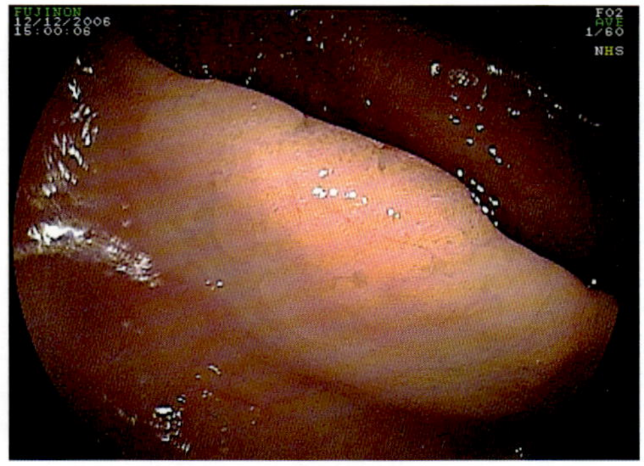

3

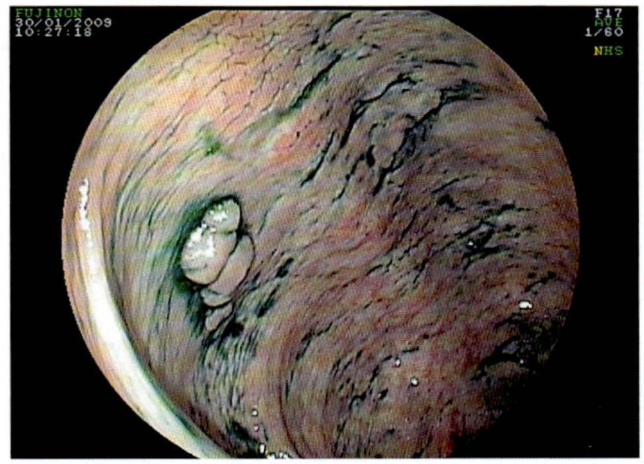

5

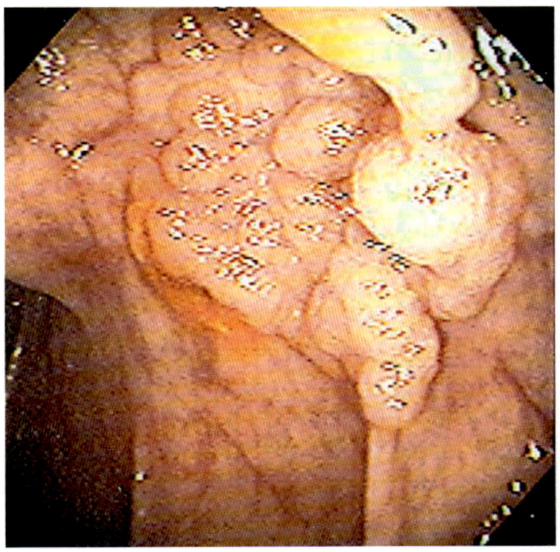

4

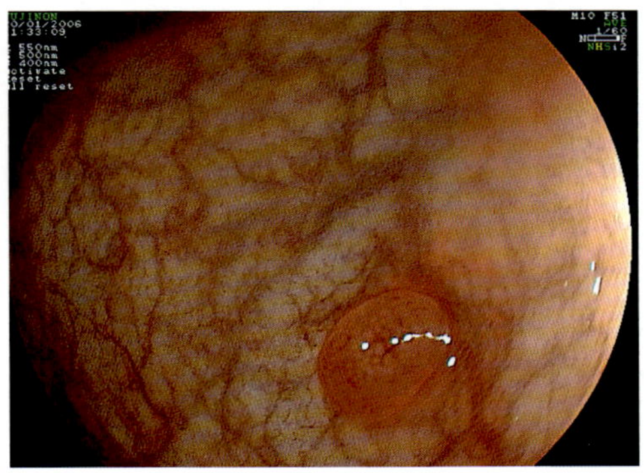

6

Fig. 2. Sessile polyp locate in the transverse colon. **Fig. 3.** Flat polyp located on top of a fold. Due to their shape (flat) and location (top of fold) these flat polyps can be easily overseen. **Fig. 4.** Large carpet-shaped polyp. This type of polyp is also called 'laterally spreading type (LST) lesion'. The Paris-Kyoto classification categorizes this polyp as a flat, mixed type, superficial ('non-elevated'), polypoid lesion (0–Isp). However, the polyp is also a superficial, non-polypoid lesion, slightly elevated (type 0–IIa). Whether using this classification enables the endoscopist to better predict the polyp biology is unclear. For practical purposes, whether the polyp ('lesion') is 'non-polypoid' or 'polypoid' or mixed ('non-polypoid' and 'polypoid') or flat is less important. The main objective of the colonoscopist is to provide a detailed description of the polyp and to determine whether an endoscopic polypectomy is feasible. **Fig. 5.** Chromoendoscopy with indigo carmine. Note that the borders of the polyp are clearly demarcated from the surrounding mucosa. The pit pattern can also be better appreciated. **Fig. 6.** Virtual chromoendoscopy using Fujinon intelligent chromoendoscopy (FICE). The vascular pattern becomes more visible.

Table 2. Snares available for polypectomy

Monofilament, braided and coiled wire snares (diameter: mini <11 mm, standard 15–45 mm) • Mini oval • Standard oval • Hexagonal • Crescent • Spiral • Mini barbed • Needle tip anchored • With heat-resistant net (Nakao net)
Combination: needle/snare
Rotatable snares

Table 3. Technical pearls to deal with various types of colon polyps

	Type of polyp	Technical advice
Shape	Sessile >10–15 mm	Use IAP and EMR
	Flat, on top of folds, carpet-shaped (LST) or villous	Use IAP and EMR
Size	>15 mm	Resect in toto (except cecum)
	Large, >30 mm	Use IAP and perform piecemeal polypectomy Use APC to eliminate remaining tissue
	Big head	Inject diluted epinephrine in head to reduce the volume of the polyp and decrease the chance of bleeding
	Thick pedicle	Use IAP, clips or loops before resecting the polyp. Grasp the pedicle in the middle. Use coagulation current for resection
Number	Multiple polyps	Send to pathologist separately; resect when going in (if small) or when going out (if large). If more than 10 polyps, resect on separate occasions (≥1 colonoscopy)
Location	Right colon and cecum	Do not use hot biopsy Take air out before catching or snaring the polyp
	Behind folds	Inject distally first
	Difficult endoscope position	Change position: 5–6 o'clock position
		Use abdominal compression
		Have assistant hold the endoscope
	Suspicious appearing polyp or large, incompletely resected	Mark the polyp site (e.g. tattoo with india ink)

IAP = Injection-assisted polypectomy or submucosal cushion, EMR = endoscopic mucosal resection. Reproduced with permission from Mönkemüller et al. [1].

Remember that the accessories exit the colonoscope at the 5 or 6 o'clock position, depending on the colonoscope type used [1, 5] (fig. 7, 8). Thus, a polyp should be placed in the lower field of endoscopic view, between the 5 and 6 o'clock position. In addition, it is useful to remove any residuals from the targeted area in order to improve visualization. Taking out the air before introducing the snare into the accessory channel will also decrease tension on the wall and allow better ensnaring of the polyp. Table 3 lists some technical pearls to deal with various types of colon polyps.

Placing the Snare around the Polyp

The feasibility of polypectomy depends mainly on the following aspects: morphology of the polyp, size and location. Practically all pedunculated polyps can be resected endoscopically, whereas large, sessile polyps located in the cecum should be resected surgically.

Once the polyp is 'en face', the polyp should be placed at the 5–6 o'clock position. Then the closed snare should be advanced out of the accessory channel, passed the polyp. The snare is then opened by the assistant and the endoscopist pulls it back and places the extended snare over the polyp (fig. 9). While the assistant closes the snare it is important for the endoscopist to advance the snare into the lumen, perfectly grasping the polyp base, below the polyp head (fig. 10). When the polyp is stalked, then the snare should be placed around the middle of the pedicle. For sessile polyps it is important to include a small amount of normal-appearing mucosa at the polyp base, in order to allow adequate resection margin (fig. 11). For sessile polyps of >15 mm we always recommend using injection-assisted polypectomy ('submucosal cushion') as this will enable resection of more neoplastic tissue in toto and potentially decrease the chances of perforation [see Injection-assisted polypectomy, p 263]. Before applying electrosurgical current, it is important to pull the polyp towards the center of the lumen (i.e. 'tent' the polyp; fig. 7, 8). Avoid touching the mucosa in order to avoid transmission of electrosurgical energy through the mucosal wall which can result in perforation. Remember that polypectomy is a curative procedure when neoplasia is limited to the mucosa and this is entirely resected during polypectomy. If the polyp cannot be placed at the 5 o'clock position, then the 'reverse' snare position (hypomochlion or fulcrum technique) can be used: the snare is advanced and opened while the tip is 'anchored' at the mucosa in front of the polyp; then the endoscopist pushes the snare out, which turns on itself while remaining anchored, and the opened snare falls on top of the polyp. While closing the snare it is important to simultaneously advance the snare further out of the scope it in order to fully grasp the polyp base.

Polyp Shape and Size

There are no set rules for limiting endoscopic polypectomy [see also chapters by Pachlewski and Regula, p 269, and Yamamoto, p 287]. However, polyps that extend more than half of the luminal circumference (1/3) in the cecum, or extend in between and beyond two folds should not be removed endoscopically [1, 5]. Nevertheless, some polyps may appear very large, but once intercepted the endoscopist may decide to resect them endoscopically (fig. 12, 13). Also, large ulcerated polyps located in any part of the colon or large villous polyps located in the cecum should be removed surgically. In general, polyps larger than 15 mm should be resected using the piecemeal technique, unless they are pedunculated or located in the distal colon where the wall is thicker. If the pedicle of the polyp is thick or very long it is useful to inject it beforehand with a

7 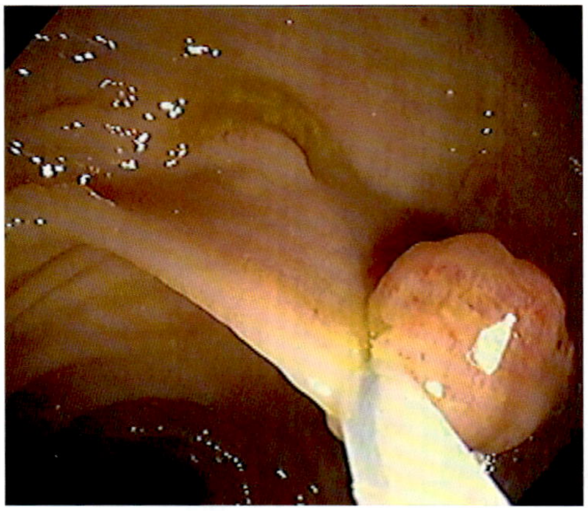 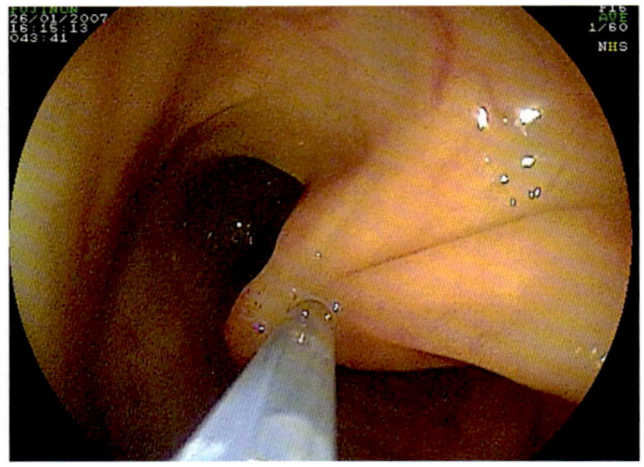 8

9 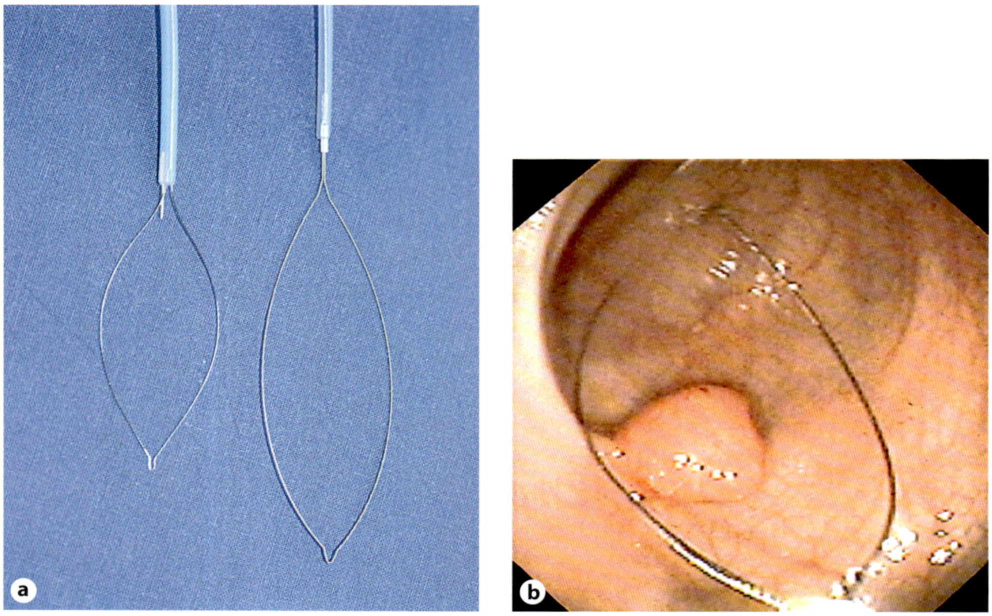

Fig. 7. In colonoscopes the accessories exit the working channel at 5 o'clock. **Fig. 8.** For polyps in difficult positions it may be useful to use a gastroscope to resect them because the snare exits the working channel at the 7 o'clock position. **Fig. 9.** **a** Polypectomy snares. **b**. Open the snare on top of the polyp.

saline-epinephrine mixture or apply clips or endoloops in order to decrease the chances of bleeding. However, there are no large studies demonstrating any benefit of 'prophylactic' clipping or endolooping. Many endoscopists remove the polyp first and then inspect the site and determine whether there is need to provide any type of active or prophylactic hemostatic therapy. In our experience, it is always better to provide prophylaxis if the polyp is located in a difficult position, because after resection it may be difficult to adequately place clips or inject the polyp base.

If multiple polyps are present these can be collected as they are resected using a Roth's net (fig. 14). While retrieving the colonoscope it is still possible to inspect the mucosa and find additional polyps (fig. 15). However, when collecting many polyps, the location of each polyp cannot be transmitted to the pathologist. Even small polyps can harbor an invasive carcinoma [17]. Some endoscopists send all the polyps separately, whereas others categorize them into polyps from the right colon and polyps from the left colon, anticipating that the surgeon can perform a right or left hemicolectomy. It is our recommendation to send polyps separately, labeling their exact location.

Be Careful with Polyps Located in the Cecum

The most dangerous site to remove polyps is the cecum, mainly because of the thinness of its wall, especially if the colon is insufflated with air. Therefore, always pay special attention when resecting these polyps. Avoid the hot biopsy technique in the cecum, as transmural burns can occur more easily.

Hot versus Cold Biopsy

Biopsy 'removal' should be employed for polyps of <5 mm (this is the common diameter of an extended forceps) [18]. Larger polyps should be either cold-snared or snared with electrocautery [19, 20]. The hot biopsy technique offers the potential advantage of tissue 'cauterization' and polyp elimination [21]. However, even after adequate hot biopsy there is residual neoplastic tissue left in situ in at least 15% of cases [18]. In addition, we have shown that the interpretation of polyps resected using hot-biopsy techniques is severely hampered by the presence of cauterized tissue [18].

Electrosurgical Currents

Polyps can be snared using various types of electrosurgical current: coagulation, blended and cut [22]. Interestingly, the use of electrosurgical currents for colon polypectomy is not standardized. A recent survey of US endoscopists revealed that there is no preferred electrosurgical current for polypectomy, pure coagulation being used by 46% of the endoscopists, 46% use blend and 3% use pure cut [23]. Regardless of electrosurgical current used it is always imperative to inspect the surrounding polyp area to make sure that no normal tissue has been accidentally caught. Also, make sure that the tip of the snare is not toughing the contralateral wall, as perforation can occur during application of the electrosurgical currents.

Hypothetically, pure cutting currents produce less tissue damage than coagulation currents [22]. However, immediate bleeding is more when using cutting currents [24]. On the other hand, the rate of transmural burn and perforation appears to be more frequent with coagulation current [24, 25]. The currents employed for polypectomy may also influence the histologic ability to evaluate the polyps. In one study the tissue margin was less evaluable when using a blended current with Valleylab® generators than when using computerized blended current with Erbe® generators [26]. Remember, that the pathologist will only be able to determine the adequacy of polyp resection if the entire margin can be adequately assessed. Thus, histopathologic examination will be the primary determinant of whether the polypectomy was therapeutic or not.

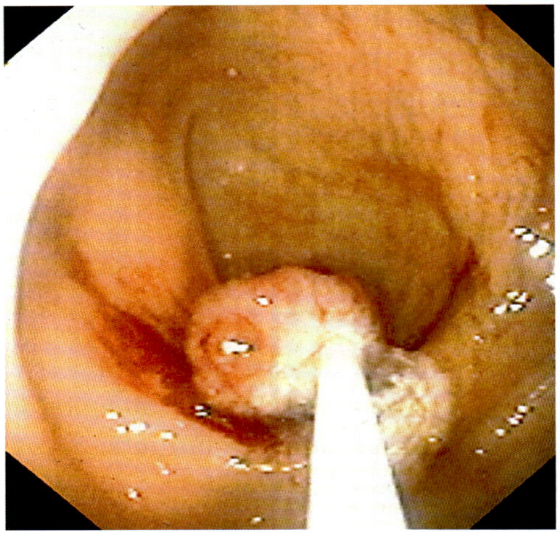

10

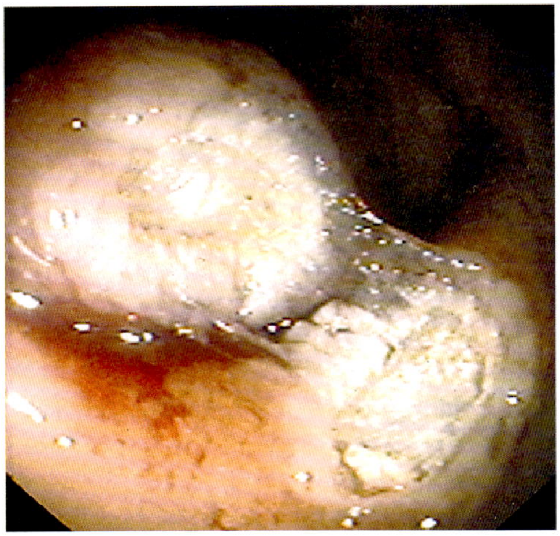

11

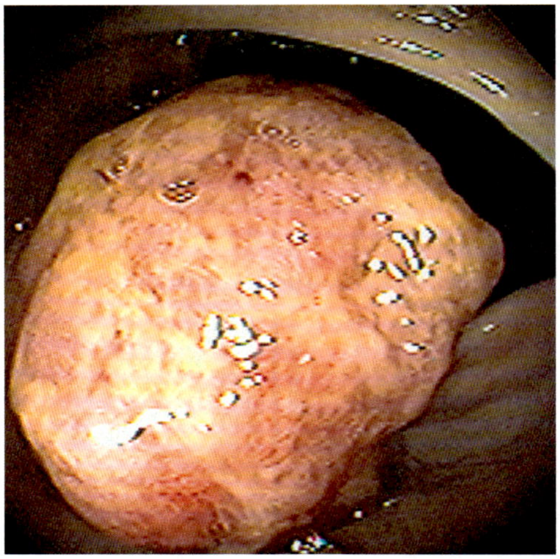

12

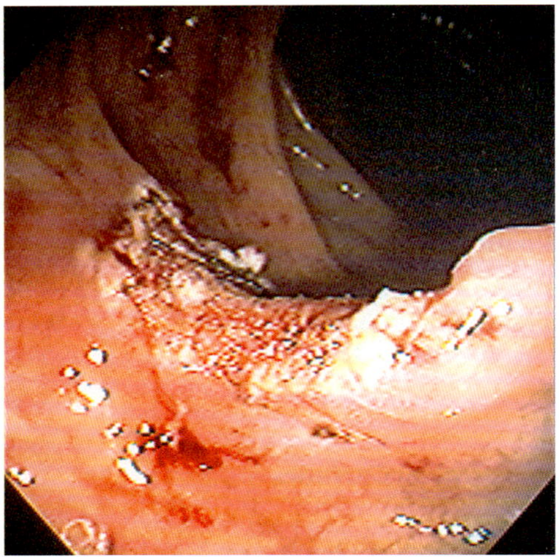

13

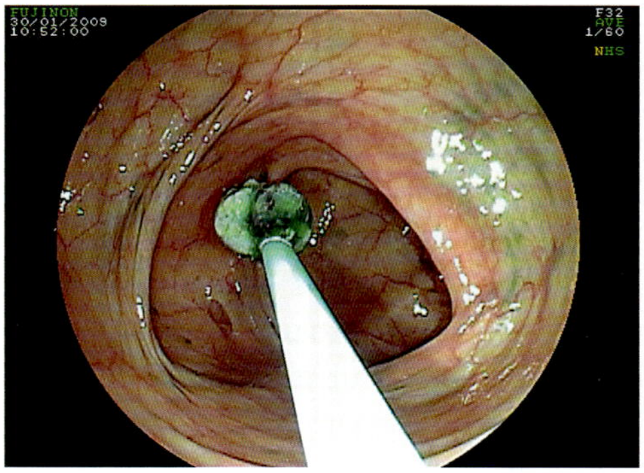

14

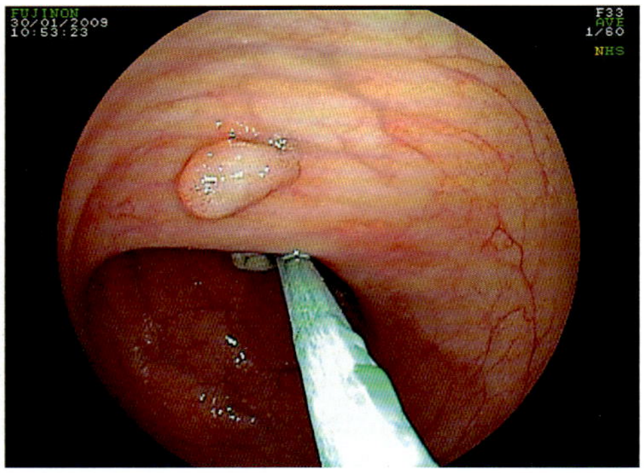

15

Fig. 10. Grasp the polyp at the base of its head, trying to ensnare some normal tissue. **Fig. 11.** Post-polypectomy site of polyp shown in figures 9 and 10. **Fig. 12.** Large polyp, partially occluding the lumen. **Fig. 13.** Careful inspection revealed that the polyp base was not too large and a decision to resect the polyp after the creation of a submucosal cushion was taken. After removal of 80% of the polyp a nice mucosectomy of the remaining tissue 'stump' was performed. The rim was then treated with argon plasma coagulation to remove any potential residual neoplastic tissue. **Fig. 14.** The polyp resected in the ascending colon has been grabbed with a Roth's® net. **Fig. 15.** While keeping the polyp held inside the Roth's® net, careful inspection of the remaining colon mucosa was performed and a new polyp was found in the sigmoid colon.

Measures to Prevent Complications (Bleeding and Perforation)

Tables 3 and 4 list useful measures to prevent complications during colonoscopy.

Use Submucosal Cushion (Injection-Assisted Polypectomy)

The use of injection-assisted polypectomy (IAP) is advocated for polyps of >10–15 mm, flat lesions, carpet-shaped polyps, and polyps located in the right colon [27] (fig. 3, 4, 12). There are multiple substances available on the market to perform IAP. These include saline, saline-diluted epinephrine mix, saline and dextrose 50% mix (50/50), Normal saline and methylene blue mixture, sodium hyaluronidase, fibrinogen and hydroxypropylmethyl cellulose [27, 28]. In our experience saline is best used in the cecum, whereas a mixture of saline and epinephrine (1:10,000) is best suited for all other colon parts, especially the rectum with its rich vascular supply. Newer data demonstrate that saline and dextrose 50% provide a longer-lasting cushion than saline or saline/epinephrine [28] (fig. 16–19). Due to its vasoconstrictive capabilities diluted epinephrine is not only used to create submucosal cushions, but has also been described as in intrapolyp injection method aimed at decreasing the size of the polyp head and, due to its vasoconstrictive effects, also decreases the chances of bleeding [29]. By 'shrinking' the polyp head a piecemeal resection is thus facilitated.

The creation a submucosal cushion should follow a standardized approach:

(a) Always inject in the proximal part of the polyp base (i.e. behind polyp) in order to let the polyp bulge towards the endoscopist.

(b) The tip of the needle should just barely penetrate the mucosa.

(c) Penetrate the submucosa at an angle of <30°, if possible almost tangential. This will allow a larger below-the-polyp diffusion of the injected agent. Injections close to the 90° angle will not raise the polyp and the endoscopist runs the risk of penetrating with the entire needle through the entire colon wall, thus injecting freely into the peritoneum.

(d) Pay attention not to inject too much material, as occasionally the polyp may lift too much and becomes very difficult to entrap with the snare. In some instances a polyp will not rise despite adequate and sufficient submucosal injection ('non-lifting sign'). This is a warning sign and is often due to the presence of invasive cancer which has rooted itself into or through the submucosa [1, 5].

In order to minimize the risk of bleeding additional measures can be taken for polyps with a thick stalk. An important precondition for a successful and safe polypectomy or mucosal resection is elevation of the polyp so that it stands out clearly from the muscularis propria (lifting sign) using the electrosurgical snare. The snare should be placed around the lesion parallel to the intestinal wall, pressing lightly against the wall; the snare should then be closed slowly and lifted up parallel to the intestinal wall. It is important to avoid one-sided tissue contact of the snare tip to the intestinal wall. Additional options to minimize the risk of bleeding include prophylactic injection of diluted epinephrine, or placement of an endoloop or hemoclip on the polyp stalk. Regarding the injection, a small amount of diluted epinephrine can be injected into the polyp base (stalk) and/or polyp base and polyp itself and wait for about a minute or two. This will not only produce vasoconstriction and create cushion at the base of the polyp but will in most cases shrink the polyp to a size which should enable easier snaring.

Table 4. Tips to prevent complications during colonoscopy and polypectomy

1	Carefully inspect the lumen while advancing the colonocope
2	Be aware and respectful of diverticula
3	Do not push the scope forcefully
4	Know your accessories
5	Know your electrosurgery unit. It is your responsibility (and not that of the staff) to ensure that the equipment works well
6	Before attempting polypectomy it is important to know exactly where the pedal of the electrosurgical unit is located. The worst situation is to start looking for the pedal while the polyp is already snared. In analogy, you do not look for the gas pedal while driving! When performing polypectomy it is important to keep the eyes on the video monitor
8	The opening of the snare should occur under direct vision (i.e. not blindly behind a curve or fold)
9	It is better to use the submucosal cushion than having doubts about too deep a resection (avoid ensnaring the deeper muscle layers). Excessive transmission of thermal energy through the bowel wall can result in perforation
10	Use the tenting technique to pull the polyp away from its base
11	Coordinate the polypectomy with the assistant
12	Hemoclips, epinephrine and thermocoagulation devices should always be readily available
13	Avoid heroic resection of large or difficult lesions. Remember that laparoscopic resection is always an option for large polyps located in weird locations.
14	When in doubt, get a second opinion or refer the patient to a more experienced colonoscopist. The patient will always prefer to undergo a second colon preparation than having emergency surgery for perforation

Management of Complications

The two most frequent complications of advanced colon polypectomy are bleeding and perforation [30, 31]. The incidence of bleeding after polypectomy varies from 0.85 to 24% [24, 25, 30–32]. Post-polypectomy bleeding can occur immediately or be delayed. Immediate bleeding is more common when using pure-cut currents and delayed bleeding occurs more frequently when using coagulation currents [1, 5]. The incidence of bleeding also varies based on the resection technique used. The bleeding rate after mucosectomy or piecemeal resection has been reported to be as high as 24% [33–37]. The risk of bleeding also correlates with the type and size of polyp, occurring more frequent in sessile polyps of >10 mm or polyps with a thick stalk [1, 5].

If bleeding occurs, the first measure should be to attempt to re-snare the stalk and hold the snare firmly closed for at least a minute trying to facilitate the natural coagulation while you decide what to do next (injection, hemoclip or argon plasma coagulation). Generally, if the patient has intact hemostatic mechanisms, the bleeding will partially stop, and you will have enough time to obtain definite hemostasis in calmer manner. The most well-known hemostatic method is the induction of tamponade and arterial spasm by injection of diluted epinephrine. Contact thermal methods such as a heater probe or non-contact tools such as argon plasma coagulation should only be used if the mucosectomy is not deep, as its application can lead to a transmural burn. Currently, the most practical method to stop bleeding is the use of hemoclips (fig. 20). Various types of clips are currently available. Clipping devices are single-use or reusable. We prefer to use the reusable devices. In cases of bleeding frequently only one clip is sufficient to achieve hemostasis, whereas for perforation multiple clips are required to close the mucosal defect. When resecting polyps with a large or thick stalk or performing mucosectomy, some experts prefer to use the clip prophylactically, either before or after polypectomy, whereas

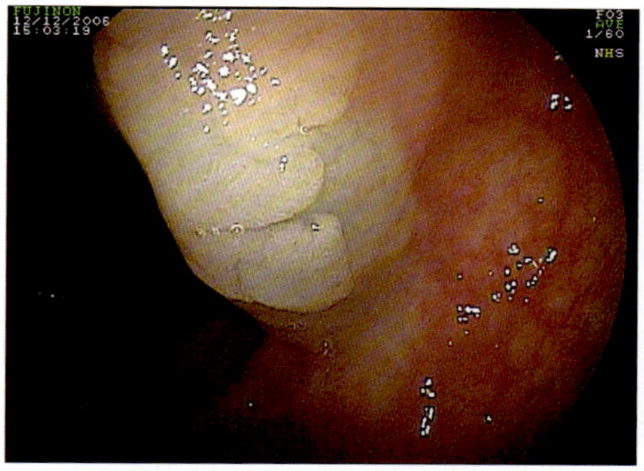

16

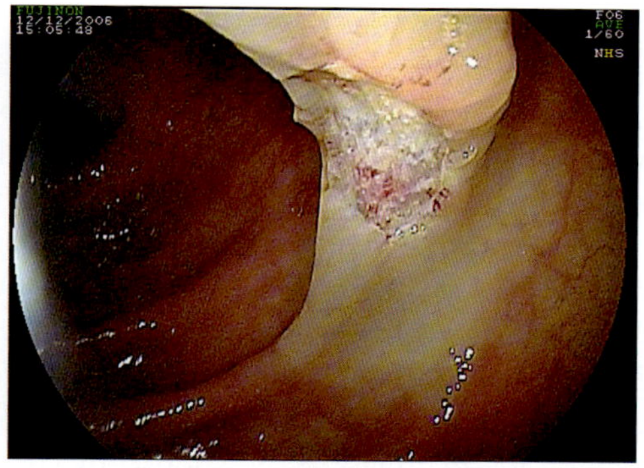

17

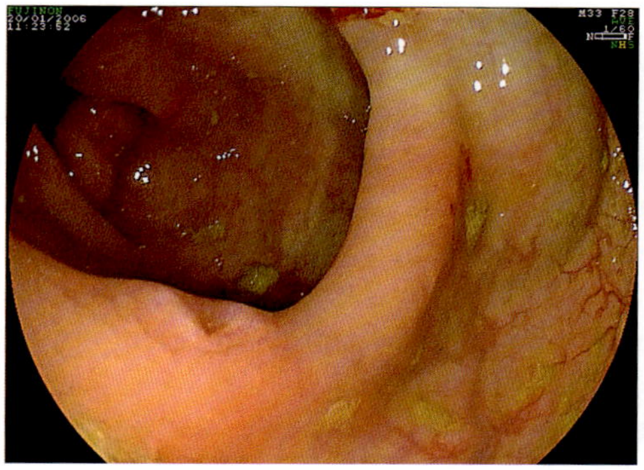

18

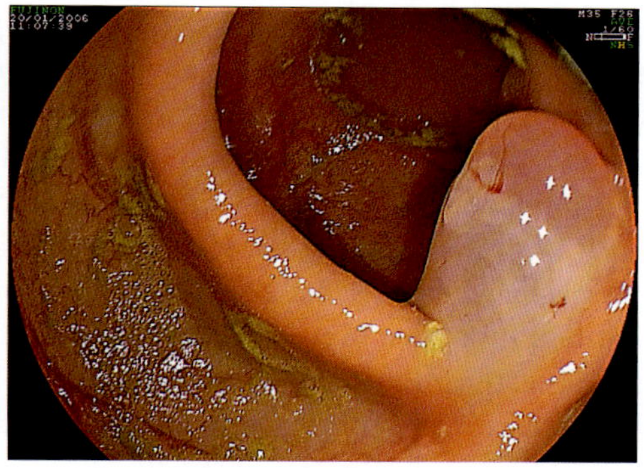

19

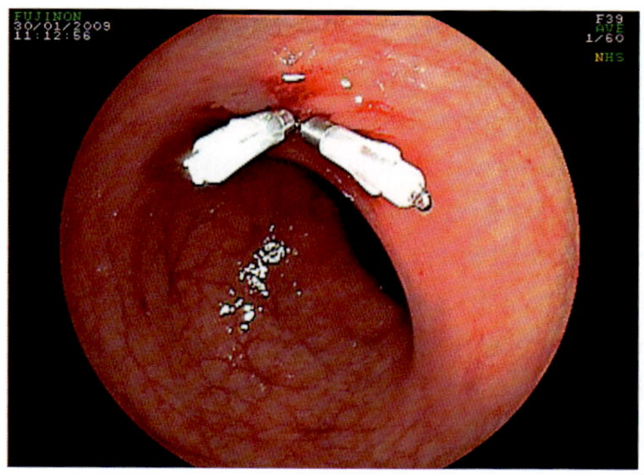

20

Fig. 16. Note the adequate submucosal rise of the flat polyp located on top of a mucosal fold (fig. 3). The mucosa below the polyp has a white discoloration due to the vasoconstrictive effect of epinephrine.

Fig. 17. Post-polypectomy (mucosectomy) site. Histologically this was an adenoma with high-grade dysplasia. The lesion was resected in toto.

Fig. 18. Small flat polyp with depressed center located on top of a fold. Polyps with indentation are highly suspicious for containing advanced neoplasia or invasive carcinoma.

Fig. 19. Injection of saline-epinephrine mixture resulted in an adequate rise of this polyp, therefore decreasing the possibilities of having invasive components. This polyp was resected in toto using a snare.

Fig. 20. Two clips were placed at the bleeding base of a resected polyp. Adequate hemostasis was achieved.

other experts place clips only if there is evidence of bleeding. When using clips to achieve hemostasis, careful attention should be placed on grasping the bleeding stump of the vessel.

The second most common complication is perforation [24, 25, 30–32]. Perforation may result from mechanical forces against the bowel wall, barotrauma or as a direct result of therapeutic interventions. Colon perforation after polypectomy occurs more commonly in the right colon, but it can occur following any type of endoscopic resection, occurring in up to 14% after endoscopic submucosal dissection [34–37]. Perforation can be small (partially covered with serosa), frank and large. Although surgery has been the standard practice to manage perforations, application of clips and loops have emerged as useful options to close lesions of <10–15 mm in size. If a perforation is suspected, immediate administration of intravenous broad-spectrum antibiotics should be instituted in the endoscopy suite. The most common pathogenic bacteria of the colon are Enterobacteriacea and *Bacteroides* spp., *Pseudomonas aeruginosa* and enterococci may also be present. Thus, antibiotics covering these organisms should be used, such as piperacillin-tazobactam, ampicilllin-sulbactam or quinolones plus metronidazole. If endoscopic closure of the defect is attempted, careful attention should be paid to avoid air insufflation into the colon because the air will penetrate through the colonic defect into the peritoneal cavity and remain trapped based on the non-escape valve mechanism. Experts can accomplish successful endoscopic closure of a perforation in about 50% of cases [32–34]. Thus, the surgeon should always be notified immediately about the perforation and, if possible, discuss the treatment options at bedside (i.e. the endoscopy table).

When closing the perforation hemoclips should be placed at the ends of the tear and then proceed to close the central part with subsequent clips. If the perforation is detected after the patient has left the endoscopy suite, an operative intervention is always mandatory, with the exception of transmural burns or post-polypectomy syndrome, where the perforation can be managed conservatively.

The transmural burn syndrome (also called 'post-polypectomy coagulation syndrome') usually occurs when thermal energy administered during snare electrocoagulation extends into the muscularis propria and serosa without leading to a free perforation [1, 5]. Its incidence ranges from 0.5 to 2% of polypectomies [1, 5]. This complication usually presents 2 days after colonoscopy, ranging from 4 hours to 7 days. Treatment of transmural burn syndrome implies bowel rest and the administration of intravenous fluids and broad spectrum antibiotics.

Conclusions

Colonoscopic polypectomy is the standard approach for the prevention of CRC. Polyps are classified based in endoscopic and histologic appearance. Various endoscopic polyp resection techniques exist. The most common method to remove polyps is with the electrosurgical snare. Adequate endoscopic training is of utmost importance for acquiring the necessary knowledge and skills to resect colon polyps. Minor and major complications occur in about 10% of advanced polypectomies. Every effort should be given to focus on prevention of these complications.

References

1 Mönkemüller K, Neumann H, Malfertheiner P, Fry LC: Advanced colon polypectomy. Clin Gastroenterol Hepatol 2009;7:641–652.

2 Maratka Z: Terminology, Definitions and Diagnostic Criteria in Digestive Endoscopy, ed 3. Bad Homburg, Normed Verlag, 1994, vol 1, pp 14–19.

3 Bond JH: Colon polyps and cancer. Endoscopy 2001; 33:46–54.

4 Paris Workshop Participants: The Paris endoscopic classification of superficial neoplastic lesions: esophagus, stomach and colon. Gastrointest Endosc 2002;58:3–43.

5 Mönkemüller K, Neumann H, Fry LC, Ivekovic H, Malfertheiner P: Polypectomy techniques for difficult colon polyps. Dig Dis 2008;26:342–346.

6 Kudo S, Lambert R, Allen JI, et al: Non-polypoid neoplastic lesions of the colorectal mucosa. Gastrointest Endosc 2008;68:3–47.

7 Levin B, Lieberman DA, McFarland B, et al: Screening and surveillance for the early detection of colorectal cancer and adenomatous polyps, 2008: a joint guideline from the American Cancer Society, the US Multi-Society Task Force on Colorectal Cancer, and the American College of Radiology. CA Cancer J Clin 2008;58:130–160.

8 Fu KI, Sano Y, Kato S, et al: Chromoendoscopy using indigo carmine dye spraying with magnifying observation is the most reliable method for differential diagnosis between non-neoplastic and neoplastic colorectal lesions: a prospective study. Endoscopy 2004;36:1089–1093.

9 Lapalus MG, Helbert T, Napoleon B, et al: Does chromoendoscopy with structure enhancement improve the colonoscopic adenoma detection rate? Endoscopy 2006;38:444–448.

10 Bianco MA, Rotondano G, Marmo R, et al: Predictive value of magnification chromoendoscopy for diagnosing invasive neoplasia in nonpolypoid colorectal lesions and stratifying patients for endoscopic resection or surgery. Endoscopy 2006; 38:470–476.

11 Hurlstone DP, Cross SS, Drew K, et al: An evaluation of colorectal endoscopic mucosal resection using high-magnification chromoscopic colonoscopy: a prospective study of 1000 colonoscopies. Endoscopy 2004;36:491–498.

12 Pohl J, May A, Rabenstein T, et al: Computed virtual chromoendoscopy: a new tool for enhancing tissue surface structures. Endoscopy 2007;39:80–83.

13 Tischendorf JJ, Wasmuth HE, Koch A, et al: Value of magnifying chromoendoscopy and narrow band imaging (NBI) in classifying colorectal polyps: a prospective controlled study. Endoscopy 2007;39: 1092–1096.

14 Rex DK, Cutler CS, Lemmel GT, Rahmani EY, Clark DW, Helper DJ, Lehman GA, Mark DG: Colonoscopic miss rates of adenomas determined by back-to-back colonoscopies. Gastroenterology 1997;112:24–28.

15 Zuckerman MJ, Hirota WK, Adler DG, et al: ASGE guideline: the management of low-molecular-weight heparin and nonaspirin antiplatelet agents for endoscopic procedures. Gastrointest Endosc 2005;61: 189–194.

16 Veitch AM, Baglin TP, Gershlick AH, Harnden SM, Tighe R, Cairns S; British Society of Gastroenterology; British Committee for Standards in Haematology; British Cardiovascular Intervention Society: Guidelines for the management of anticoagulant and antiplatelet therapy in patients undergoing endoscopic procedures. Gut 2008; 57:1322–1329.

17 Stolte M, Bethge B: Colorectal mini/de novo carcinoma: a reality in Germany too. Endoscopy 1995;27: 286–290.

18 Mönkemüller KE, Fry LC, Jones BH, et al: Histological quality of polyps resected using the cold versus hot biopsy technique. Endoscopy 2004; 36:432–436.

19 Deenadayalu VP, Rex DK: Colon polyp retrieval after cold snaring. Gastrointest Endosc 2005;62:253–256.

20 Carpenter S, Petersen BT, Chuttani R, et al: Polypectomy devices. Gastrointest Endosc 2007;65: 741–749.

21 Vanagunas A, Jacob P, Vakil N: Adequacy of 'hot biopsy' for the treatment of diminutive polyps: a prospective randomized trial. Am J Gastroenterol 1989;84:383–385.

22 Slivka A, Bosco JJ, Barkun AN, et al: Electrosurgical generators. Gastrointest Endosc 2003;58:656–660.

23 Singh N, Harrison M, Rex DK: A survey of colonoscopic polypectomy practices among clinical gastroenterologists. Gastrointest Endosc 2004;60:414–418.

24 Van Gossum A, Cozzoli A, Adler M, Taton G, Cremer M: Colonoscopic snare polypectomy: analysis of 1485 resections comparing two types of current. Gastrointest Endosc 1992;38:472–475.

25 Parra-Blanco A, Kaminaga N, Kojima T, Endo Y, Tajiri A, Fujita R: Colonoscopic polypectomy with cutting current: is it safe? Gastrointest Endosc 2000; 51:676–681.

26 Fry LC, Lazenby AJ, Mikolaenko I, Lazenby A, Rickes S, Mönkemüller K: Diagnostic quality of polyps resected by snare polypectomy: does the type of electrosurgical current used matter? Am J Gastroenterol 2006;101:2123–2127.

27 Dobrowolski S, Dobosz M, Babicki A, et al: Prophylactic submucosal saline-adrenaline injection in colonoscopic polypectomy: prospective randomized study. Surg Endosc 2004;18:990–993.

28 Varadarajulu S, Tamhane A, Slaughter RL: Evaluation of dextrose 50% as a medium for injection-assisted polypectomy. Endoscopy 2006;38:907–912.

29 Hogan RB, Hogan RB 3rd: Epinephrine volume reduction of giant colon polyps facilitates endoscopic assessment and removal. Gastrointest Endosc 2007;66: 1018–1022.

30 Webb WA, McDaniel L, Jones L: Experience with 1000 colonoscopic polypectomies. Ann Surg 1985;5: 626–632.

31 Heldwein W, Dollhopf M, Rösch T, et al: The Munich Polypectomy Study (MUPS): prospective analysis of complications and risk factors in 4000 colonic snare polypectomies. Endoscopy 2005;37: 1116–1122.
32 Sawhney MS, Salfiti N, Nelson DB, et al: Risk factors for severe delayed postpolypectomy bleeding. Endoscopy 2008;40:115–119.
33 Ahmad NA, Kochman ML, Long WB, et al: Efficacy, safety, and clinical outcomes of endoscopic mucosal resection: a study of 101 cases. Gastrointest Endosc 2002;55:390–396.
34 Yamamoto H, Yahagi N, Oyama T: Mucosectomy in the colon with endoscopic submucosal dissection. Endoscopy 2005;37:764–768.
35 Fujishiro M, Yahagi N, Nakamura M, et al: Endoscopic submucosal dissection for rectal epithelial neoplasia. Endoscopy 2006;38:493–497.
36 Onozato Y, Kakizaki S, Ishihara H, et al: Endoscopic submucosal dissection for rectal tumors. Endoscopy 2007;39:423–427.
37 Rösch T, Sarbia M, Schumacher B, et al: Attempted endoscopic en bloc resection of mucosal and submucosal tumors using insulated-tip knives: a pilot series. Endoscopy 2004;36:788–801.

Klaus Mönkemüller, MD, PhD, FASGE
Department of Gastroenterology, Hepatology and Infectious Diseases, Otto-von-Guericke University
Josef-Albers-Strasse 70
DE–46236 Bottrop (Germany)
Tel. +49 2041 106 1000, Fax +49 2041 106 1009, E-Mail klaus.moenkemueller@mhb-bottrop.de

Mönkemüller K, Wilcox CM, Muñoz-Navas M (eds): Interventional and Therapeutic Gastrointestinal Endoscopy.
Front Gastrointest Res. Basel, Karger, 2010, vol 27, pp 269–286

Endoscopic Mucosal Resection for Colorectal Polyps

Jacek Pachlewski · Jaroslaw Regula

Department of Gastroenterology and Hepatology, Medical Center for Postgraduate Education and the Maria Sklodowska-Curie Memorial Cancer Center and Institute of Oncology, Warsaw, Poland

Abstract

Endoscopic mucosal resection (EMR) is the method of choice for removal of lesions that are histologically adenomas or early cancers that infiltrate a maximum of one-third of the submucosal layer as well as for removal of large, flat lesions called laterally spreading tumors. Efficiency, positive final outcomes and safety depend mainly on patient selection, experience and skills of endoscopic team in applying technical approaches. The most popular approaches are injection-assisted EMR and EMR without injection. The decision of whether to remove large flat lesions may use simple measures, e.g. careful assessment in white light with chromoendoscopy and assessment of lifting after injection. Endoscopic and histopathologic assessment of completeness of adenoma removal is crucial and requires perfect job at each step of EMR procedure.

Endoscopic mucosal resection (EMR or mucosectomy), described for the first time by Deyhle et al. [1] in 1973 for adenomas and Karita et al. [2] in 1991 for early colorectal cancers, allows for non-surgical removal of sessile and flat neoplastic lesions in the large bowel. This terminology, however, is not precise and does not reflect reality, as this method allows for removal not only of mucosa, but also of submucosa down to the level of muscularis propria.

Endoscopic removal of pedunculated polyps, even large polyps, is usually technically simple, safe and complete. In contrast, safe and complete removal of non-pedunculated and flat polyps, even small ones and particularly those in the right colon, is difficult. These lesions require experience of the endoscopist and additional accessories. Difficulty of removal depends on the size, configuration and localization of the lesion. An extremely careful assessment of polyp borders and surface, even without special visualization techniques, as well as mobility in relation to the bowel wall, sometimes with a trial injection under the lesion, allows for proper assessment of possibility for endoscopic removal.

EMR is the method of choice for removal of lesions that are histologically adenomas or early cancers that infiltrate a maximum of one-third of the submucosal layer (sm1), usually morphologically 0-Is or 0-II in the Paris classification [3]. Also amenable to removal are large, flat lesions (previously called 'carpet-like') that are currently known as laterally spreading tumors (LSTs). According to classical definition, flat adenomas (0-II lesions) are not larger than 10 mm, with a

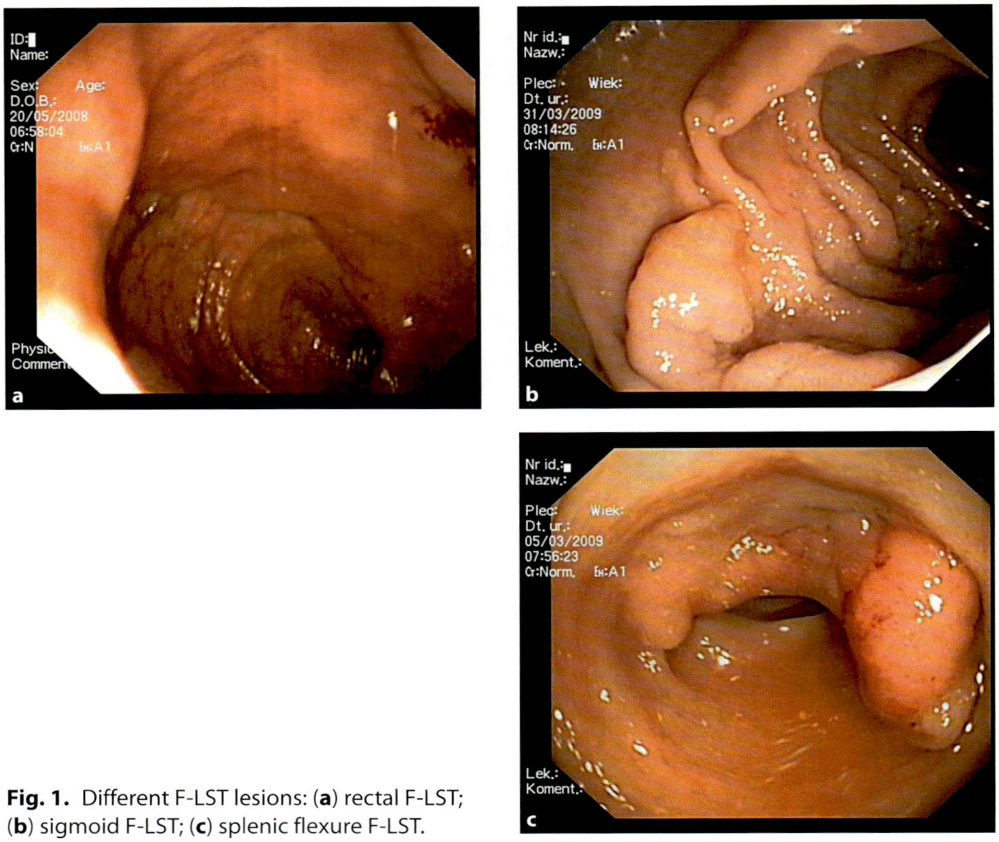

Fig. 1. Different F-LST lesions: (**a**) rectal F-LST; (**b**) sigmoid F-LST; (**c**) splenic flexure F-LST.

height less than double the thickness of the surrounding normal mucosa, as assessed by the histopathologist [4]. According to the Paris classification, flat lesions are defined as lesions with a height less than the diameter of closed biopsy forceps (approx. 2.5 mm) [3]. Another simple definition describes flat lesions as exhibiting a width that is at least two times larger than the height.

LSTs are usually extensive, flat and cover the large part of the circumference of the bowel wall at a distance of several centimeters. These lesions can be either uniformly flat without irregularities on the surface *(*F-LST*)* or have visible granules on the surface (G-LST) [5, 6]. The former pose a higher risk of high-grade dysplasia or cancer, while the risk for the latter is lower [7]. These lesions can also have protrusions surrounded by flat areas. LST examples are presented in figures 1 and 2.

Technique

Correct grasping of the lesion by the endoscopic snare is the critical maneuver of the EMR procedure that determines its safety and effectiveness. The types of EMR differ mostly according to the various methods of preparing the lesion for grasping. The most popular approaches are injection-assisted mucosectomy and mucosectomy without injection. Other techniques

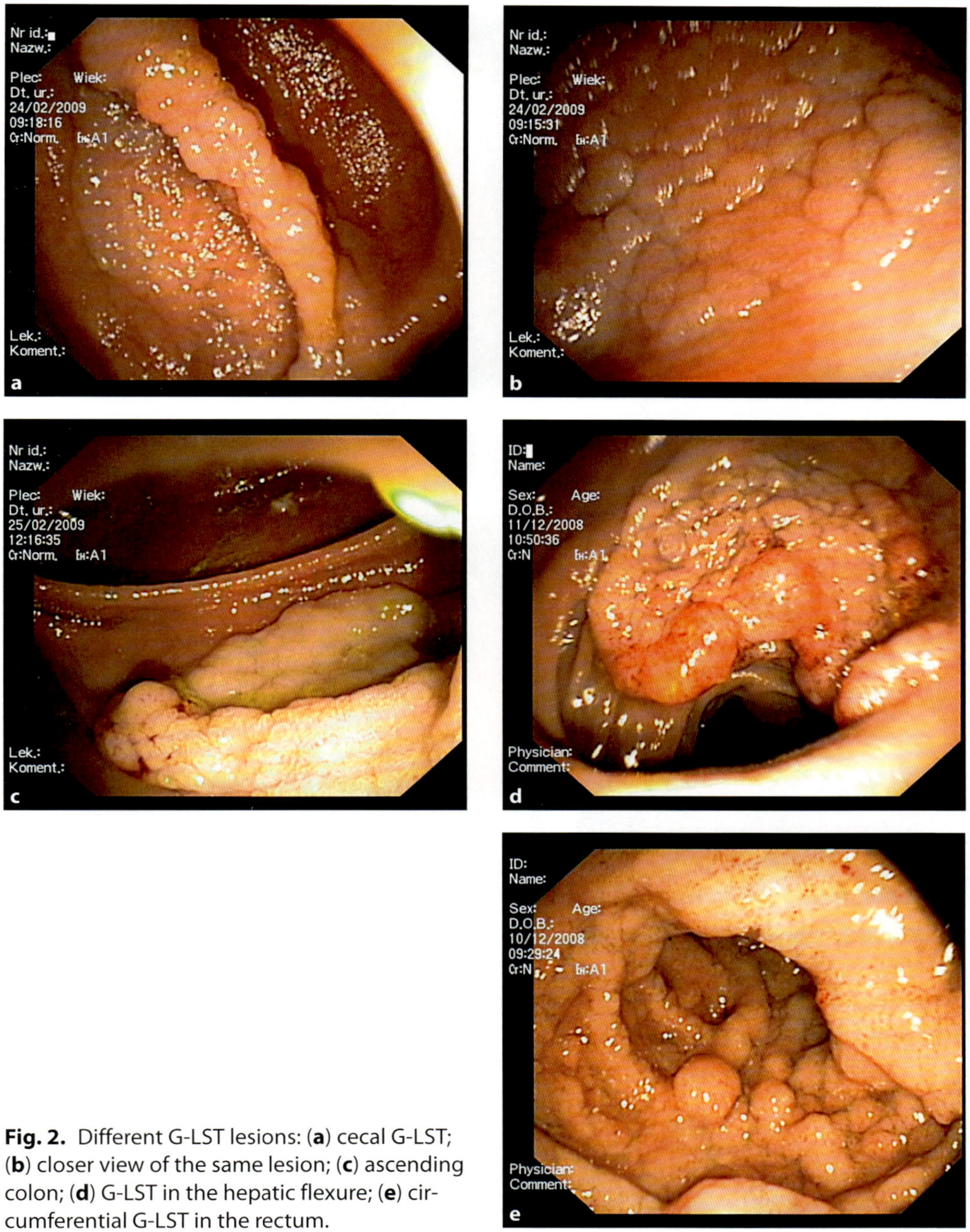

Fig. 2. Different G-LST lesions: (**a**) cecal G-LST; (**b**) closer view of the same lesion; (**c**) ascending colon; (**d**) G-LST in the hepatic flexure; (**e**) circumferential G-LST in the rectum.

require additional accessories, including a transparent cap attached to the tip of the endoscope (EMR-cap) or a ligation device (EMR-ligation). Some experts prefer using colonoscopes with an additional channel to assist mucosectomy using lifting forceps [8]. No studies have formally compared the different types of EMR; therefore experience and preference of the endoscopist, as well as the accessories available, influence the choice of method.

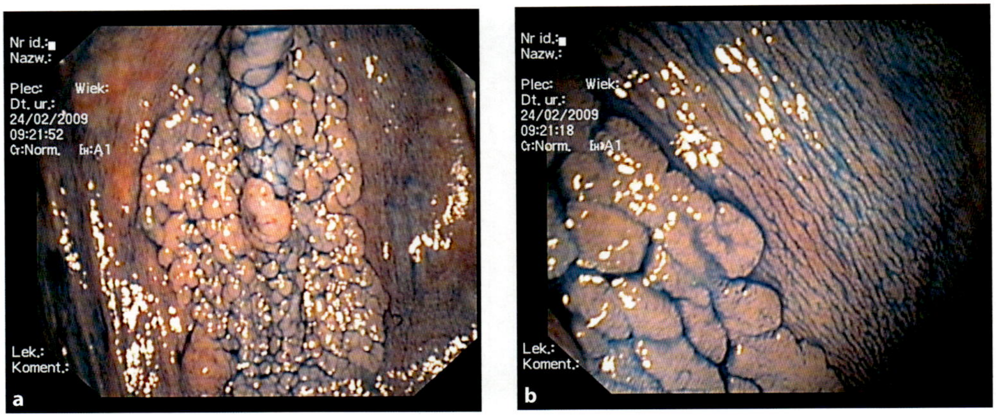

Fig. 3. Chromoendoscopy: (**a**) G-LST indigocarmine staining; (**b**) closer view of the same lesion.

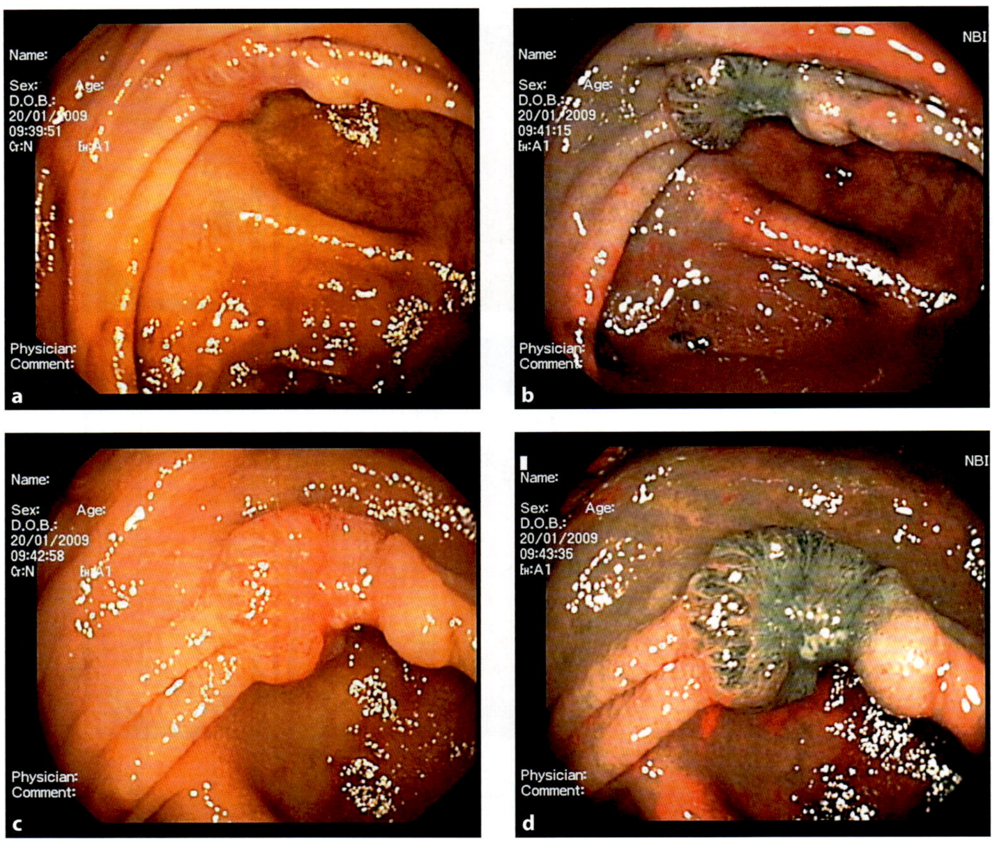

Fig. 4. NBI for visualization of surface and borders: (**a**) cecal 0-IIa+c lesion; (**b**) corresponding NBI picture; (**c**) closer look; (**d**) corresponding NBI picture.

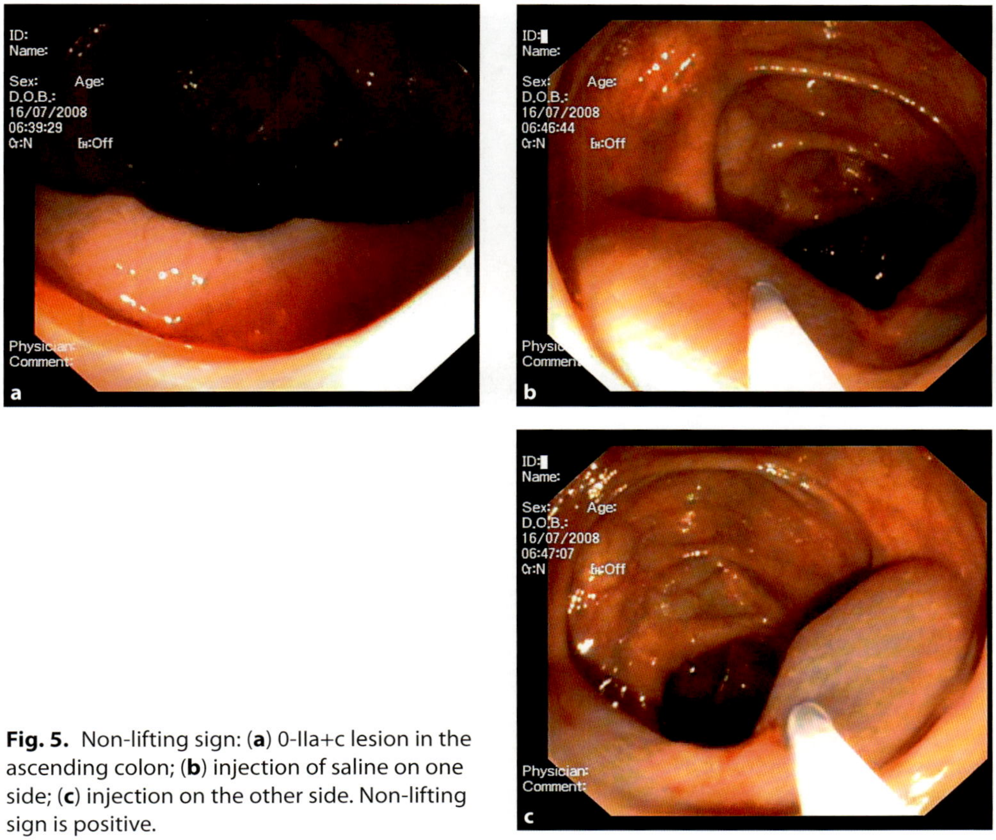

Fig. 5. Non-lifting sign: (**a**) 0-IIa+c lesion in the ascending colon; (**b**) injection of saline on one side; (**c**) injection on the other side. Non-lifting sign is positive.

Flat and non-pedunculated adenomas up to 2 cm in diameter can be safely removed in one piece. Endoscopic completeness in the vertical plane is ensured by exposing the muscularis propria, while completeness in the horizontal plane (within lateral borders) is ensured by careful endoscopic grasping of the lesion as well as the normal mucosa margins. Histopathology can confidently confirm completeness only if the polyp is removed in one piece.

Polyps of up to 2 cm in diameter located in the rectum or left colon without any obvious malignant appearance may be removed by the snare without injection; however, careful assessment of the size of the entrapped tissue as well as mobility in relation to bowel wall is necessary before cutting. Conversely, irrespective of localization, even small flat polyps that show rigidity (immobile parts) with a non-granular amorphic surface with central depression or ulceration may only be removed after injection, e.g. after successful lifting of the lesion with injected fluid.

The surface of the polyps may be better visualized using chromoendoscopy with indigocarmine (0.2–0.5%) or crystal violet (0.05%) as well as with help of narrow band imaging (NBI) (fig. 3, 4). This is necessary for pre-procedural differential diagnosis between adenoma and cancer and for indirect assessment of depth of invasion. Pre-procedure endosonography using high-frequency mini-sondes theoretically could provide information on depth of invasion, but in practice, this approach is used rarely and only for lesions located in the rectum and sigmoid colon. It must be stressed, then, that the decision of whether to remove large flat lesions may use

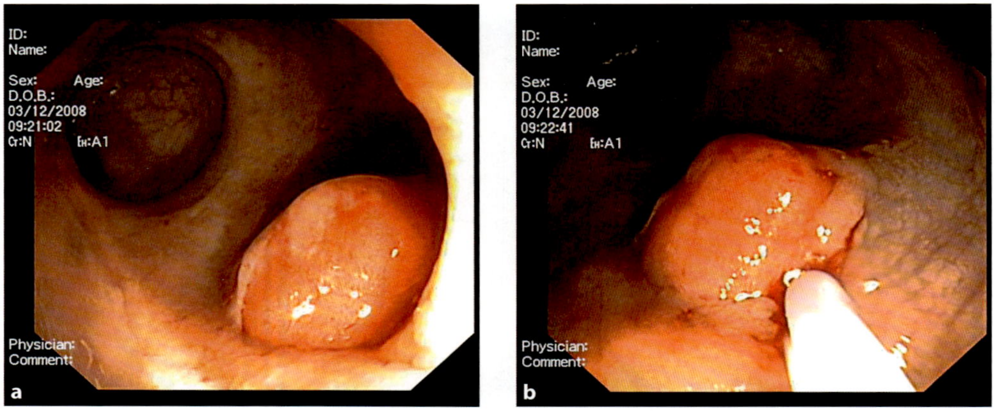

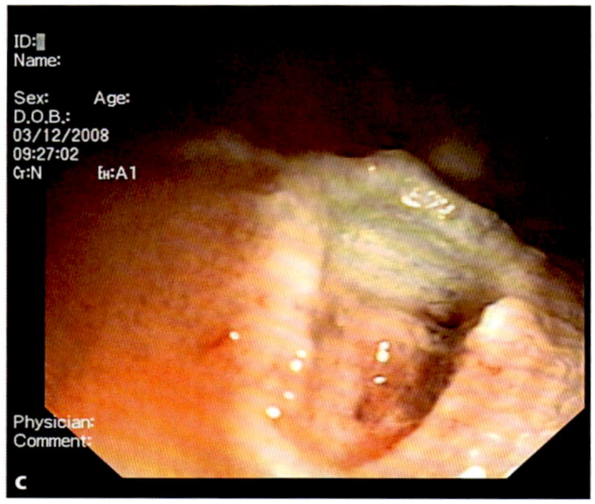

Fig. 6. O-Is lesion. Problematic successful injection: (**a**) macroscopically suspicion of deep invasion; (**b**) successful injection; (**c**) proximal part removed completely, distal is not.

simple measures, e.g. careful assessment in white light with chromoendoscopy and assessment of lifting after injection.

A non-lifting sign after proper injecting of 5–10 ml of fluid under the polyp is an important assessment for depth of invasion, and if positive is a clear contraindication for endoscopic removal. However, it should be noted that a non-lifting sign can be also observed after previous unsuccessful polyp removal, and even in site of diagnostic forceps biopsy; in these cases, such a sign indicates higher risk of procedure and smaller chances for full completeness. This may also be a false positive in cases of improper injection technique. Positive non-lifting sign is presented in figure 5. False negative sign is presented in figure 6, where injection looked successful but resection was incomplete.

Non-pedunculated and flat polyps measuring >2 cm in diameter occur in 0.8–5.2% of colonoscopies [9–11]. Such polyps should be removed using a piecemeal technique even if it appears to be possible to place the snare around the entire polyp [5, 12]. The first injection should be performed in the proximal part of the polyp in order to maintain visibility of the lesion. The removed fragments should not be >10–15 mm. The basic indication of complete removal is full exposure of the muscularis propria, but also obtaining as small a number as possible of resected fragments to facilitate histopathologic assessment.

Extensive LSTs may be endoscopically removed and usually in multiple fragments; the removal does not require special equipment, but only sufficient experience of the endoscopist, patience and sufficient time. Removal should be performed in a specific order, starting from one border and moving towards the center. The first fragment should include a small margin of the normal mucosa, and the next piece should include a border of the previously removed fragment. Proper grasping requires bowel decompression (desufflation) simultaneous with closing the snare. The air should be insufflated again after checking that the snare is closed in order to see the lesion. The snare and entrapped lesion should be then drawn into the direction of the bowel lumen, and only after this is completed can the current application be initiated. Complete removal of even extensive adenomas is optimally performed within one session, as performing the procedure in more than one session makes it difficult or even impossible to clearly delineate borders and decreases the chances for completeness. Different EMR procedures with the special caution paid to proper technique are presented in figures 7–13.

Endoscopic assessment of completeness of adenoma removal is very important, and requires careful visualization of the borders of the removed polyp as well as the clearly visible and exposed muscularis propria. This assessment may be performed using so-called 'underwater visualization', which is obtained by instillation of enough water to go 'submarine' (fig. 14). Alternatively, borders can be visualized by the addition of methylene blue into the injected fluid or with NBI. Adenoma remnants are best removed by additional snare grasping, however this may not be possible, especially in the central part of the removal field where injection may not sufficiently lift the lesion. Leaving fragments or unevenly exposed muscularis propria is unacceptable, as this may result in failure of endoscopic therapy. Small remnants may also be destroyed using argon plasma coagulation (APC). APC should preferably be performed during the same session or occasionally the day after sloughing of necrotic tissue. APC use in the presence of exposed muscularis propria should occur with caution, particularly in the right colon (fig. 15). Power settings in the right colon should be as low as 20 W as compared to 60 W when the procedure is performed in the rectum. Prophylactic border APC coagulation without observing remnants is not an accepted practice.

All removed fragments should be counted during the procedure and then removed using a standard snare or so-called Roth net. Small fragments can also be suctioned with fluid to a special collection bottle attached at the end of suction channel.

Prophylactic APC coagulation of superficial vessels at the area of exposed muscularis propria may decrease the risk of late bleeding (fig. 16). Tattooing of the removal site may facilitate endoscopic surveillance, and if necessary surgical resection; this should be performed using 1–2 ml of ink injected at least at two opposite sites of the removed lesion (fig. 17).

Adenomas without the malignancy removed en bloc with endoscopic and histopathologic completeness do not require special surveillance. Large lesions removed in fragments without confirmed completeness require re-examination in 2–6 months. At that time, a clean removal site without recurrence on chromoendoscopy and without dysplasia on biopsy allows to call endoscopic therapy successful. A clean base visualized only in white light without obtaining biopsies does not exclude recurrence and suggests it is necessary to re-examine the patient in 12 months. If the post-removal base is clean at 12 months, further special surveillance is not needed unless indicated by general rules applied to post-polypectomy patients (fig. 18). Presence of post-removal inflammatory reaction or ulceration at the EMR site makes it difficult or impossible to sufficiently assess the post-removal base and may delay the planned follow-up examinations for approximately 4–6 weeks [12, 13].

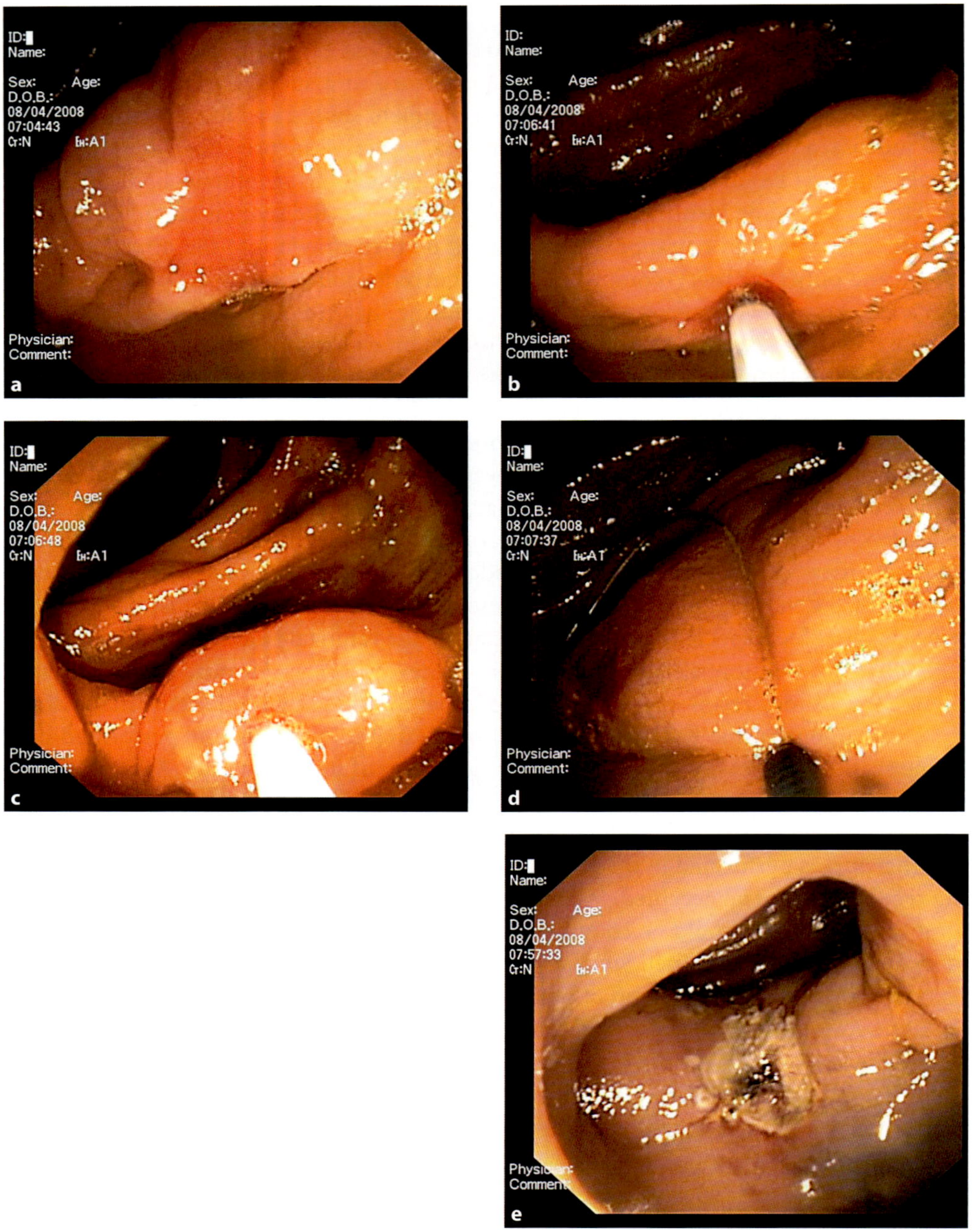

Fig. 7. IIc lesion for EMR: (**a**) discoloration and depression show borders of the lesion; (**b**) needle puncture; (**c**) successful injection and lifting of the lesion; (**d**) placing the snare and pressing it around lesion; (**e**) successful EMR.

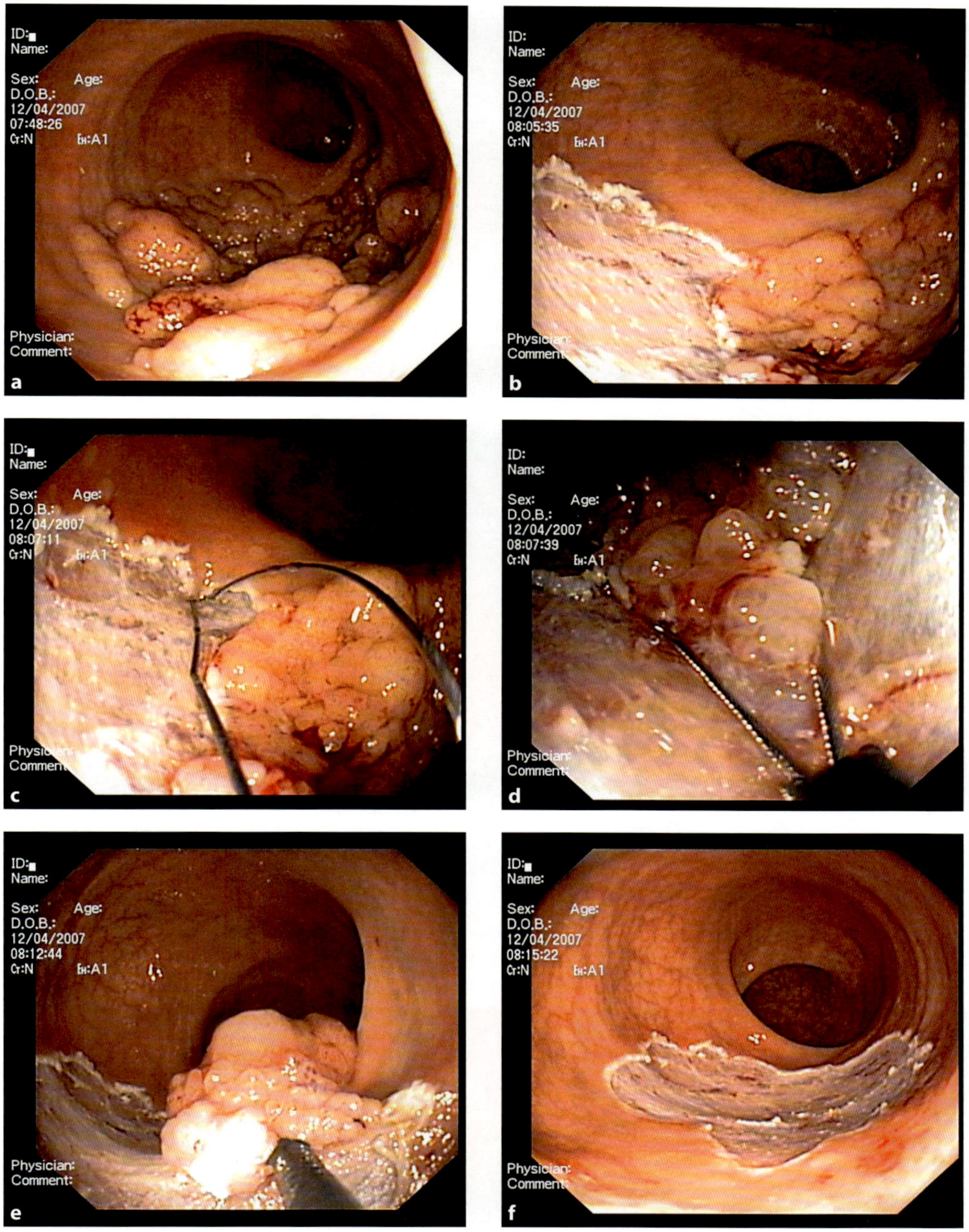

Fig. 8. G-LST, piecemeal EMR: (**a**) large rectal G-LST; (**b**) planned systematic procedure. First cuts included normal mucosa margins: (**c**) placing the snare for next cuts; (**d**) closing snare with simultaneous desufflation; (**e**) obtaining good vision by re-insufflation before final cut; (**f**) final picture; note clean, even base and precisely delineated border.

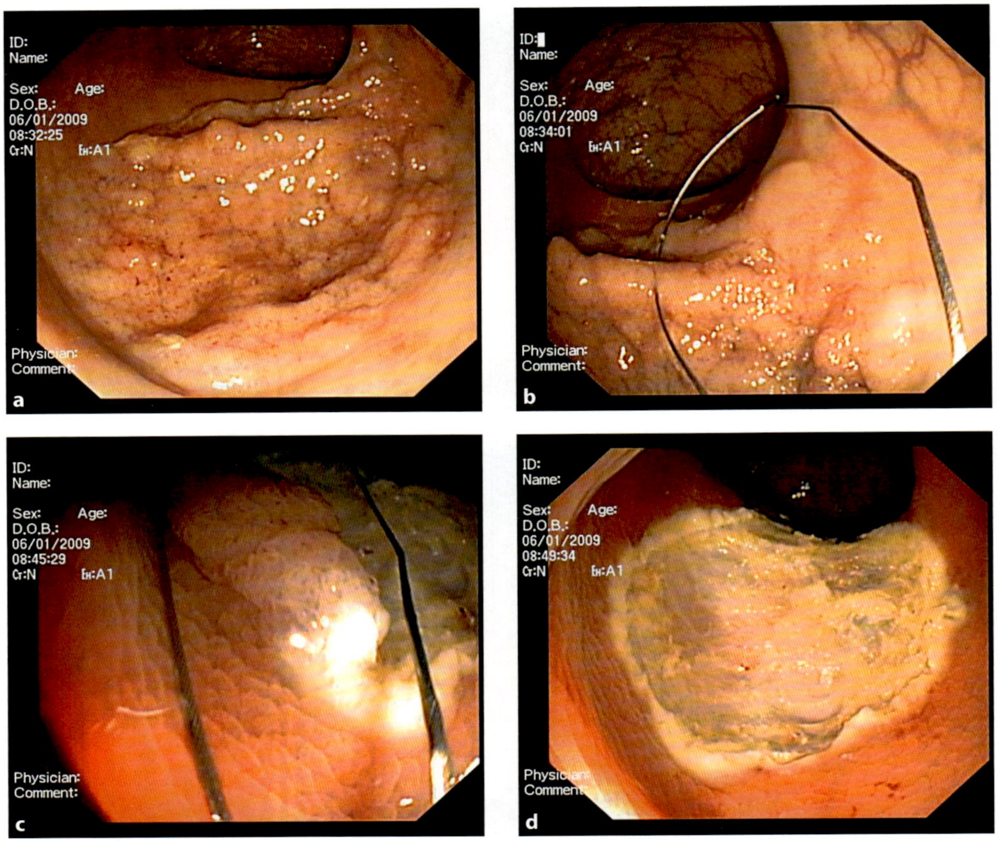

Fig. 9. Rectal LST, piecemeal EMR: (**a**) LST in the rectum; (**b**) precise placing snare for the first cut; (**c**) the last cut; (**d**) final picture.

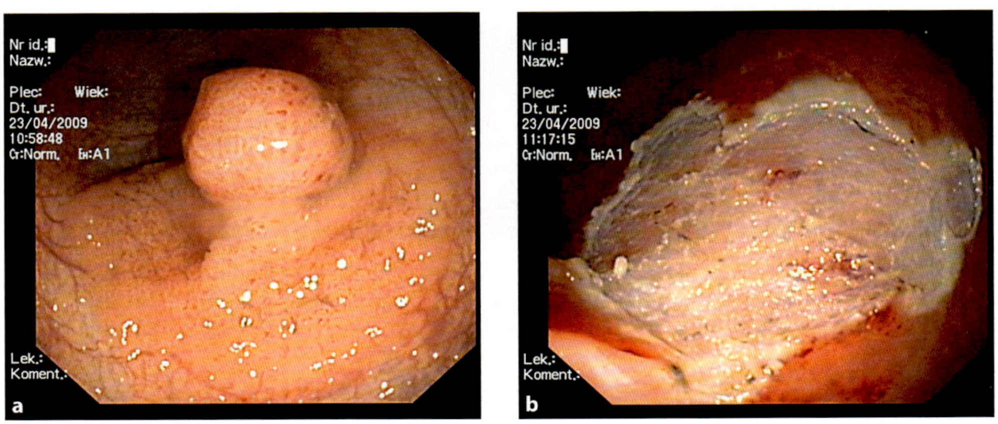

Fig. 10. EMR of flat adenoma with central protrusion: (**a**) flat adenoma with central protrusion; (**b**) view immediately after EMR.

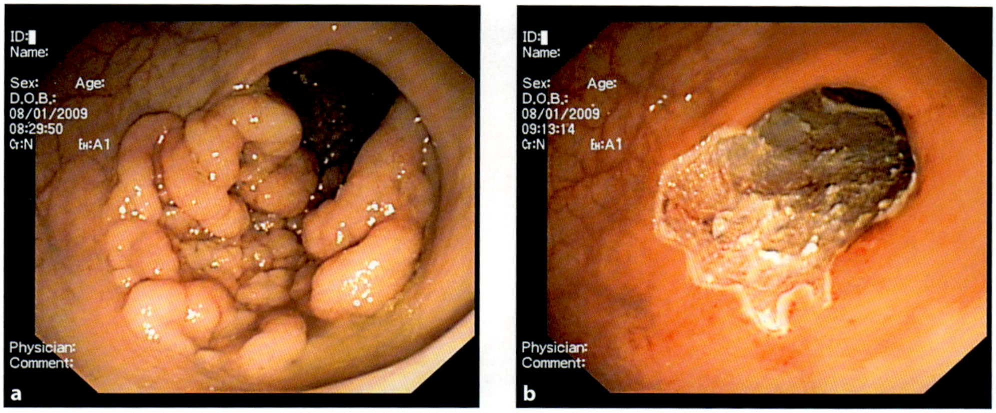

Fig. 11. EMR of G-LST in rectosigmoid: (**a**) large G-LST before removal; (**b**) final picture 45 min later.

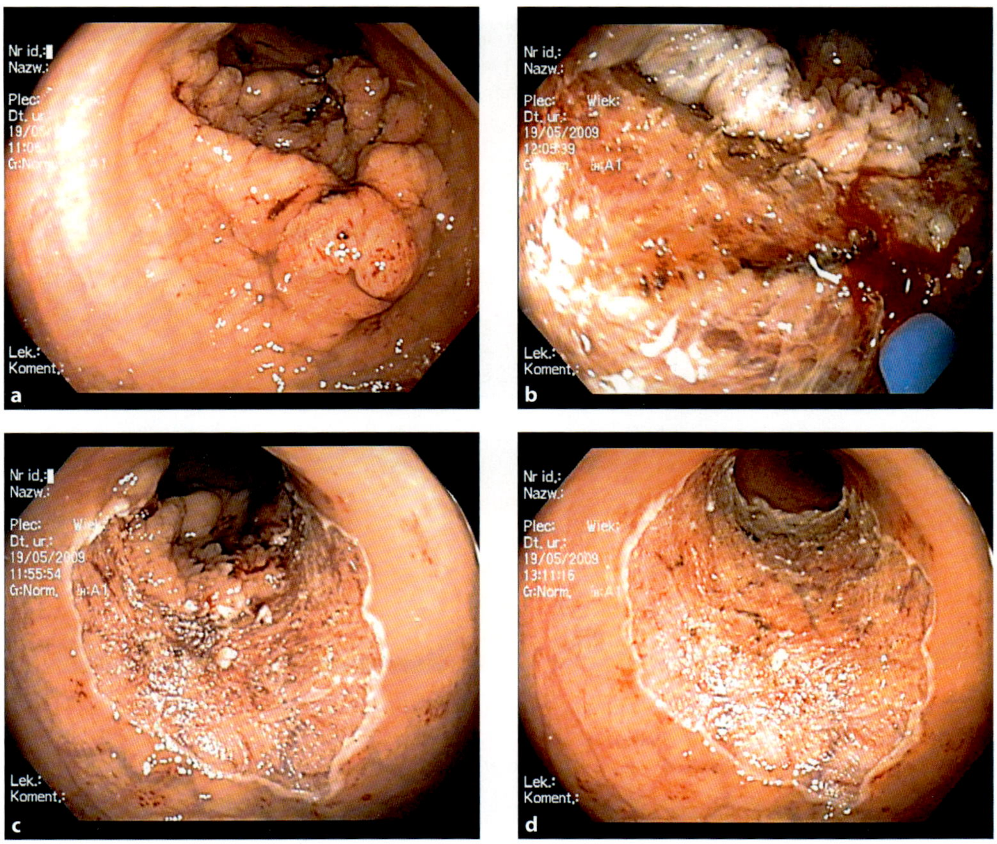

Fig. 12. G-LST, EMR piecemeal: (**a**) rectal G-LST before removal; (**b**) intraprocedural bleeding stopped by APC; (**c**) EMR halfway; note precise border cuts; (**d**) final results.

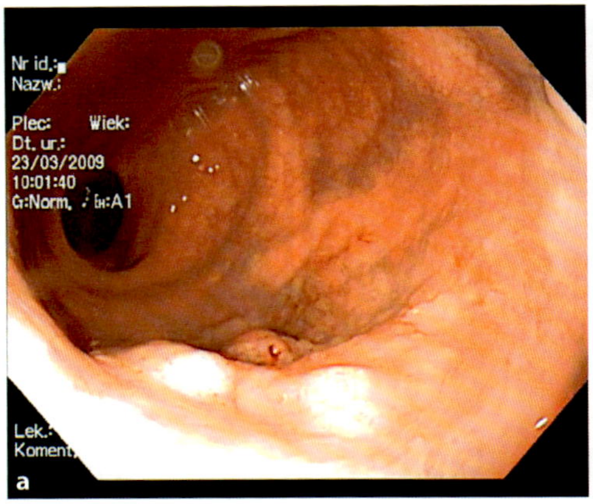

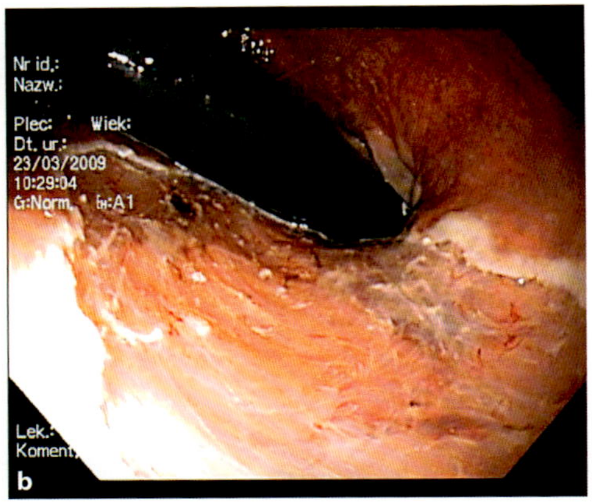

13

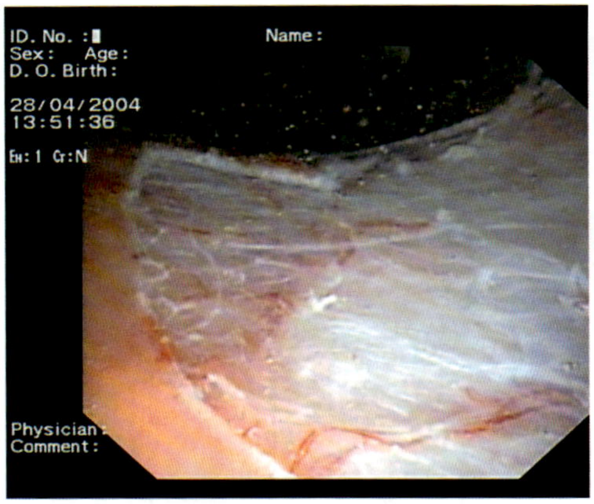

14

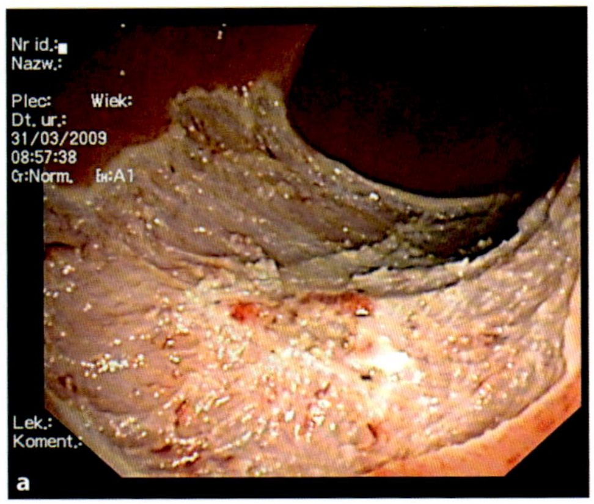

15

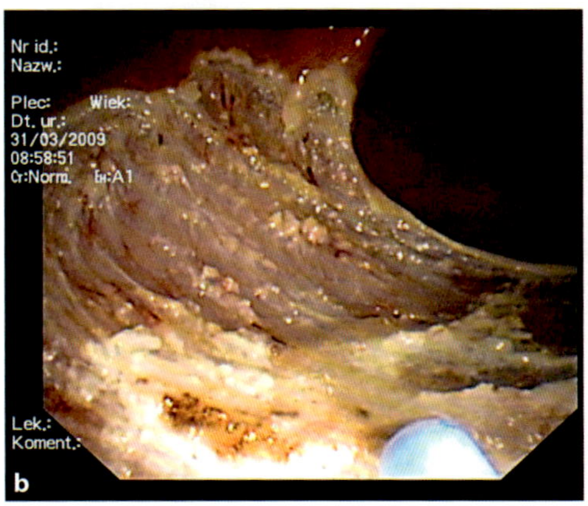

15

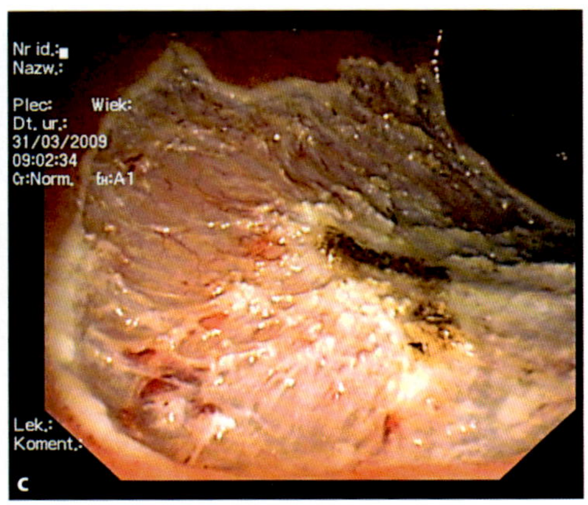

Fig. 13. EMR in retroflexion: (**a**) large LST in distal rectum; (**b**) retroflexion view of post-EMR scar.
Fig. 14. Underwater view to better visualize post-EMR borders. **Fig. 15.** EMR+APC: (**a**) small residual tissue in place of previous biopsy site; (**b**) APC of residual tissue within post-EMR scar; (**c**) picture following APC.

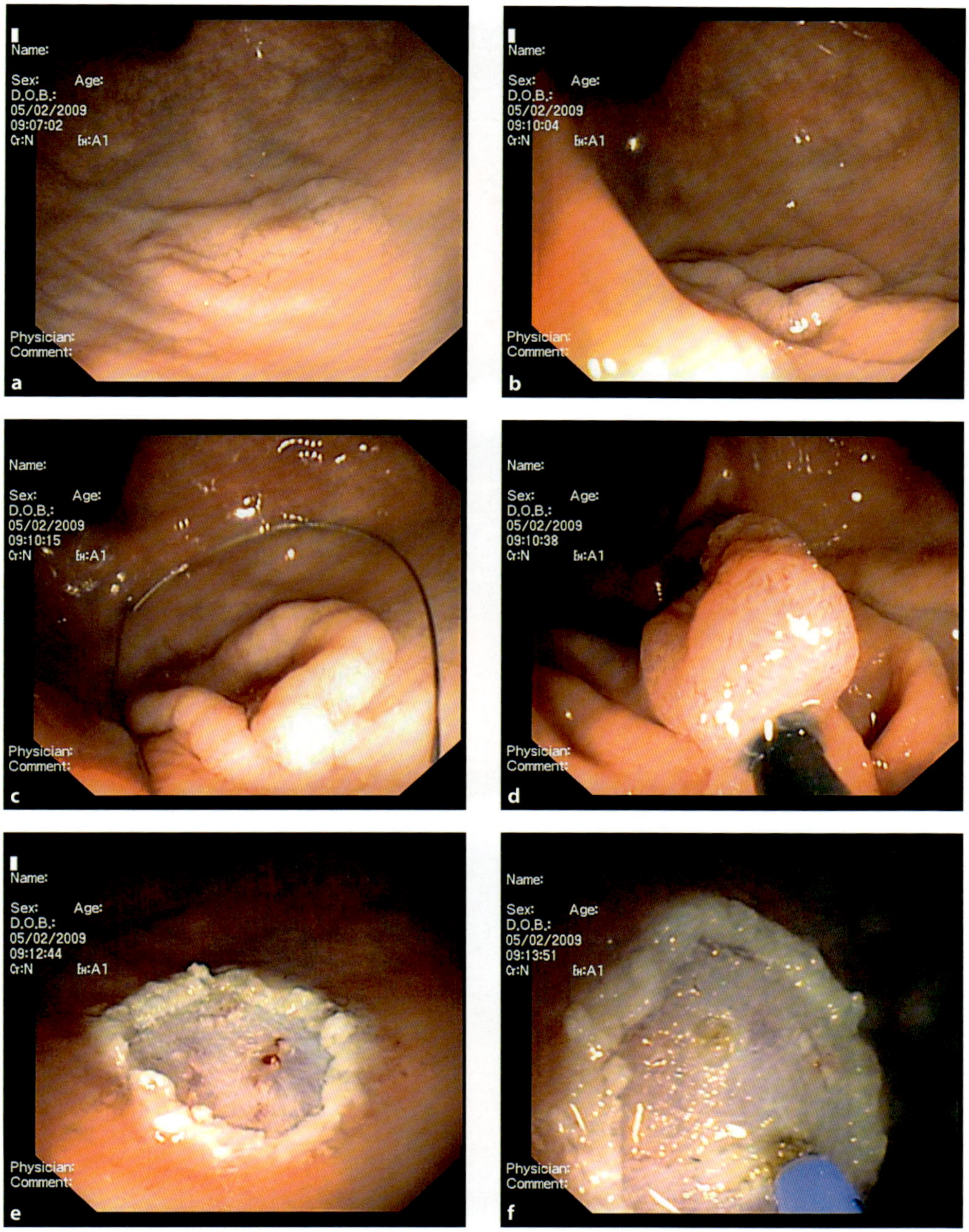

Fig. 16. Flat adenoma; EMR with visible vessel afterwards: (**a**) flat adenoma – initial view; (**b**) pseudodepression on desufflation; (**c**) placing the snare; (**d**) closing the snare; (**e**) post-EMR base with visible vessel; (**f**) successful APC of visible vessel.

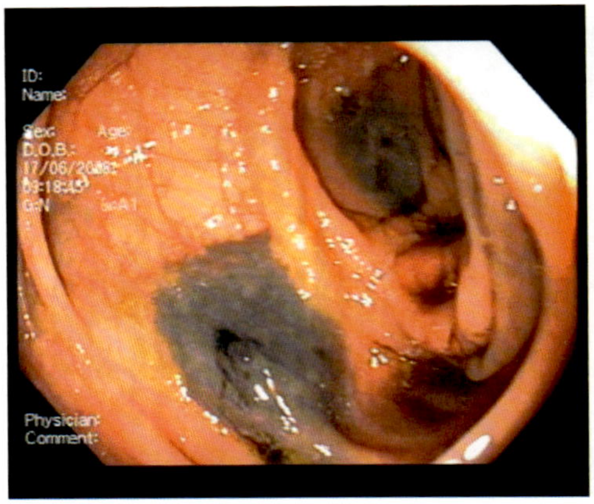

17

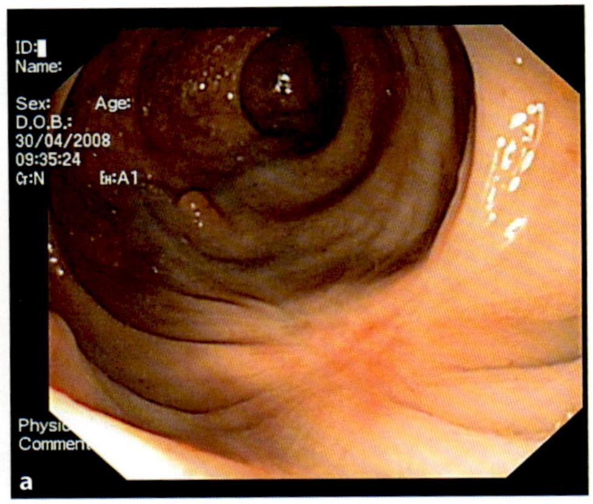

18

18

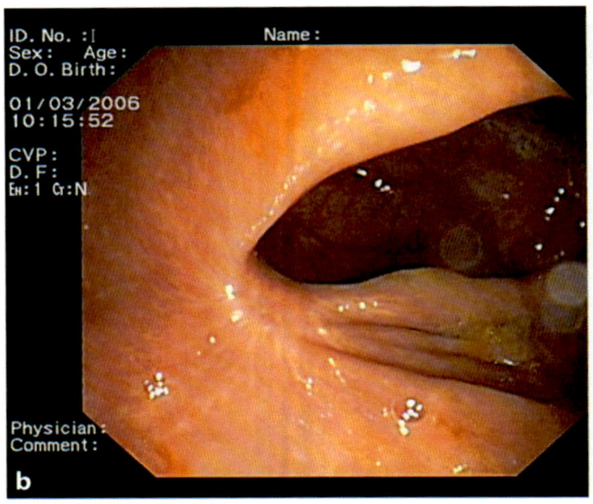

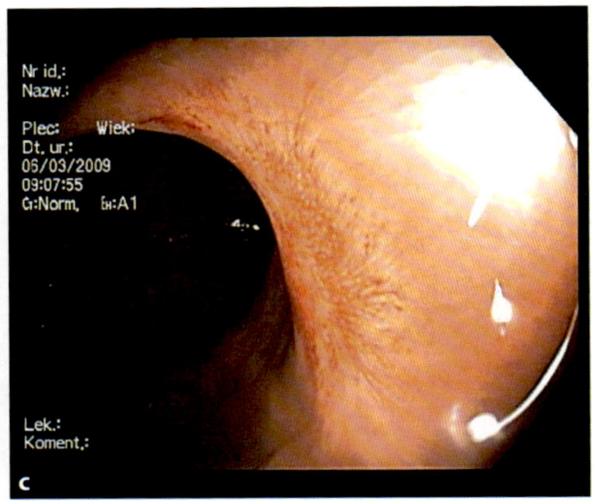

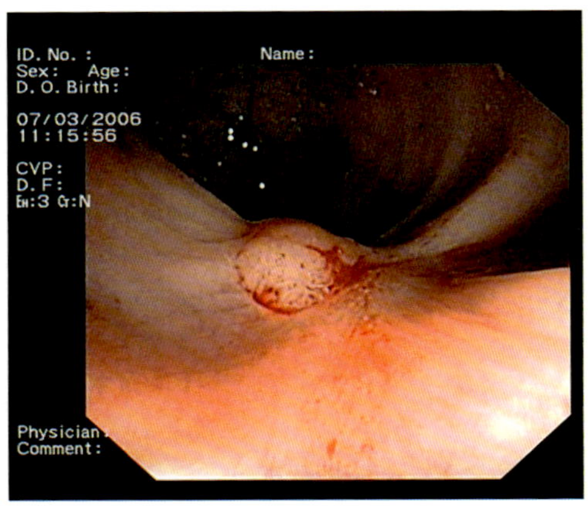

19

Fig. 17. Tattoo proximally and distally to lesion.

Fig. 18. Post-EMR scars: (**a**) clean post-EMR scar in ascending colon; (**b**) clean post-EMR scar in ascending colon; (**c**) clean post-EMR scar in rectum.

Fig. 19. Adenoma recurrence following unsuccessful EMR.

Adenoma recurrence may be removed by snare or destroyed by APC (fig. 19). In such cases, special care has to be taken, as the risk of undetected malignancy increases. Surveillance should be closer and the nearest examination should be repeated in 8–12 weeks. Procedures can be repeated until the adenoma is eradicated.

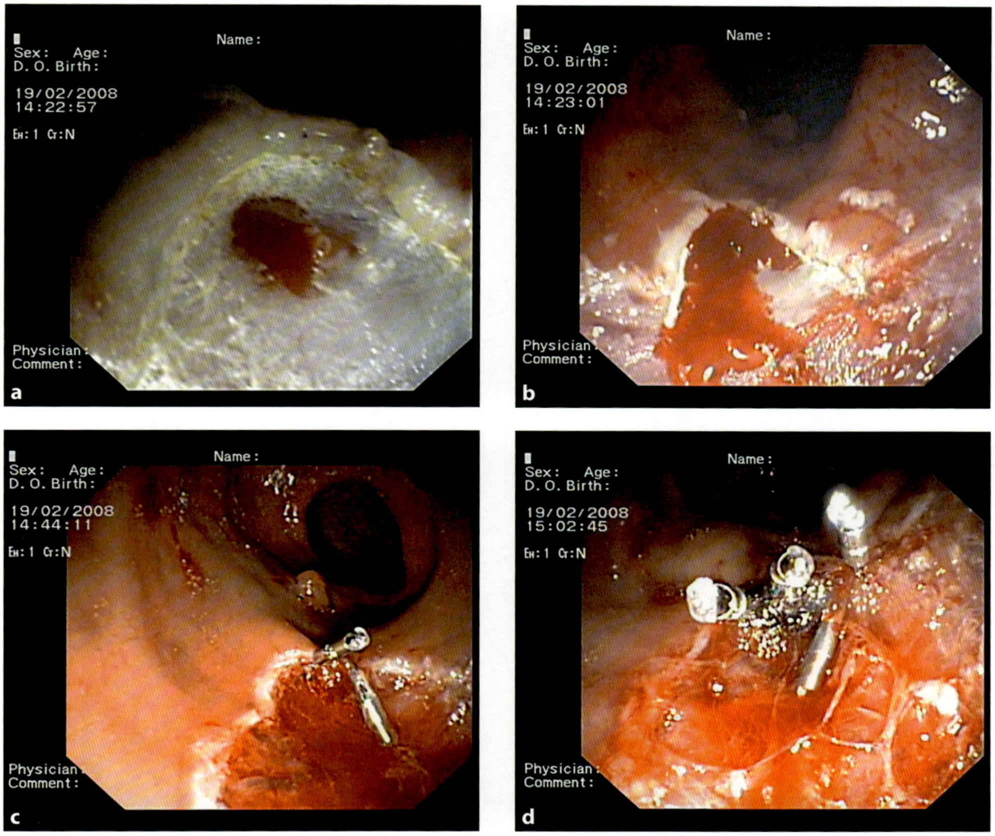

Fig. 20. Clips for bleeding: (**a**) start of bleeding immediately after EMR; (**b**) bleeding increases within seconds; (**c**) first two clips successfully placed; (**d**) final picture after placing four clips.

Accessories

The accessories necessary to perform inject-cut EMR are mostly basic equipment in the standard endoscopy unit: standard diathermic snares, biopsy forceps, APC sondes, hemostatic clips, injection needles and injection fluid, catheter and stains for chromoendoscopy and tattooing, Roth net and bottle for collection of small fragments through the biopsy channel. Endoscopes should preferably be HD standard, and NBI is useful. There is no standard set of accessories, and choice depends on individual preference and experience.

Solutions for submucosal injection differ mainly according to time of disappearance and potential adverse reactions. Injection of hyaluronic acid shows the longest persistence (up to 22 min), however it may induce local inflammation and may possibly also induce the growth of neoplastic cells [14]. The shortest time of persistence is with physiologic saline (approx. 2.5 min), although this is the least expensive solution and is completely neutral, without any possible chemical adverse effects. Similarly, dextrose 30–50% solution also shows a persistence time of approximately 4.7 min [15]. Despite all research, physiologic saline solution that can be frequently re-injected is most often used in practice. Usually, saline is supplemented with

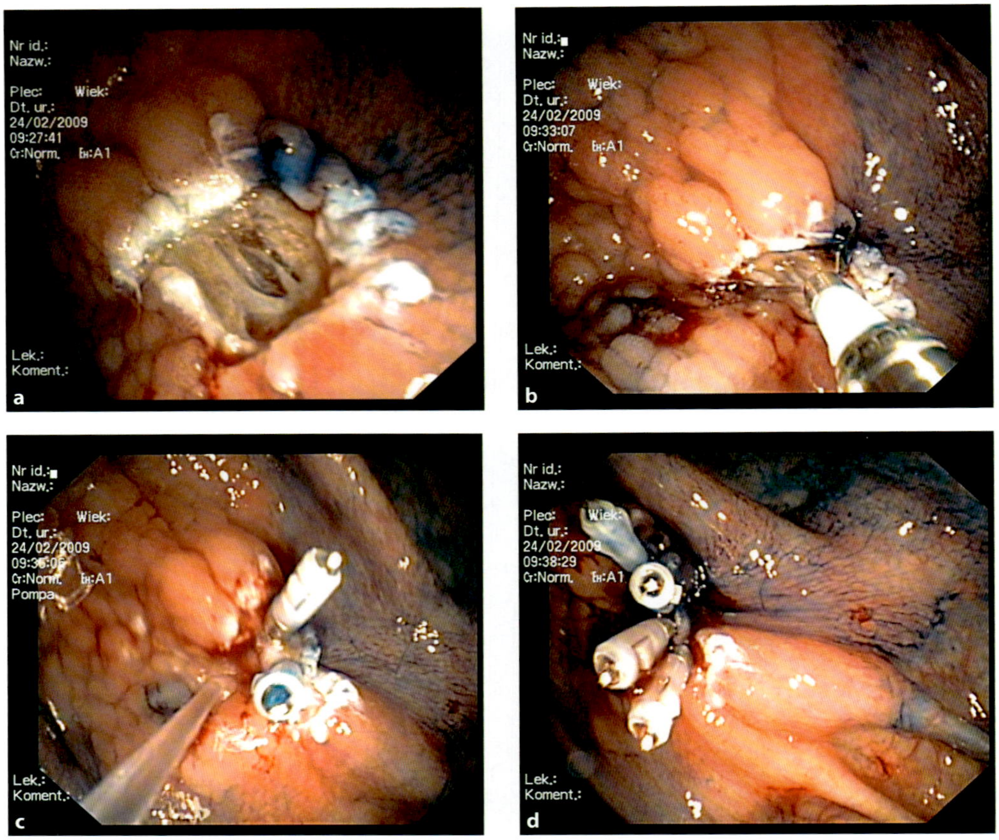

Fig. 21. Clips placement due to perforation suspicion in the cecum: (**a**) post-EMR view – suspicion of perforation; (**b**) preventive clip application; (**c**) two clips placed; (**d**) final view with four clips.

adrenaline, at concentration of 1:10,000–1:40,000, as well as with methylene blue. Tattooing can use special ink injected through bacteriological microfilters or sterilized before use. Also, pure carbon black ink (Spot – endoscopic marker) is commercially available. The most effective size for injection needles is 23 G.

Outcomes

Results of published studies using EMR; its efficiency and positive outcomes depend mainly on patient selection, experience and skills of endoscopic team in applying technical approaches. Selected papers are presented in table 1.

EMRs performed by expert endoscopists should be safe procedures. The most frequent complication is bleeding during the EMR, however this can almost always be successfully treated endoscopically and therefore is rarely clinically important and does not require a blood transfusion (fig. 20). Late bleeding occurring up to 14 days after the procedure is much more dangerous, and usually requires hospitalization and endoscopic intervention. It may also spontaneously stop and does not usually require urgent surgery. Perforation is rare (up to 3%), but is regarded

Table 1. Results of main studies using EMR

Reference (first author)	Polyps n	Mean diameter mm[a]	Follow-up months	Recurrence %	Complications, %	
					bleeding	perforation
Regula [11]						
APC(+)[b]	68	29	38	14	14	0
APC(–)	14	26	32	14	7	0
Zlatanic [16]						
APC(+)	30	32	5.5	50	3.3	0
APC(–)	37	28	7.1	46	12.5	3.1
Conio [17]	139	20 (P), 30 (D)	12.3	21.9	11	0
Church [18]	48	45	3	43	6.3	0
Doniec [19]	141	47	40	4.3	2.8	0.7
Stergiou [20]	68	>30	3	29	22	0
Bergmann [21]	71	25	18	3.1	1.5	1.5

[a] P = diameter for proximal polyps, D = diameter for distal polyps.
[b] APC(+) = EMR with APC; APC(–) = EMR without APC.

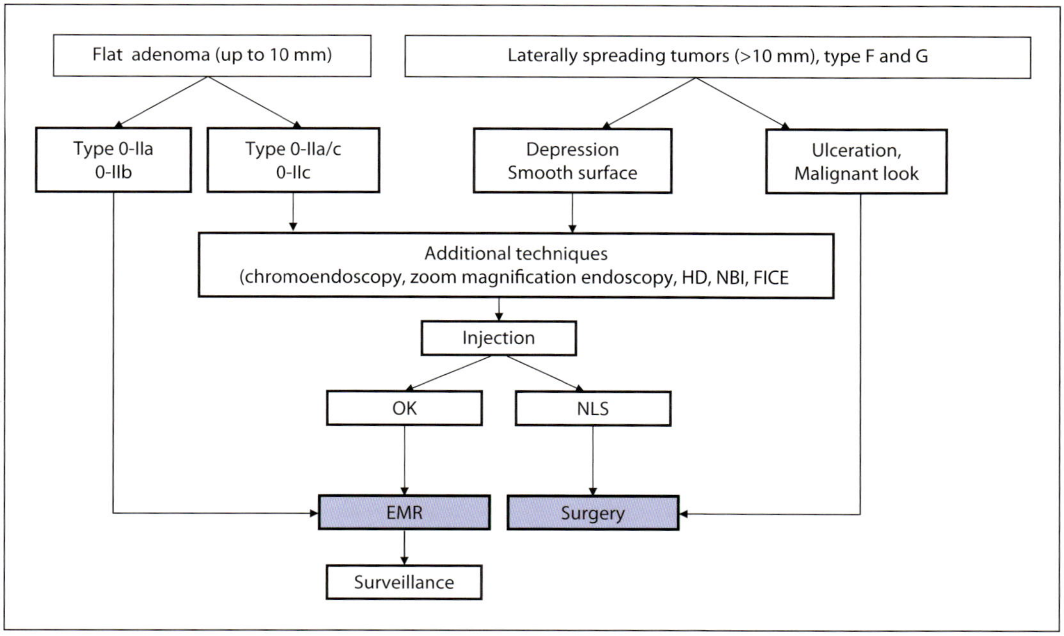

Fig. 22. Decision tree concerning EMR. In G-LST without depression and smooth surface especially in rectum, injection is not obligatory.

as the most serious complication of EMR, usually requiring surgery. When diagnosed during the procedure, it may be clipped successfully without needing operation (fig. 21).

Figure 22 presents an algorithm that can be applied in most endoscopic centers with the interest of advanced therapy of large colorectal adenomas.

References

1 Deyhle P, Largader F, Jenny S, et al: A method for endoscopic electroresection of sessile colonic polyps. Endoscopy 1973;5:38–40.

2 Karita M, Tada M, Okita K, et al: Endoscopic therapy for early colon cancer: the strip biopsy resection technique. Gastrointest Endosc 1991;37:128–132.

3 Participants in the Paris Workshop: The Paris endoscopic classification of superficial neoplastic lesions: esophagus, stomach, and colon. Gastrointest Endosc 2003;58:S3–S43.

4 Muto T, Kamiya J, Sawada T, et al: Small 'flat adenoma' of the large bowel with special reference to its clinicopathologic features. Dis Col Rectum 1985;28: 847–851.

5 Kudo S, Kashida H, Tamura T, et al: Colonoscopic diagnosis and management of nonpolypoid colorectal cancer. World J Surg 2000;24:1081–1090.

6 Okamoto T, Tanaka S, Haruma K, et al: Clinicopathological evaluation on colorectal laterally spreading tumor. Nippon Geka Gakkai Zasshi 1996; 93:83–89.

7 Saito Y, Fujii T, Kondo H, et al: Endoscopic treatment for laterally spreading tumors in the colon. Endoscopy 2001; 33:682–686.

8 Soetikno R, Gotoda T, Nakanishi Y, et al: Endoscopic mucosal resection. Gastrointest Endosc 2003;57:567–579.

9 Iishi H, Tatsuta M, Iseki K, et al: Endoscopic piecemeal resection with submucosal saline injection of large sessile colorectal polyps. Gastrointest Endosc 2000;51:697–700.

10 Kudo SE, Kashida H: Flat and depressed lesions of the colorectum. Clin Gastroenterol Hepatol 2005;3:S33–S36.

11 Regula J, Wronska E, Polkowski M, et al: Argon plasma coagulation after piecemeal polypectomy of sessile colorectal adenomas: long-term follow-up study. Endoscopy 2003;35:212–218.

12 Hurlstone DP, Sanders DS, Cross SS, et al: Colonoscopic resection of lateral spreading tumours: a prospective analysis of endoscopic mucosal resection. Gut 2004; 53:1334–1339.

13 Rusche M, Chadalawada V, Bratcher LL, et al: Negative scar biopsy after large polypectomy at 3 months predictive of cure. Am J Gastroenterol 2005;100:S393.

14 Matsui Y, Inomata M, Izumi K, et al: Hyaluronic acid stimulates tumor cell proliferation at wound sites. Gastrointest Endosc 2004;60:539–543.

15 Varadarajulu S, Tamhane A, Slaughter RL. Evaluation of dextrose 50% as a medium for injection-assisted polypectomy. Endoscopy 2006;38:907–912.

16 Zlatanic J, Way JD, Kim PS, et al: Large sessile colony adenomas: use of argon plasma coagulator to supplement piecemeal snare polypectomy. Gastrointest Endosc 1999;49:731–735.

17 Conio M, Repici A, Demarquay JF, et al: EMR of large sessile colorectal polyps. Gastrointest Endosc 2004; 60:234–241.

18 Church JM: Avoiding surgery in patients with colorectal polyps. Dis Colon Rectum 2003;46:1513–1516.

19 Doniec JM, Lohnert MS, Schniewind B, et al: Endoscopic removal of large colorectal polyps: prevention of unnecessary surgery? Dis Colon Rectum 2003;46:340–348.

20 Stergiou N, Riphaus A, Lange P, et al: Endoscopic snare resection of large colonic polyps: how far can we go? Int J Colorectal Dis 2003;18:131–135.

21 Bergmann U, Beger HG: Endoscopic mucosal resection for advanced non-polypoid colorectal adenoma and early stage carcinoma. Surg Endosc 2003;17: 475–479.

Jaroslaw Regula, MD
Department of Gastroenterology and Hepatology, Institute of Oncology
Roentgen Street 5, PL–02-781 Warsaw (Poland)
Tel. +48 22 546 23 28, Fax +48 22 546 30 35, E-Mail jregula@coi.waw.pl

Mönkemüller K, Wilcox CM, Muñoz-Navas M (eds): Interventional and Therapeutic Gastrointestinal Endoscopy.
Front Gastrointest Res. Basel, Karger, 2010, vol 27, pp 287–295

Endoscopic Submucosal Dissection for Colorectal Tumors

Hironori Yamamoto

Jichi Medical University, Tochigi, Japan

Abstract

Endoscopic submucosal dissection (ESD) is a resection technique for superficial neoplastic lesions of the gastrointestinal tract without the use of snaring. It was developed for en bloc resection of large superficial mucosal tumors and initially used in the stomach, then later in the esophagus and colon and rectum as well. ESD provides a reliable en bloc resection of the lesions with a high complete resection rate and a low recurrence rate. However, it can be curative only when the tumors are localized without metastases. Staging of the tumor with precise endoscopic examination is important to select tumors appropriate for ESD. Moreover, a complete curative resection should be confirmed by detailed pathological examination of the resected tissue. The techniques of ESD for colorectal tumors are described in detail here.

Superficial mucosal tumors of the gastrointestinal tract can be cured by endoscopic resection regardless of their size as long as the tumors are localized and without metastases. However, the application of conventional endoscopic mucosal resection (EMR) with snaring is somewhat limited by the size of the tumor. We started using a new endoscopic resection technique using sodium hyaluronate and a needle knife in 1998 [1]. En bloc resection of a large superficial gastric neoplasm without the use of snaring was first reported by us in 2001 [2]. Similar techniques using different devices for the same purpose were developed by others as well [3, 4]. The dissecting technique developed for en bloc resection of large superficial mucosal tumors was then referred to as endoscopic submucosal dissection (ESD), which was initially used in the stomach, then later in the esophagus and colon and rectum as well [4–6].

Basic Principles

Endoscopic resection is less invasive than surgical resection. However, it has limited applications. Lymph node dissection cannot be performed with the currently available endoscopic techniques, including ESD. Therefore, endoscopic therapy for gastrointestinal neoplasms can be curative only when the tumors are localized and without metastases.

The risk of lymph node metastases strongly correlates with the depth of invasion of the tumor, the histopathologic type of the lesion and the presence of lymphatic or vascular involvement. Therefore, precise examination of the tumor for staging with pit pattern diagnosis using a magnifying endoscope is important to select tumors appropriate for endoscopic resection. Moreover, detailed pathological examination of the resected tissue is also important because it provides precise information regarding whether the neoplasms have been completely resected, allowing appropriate decisions regarding the need for additional surgery. Endoscopic resection can be considered curative by confirmation of negative resection margins, differentiated histopathologic type, depth of submucosal invasion to be <1,000 μm and no lymphatic or vascular involvement. For the accurate histopathologic assessment of the resected specimen, en bloc resection of the entire lesion is required.

ESD is superior to EMR for a more reliable en bloc resection of a targeted area of the mucosa. It also provides a higher complete resection rate with a lower recurrence rate compared with piecemeal EMR [7].

The drawbacks of ESD include the fact that it is a time-consuming procedure, has greater technical demands, and a higher rate of perforation.

Technique

ESD for colorectal tumors is considered more technically demanding than ESD in the stomach for a variety of reasons including: (1) the colonic wall is thinner and softer than the gastric wall; (2) endoscopic control is difficult in some parts of the colon because of paradoxical movement; (3) there are limitations in the retroflex approach due to the narrow lumen of the colon, and tumors can be located on or behind a prominent fold of the colon, and (4) moreover, perforation of the colon has a higher risk of diffuse peritonitis necessitating surgical repair compared with perforation of the stomach.

In order to overcome the above-mentioned difficulties, several devices have been applied to ESD in the colon and rectum. For ESD in the colon, it is important to use a dissecting technique that allows direct visualization of the submucosal tissue, and to use a long-lasting injecting fluid [8].

Determination of Tumor Extent

Mucosal neoplasms in the colon and rectum typically have clear margins which become even clearer after submucosal injection. Therefore, placing marks around the tumor is not necessary in most cases. Chromoendoscopy with indigo carmine spray is useful to enhance the borders of the tumors. New imaging techniques, such as narrow band imaging and flexible spectral imaging color enhancement, are also useful to determine the borders of these tumors.

Submucosal Injection

Creation and maintenance of sufficient mucosal elevation with submucosal injection is essential for safe mucosal incisions and submucosal dissection. As long as thickening of the submucosal layer is maintained throughout the ESD procedure, one of the difficulties associated with ESD in the colon, namely the thin colonic wall, can be overcome. For these purposes, 0.4% sodium hyaluronate solution (MucoUp; Seikagaku Corp, Tokyo, Japan) is the best injection fluid for ESD. Submucosal injection of sodium hyaluronate creates a long-lasting mucosal protrusion that usually lasts more than 1 h [9–11].

Strategy and Technique for Mucosal Incisions and Submucosal Dissection

For successful ESD, it is mandatory to have a good strategy considering the angle of approach to the lesion, and the direction of gravity in relation to the location of the lesion. The position of the patient should be selected to locate the lesion at the top of the colonic lumen with regard to gravity. If the lesion is located at the top, the dissected part of the lesion is naturally pulled down by gravity, which allows sufficient opening of the incised wound with good visualization of the submucosal tissue during the procedure. In cases of unfavorable events such as bleeding and perforation, this positioning is beneficial to avoid or minimize further complications. In the case of bleeding, blood flows down from the bleeding point by gravity. If bleeding occurs at the bottom of the lumen with regard to gravity, the bleeding point is immediately covered by a pool of blood which hampers appropriate hemostatic procedures. Conversely, if the bleeding point is at the top of the lumen, hemostasis can be performed reliably with accurate identification of the bleeding point because blood flows away from the bleeding point by gravity. Even in cases of perforation, if the perforation occurs at the top of the lumen with regard to gravity, identification and closing of the perforation is easier, maintaining a good view of the site of perforation. Only air, not infected intestinal fluid, will flow out from the lumen to the abdominal cavity before closing the perforation, which is important to prevent diffuse peritonitis.

It is also important to maintain sufficient elevation of the mucosa from the muscle layer throughout the ESD procedure because the wall of the colon is so thin that it becomes very difficult to dissect if submucosal thickening disappears. The operator should elevate the mucosal area to be dissected by injecting a sufficient amount of sodium hyaluronate into the submucosa. The mucosal incision is made only in the area to be dissected and then dissection of the submucosa from the incised part is promptly started. If the operator performs a circumferential mucosal incision and postpones submucosal dissection, even viscous sodium hyaluronate will eventually drain from the incised wound, resulting in loss of submucosal thickening, which makes completion of the procedure difficult.

The mucosal incision is made with a short FlushKnife (1.5 mm; DK2618JN15; Fujifilm Corp., Tokyo, Japan) after sufficient protrusion of the mucosa is obtained. Only the needle part should be used for the incision, keeping the tip of the sheath touching the surface of the mucosa without pushing the sheath into the submucosal layer. The Endo Cut mode is used for the mucosal incision.

Submucosal dissection can be performed safely with a FlushKnife as long as adequate thickening of the submucosal layer, as a safety margin away from the muscle layer, is maintained. The dissection should be done parallel to the muscular layer, by sliding the knife from the center of the tumor toward the mucosal incision on the side, while hooking submucosal fibers with the knife.

Recently, we have often used a tunneling method to dissect the submucosal layer. With this method, after mucosal incision and submucosal dissection at the proximal edge of the colonic tumor, the mucosal incision and submucosal dissection are then performed from the distal edge of the tumor. Submucosal dissection is continued to make a tunnel in the submucosal layer by inserting the tip of the endoscope with a transparent hood under the mucosal tumor. The tunneling dissection is continued, to reach the mucosal incision at the proximal edge. After penetration of the tunnel from the distal edge to the proximal edge of the tumor, the tunnel is widened on both sides laterally. Finally, the mucosa on both sides of the tumor is incised laterally and then dissection of the submucosa on both sides is also performed to complete the resection (fig. 1). By making a submucosal tunnel, the endoscope tip is stabilized allowing precise control of the knife for dissection. It also opens the dissected wound with the hood at the endoscope tip providing

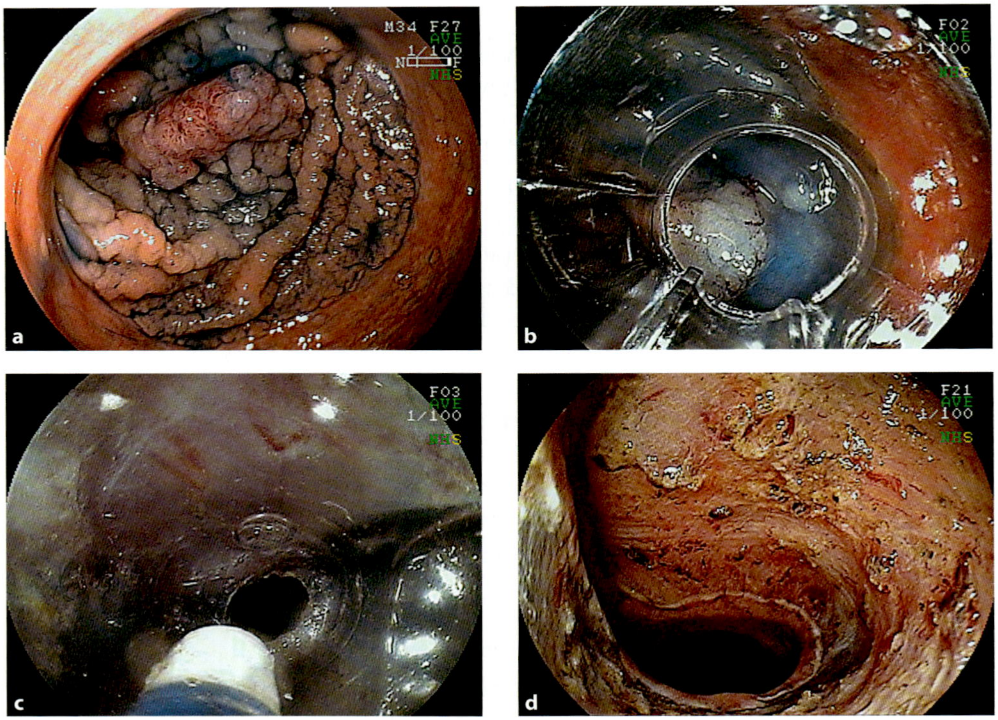

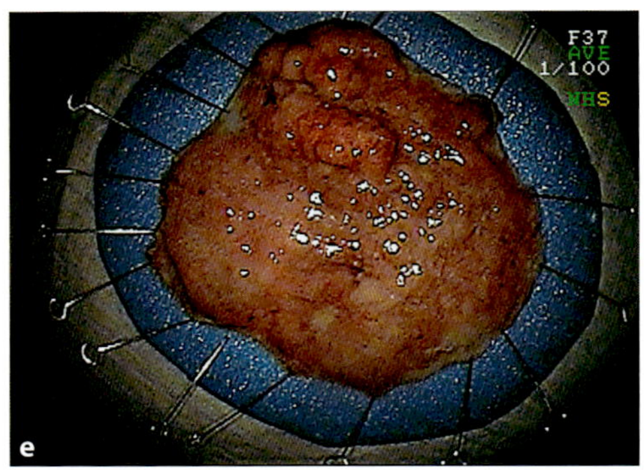

Fig. 1. ESD using a tunneling method. **a** A large granular laterally spreading tumor in the rectum. **b** Distal edge of the tumor after submucosal injection of sodium hyaluronate solution. **c** Penetration of the tunnel in the submucosal layer. **d** Mucosal defect after the completion of ESD. **e** En bloc resection of the entire lesion (68 × 62 mm in diameter). Histopathologic examination confirmed complete curative resection (adenocarcinoma in adenoma, no invasion to submucosa, no lymphatic or vascular involvement).

a good safety margin for further dissection by stretching the submucosal tissue. Adjusting the approach angle of the knife to be tangential to the wall also is easy with this method because an adjusting force with the endoscope tip can be applied in either direction by pushing the mucosa up or pushing the muscle wall down with the tip of the hood. The tunneling method is particularly useful for large lesions, lesions with fibrosis, and lesions located on a curved wall.

Endoscopes

ESD procedures require precise control of the endoscope tip. Therefore, a thin endoscope is preferred over a robust therapeutic colonoscope. For this reason, some operators select a single-channel upper endoscope for ESD in the distal colon or rectum. We use a specifically designed colonoscope (EC-450RD5; Fujifilm Corp., Tokyo, Japan; fig. 2) for ESD in the colon and rectum. This colonoscope is a single-channel scope with a thin upper endoscope tip size (9.8 mm) and a regular colonoscope shaft size (12.8 mm). The retroflex approach is available in any part of the colon and rectum using this scope because the bending section of the endoscope tip is thin and short with good angulation ability. A relatively large accessory channel of 3.2 mm and a water jet function with good targeting direction make this scope suitable for ESD.

When a lesion for ESD is located in an unstable part of the colon and paradoxical movements with a standard colonoscope hamper the reliable performance of the ESD procedure, we select a double-balloon colonoscope (EC-450BI5, Fujifilm, Japan; fig. 3). The double-balloon colonoscope provides precise control of the endoscope tip, even in this situation (fig. 4).

Accessories

Injection Needle
For the injection of sodium hyaluronate solution, a high-flow injection needle with a large inner lumen should be used to minimize injecting resistance.

Electrosurgical Knife
Several kinds of electrosurgical knives have been developed for ESD. Among the currently available knives, we usually use a FlushKnife for ESD in the colon. A FlushKnife is a special needle knife featuring the water jet function through the knife sheath. This water jet function can be used to cleanse the surface of the mucosa and the needle itself. It can also be used for fluid injections directly into the submucosal layer through the FlushKnife after mucosal incision. Because a FlushKnife can be used for both injection and dissection, submucosal dissection can be performed immediately after the injection without changing the devices, which makes the procedure efficient. For this knife, the appropriate length of the needle can be selected from among 1, 1.5, 2, 2.5 and 3 mm sizes, based on the specific situation (fig. 5).

Hood
A transparent hood attached to the tip of the endoscope is useful to open the incised wound and to maintain a good endoscopic view during the procedure. It also allows precise control of the knife by stabilizing the target with its tip. Use of a hood is substituted for the triangulation used during surgical procedures, which is difficult to apply in endoscopic procedures. We mainly use a transparent hood with a small-caliber tip (ST hood; DH-15GR, DH-16CR; Fujifilm, Japan; fig. 6) for colonic ESD. The ST hood has an aperture small enough to make it easy to widen an incised wound using the edge of the hood, and to allow more accurate adjustment of the depth of incision by the knife point. Using the ST hood, it is easy to create a submucosal tunnel proceeding with submucosal dissection by inserting the tip of the hood into the submucosal layer, which is a useful strategy for effective ESD.

Electrosurgical Current Generator
It is important to select the appropriate high-frequency electrosurgical current generator and to set it appropriately for a reliable incision with effective control of bleeding and minimum tissue damage. We mainly use the ERBE VIO 300 D (Erbe, Tubingen, Germany). It is set to 'Endo Cut

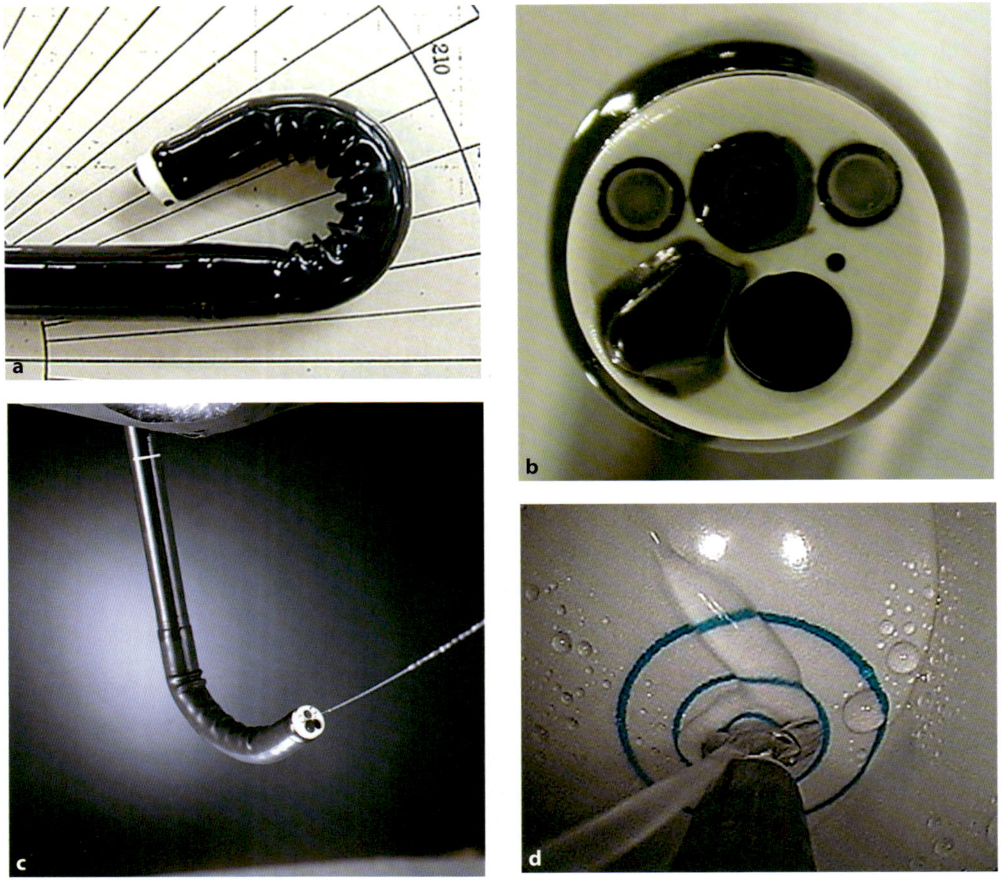

Fig. 2. Colonoscope for ESD (EC-450RD5; Fujifilm Corp.). **a** The bending section of the endoscope tip is thin and short with good angulation capability. **b** A large accessory channel and a water jet channel are situated close to each other. **c** Water jet function of the scope. **d** Good targeting direction of the water jet to the tip of an accessory device.

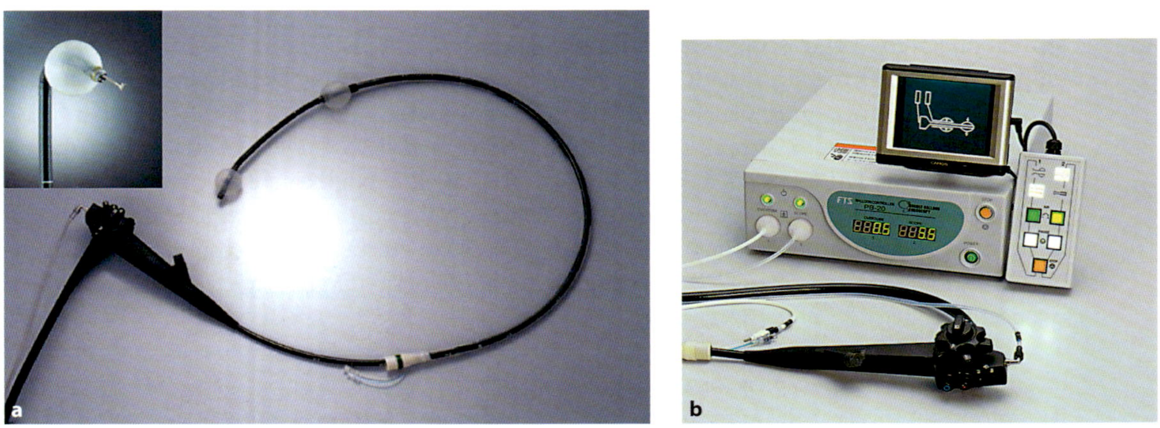

Fig. 3. Double-balloon colonoscope (EC-450BI5, Fujifilm Corp.). **a** Soft balloons are equipped at the tip of the endoscope and the tip of the overtube. **b** A balloon controller to inflate or deflate the balloons.

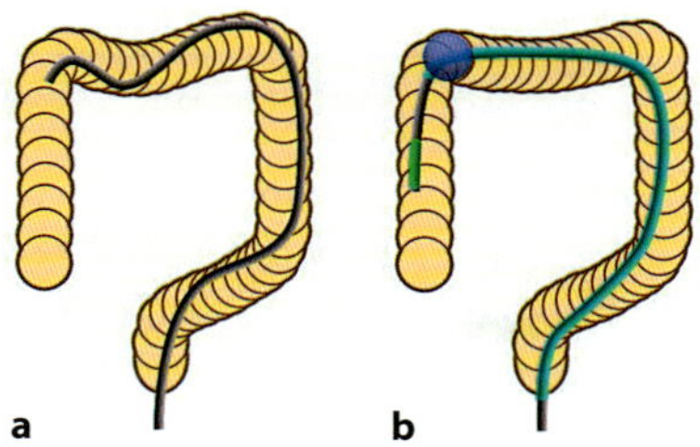

Fig. 4. **a** Paradoxical movements with a standard colonoscope. **b** Precise control of the endoscope tip provided by the double-balloon colonoscope.

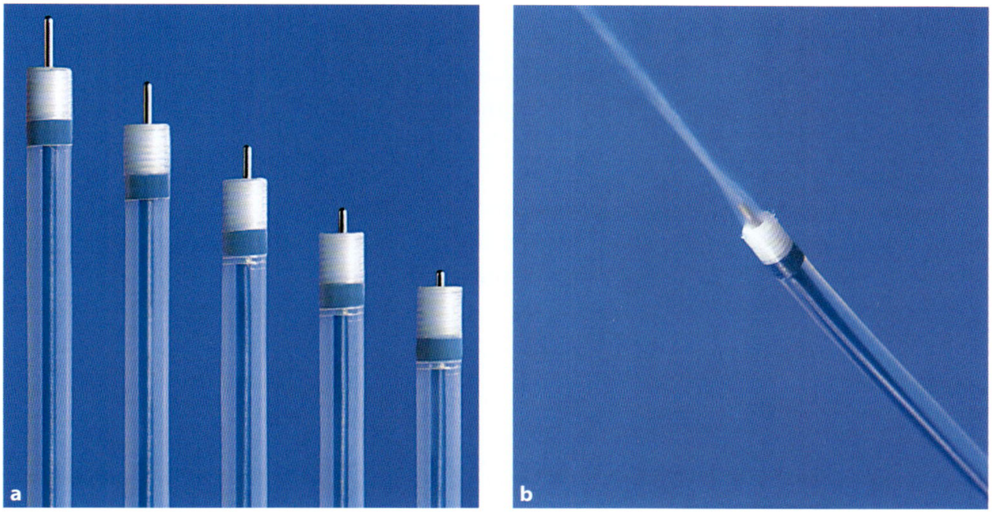

Fig. 5. Flush knife (DK2618JN10–30; Fujifilm Corp.). **a** The appropriate length of the needle can be selected from among 1, 1.5, 2, 2.5 and 3 mm sizes. **b** Water jet function through the knife sheath.

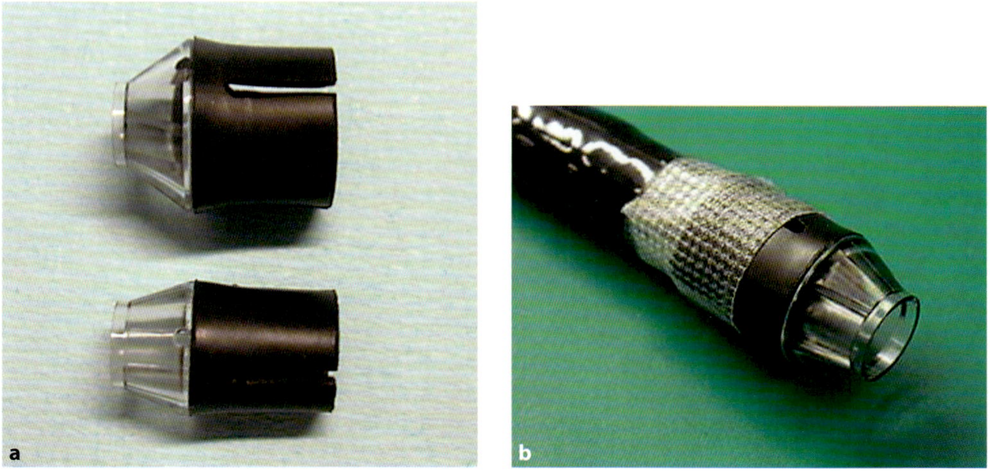

Fig. 6. ST hood (DH-15GR, DH-16CR; Fujifilm Corp.). **a** Two sizes of the hood, DH-15GR for a thin endoscope tip and DH-16CR for a standard colonoscope tip) are available. **b** ST hood attached to the endoscope.

Table 1. Output settings of ERBE VIO 300D for ESD procedures

	Device	Cut modes		Coagulation modes
Mucosal incision	Flush knife	Endo Cut I E 1/D 4/I 1	Dry Cut E 6 30 W	
Submucosal dissection	Flush knife	Dry Cut E6 30 W		Swift Coag E4 30 W
Hemostasis	Flush knife Hemostatic forceps			Spray Coag E2 5 W Soft Coag E6 80 W

I' mode for mucosal incision, and to 'swift coagulation' or 'dry cut' mode for submucosal dissection. The output settings for the procedures are summarized in table 1.

Hemostatic Forceps

Effective control of bleeding during the procedure is a vital factor for successful ESD. Minor bleeding and small blood vessels can be managed using the knife. However, more reliable hemostasis for a larger vessel can be achieved using hemostatic forceps (HDB2422W; Pentax, Tokyo, Japan). The generator is set to soft coagulation mode for the hemostatic forceps.

Outcomes

In our experience of over 500 cases of colorectal ESD, en bloc resection has been successfully performed for lesions up to 164 mm in diameter with an en bloc resection rate of 92% and a perforation rate of 4%. A perforation made by the knife is usually tiny and recognized immediately; therefore, a perforation can be closed with endoscopic clip placement and managed non-operatively.

Conclusions

Tips and tricks for ESD for colorectal tumors have been described. ESD is a reliable method for the en bloc resection of large superficial mucosal tumors. En bloc resection is important for the accurate histopathologic examination of lesions to ensure curative resection by confirming complete local resection and assessing the risk of lymph node metastases. Complete resection can be achieved using en bloc resection and a minimum risk of recurrence.

References

1 Yamamoto H, Koiwai H, Yube T, et al: A successful single-step endoscopic resection of a 40 millimeter flat-elevated tumor in the rectum: endoscopic mucosal resection using sodium hyaluronate. Gastrointest Endosc 1999;50:701–704.

2 Yamamoto H, Sekine Y, Higashizawa T, et al: Successful en bloc resection of a large superficial gastric cancer by using sodium hyaluronate and electrocautery incision forceps. Gastrointest Endosc 2001;54:629–632.

3 Kondo H, Gotoda T, Ono H, et al: Percutaneous traction-assisted EMR by using an insulation-tipped electrosurgical knife for early stage gastric cancer. Gastrointest Endosc 2004;59:284–288.
4 Oyama T, Tomori A, Hotta K, et al: Endoscopic submucosal dissection of early esophageal cancer. Clin Gastroenterol Hepatol 2005;3(suppl 1):S67–S70.
5 Ono H: Endoscopic submucosal dissection for early gastric cancer. Chin J Dig Dis 2005;6:119–121.
6 Yamamoto H: Endoscopic submucosal dissection of early cancers and large flat adenomas. Clin Gastroenterol Hepatol 2005;3:S74–S76.
7 Saito Y, Fukuzawa M, Matsuda T, et al: Clinical outcome of endoscopic submucosal dissection versus endoscopic mucosal resection of large colorectal tumors as determined by curative resection. Surg Endosc 2009 [Epub ahead of print].
8 Yamamoto H, Yahagi N, Oyama T: Mucosectomy in the colon with endoscopic submucosal dissection. Endoscopy 2005;37:764–768.
9 Yamamoto H, Yube T, Isoda N, et al: A novel method of endoscopic mucosal resection using sodium hyaluronate. Gastrointest Endosc 1999;50:251–256.
10 Yamamoto H, Yahagi N, Oyama T, et al: Usefulness and safety of 0.4% sodium hyaluronate solution as a submucosal fluid 'cushion' in endoscopic resection for gastric neoplasms: a prospective multicenter trial. Gastrointest Endosc 2008;67:830–839.
11 Fujishiro M, Yahagi N, Kashimura K, et al: Comparison of various submucosal injection solutions for maintaining mucosal elevation during endoscopic mucosal resection. Endoscopy 2004;36: 579–583.

Hironori Yamamoto, MD, PhD
Department of Endoscopic Research and International Education, Jichi Medical University
3311–1 Yakushiji, Shimotsuke
Tochigi 329–0498 (Japan)
Tel. +81 285 58 7539, Fax +81 285 44 0047, E-Mail yamamoto@jichi.ac.jp

Mönkemüller K, Wilcox CM, Muñoz-Navas M (eds): Interventional and Therapeutic Gastrointestinal Endoscopy.
Front Gastrointest Res. Basel, Karger, 2010, vol 27, pp 296–302

Colonic Stents for Malignant Colonic Obstruction

Davor Štimac

Division of Gastroenterology, University Hospital Rijeka, Rijeka, Croatia

Abstract

Colorectal self-expanding metal stents are a pillar for the palliative treatment of patients with advanced colon malignancies. The placement of stents can be fluoroscopic or non-fluoroscopic-guided. The use of stents is associated with significant reduction in hospital duration, mortality and medical complications compared to surgery. The most frequent complications are stent malposition and migration, bleeding, colonic perforation and tumor ingrowth and/or overgrowth.

Self-expanding metal stents (SEMS) were initially used in interventional endoscopy to overcome problems of occlusion of plastic biliary stents and problems of esophageal perforation during the placement of plastic stents. Later they were used in the stomach, duodenum, jejunum and colon to palliate obstructive symptoms in patients with advanced cancer [1]. The first report on the use of SEMS in palliative treatment of malignant colorectal stenosis was published in 1991 [2]. Since then, colorectal stenting is revolutionizing the way in which patients with obstructive pathology due to colorectal diseases are managed.

Indications

The clinical indications for colorectal stenting with SEMS can be divided into absolute and relative [1–3]. The malignancies causing large bowel obstruction are listed in table 1. Absolute indications are palliation of advanced malignancy and preoperative decompression. Palliative therapy with SEMS is used in patients with primary or recurrent colorectal cancer and colonic obstruction who have extensive local or metastatic disease, but also in patients with potentially resectable disease who are not operative candidates because of age or comorbidity. Colonic obstruction also occurs in patients with invasive extrinsic tumors like local pelvic tumors (mostly ovarian cancer) or metastatic disease to the pelvis [4]. Curative surgery in this group of patients is nearly impossible and most patients are unresectable [5].

Table 1. Malignancies causing large bowel obstruction

Intrinsic	
	Primary rectal
	Primary colonic
Extrinsic	
	Gynecologic
	Urinary
	Metastatic

Almost 30% of patients with colorectal cancer present with acute colon obstruction [6, 7]. Because of uncleansed colon proximal to the obstruction, the risk for breakdown of colonic anastomosis is high. These patients cannot undergo a one-stage operative resection and the current standard of care for acute malignant colonic obstruction is surgical decompression via formation of a colostomy with resection of the primary tumor either by open surgery or laparoscopically. Reanastomosis is performed at least 8 weeks later, but many patients with advanced age and comorbidities remain permanently with colostomy [8, 9]. Preoperative SEMS decompression helps in clinical stabilization of patients allowing a one-stage operation and thus avoidance of colostomy [9]. SEMS also allows for preoperative chemoradiation and has been advocated for use as a 'bridge to surgery' for those with resectable disease [8]. The SEMS remains in the colon until surgery, when is it resected with the tumor [9]. Colonic resection after SEMS decompression can be done by open surgery or laparoscopically [10].

Relative indications include stenting of malignant fistulas from the colon to the vagina or bladder. For this indication, covered stents have been used [11]. Case reports about successful placement of SEMS for double colorectal cancers have also been also published [12]. Recently, some papers have been published about SEMS placement for benign colorectal obstructions. The etiologies of the strictures were Crohn's disease, diverticulitis, radiation, postsurgical, colocutaneous fistulas and undefined benign diseases. Conversion of high-grade benign colonic obstruction can be achieved, but a high grade of delayed complications was observed, therefore mandating further investigations on this topic [13, 14].

Current Techniques

Before insertion of colorectal SEMS, patients with subtotal obstruction in the distal colon should be prepared with cleansing enemas; those with obstruction in the proximal colon should undergo a cautious colonoscopy bowel preparation. Standard intravenous conscious sedation is usually administered. The SEMS should be 3–4 cm longer than the stricture length. A preprocedural plain radiograph and CT scan are mandatory to monitor possible colonic perforation and additional sites of colonic obstruction [8]. Administration of retrograde contrast before the procedure or through the catheter at the time of procedure is helpful to better understand the anatomy of the stricture. SEMS placement can be either fluoroscopic or non-fluoroscopic-guided. In the fluoroscopic technique, a hydrophilic guidewire is used to traverse the stricture, and its position is recognized fluoroscopically before the catheter is advanced over the guidewire through the lesion. Water-soluble radiographic contrast is injected to confirm the position and luminal

Table 2. Currently available colorectal stents

Stent name	Manufacturer	Delivery system	Material
Colonic Z Stent	Cook, USA	OTW	Stainless steel
Wallstent	Boston Scientific, USA	TTS	Elgiloy
Wallflex	Boston Scientific, USA	TTS	Nitinol
Ultraflex Precision	Boston Scientific, USA	OTW	Nitinol
Niti S Colorectal Stent	Taewoong, South Korea	OTW/TTS	Nitinol
Bonastent	Standard SciTech, South Korea	OTW/TTS	Nitinol
Hanarostent Colorectal	M.I. Tech Co., South Korea	OTW/TTS	Nitinol

1 2

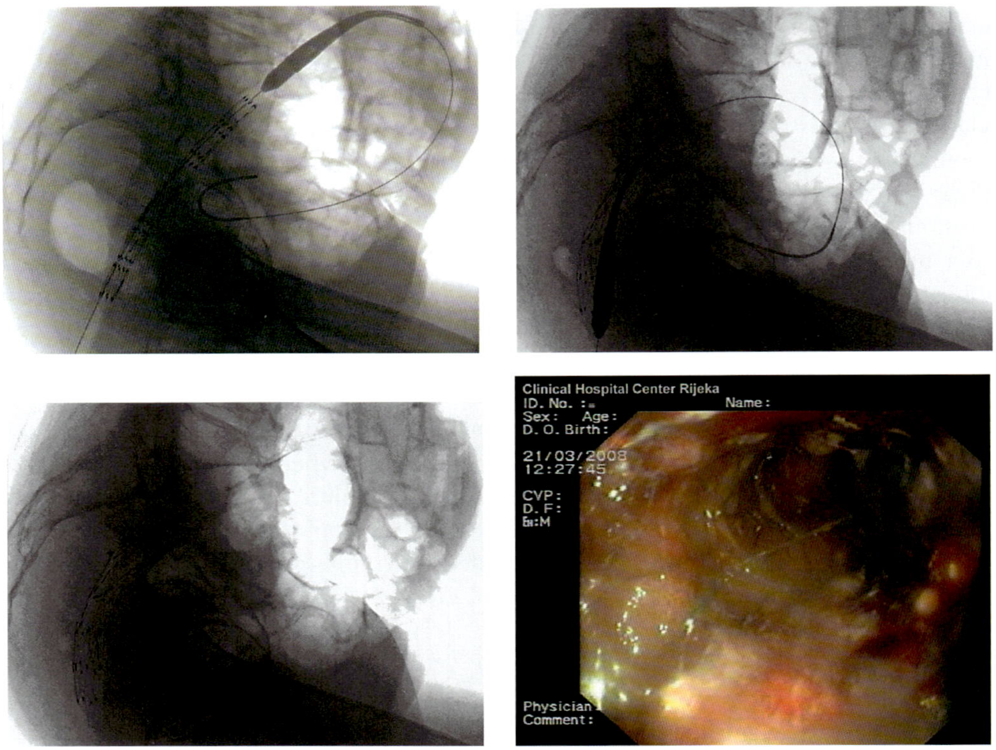

3 4

Fig. 1–3. Fluoroscopic-guided SEMS placement. **Fig. 4.** Endoscopic view of SEMS in the rectosigmoid.

patency. After that, the guidewire is exchanged for a stiff guidewire and the stent is deployed [4] (fig. 1–4).

The non-fluoroscopic-guided SEMS placement technique can be performed with non-TTS (*through the scope*), also called the OTW (*over the wire*) technique, but also with the TTS technique. In these cases, the diameter of the working channel should be large enough to permit the passage of the stent-deploying device. For distal obstructions it is possible to assess the complete lesion with the endoscope, in some cases after balloon dilatation. After that, undeployed SEMS

Table 3. Complications related to colonic SEMS

	Intraprocedural	Early	Late
Malposition	+		
Bleeding	+	+	+
Perforation	+	+	
Failure to expand	+	+	
Migration		+	+
Occlusion by stool		+	+
Tumor ingrowth/overgrowth			+
Fecal incontinence			+
Death	+	+	+

is passed through stenosis and the endoscope is used for verification of the exact position of the distal SEMS end before and during deployment. *Through the scope* SEMS are preferred for proximal strictures. Once the SEMS passes through the endoscopic channel, the endoscope is positioned below the distal stricture margin during SEMS deployment [4].

A large number of dedicated colonic SEMS are currently available [8, 15, 16] (table 2). The ideal SEMS would be with a small diameter delivery system that is easy to insert through the colonoscope, flexible enough to conform curvatures and with a strong expansible force to expand to the caliber of the colon [17, 18].

Complications

Complications can be intraprocedural, early and late [4, 9]. Intraprocedural complications are SEMS migration, stool impaction, malposition, bleeding and perforation. The most devastating is free perforation because if it is not endoscopically managed it will inevitably result in diffuse peritonitis. Stent migration is generally distal and can be asymptomatic or may result in tenesmus or rectal bleeding. Late complications include stent migration, perforation and obstruction. Tumor ingrowth is the principal cause of late obstruction and can be treated by argon plasma coagulation, laser or restenting ('stent-in-stent') [9]. Patients with SEMS placed in the rectum may feel tenesmus, rectal pain or fecal incontinence if SEMS is placed <2 cm proximal to the upper end of anal canal. Meta-analyses have shown incidence rates for major complications like perforation, stent migration and reobstruction of 4, 11 and 7%, respectively [18, 19]. The most frequent complications are presented in table 3.

Outcomes

A large meta-analysis published in 2007 showed that SEMS insertion leads to reduction for stoma formation both in a palliative setting and in those where it is performed as 'bridge to surgery' [20]. The use of stents is associated with a significant reduction in hospital stay, mortality rate and medical complications. The use of SEMS has not been shown to adversely affect long-term survival in potentially curable lesions, while in the palliative group patients it leads to rapid symptom relief and less need of stoma formation in the terminal phase [20]. An older systematic review of all colorectal stent placements up to 2000 showed that stent placement prevented colostomy in 90% of cases [21]. In two recent papers published in 2008, European experience with uncovered woven nitinol stents (Ultraflex and Wallflex) was presented. In the first study, all 36 SEMS were used as a 'bridge to surgery' with technical success of 97% and clinical success of 81%. Complications were colonic perforation in 8.3%, bowel obstruction in 5.6% and stent migration in 2.8% [16]. In the second study, 42 SEMS were used in a variety of malignant colonic obstructions with a technical success of 93% and a clinical success of 95%. All 19 patients with operable tumors were bridged to surgery with success. Stent occlusion occurred in 9.6%, perforation in 2.4%, and migration in 2.4% [17].

Limitations

The limitations for colorectal stenting are technical and financial. Technical limitations include the inability to pass a guidewire through the stricture and some anatomic difficulties like angulated colon, but also clinically unsuccessful stent placement because of other unidentified sites of malignant obstruction [4]. Use of stents causes a significant reduction in total hospital stay compared to colostomized patients or when used as 'bridge to surgery', especially when postinterventional care is included in the calculations [8, 22, 23]. The main limitation in many hospitals is the lack of trained personnel needed for colonic stent insertion or personnel is not available outside of regular working hours [8, 19]. However, a study performed in 13 Spanish hospitals has shown that the procedure is feasible even in general endoscopic practice settings, without substantial differences in outcome as compared to specialized centers [24].

Controversies

Despite having being used for more than 10 years, several controversies remain unresolved. It is clear that SEMS is a viable alternative to colostomy for the palliative treatment of patients with inoperable colon cancers [18, 25]. The role of SEMS as a bridge to surgery is more controversial, because in most centers surgical decompression is still the preferred management of acute colonic obstruction. However, morbidity and mortality rates are significantly higher for colorectal surgery in emergency than for elective operations. A decision analysis study has shown that early placement of colonic stent is more effective than the traditional emergency surgery for treatment of patients with acute malignant obstruction [18]. Moreover, many patients are unable to undergo planned reversal of the colostomy because of age, comorbidities and other reasons, and thus remain with permanent stoma [8]. Some surgeons perform a one-stage resection with primary anastomosis, but this approach is associated with a high risk for complications [26]. An Italian study has shown that SEMS placement does not exclude laparoscopic resection as a second step and this approach offers a faster recovery [10]. Although there are no randomized trials about quality of life, it could be argued that SEMS placement may be better than a colostomy because of the burden associated with surgical recovery and learning to manage a stoma [22].

The effectiveness of covered stents for restricture prevention is another controversial question because of a higher rate of stent migration [22, 27]. In a recently published prospective study from Korea, covered and uncovered stents were similarly effective treatment for malignant colorectal obstruction according to the rates of clinical success, early migration and other early complications, but late stent migration was more common in the covered stent group [28]. Because of the development of many new agents for advanced colorectal disease the tumor-shrinking effect of chemotherapy can have an impact on stent patency, however further prospective randomized trials are needed [27]. Because of short life expectancy, palliative SEMS is a controversial issue in extrinsic malignant diseases. Although there several studies with results in this group of patients, recent research [5, 29] supports SEMS as a feasible option for such cases to avoid major surgery.

A recent study reports the first comparative analysis of different metal stents in the colon. Newer design TTS stents made of nitinol alloy had fewer major stent-related complications and thus less need for reinterventions. Prospective, randomized studies comparing different stent types will offer further insight into better designed SEMS for longer-term palliation of colon malignancies [17].

References

1 Adamsen S, Meisner S: Expandable metal stents for malignant colorectal obstruction. Tech Gastrointest Endosc 2001;3:103–107.

2 Dohmoto M: New method: endoscopic implantation of rectal stent in palliative treatment of malignant stenosis. Endosc Dig 1991;3:1507–1512.

3 Baron TH: Expandable metal stents for the treatment of cancerous obstruction of the gastrointestinal tract. N Engl J Med 2001;3441681–1687.

4 Baron TH, Harewood GC: Enteral self-expandable stents. Gastrointest Endosc 2003;58:421–433.

5 Shin SJ, Kim TI, Kim BC, Lee YC, Song SY, Kim WH: Clinical application of self-expandable metallic stent for treatment of colorectal obstruction caused by extrinsic invasive tumors. Dis Colon Rectum 2008; 51:578–583.

6 Deans GT, Krukowski ZH, Irwin ST: Malignant obstruction of the left colon. Br J Surg 1994;81:1270–1276.

7 Wang HS, Lin JK, Mou CJ, Lin TC, Chen WS, Jiang JK, Yang SH: Long-term prognosis of patients with obstructing carcinoma of the right colon. Am J Surg 2004;187:497–500.

8 Farrell JJ: Preoperative colonic stenting: how, when and why? Curr Opin Gastroenterol 2007;23:544–549.

9 Baron TH, Kozarek RA: Endoscopic stenting of colonic tumours. Best Pract Res Clin Gastroenterol 2004;18:209–229.

10 Stipa F, Pigazzi A, Bascone B, Cimitan A, Villotti G, Burza A, Vitale A: Management of obstructive colorectal cancer with endoscopic stenting followed by single-stage surgery: open or laparoscopic resection? Surg Endosc 2008;22:1477–1481.

11 Repici A, Reggio D, De Angelis C, Barleti C, Marchesa P, Musso A, et al: Covered metal stents for management of inoperable malignant colorectal strictures. Gastrointest Endosc 2000;52:735–740.

12 Abe T, Maetani I, Kakemura T, Fujinuma S, Sakai Y: Successful placement of self-expandable metallic stents for double colorectal cancers. Dig Endosc 2006;18:298–302.

13 Small AJ, Young-Fadok TM, Baron TH: Expandable metal stent placement for benign colorectal obstruction: outcomes for 23 cases. Surg Endosc 2008;22: 454–462.

14 Geiger TM, Miedema BW, Tsereteli Z, Sporn E, Thaler K: Stent placement for benign colonic stenosis: case report, review of literature and animal pilot data. Int J Colorectal Dis 2008;

15 Fregonese D, Naspetti R, Ferrer S, Gallego J, Costamagna G, Dumas R, et al: Ultraflex precision colonic stent placement as a bridge to surgery in patients with malignant colon obstruction. Gastrointest Endosc 2008;67:68–73.

16 Repici A, De Caro G, Luigiano C, Fabbri C, Pagano N, Preatoni P, et al: WallFlex colonic stent placament for management of malignant colonic obstruction: a prospective study at two centres. Gastrointest Endosc 2008;67:77–84.

17 Small AJ, Baron TH: Comparison of Wallstent and Ultraflex stents for palliation of malignant left-sided colon obstruction: a retrospective case-matched analysis. Gastrointest Endosc 2008;67:478–488.

18 Targownik LE, Spiegel BM, Sack J, Hines OJ, Dulai GS, Gralnek IM, Farrell JJ: Colonic stent vs. emergency surgery for management of acute left-sided malignant colonic obstruction: a decision analysis. Gastrointest Endosc 2004;60:865–874.

19 Sebastian S, Johnston S, Geoghegan T, Torreggiani W, Buckley M: Pooled analysis of the efficacy and safety of self-expanding metal stenting in malignant colorectal obstruction. Am J Gastroenterol 2004;99: 2051–2057.

20 Tilney HS, Lovergrove RE, Purkayastha S, Sains PS, Weston-Petrides GK, Darzi AW, et al: Comparison of colonic stenting and open surgery for malignant bowel obstruction. Surg Endosc 2007;21:225–233.

21 Khot UP, Lang AW, Murali K, Parker MC: Systematic review of the efficacy and safety of colorectal stents. Br J Surg 2002;89:1096–1102.

22 Saida Y, Nagao J, Nakamura YA, Nakamura YO, Katagiri M, Enomoto T, et al: Self-expandable metallic stent for patients with non-resectable malignant colorectal stricture: review of 102 cases in the Japanese literature. Digest Endosc 2007;19:59–64.

23 Vandervoort J, Tham TCK: Colonic stents for malignant obstruction-not a bridge too far. Gastrointest Endosc 2006;64:921–924.

24 Garcia-Cano J, Gonzales Huix F, Juzgado D, Igea F, Perez-Miranda M, Lopez-Roses L, et al: Use of self-expanding metal stents to treat malignant colorectal obstruction in general endoscopic practice. Gastrointest Endosc 2006:64:914–920.

25 Xinopoulos D, Dimitroulopoulos D, Theodosopoulos T, Tsamakidis K, Bitsakou G, Plataniotis G, et al: Stenting or stoma creation for patients with inoperable malignant colonic obstructions? Surg Endosc 2004;18:421–426.

26 Tan SG, Nambiar R, Rauff A, Ngoi SS, Goh HS: Primary resection and anastomosis in obstructed descending colon due to cancer. Arch Surg 1991; 126:748–751.

27 Im JP, Kim SG, Kang HW, Kim JS, Jung HC, Song IS: Clinical outcomes and patency of self-expanding metal stents in patients with malignant colorectal obstruction: a prospective single-center study. Int J Colorectal Dis 2008;23:789–794.

28 Lee KM, Shin SJ, Hwang JC, Cheong JY, Yoo BM, Lee KJ, et al: Comparison of uncovered stent with covered stent for treatment of malignant colorectal obstruction. Gastrointest Endosc 2007;66:931–936.

29 Caceres A, Zhou Q, Iasonos A, Gerdes H, Chi DS, Barakat RR: Colorectal stents for palliation of large bowel obstructions in recurrent gynaecologic cancer: an updated series. Gynecol Oncol 2008;108:482–485.

Davor Štimac, MD, PhD
Division of Gastroenterology, University Hospital Rijeka
Krešimirova 42, HR–51000 Rijeka (Croatia)
Tel. +385 51 658 122, Fax +385 51 658 826, E-Mail davor.stimac@ri.t-com.hr

Mönkemüller K, Wilcox CM, Muñoz-Navas M (eds): Interventional and Therapeutic Gastrointestinal Endoscopy.
Front Gastrointest Res. Basel, Karger, 2010, vol 27, pp 303–310

Endoscopic Retrograde Cholangiography

Todd H. Baron

Division of Gastroenterology and Hepatology, Mayo Clinic, Rochester, Minn., USA

Abstract

While endoscopic retrograde cholangiopancreatography has become almost exclusively a therapeutic procedure, obtaining high-quality cholangiograms is still an integral part of endoscopic retrograde cholangiopancreatography. Optimal methods of performing cholangiography include recognition of normal anatomy, complete opacification of ducts in some situations while minimizing contrast injection in other situations, avoiding introduction of air, removal of preexisting pneumobilia, and rotation of fluoroscopic images and/or patient position as needed. This chapter will describe the methods used to optimize endoscopic retrograde cholangiographic images.

Endoscopic retrograde cholangiopancreatography (ERCP) has shifted from a diagnostic procedure to a therapeutic procedure. Nonetheless, cholangiography and techniques to optimize the acquisition of cholangiographic images during ERCP is important so that appropriate decisions for intervention can be made. This chapter provides practical advice for performing optimal cholangiography.

Important First Step: Review Previous Imaging

The review of prior CT, MRCP, and operative or endoscopic cholangiograms often provides information. Being able to accurately determine, for example, the location of a stricture in reference to the hepatic bifurcation can sometimes be made much easier during ERCP if imaged on MRCP.

Prior to Injection of Contrast: Obtain Scout Radiographs

Scout radiographs are baseline images that are taken prior to the injection of contrast. These images allow documentation of indwelling devices present prior to the procedure and allow one to avoid confusion as to what abnormalities or radiographic findings were present prior to contrast injection. Baseline radiopacities that need to be identified prior to ERCP include pneumobilia, presence of surgical clips or contrast from recent CT scanning, rib calcifications, and pancreatic calcifications in the area of the distal bile duct. These scout radiographs are taken immediately prior to performing the procedure. Some recommend the images should be obtained without the endoscope and views of the entire abdomen be obtained. However,

1
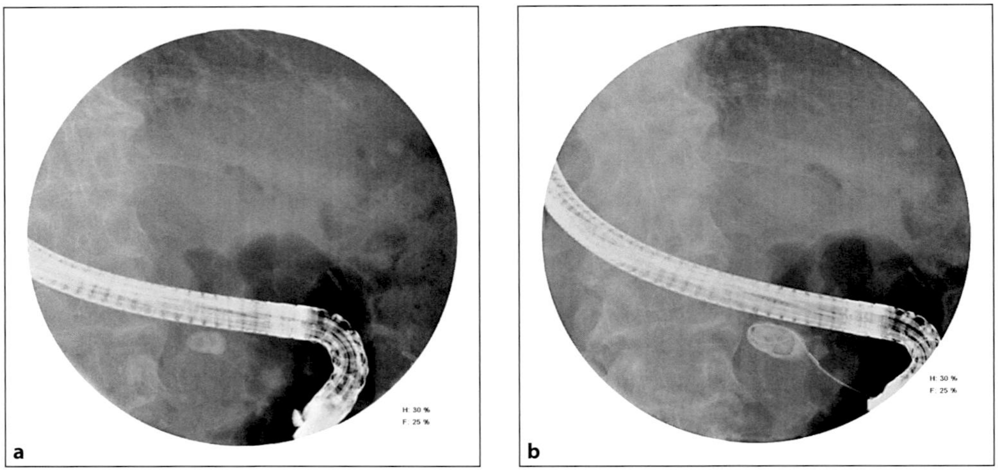

Fig. 1. **a** Scout radiograph taken prior to cholangiography in a patient with a distal common bile duct remnant following end-to-side hepaticojejunostomy. Note a solitary calcification below the endoscope. **b** After injection of contrast into distal CBD remnant. The filling defect is not seen in the distal CBD.

Fig. 2. Normal retrograde cholangiogram. Note small caliber bile duct with patent cystic duct.

Fig. 3. **a** Hilar cholangiocarcinoma. The bifurcation strictures are not well visualized with patient in the prone position. **b** After rotation of the patient into the supine position bifurcation strictures are well defined (arrows).

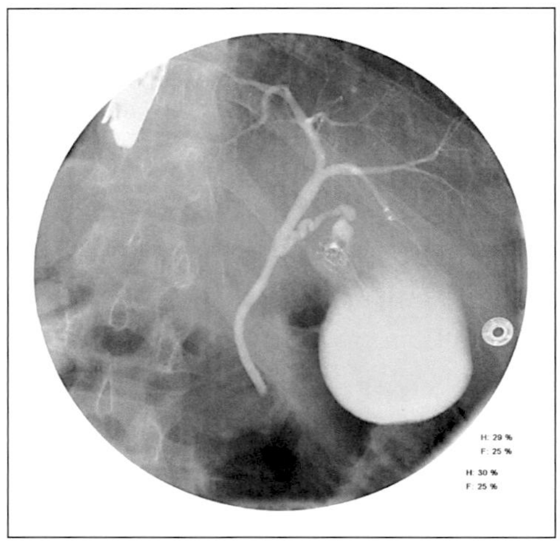

2

3
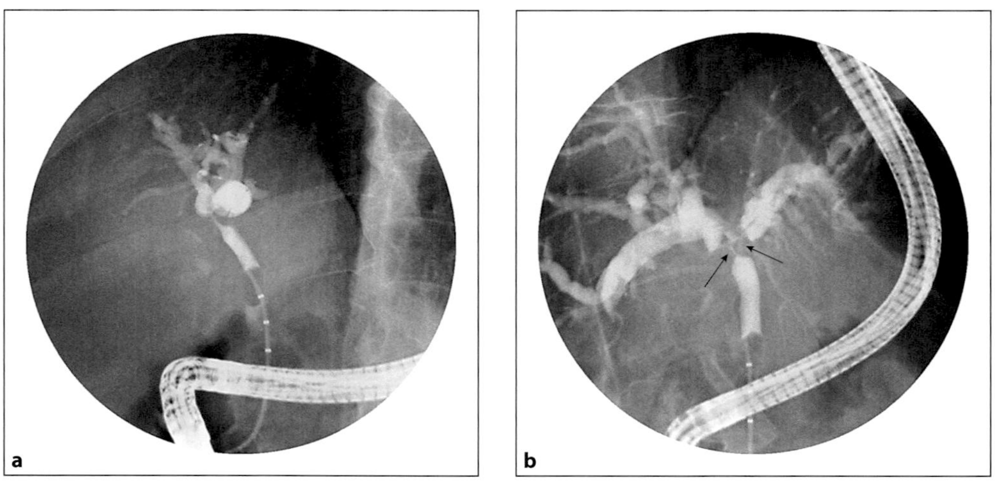

obtaining an image centered over the intended area of interest with the duodenoscope in position prior to cannulation allows a better reference when films are obtained when the procedure is performed (fig. 1a, b).

Prevention of Air Introduction

The presence of air in the bile duct can create filling defects that mimic stones. To ensure that air is not inadvertently introduced during injection, the assistant must flush the injection lumen of the catheter with contrast and be sure there is no air in the contrast syringe.

Understanding of Biliary Anatomy

In order to properly interpret cholangiography, one should be thoroughly familiar with normal hepatobiliary anatomy (fig. 2). This includes recognition of the common hepatic, cystic and common bile ducts on cholangiography. It is important to realize that proximal to the hepatic bifurcation, the right hepatic duct is formed by two main tributaries in the majority of patients – the right posterior and the right anterior hepatic ducts [1, 2]. The right posterior duct usually passes posteriorly to the anterior duct, joining it at the left medial side to form the right hepatic duct. The left hepatic duct is formed by smaller tributaries. In 16% of patients, however, the right posterior duct drains directly into the left hepatic duct proximally to the bifurcation, and in 12% of patients, the right anterior, right posterior, and left hepatic ducts form a 'triple confluence' at the common hepatic duct.

Fluoroscopic Imaging

Having a dedicated ERCP suite allows the endoscopists, radiology technicians, nurses, and support staff to become familiar with the imaging equipment. Optimal images are obtained with the aid of 180° rotatable C-arm which provides for a wide variety of fluoroscopic projection angles. The ability to rotate the fluoroscopy is helpful in defining ductal strictures, 'opening up' the bifurcation, rotating the cystic duct off the bile duct, and assessing takeoff of ductal systems since pathology can be missed when performing cholangiography in only one plane. Easy manipulation of magnification and rapid image sequence acquisition are possible with digital systems. In those instances where conventional, non-rotatable fluoroscopic tables are used, rotation of the patient can performed, when necessary to obtain optimal images. In some instances, this may involve rotating the patient into the supine position to better visualize the bifurcation (fig. 3a, b).

Contrast Strength

Most endoscopy units use full-strength, undiluted contrast, irrespective of the suspected underlying pathology. Diluted contrast can be helpful in identifying small stones, since very dense contrast can obscure the detection of small stones. However, full-strength contrast allows one to detect inadvertent pancreatography earlier and thus limit the volume injected and decrease the risk of pancreatitis.

Fig. 4. After passing catheter above the level of the cystic duct and into the intrahepatic system changes of intrahepatic PSC are seen (arrow).

Fig. 5. **a** Cholangiogram obtained for biliary obstruction. **b** After advancing the endoscope into the long position the stricture margins are better identified.

Fig. 6. **a** Suspected leak after recent cholecystectomy. Note surgical drain. Filling of the intrahepatic system is seen but a leak is not identified. **b** With increasing contrast injection under pressure a leak is identified (arrow).

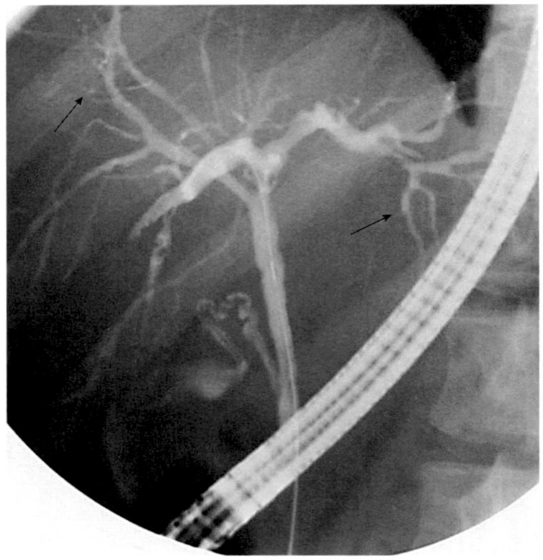

4

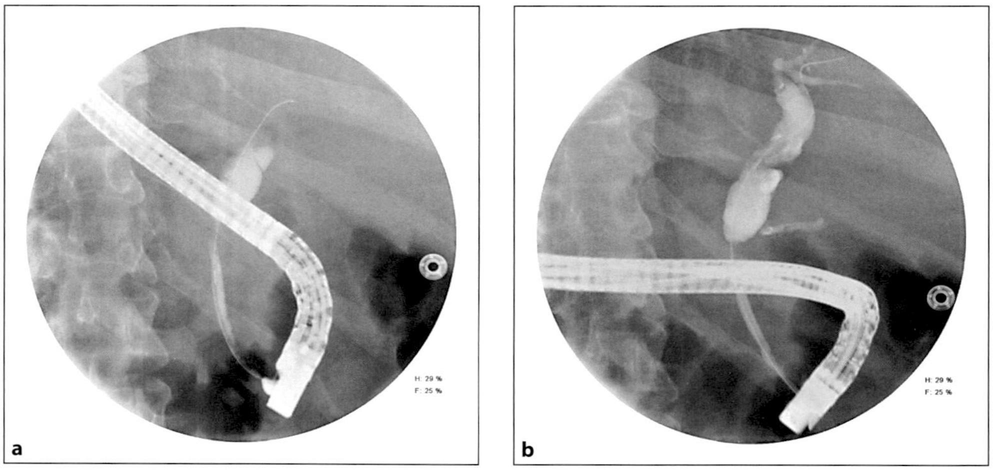

5 a b

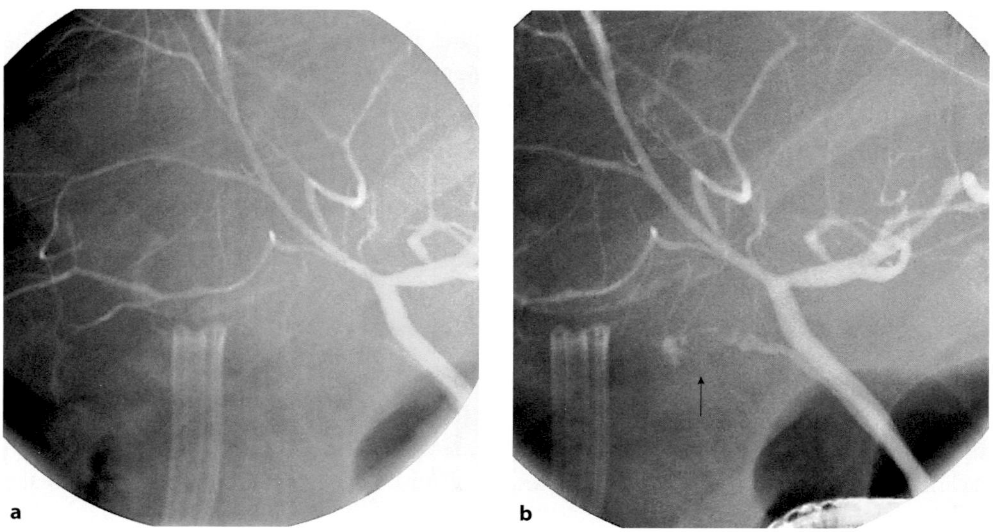

6 a b

Understanding the Effect of Patient Position on Contrast Distribution

When patients are in the prone or left lateral decubitus position during ERCP it is important to recognize that the left lobe of the liver as well as the caudate lobe, which are anatomically located anteriorly, are in the dependent position. As a result, the left lobe fills earlier and to a much greater degree than the right lobe. This has two ramifications: (1) If the right system is not visualized during cholangiography, one cannot imply or exclude underlying pathology. To adequately fill the right intrahepatic system often requires greater force to fill the branches of the right hepatic ducts in comparison with the left hepatic system. In the event that the right system needs to be visualized, a catheter can be passed deeply over a wire directly into the right intrahepatic system. Alternatively, an occlusion balloon can be inflated below the bifurcation but above the cystic duct (when the gallbladder is intact) to allow filling of the right intrahepatic system. (2) If the right system is seen initially without contrast seen in the left system, it may imply obstruction of the left system. Important pathology of the right system, such as subtle primary sclerosing cholangitis, can be easily overlooked unless appropriate filling of the intrahepatics has been achieved. Adequate filling is assured with delineation of the tertiary segments (fig. 4).

If adequate filling of the right system cannot be assured using the occlusion balloon, the patient can be placed supine or in the right lateral decubitus position, which allows preferential right-sided filling.

Obscuring of the Bile Duct with the Duodenoscope

Visualization of the entire distal common bile duct is not possible because the opaque duodenoscope passes between the bile duct and the x-ray beam. The duodenoscope can hide potential pathology, including malignant strictures. In order to visualize this area the duodenoscope should be advanced into the 'long position' so that the entire cholangiogram can be visualized and fluoroscopic images be obtained (fig. 5a, b). If the distal segment cannot be completely evaluated with the duodenoscope in the 'long position', withdrawing the duodenoscope into the stomach after contrast injection can be performed, though this results in loss of cannulation.

Obtain Early Injection Cholangiograms

The initial cholangiographic images prior to excessive contrast injection are among the most important, especially when evaluating the extrahepatic bile duct. During these first images, common bile duct stones are found in their 'undisturbed state' and are often most amenable to visualization. Once contrast has been injected under pressure into the bile duct, extrahepatic stones may flushed retrograde into the more proximal duct, where they can be more difficult to identify. In addition, small stones can be obscured by dense contrast unless early films are taken.

Likewise, early images of the bifurcation are also important, since with extensive filling of dilated intrahepatics above a hilar lesion can then overly and obscure the bifurcation.

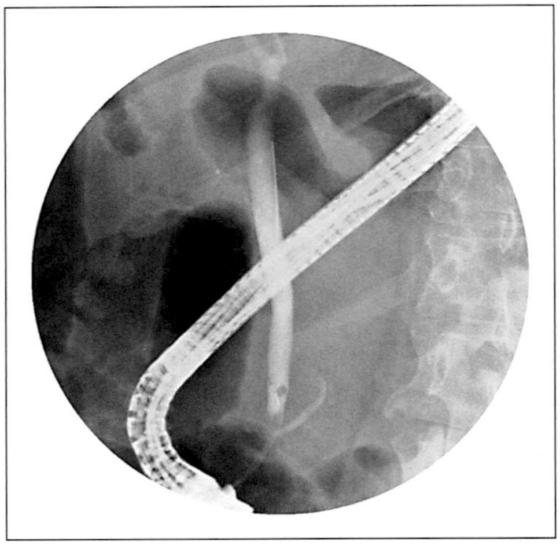

Fig. 7. Small filling defect in the distal bile duct. Features consistent with stone are that it is mildly oblong and not perfectly round and the catheter (adjacent) was aspirated and the filling defect remained.

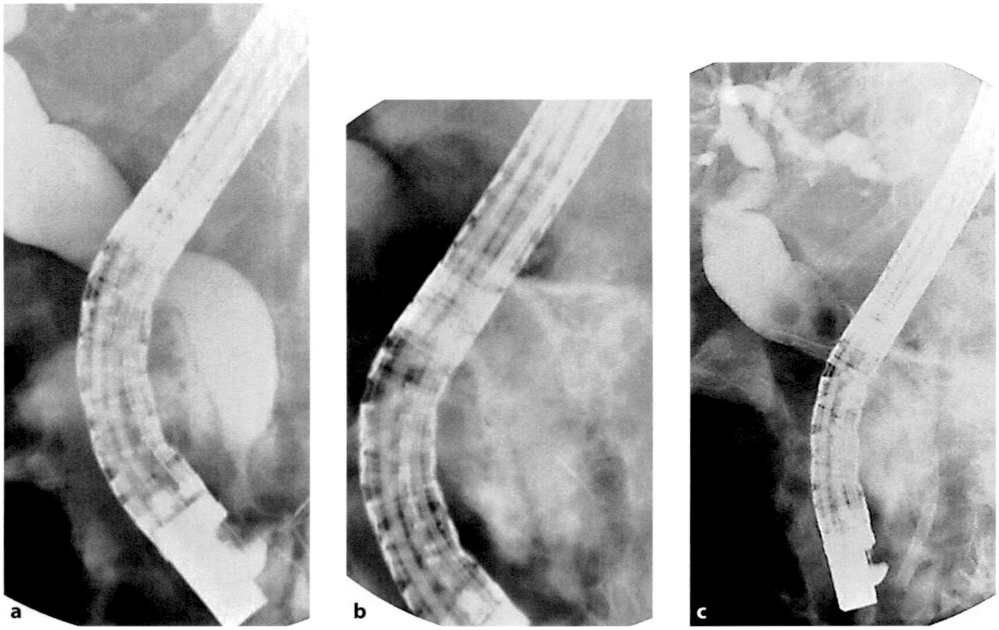

Fig. 8. a, **b** After biliary sphincterotomy the bile duct was initially recannulated with an occlusion balloon without the use of a guidewire. This resulted in false passage and extravasation of contrast. **c** A biliary stent was placed and prevented clinical manifestations of a bile leak.

Look for Intrahepatic Duct Leaks

The ducts of Luschka originate from the inferior right hepatic lobe and course along the gallbladder and usually empty into the extrahepatic common bile duct. They are the second most common site of postcholecystectomy bile leaks, and should be carefully evaluated when performing cholangiography for postoperative bile injury [3]. Since they originate from the right system, the leak is often seen draining in the region of the resected gallbladder fossa. These leaks can therefore be confused with leaks from the cystic duct remnant, which often drain in the same location. To minimize the chance of misdiagnosis, initial cholangiography of the right system can be performed with an occlusion balloon positioned just above cystic duct takeoff. This allows relative isolation of the right system, and allows one to target the ducts of Luschka.

Smaller bile leaks may not be identified until after contrast has been injected under pressure in the vicinity of the leak. Thus, in patients in whom there is a strong suspicion of intrahepatic duct leaks, advancing a catheter into the area of suspicion often allows the leak to be identified (fig. 6a, b).

Removal of Preexisting Pneumobilia

Pneumobilia is invariably present in patients with previous biliary sphincterotomy, biliary enteric anastomoses, and those patients undergoing ERCP immediately after removal of biliary stents. Air may interfere with cholangiographic interpretation. Therefore, in such patients, an occlusion balloon should be passed to just below the hepatic bifurcation. After inflation of the balloon, air is aspirated from the intrahepatics through the contrast or wire lumen port until bile is seen in the aspirating syringe. This maneuver should be performed prior to the installation of contrast to avoid further proximal displacement of air. Contrast is then injected as the occlusion balloon is withdrawn towards the distal duct to obtain images free from air.

Differentiating Air from Stones

Inadvertent injection of air cannot be avoided completely. Thus, in patients with round filling defects suspected of being air bubbles there are several ways to distinguish them from stones. One way is to elevate the head of the table which causes stones to move distally and air to move proximally within the bile duct. Secondly, air bubbles are almost always perfectly round whereas stones tend to be faceted (fig. 7). Air bubbles may change shape during time or break into smaller bubbles. Finally, placing a catheter alongside a bubble while aspirating will often cause bubbles to change shape or disappear while stones will remain constant in configuration.

Minimizing Contrast Injection in Selected Situations

In patients with malignant hilar biliary obstruction, adequate palliation can be achieved with unilateral drainage. Thus it is not necessary to fill both systems and when both systems are filled, both require drainage to avoid cholangitis. Unilateral drainage can be achieved by limiting contrast injection to the initial cannulation below the hepatic bifurcation. After a guidewire is passed into the intended intrahepatic system, contrast and stent placement are performed.

Another circumstance in which contrast should be limited is in the presence of purulent cholangitis so as to prevent sepsis since high-volume and high-pressure injection promotes bacteremia. Once the duct is decompressed with sphincterotomy and stone extraction a full cholangiogram can be obtained to ensure complete ductal clearance.

Recognition of Complications

A variety of complications can occur following ERCP. Recognition of these complications during cholangiography allows prompt treatment. For example, false passage of a catheter may result in localized perforation (fig. 8a–c).

Communicate with Radiology Colleagues

Recent publications have suggested that postprocedure interpretation of ERCP spot images by radiologists is not beneficial [4, 5]. However, radiology interpretation is still commonly performed. So that a consistent interpretation can be achieved between the endoscopist and radiologist it is important that the spot radiographs document in stepwise manner the procedure being performed. If therapeutic procedures are performed they should be clearly communicated to the radiologist interpreting the images. Our experience is that radiologists are most helpful when commenting on subtle changes of the secondary or tertiary segments when trying to distinguish between primary sclerosing cholangitis, cholangiocarcinoma and/or normal anatomic variants. Radiology interpretation seems to be less helpful when commenting on filling defects such as seen with choledocholithiasis.

Conclusion

These practical recommendations are aimed to assist endoscopists of all skill levels in order to optimize their ability to perform cholangiography. As MRCP increasingly replaces diagnostic ERCP, it is essential that endoscopists be able to obtain accurate, relevant cholangiograms.

References

1 Gazelle GS, Lee MJ, Mueller PR: Cholangiographic segmental anatomy of the liver. Radiographics 1994;14:1005–1013.

2 Yang WL, Zhang XC, Zhang DW, Tong BF: Diagnosis and surgical treatment of hepatic hilar cholangiocarcinoma. Hepatobiliary Pancreat Dis Int 2007;6:631–635.

3 Spanos CP, Syrakos T. Bile leaks from the duct of Luschka (subvesical duct): a review. Langenbecks Arch Surg 2006;391:441–447.

4 Khanna N, May G, Bass S, Cole M, Romagnuolo J: Postprocedural interpretation of endoscopic retrograde cholangiopancreatography by radiology. Can J Gastroenterol 2008;22:55–60.

5 Kucera S, Isenberg G, Chak A, et al. Postprocedure radiologist's interpretation of ERCP x-ray films: a prospective outcomes study. Gastrointest Endosc 2007;66:79–83.

Todd H. Baron, MD
Division of Gastroenterology and Hepatology, Mayo Clinic
200 First Street SW, Charlton 8A, Rochester, MN 55905 (USA)
Tel. +1 507 266 6931, Fax +1 507 266 3939, E-Mail baron.todd@mayo.edu

Mönkemüller K, Wilcox CM, Muñoz-Navas M (eds): Interventional and Therapeutic Gastrointestinal Endoscopy.
Front Gastrointest Res. Basel, Karger, 2010, vol 27, pp 311–318

Prevention of ERCP-Induced Pancreatitis

Gianpiero Manes

Department of Gastroenterology, University Hospital L. Sacco, Milan, Italy

Abstract

Among the various complications, pancreatitis represents both the most frequent and insidious complication of endoscopic retrograde cholangiopancreatography (ERCP). In about 25% of cases pancreatitis has a moderate/severe course and mortality is described. To reduce the occurrence of pancreatitis different strategies are usually adopted, from the identification of the different risk factors to the avoidance of risky procedures during ERCP, from the insertion of a pancreatic stent, to the administration of some drugs potentially able to interfere with its pathogenesis. Every attempt to reduce the occurrence of pancreatitis is a multistep process which starts before ERCP and continues during and immediately after the procedure. Exact knowledge of the mechanisms that are at the basis of the pathogenesis of post-ERCP pancreatitis is thus fundamental and should guide what the endoscopist does.

Endoscopic retrograde cholangiopancreatography (ERCP) is associated with the development of complications in about 5–10% of cases. Among the various complications, post-ERCP pancreatitis (PEP) represents both the most frequent and insidious complication [1]. Once PEP develops its course is largely unpredictable and may be only partly influenced by the available treatments. In 75% of cases PEP has a benign self-limiting course, but in the remaining 25% the course is moderate/severe and even mortality has been described [1]. Reducing the occurrence of PEP represents a primary problem for endoscopists who perform ERCP and different strategies are usually adopted to achieved this aim. These include the identification of different factors associated with the development of PEP, the administration of some drugs potentially able to interfere with the pathogenic mechanism of PEP at different levels, and attempts to reduce the use of dangerous maneuvers and use safe approaches during ERCP. Every attempt to reduce the occurrence of PEP is a multistep process which starts before ERCP and continues during and immediately after the procedure. The exact knowledge of the mechanisms that are at the basis of the pathogenesis of PEP is thus fundamental and should guide what the endoscopist does.

Pathogenesis of Post-ERCP Pancreatitis

Attempts to cannulate the papilla can cause trauma and edema, which may narrow the papillary orifice and create an obstacle to the flow of pancreatic juice. Moreover, injection pressure and the amount of contrast media in the pancreatic duct contribute to ductal epithelial or acinar injury. Contrast agents have been considered a possible cause of pancreas damage when injected into the pancreas, but new low osmolarity, non-ionic agents are unlikely to be in themselves toxic to the pancreas. Acinarization occurs when the volume injected into the pancreatic duct exceeds the ductal capacity. Increases in intraductal pressure and filling of side branches may result in leakage of pancreatic secretions into the circulation. Cannulation maneuvers can carry activated intestinal enzymes into the pancreatic duct which could promote autodigestion.

Once pancreatic enzymes have been inappropriately activated in the pancreatic cell and interstitium, the subsequent phases of PEP are common for different etiologies and include activation of the cytokine cascade which determines the possible evolution of the disease from a local event to a systemic disease with involvement of several other organs and systems, and development of local and systemic complications [2].

Attempts to prevent PEP have been oriented to each phase of its pathogenesis, from papillary trauma to different mediators of the systemic inflammatory response syndrome.

Pre-ERCP Phase

The only way to completely prevent PEP is to avoid the procedure. This is of course not possible but it is mandatory to try to perform ERCP only if absolutely indicated. With the availability of new accurate imaging procedures, such as magnetic resonance cholangiopancreatography and endoscopic ultrasound, ERCP should be used exclusively with therapeutic purpose. This refers particularly to patients with obscure abdominal pain also including patients with sphincter of Oddi dysfunction (SOD) who are at the highest risk of developing PEP [3].

Recognition of Patient-Related Risk Factors for PEP

The risk of developing PEP is increased in some individuals and may be correlated to some demographic, anatomic and pathologic factors. The risk of PEP is greater in young patients and women [4]. In patients with suspected SOD, the risk of developing PEP is 4-fold higher than in other individuals, and this risk is even higher [5] if the procedure is performed in young females with SOD. An history of previous acute pancreatitis, recurrent pancreatitis and PEP is also associated in most studies with an increased risk of PEP [4]. A thin, not dilated bile duct as well as normal bilirubin and cholestase serum levels have been described in some studies to represent an independent risk factor for pancreatitis [4]. We have recently demonstrated that a 'non-dilated' bile duct represents a risk factor for PEP and other post-ERCP complications when pre-cut is performed [6]. High-risk patients may develop PEP independent of the type of endoscopic procedure performed; moreover, the risk of pancreatitis escalates when multiple risk factors occur in the same patient or technique-related risk factors occur during the procedure.

When performing ERCP in patients with a potentially pre-procedure high risk of developing pancreatitis the correct indications should be accurately evaluated. When ERCP is clearly indicated, the high-risk patients should be informed about the specific risk of post-procedure pancreatitis and the potential measures to decrease risks. ERCP should be performed by the most expert endoscopist. Administration of pharmacologic prophylaxis (if you believe that it works) could be considered. Nevertheless, the most important factor is probably to try to perform ERCP in a safe way which means to limit the use of dangerous approaches during the procedure and to adopt different measures that are likely to reduce the occurrence of complications.

During ERCP

Dangerous Maneuvers: Procedure-Related Risk Factors
Several maneuvers performed during ERCP are likely to be associated with a higher risk of developing pancreatitis and other complications. This has two important implications: (1) every attempt should be made to reduce the use of traumatic procedures during ERCP, and (2) the real risk of developing pancreatitis can be assessed only at the end of ERCP, combining the different patient-related and procedure-related risk factors recognized for that patient.

Pancreatitis occurs more frequently after repeated attempts to cannulate the papilla and after repeated injection of contrast into the pancreatic duct and acinarization [7, 8]. Moderate-to-difficult cannulation is an independent risk factor of PEP in prospective, multicenter studies [4].

Balloon dilation of the papilla, a technique used to preserve the sphincter while removing stones, has been demonstrated to quadruple the risk of PEP in several controlled studies [9]. Pancreatitis occurs in about 15–16% of patients undergoing balloon dilation [9, 10]. We usually reserve balloon dilation only to special circumstances such as patients with coagulopathy when the risk of performing conventional sphincterotomy exceed that of balloon dilation.

Sphincter manometry is another *nonconventional* procedure which has been associated with a higher risk of PEP. Manometry is usually performed in patients with suspected SOD, a real risk factor for PEP [5], and this could lead to an overestimation of its role in the development of pancreatitis. The recent use either of the aspiration technique together with perfusion catheter or microtransducer non-perfusion catheters has significantly reduced the risk of developing PEP [11] so that the present opinion is that SOD and not manometry should be regarded as a risk factor. In SOD patients the suggestion is to avoid the use of simple perfusion catheters for sphincter manometry and to couple the procedure with pancreatic sphincterotomy or, better, pancreatic stent placement to reduce the risk of PEP [12].

Performance of biliary sphincterotomy has been advocated in the past as a possible cause of PEP. It is, however, difficult to evaluate whether pancreatitis has occurred as a consequence of sphincterotomy or of any maneuvers performed prior to cutting the papilla, i.e. any attempts to cannulate the papilla, or after cutting the papilla. Sphincterotomy can determine the development of PEP from inadvertent cutting of the pancreatic orifice or its edema. The coagulation current can cause edema of the pancreatic orifice. When correctly performed sphincterotomy is unlikely to represent a risk factor for PEP [4] and some authors empirically suggest that cutting the biliary sphincter may also reduce the pressure in the pancreatic duct and thus even reduce the occurrence of pancreatitis [13].

Precut access sphincterotomy is used when standard cannulation fails and several techniques have been developed. Use of precut is contentious. Several uncontrolled mainly retrospective studies suggest that precut is successful and safe when used for good indications by experienced endoscopists [14, 15]. However, There is, ample evidence arising mainly from large multicenter studies that precut is an independent risk factor for complications such as acute pancreatitis, hemorrhage and perforation, independentof the operator's skill [4, 5]. Some authors have suggested that precutting carries an increased risk of complications mainly because it is usually used as a last resort after many manipulations causing papillary trauma, repeated pancreatic injections of contrast and sometimes acinarization; 2 recent controlled randomized studies have demonstrated this concept [5, 16]. It should be emphasized that precut can be a safe procedure only when performed in large-volume centers by experienced endoscopists.

How to Perform Non-Traumatic Low-Risk ERCP

During cannulation, papillary trauma should be reduced to a minimum, although it is probably not completely avoidable. Gentle probing, soft manipulation of the papilla and use of appropriate instruments (soft, tapered tipped cannulas, sphincterotomes and hydrophilic wires) are advocated. Prolonged probing in an unsuccessful direction and repeated cannulation or injection of the pancreas should be avoided. Avoidance of blind contrast injection is suggested. Contrast should be injected only if sure of deep cannulation of the desired duct; alternatively, when probing for a duct, the injection should be gentle and minimal to avoid injury to the pancreas. Placement of a pancreatic guidewire or stent may assist biliary cannulation providing the correct orientation for biliary cannulation. Guidewire-assisted cannulation is associated with a significantly lower likelihood of PEP when compared to the standard cannulation technique [17]. According to our experience, use of hydrophilic or hydrophilic-tipped wires is particularly useful when approaching a difficult papilla, allowing cannulation in a non-traumatic way in the most cases. If cannulation is not achieved after proper attempts, the endoscopist must balance the need for deep cannulation and use of more aggressive techniques such as precutting against the possible provocation of complications. Also, consideration should be given to terminate non-urgently indicated procedures and to schedule a second ERCP which is found to be associated with a high success rate.

Pancreatic Stenting

According to several studies, pancreatic stenting probably represents the most effective way to prevent PEP [18]. Pancreatic stents maintain the flow of pancreatic juice in spite of either papillary or pancreatic trauma. Moreover, a pancreatic stent protects the pancreas from inadvertent cannulation and injection. Placement of a pancreatic stent requires a high level of expertise and attempts to cannulate the pancreas could by itself be a cause of complications. Because of this, pancreatic stent placement should be considered if pancreatic duct anatomy is suitable, appropriate equipment is available, and the endoscopist is familiar with the technique. Pancreatic stent placement should only be considered for higher risk patients, i.e. before or after sphincterotomy in SOD patients, in case of pancreatic sphincterotomy, papillectomy, manometry, sphincter balloon dilation, and pancreatic brushing. In case of difficult cannulation and/or repeated pancreatic injections or cannulations, pancreatic stenting could be indicated for several reasons: to reduce the risk of pancreatitis, to avoid inadvertent cannulation of the pancreas, and to provide correct orientation and protection of the pancreatic duct from injuries when performing precut sphincterotomy. When the endoscopist realizes that cannulation is difficult and the pancreatic duct is accessed first, we suggest stent placement early in the procedure.

The available pancreatic stents are different with regard to material, shape, and caliber (fig. 1). We usually use double-flanged 5-Fr pancreatic stents. Although also 7-Fr stents can be placed, authors usually suggest using small-caliber stents, 3–5 Fr, to minimize pancreatic ductal damage. As a further benefit, small caliber stents, usually without internal flanges, pass spontaneously into the duodenum and do not require endoscopic removal. The length of the stent should be chosen according to the pancreatic duct anatomy: We usually prefer >5- to 6-cm-long stents which are able to maintain a stable, straight position in the pancreas. Shorter stents, 2–3 cm long, are used if the pancreatic duct contour does not permit deep cannulation with a guidewire. In this case the presence of a inner flange is needed to avoid premature stent migration. The stent should generally be left in place for a minimum of 2–3 days and should be removed endoscopically within 2–3 weeks if spontaneous passage is not documented by a plain abdominal radiograph.

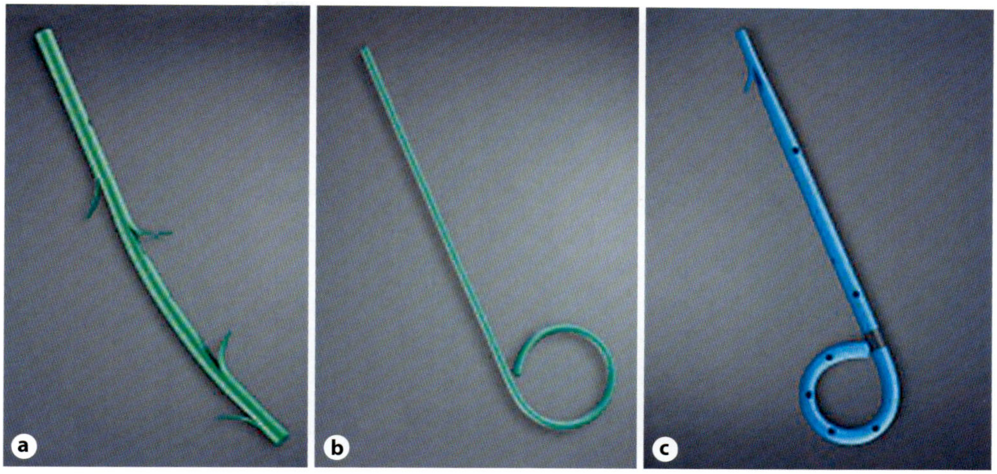

Fig. 1. Pancreatic stents of different design and shape. **a** Geenen double inner flanged polyethylene stent (Geenen pancreatic stent, Cook Endoscopy). **b** Zimmon unflanged polyethylene stent with duodenal pigtail to avoid inward migration (Zimmon pancreatic stent, Cook Endoscopy). **c** Zimmon single inner flanged polyethylene stent with duodenal pigtail (Zimmon pancreatic stent, Cook Endoscopy).

Post-ERCP Phase

We usually prescribe post-ERCP laboratory controls, amylasemia and blood count, about 4–6 h after the procedure. We also suggest fasting for the first 6–12 h both for inpatients and outpatients, although a recent study suggests that early refeeding is not detrimental [19]. Outpatients usually remain in the clinic under observation for at least 6 h before being discharged. Early laboratory testing would enable identification of those patients who need to be hospitalized. Decision to perform ERCP in an outpatient or inpatient setting depends mainly on the presumed pre-ERCP risk of complications. In case of a difficult and traumatic procedure patients remain under observation during the night.

Symptoms of PEP develop usually 4–12 h after the end of the procedure. Pain that appears in the first minutes or hours after the procedure is usually due to excessive air insufflation or perforation. It is important to recognize acute pancreatitis early and distinguish it from other possible complications, mainly perforation and hyperamylasemia. According to the consensus workshop [20], PEP is defined as an at least threefold increase in serum amylase after 24 h with typical pain and symptoms impressive enough to require admission to hospital (or extension of an existing admission). Hyperamylasemia is defined as any increase in amylase levels above the normal limit, without other symptoms. Abdominal pain is defined as a pain lasting more than 60 min not associated with a significant increase in amylase levels. Perforation can be suspected either during ERCP by demonstrating a leak of air or contrast in the retroperitoneal space or after the procedure when patients complain of pain. CT scan of abdomen is the technique to be performed to demonstrate retroperitoneal air.

The spectrum of severity and treatment of patients with PEP is the same as for spontaneous pancreatitis.

Table 1. Pharmacological prevention of post-ERCP pancreatitis: targeted mechanisms, drugs tested, and overall results

Mechanism	Drug	Efficacy	References
Sphincter spasm	Ca^{2+} blocker (nifedipine)	Ineffective	26, 27
	Nitroglycerine	Controversial	29, 30
	Topical lidocaine spray	Ineffective	28
Trypsin activation	Gabexate mesylate	Controversial	21–24
	Ulinastatin	Ineffective	31
Pancreatic secretion	Somatostatin	Controversial	32
	Octeotride	Ineffective	33
Inflammation and cytokine cascade	Corticosteroids	Ineffective	34
	Allopurinol	Ineffective	35
	IL-10	Ineffective	36
	Heparin	Ineffective	37
	NSAID (diclofenac, indomethacine)	Controversial	25
	MAPK inhibitor (semapimod)	Ineffective	38

MAPK = Mitogen-activated protein kinase; IL-10 = interleukin-10; NSAID = non-steroidal anti-inflammatory drug.

Pharmacological Prophylaxis of PEP

Pharmacological prevention of pancreatitis after ERCP has been studied extensively. Moreover PEP represents in ideal 'experimental model' of human acute pancreatitis which has been used to test new drugs in a way that resembles what is usually done in animal models, i.e. administration of the drug before pancreatitis induction. The list of tested drugs is long and the results disappointing: an ideal drug should be effective, cheap, and easy to administer before or immediately after ERCP. A large number of these drugs do not meet these prerequisites. Nevertheless, the vast majority of the performed studies present several biases, mainly with regard to sample size and selection criteria, i.e. the risk level for developing PEP (average-risk patients are usually enrolled in these studies), so that the available results may not be conclusive.

Table 1 reports the drugs that have been tested in the prophylaxis of PEP and are likely to act on the different mechanisms involved in the pathogenesis of PEP: relaxing the sphincter of Oddi, reducing pancreatic secretion, preventing the intra-acinar trypsinogen activation, and interrupting the inflammatory cascades. In spite of the large number of studies available, no drug can be regarded as absolutely effective in the prevention of PEP although data on gabexate and non-steroidal anti-inflammatory drugs (NSAIDs) are promising.

Gabexate mesylate is a synthetic broad-spectrum protease inhibitor. Its efficacy in preventing PEP has been demonstrated in previous studies [21, 22]. Nevertheless, it is not widely used since some reports have not confirmed its efficacy [23], it is not available in the USA, and administration at a dose of 500–1,000 mg in each patient may be costly and requires prolonged (6–12 h) infusion [21, 22]. Because of this, its generalized use may be unpractical and probably not justified in terms of cost-effectiveness. Based on these data administration of gabexate prior to ERCP in every patient undergoing the procedure is likely to be not useful since the majority of patients will not develop pancreatitis. In a recent controlled multicenter trial we have demonstrated that administration of gabexate immediately after the end of ERCP is as effective as pre-ERCP administration [24]. These data, which deserve further confirmation, offer a valuable opportunity to administer the drug only in high-risk patients, i.e. those patients who, at the end of ERCP, are judged by the endoscopist as being highly likely to develop PEP by combining the patient-related and procedure-related risk factors. The cascade of events triggered by ERCP that can lead to PEP is likely to take some hours to develop completely. This provides a therapeutic window of some hours for gabexate mesylate to work in ERCP. This would represent the theoretical basis for the efficacy of post-ERCP administration of the drug in reducing the incidence of pancreatitis. Administration of gabexate after ERCP to a very selected high-risk group of patients would result in an effective and cheap prophylaxis of PEP.

NSAIDs, namely diclofenac and indomethacin, represent another group of drugs which in the last years have been extensively tested in the prevention of PEP, administered both pre- and post-ERCP. Interest for these drugs has increased as they are very cheap and easy to administer. A recent meta-analysis concluded that the efficacy of prophylactic NSAIDs applies to both standard- and high-risk patients, with a similar relative risk reduction, while high-risk cases enjoy the greatest benefit. Meta-analysis showed that a single rectal dose of NSAID, either immediately before or after ERCP, tended to reduce the frequency and severity of PEP [25].

In our everyday activity we do not routinely use any pre-procedure administration of drugs unless the patient is presumed to have a high risk of pancreatitis before the procedure. We administer 500 mg gabexate over 6 h starting immediately after ERCP only in those patients who we recognize as being at high risk of developing pancreatitis according to the presence of a constellation of patient-related and procedure-related risk factors.

References

1 Freeman ML: Adverse outcome of ERCP. Gastrointest Endosc 2002;56(suppl):S273–S282.
2 Pandol SJ, Saluja AK, Imrie CW, et al: Acute pancreatitis: bench to bedside. Gastroenterology 2007; 132:1127–1151.
3 Cohen S, Bacon BR, Berlin IA, et al: National Institutes of Health State-of-the-Science Conference Statement: ERCP for diagnosis and therapy, 14–16 January. Gastrointest Endosc 2002;56:809.
4 Freeman ML, DiSario JA, Nelson DB, et al: Risk factors for post-ERCP pancreatitis: a prospective, multicenter study. Gastrointest Endosc 2001;54: 535–536.
5 Masci E, Mariani A, Curioni S, et al: Risk factors for pancreatitis following endoscopic retrograde cholangiopancreatography: a meta-analysis. Endoscopy 2003;35: 830–834.
6 Manes G, di Giorgio P, Repici A, et al: An analysis of the factors associated to the development of complications in patients undergoing precut sphincterotomy: a prospective, controlled, randomized, multicenter study. Am J Gastroenterol 2009 [Epub ahead of print].
7 Freeman ML, Guda NM: Prevention of post-ERCP pancreatitis: a comprehensive review. Gastrointest Endosc 2004;59:845–864.
8 Johnson GK, Geenen JE, Johnson P, et al: Evaluation of post-ERCP pancreatitis: potential causes noted during controlled study of different contrast media. Gastrointest Endosc 1997;46:217–222.
9 Freeman ML, DiSario JA, Nelson DB, et al: Risk factors for post-ERCP pancreatitis: a prospective, multicenter study. Gastrointest Endosc 2001;54:425–434.
10 Baron TH, Harewood GC: Endoscopic balloon dilation of the biliary sphincter compared to endoscopic biliary sphincterotomy for removal of common bile duct stones during ERCP: a metaanalysis of randomized, controlled trials. Am J Gastroenterol 2004; 99:1455–1460.
11 Sherman S, Troiano FP, Hawes RH, et al: Sphincter of Oddi manometry: decreased risk of clinical pancreatitis with use of a modified aspirating catheter. Gastrointest Endosc 1990;36:462–466.
12 Fogel EL, Eversman D, Jamidar P, et al: Sphincter of Oddi dysfunction: pancreaticobiliary sphincterotomy with pancreatic stent placement has a lower rate of pancreatitis than biliary sphincterotomy alone. Endoscopy 2002;34:280–285.
13 Akashi R, Kiyozumi T, Tanaka T, Sakurai K, Oda Y, Sagara K: Mechanism of pancreatitis caused by ERCP. Gastrointest Endosc 2002;55:50–54.

14 de Weerth A, Seitz U, Zhong Y, et al: Primary precutting versus conventional over-the-wire sphincterotomy for bile duct access: a prospective randomized study. Endoscopy 2006;38:1235–1240.
15 Tang SJ, Haber GB, Kortan P, et al: Precut papillotomy versus persistence in difficult biliary cannulation: a prospective randomized trial. Endoscopy 2005; 37:58–65.
16 Cennamo V, Fuccio L, Repici A, et al: Timing of precut procedure does not influence success rate and complications of ERCP procedure: a prospective randomized comparative study. Gastrointest Endosc. 2009;69:473–479.
17 Artifon ELA, Sakai P, Cunha JEM, et al: Guidewire cannulation reduces risk of post-ERCP pancreatitis and facilitates bile duct cannulation. Am J Gastroenterol 2007; 102:2147–2153.
18 Freeman ML: Pancreatic stents for prevention of post-endoscopic retrograde cholangiopancreatography pancreatitis. Clin Gastroenterol Hepatol 2007; 5:1354–1365.
19 Barthet M, Desieux A, Gasmi M, et al: Early refeeding after endoscopic biliary or pancreatic sphincterotomy: a randomized prospective study. Endoscopy 2002;34:546–550.
20 Cotton PB, Lehman G, Vennes J, et al: Endoscopic sphyncterotomy complications and their management: an attempt at consensus. Gastrointest Endosc 1991;37: 383–393.
21 Cavallini G, Tittobello A, Frulloni L, et al: Gabexate for the prevention of pancreatic damage related to endoscopic retrograde cholangiopancreatography. N Engl J Med 1996;335:919–923.
22 Masci E, Cavallini G, Mariani A, et al: Comparison of two dosing regimens of gabexate in the prophylaxis of post-ERCP pancreatitis. Am J Gastroenterol 2003;98:2182–2186.
23 Andriulli, A, Clemente R, Solmi L, et al: Gabexate or somatostatin administration before ERCP in patients at high risk for post-ERCP pancreatitis: a multicenter, placebo controlled, randomized clinical trial. Gastrointest Endosc 2002;56:488–495.
24 Manes G, Ardizzone S, Lombardi G, et al: Efficacy of postprocedure administration of gabexate mesylate in the prevention of post-ERCP pancreatitis: a randomized, controlled, multicenter study. Gastrointest Endosc 2007;65:982–987.
25 Elmunzer BJ, Waljee AK, Elta GH, et al: A metaanalysis of rectal NSAIDs in the prevention of post-ERCP pancreatitis. Gut 2008;57:1262–1267.
26 Prat F, Amaris J, Ducot B, Bocquentin M, et al: Nifedipine for prevention of post-ERCP pancreatitis: a prospective, double-blind randomized study. Gastrointest Endosc 2002;56:202–208.
27 Sand J, Nordback I: Prospective randomized trial of the effect of nifedipine on pancreatic irritation after endoscopic retrograde cholangiopancreatography. Digestion 1993;54:105–111.
28 Schwartz JJ, Lew RJ, Ahmad NA, et al: The effect of lidocaine sprayed on the major duodenal papilla on the frequency of post-ERCP pancreatitis. Gastrointest Endosc 2004;59:179–184.
29 Sudhindran S, Bromwich E, Edwards PR: Prospective randomized double-blind placebo-controlled trial of glyceryl trinitrate in endoscopic retrograde cholangiopancreatography-induced pancreatitis. Br J Surg 2001; 88:1178–1182.
30 Moreto M, Zaballa M, Casado I, et al: Transdermal glyceryl trinitrate for prevention of post-ERCP pancreatitis: A randomized double-blind trial. Gastrointest Endosc 2003;57:1–7.
31 Yoo JW, Ryu JK, Lee SH, et al: Preventive effects of ulinastatin on post-endoscopic retrograde cholangiopancreatography pancreatitis in high-risk patients. A prospective, randomized, placebo-controlled trial. Pancreas 2008; 37:366–370.
32 Andriulli A, Caruso N, Quitadamo M, et al: Antisecretory vs. antiproteasic drugs in the prevention of post-ERCP pancreatitis: the evidence-based medicine derived from a meta-analysis study. JOP 2003;4:41–48.
33 Testoni PA, Lella F, Bagnolo F, et al: Long-term prophylactic administration of octreotide reduces the rise in serum amylase after endoscopic procedures on Vater's papilla. Pancreas 1996;13:61–65.
34 De Palma GD, Catanzano C: Use of corticosteriods in the prevention of post-ERCP pancreatitis: results of a controlled prospective study. Am J Gastroenterol 1999; 94:982–985.
35 Zheng M, Chen Y, Bai J, et al: Meta-analysis of prophylactic allopurinol use in post-endoscopic retrograde cholangiopancreatography pancreatitis. Pancreas 2008;37: 247Y253.
36 Rongione AJ, Kusske AM, Kwan K, et al: Interleukin 10 reduces the severity of acute pancreatitis in rats. Gastroenterology 1997;112:960–967.
37 Rabenstein T, Fischer B, Wiessner V, et al: Low-molecular-weight heparin does not prevent acute post-ERCP pancreatitis. Gastrointest Endosc 2004; 59:606–613.
38 van Westerloo DJ, Rauws EA, Hommes D, et al: Pre-ERCP infusion of semapimod, a mitogen-activated protein kinases inhibitor, lowers post-ERCP hyperamylasemia but not pancreatitis incidence. Gastrointest Endosc 2008; 68:246–254.

Gianpiero Manes
Divisione e Cattedra di Gastroenterologia, Ospedale Universitario L. Sacco
Via G. B. Grassi 74
IT–20157 Milan (Italy)
Tel. +39 02 39042207, Fax +39 02 39042337, E-Mail gimanes@tin.it

Mönkemüller K, Wilcox CM, Muñoz-Navas M (eds): Interventional and Therapeutic Gastrointestinal Endoscopy.
Front Gastrointest Res. Basel, Karger, 2010, vol 27, pp 319–327

Biliary Sphincterotomy Techniques

Gianpiero Manes

Department of Gastroenterology, University Hospital L. Sacco, Milan, Italy

Abstract

Biliary endoscopic sphinterotomy, which consists in opening the terminal part of the common bile duct by cutting the papilla, is performed whenever a therapeutic procedure is needed on the biliary tree and can also represent itself as a treatment. Since its first description, sphincterotomy has not significantly changed, although both the techniques and the instruments, the so-called sphincterotome or papillotome, have progressively improved. The usual approach to cut the papilla involves deep insertion of the sphinctero-tome into the bile duct followed by electrocautery to incise the sphincter. A correct position of the catheter in the papilla as well as appropriate selection of the cutting current are determinant factors to reduce the rate of complications. Appropriate selection of the patients prior to performing ERCP, mainly in terms of coagulation parameters, is also crucial. Acute pancreatitis, perforation and bleeding represent the main complications of ERCP. In some cases, sphincterotomy may itself be the cause of such complications.

Biliary endoscopic sphinterotomy (ES) consists in opening the terminal part of the common bile duct by cutting the papilla and the distal portion of the sphincter of Oddi (SOD). ES is the pre-requisite to perform several therapeutic maneuvers on the biliary tree such as stone extraction, stenting, biliary drainage by nasoductal catheter, and brushing. Although small stones may be removed after a simple balloon dilation of the papilla and small caliber stents (7–8.5 Fr) can be introduced without previous sphincterotomy, ES is in general performed whenever a therapeutic procedure is performed on the biliary tree. ES can also represent itself as a treatment when performed in patients with papillary stenosis or SOD dysfunction.

Procedural Aspects

Patient Preparation

Since sphincterotomy is performed as a part of ERCP, preparation of the patient in terms of informed consent, sedation, antibiotic prophylaxis, and pancreatitis prophylaxis is that of ERCP and are treated in another chapter of the book. As a cut is performed, particularly relevant is the evaluation of the coagulation parameters. Patients should have a full blood count and prothrombin time or international normalized ratio performed no more than 72 h prior to the procedure [1]. ES can be safely performed on patients taking aspirin and NSAIDs. In patients on anticoagulant therapy, discontinuation of therapy can be decided on the basis of the level of thromboembolism risk. Anticoagulant can be safely substituted with low-dose heparin or unfractioned intravenous heparin which do not represent a contraindication to ES. Data on newer antiplatelet therapies (such as clopidogrel) are unavailable, but at present it is recommended that, wherever possible, they should be discontinued 7–10 days prior to ES [1]. Abnormal clotting, variously defined as a platelet count <50,000 IU/l and prolonged prothrombin time, defined as an international normalized ratio >1.5, may be associated to an increased hemorrhage risk, but it is difficult to define the point at which abnormal clotting becomes an absolute contraindication to ES [1, 2]. If the patients have a critical deranged clotting, subsequent management should be performed according to the current guidelines prior to performing ERCP.

Sphincterotome

From its first description in 1973, ES has not significantly changed and also the catheters used to cut the papilla, although progressively improved, did not change substantially. The ES catheter, the so-called sphincterotome or papillotome, consists of an outer Teflon catheter of 6–7 Fr that contains a thin steel wire which exits the catheter about 3 cm before the distal end and re-enters it about 3–5 mm from the tip. The tip of the catheter without the wire is called 'nose'. It is usually tapered, sometimes with a dome shape (Cook), a caliber ranging from 3.5–5.5 Fr, and facilitates introduction into the duct system. The exposed wire functions as a cautery knife when high-frequency electrosurgical current is applied (fig. 1). The other end of the wire is insulated and connected to the electrosurgical unit.

The earliest catheters had a single lumen which allowed injection of contrast in the duct, although the contrast could leak around the port for the wire. The more recently developed sphincterotomes have two or three lumen to allow both injection of contrast and passage of a guidewire (independently in the triple lumen catheters) so that they can be used not only to cut the papilla but also to cannulate it, inject contrast, and place a guidewire into the duct. A number of different sphincterotomes with different designs and shapes are today available on the market (fig. 1): the length of the nose can vary from 0 to 30 mm: a longer nose should usually offers a more stable position in the bile duct while cutting, but is likely to make the cannulation more difficult. The length of the wire can vary from 2 to 3.5 cm: sphincterotomes with longer wires (3–3.5 cm) are usually more flexible, are more easily oriented when used to cannulate the papilla and tend to remain in a neutral position when tightened; the disadvantage is the necessity to put the tip of the endoscope away from the papilla when performing ES to avoid contact of the wire with the elevator. Catheters with shorter wires tend to be stiffer, to displace from the bile duct when tightened, and to determine excess tension on the roof of the papilla while cutting. We usually prefer a sphincterotome with a 5-Fr dome tip, a nose of 5 mm, and a wire of 2.5 cm. Other changes of the basic structure of the sphincterotome have been proposed: the Clever Cut sphincterotome from Olympus has half the length of the cutting wire coated with insulation so that an incision can be made without the cutting wire penetrating too deep into the bile duct by using the coated portion as a guide.

Cutting Technique

The usual approach to cut the papilla involves deep insertion of the sphincterotome into the bile duct followed by electrocautery to incise the sphincter. ES cannot be performed if deep cannulation of the bile duct has not been previously achieved. The sphincterotome can be used itself to cannulate the papilla and to inject contrast in the duct and, due to the possibility to bend the tip

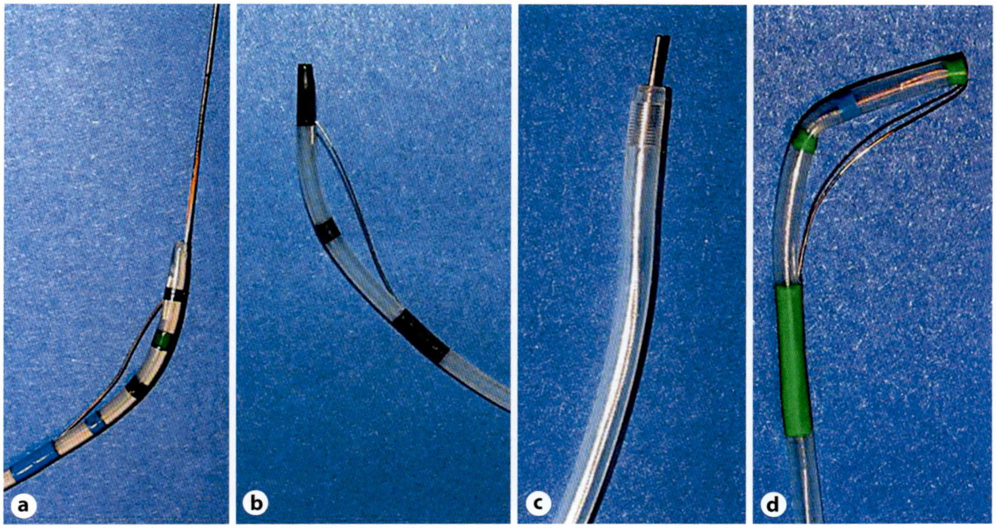

Fig. 1. Sphincterotomes of different designs and shapes. **a** Double-lumen, dome-tip, sphincterotome (FS-OMNI, Cook – the nose is 5 mm long and the wire 2.5 cm long) with Tracer Metro 0.35-inch wire (Cook) inside. **b** Thin sphincterotome with 4-Fr nose (Mini-Tome, Cook – the nose is 5 mm long and the wire 2 cm long). **c** Needle-knife precut sphincterotome (Olympus). **d** Noseless single lumen sphincterotome (Olympus).

of the catheter toward the axis of the bile duct, the cannulation process is likely to be easier than with conventional catheters. Alternatively, the sphincterotome, usually a dual or triple lumen, can be introduced over a guidewire inserted through a standard cannula into the bile duct to establish a path across the papillary orifice. If the bile duct cannot be cannulated, the papilla can be dissected with the use of a variety of techniques known altogether as 'precut sphincterotomy'. Precut is an 'access' sphincterotomy and has been described in another section of the book.

Once the sphincterotome has been deeply introduced into the bile duct and the correct position has been confirmed either by injecting contrast or by fluoroscopy, it is progressively retracted until approximately one half to two thirds of the wire is exposed outside the papilla (fig. 2). At this point the sphincterotome is gently bent to establish a contact between the wire and the papillary roof and short bursts of current are applied. The cutting of the papilla should be oriented to the 11-o'clock direction and it is achieved by exerting a slight torsion of the endoscope in the anticlockwise direction (fig. 2). The papilla is usually cut in a stepwise manner. Whitening of the mucosa indicates that the current is passing and the cut has begun (fig. 2).

A gush of bile usually indicates that the sphincter has been cut. The limit of a safe ES is the upper limit of the intraduodenal portion of the common bile duct which can be defined either by the presence of a transverse fold (fig. 2d) or by the impression of the bile duct on the duodenal wall. Extraction of large stones usually needs such a large incision. For stent insertion a smaller sphinterotomy (up to 1 cm) may be enough and it could reduce the risk of complications. The most sphincterotomies have usually an extension of 1.5–2 cm. The extent of the ES should be decided on the basis of ERCP indication as well as characteristics either of the papilla, mainly dimension and shape, or of the bile duct (a shorter cut for narrow ducts). Another factor influencing the decision to perform a shorter cut is the presence of a juxtapapillary diverticulum.

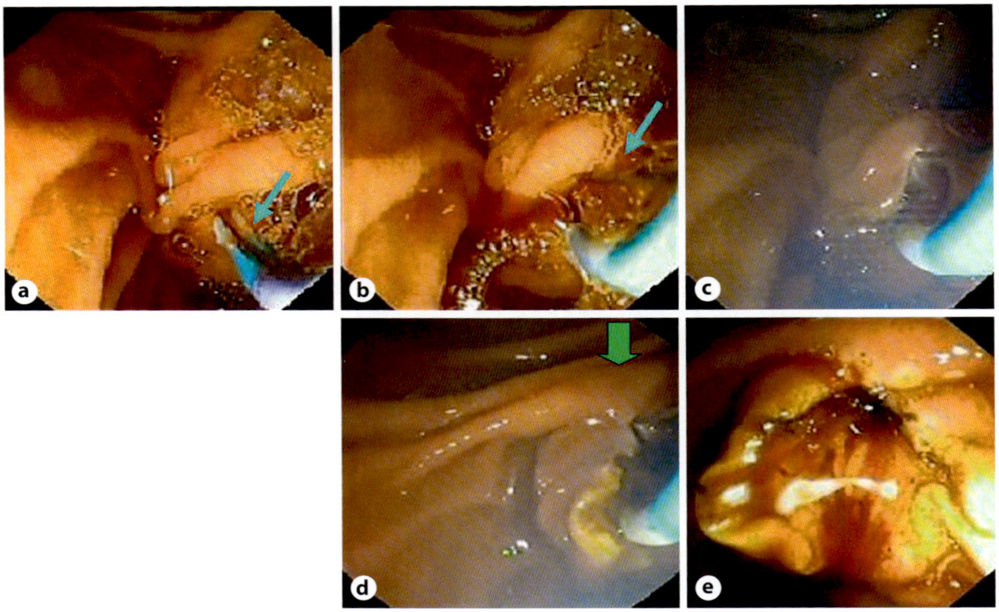

Fig. 2. **a** The sphincterotome is introduced in the biliary duct with half of the wire (arrow) exposed outside the papilla. **b** The sphincterotome is bent to establish a contact between the wire (arrow) and the roof of the papilla. **c** The papilla is cut in a stepwise manner. Whitening of the mucosa indicates that the current is passing. **d** The cutting is performed in the 11-o'clock direction until the transverse fold (arrow). **e** A gush of bile indicates that the sphincter has been cut.

Electrosurgical Unit

A diathermy unit suitable for ERCP should be able to develop pure cutting and coagulation current, as well as blended current. Several different diathermy units are available on the market. The power setting varies depending on the energy output of individual units. Pure cutting and blended (cutting and coagulation) are both usually used to perform ES according to the endoscopist's experience, clinical indications, and conditions of the patient. The unit that we usually use in our daily endoscopic activity is the Erbotom ICC 200 from ERBE (ERBE Elektromedizin, Tübingen, Germany) in the Endocut modality.

Tricks for a Good Sphincterotomy

A Good Orientation. ES should be performed in the 11-o'clock direction and in any case in the 'safety zone' between 11- and 1-o'clock (fig. 2). A deviated cut is likely to be related to an increased risk of complications such as bleeding, pancreatitis, and perforation. Most sphincterotomes tend to deviate to the right when the wire is tightened (fig. 3) which can result in a deviated cut or even in a displacement of the catheter from the duct. A catheter with a long nose maintains a more stable position in the bile duct; a catheter with a long cut wire tends to remain in a neutral position when tightened. With double or triple lumen sphincterotomes, a guidewire can be introduced in the bile duct and may serve to anchor and stabilize the sphincterotome during the cut. In some cases a displaced papilla makes it impossible to maintain the optimal axis during the cut (fig. 3). Pushing the scope into a long position may, in some cases, helps the endoscopist in obtaining an acceptable cutting axis. In some other cases a possible solution could be to cut

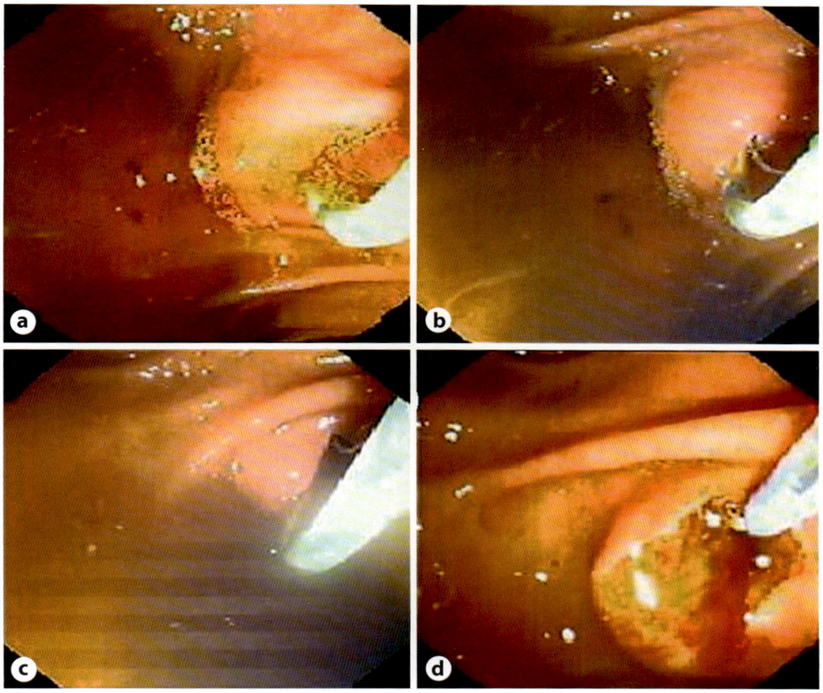

Fig. 3. a During sphincterotomy the sphincterotome tends to deviate to the right in the 1-o'clock direction. **b** A gentle torsion of the tip of the endoscope in the anticlockwise direction allows to maintain the optimal axis during the cut. **c** The result is a correct cut in the 11-o'clock direction.

the papilla while the cutting wire is not tightened but overrelaxed to form a loop on its left side which can be more easily oriented in the 11-o'clock position (fig. 4).

A Good Cutting. The contact between the wire and the tissue is determinant for the quality of the cut. An optimal contact is usually achieved when the wire is outside the papilla for one half to one third of its length. Either too little or tot much wire in contact with the tissue may produce an ineffective cut. In this case the passage of current within the wire is not followed within a few second by a whitening of the tissue. Similarly, the tension of the wire while tightening is important to determine a good and safe cut. Excess tension of the wire should be avoided to prevent an uncontrolled 'zipper cut' which could result in a perforation. Gentle movements of the elevator as well as an anticlockwise torsion of the scope may be needed during ES to maintain at the same time the right orientation of the cut and the optimal contact of the wire with the papilla.

The Best Current. ES is based on the passage of high-frequency alternating current through a poorly conductive medium, such as ampullary tissue, thereby generating heat and resulting in cutting and/or coagulation of tissue. Different types of electrosurgical current can induce different types and degrees of thermal tissue injury. ES is a technically challenging and potentially dangerous procedure and has been reported to be an independent risk factor for the development of bleeding, perforation, and post-ERCP pancreatitis.

When used during ES, pure current provides better tissue-cutting capability, whereas low-voltage coagulating current achieves better hemostasis. Pure coagulative current is never used for ES. A third form of electrosurgical current, known as mixed current, combines patterns of both pure and coagulating currents and is popular for ES. Mixed current is available in two varieties: 'blended' current, where both cutting and coagulating currents are delivered together in one waveform, and 'Endocut' current (ERBE Elektromedizin, Tübingen, Germany), where the cutting and coagulating currents are interspersed and applied one after another in short bursts, with an intermittent pause, thus achieving both effects of cutting and coagulating, similar to that achieved with blended current. Although blended and Endocut currents use different patterns for combining cutting and coagulating waveforms during ES, this difference is only of theoretical significance [3]. At the present time, there is no consensus on which type of current, used in the context of ES, is optimal with regard to maximizing safety, although some suggest that pure current may be associated to an higher rate of hemorrhage and blended current to acute pancreatitis (due to ampullary edema) [4]. In a recent meta-analysis, the incidence of post-ES pancreatitis was similar in patients undergoing ES either with pure or mixed electrosurgical current. Patients who underwent ES with pure current experienced significantly more frequent episodes of post-ES bleeding, without an accompanying increase in morbidity or mortality [5]. According to these data, we suggest that patients at high risk of bleeding should be considered for mixed current during ES and, conversely, for those at risk of developing pancreatitis pure cut should be preferred current. It has also been suggested to use a sequential combination of pure cut and blended current to reduce the risk of bleeding without increasing that of pancreatitis [6], but these data have never been confirmed by other studies so that today's state-of-the-art is that use of both pure cutting and blended current is correct provided that the operator has experience with the one or the other method.

Sphincterotomy in Patients with Distorted Anatomy

Billroth II Anatomy. In the Billroth II gastrectomy the papilla has an upside-down orientation since the afferent loop is approached by the endoscope in an antiperistaltic fashion. It means that the bile duct is oriented at 5-o'clock instead of at 11-o'clock. Conventional sphincterotomes are not suitable to perform ES in these patients since they tend to point away from the bile duct's axis and to cut the posterior wall of the duodenum instead of the roof of the papilla. The Billroth II sphincterotome consists of a catheter with a cutting wire that has a convex shape oriented at 5-o'clock when pushed out from the sheath (fig. 5). When the wire is retracted, the catheter tip is straightened and oriented in the bile duct axis and can be used to cannulate the papilla. The cut is performed in progressive steps pushing the catheter against the papilla (push sphincterotomy).

Maintaining the correct orientation of the Billroth II sphincterotome while cutting the papilla is considered difficult by several authors who prefer to introduce in the bile duct a small caliber stent that provides a correct orientation for the cut using a needle-knife sphincterotome. The endoscopist then performs a cut over the cannula emerging from the papilla in the axis and direction of the bile duct with a technique that resembles that of the precut ES. The stent would also have the function of protecting the pancreatic duct from injury.

Juxtapapillary Diverticula. Juxtapapillary diverticula are frequent findings in elderly occurring in 9–32% of ERCP [7]. The papilla can be located within the diverticulum or along its outer rim, on the left or the right side. The presence of a juxtapapillary diverticulum may represent a problem for the endoscopist since the papilla cannot be seen or can be difficult to cannulate due to a distortion in its anatomy and course. With regard to ES, it has been suggested that the diverticulum may be associated to an increased risk of bleeding [8, 9] and may be a possible contributor to perforations [10], but some studies do not support this hypothesis [7, 11]. Once the papilla has been cannulated

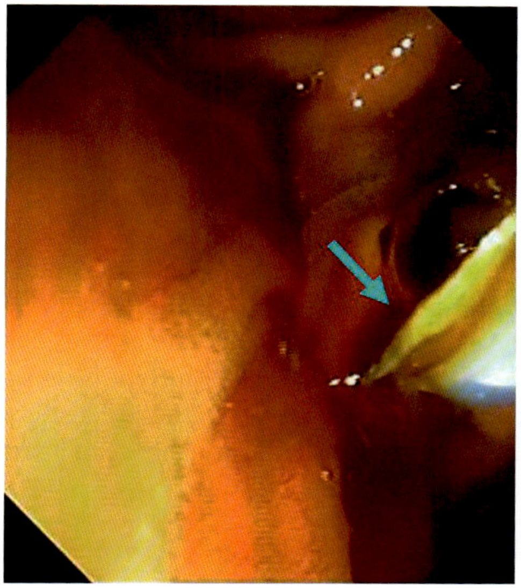

4

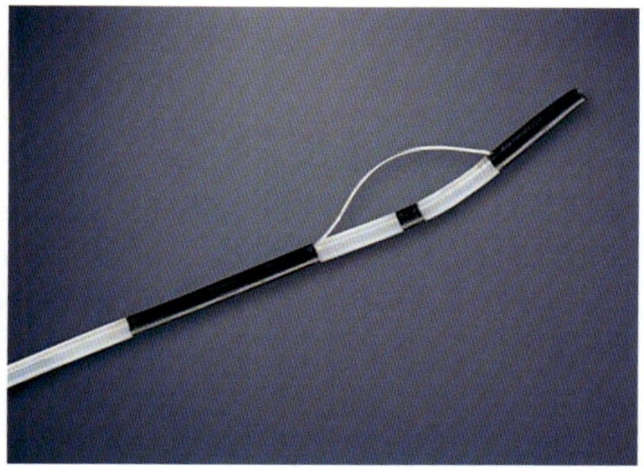

5

Fig. 4. To maintain a correct direction of the cut, the cutting wire is not tightened but overrelaxed to form a loop on the left side that is easily oriented in the 11-o'clock direction (arrow). **Fig. 5.** Billroth II sphincterotome with a 2-cm long wire (Cook).

with the help of one of the several techniques proposed (see in another section of the book), the crucial step for a safe and effective ES is to precisely demarcate the intramural segment and proper direction of the bile duct, which are endoscopically observable cephalad to the papilla. This anatomic landmark is not always endoscopically evident in some patients with a periampullary diverticulum and this could explain the potentially increased risk of perforation. Although in the most cases ES can be successfully performed in the conventional fashion, some techniques have been proposed to help in cutting the papilla within a diverticulum. This involves the introduction in the bile duct, once the papilla has been partly cut, of a retrieval balloon catheter that is inflated and then pulled toward the duodenal lumen to indicate the residual intramural segment of the duct [12]. Another technique consists in cutting the papilla using a sphincterotome with an inflated balloon at the tip (Stonetome, Microvasive) which bulges the intramural tract of the bile duct [13]. According to our experience, ES can be effectively and safely performed in the most papillas in the presence of a diverticulum. It is important to direct the catheter in the 11-o'clock position by opportunely withdrawing the endoscope in some cases (usually when the papilla is located on the floor of a large diverticulum) or pushing the scope into a long position in some other cases (to avoid contact with the cutting wire on the outer rim of the diverticulum). Another way of reducing the risk of cutting the rim of the diverticulum while performing ES is that of using a catheter with the proximal half length of the cutting wire coated with insulation (Clever Cut, Olympus).

Complications of Sphincterotomy

Biliary ES is performed during ERCP, and ERCP can be associated to the development of complications in each step of its performance, from the introduction of the endoscope in the duodenum to the cannulation of the papilla, from the sphincterotomy to the introduction of stents or other devices in the biliary tract. It is thus difficult to evaluate for each possible complication, especially for acute pancreatitis, if it has occurred as a consequence of ES or of any maneuvers performed prior to cut the papilla, i.e. the several attempts to cannulate the papilla, or after the papilla cutting. The three main complications potentially associated to ES are acute pancreatitis, bleeding and perforation.

Acute Pancreatitis

Acute pancreatitis is most often determined by repeated cannulation or injection of contrast in the pancreas which usually occurs in the cannulation process. ES can determine the development of pancreatitis from inadvertent cutting of the pancreatic orifice or its edema. Coagulation current can cause edema of the pancreatic orifice. Selection of appropriate current is thus fundamental to avoid pancreatitis (see above). Insertion of a thin stent (3-Fr) in the pancreatic duct which ensures an appropriate pancreatic drainage is likely to reduce the occurrence of pancreatitis [14, 15].

Bleeding

Bleeding is a typical complication of ES which occurs in 2–5% of cases [2]. It is defined as the clinical (not endoscopic) evidence of bleeding (hematemesis or melena) with a decrease of at least 2 g/dl in hemoglobin concentration, or need for blood transfusion [16]. Deviated cut, large ES, and coagulopathy are factors associated to the development of bleeding. Bleeding can develop immediately after ES or in the 10 days following the procedure [2, 17, 18]. The development of bleeding during the procedure is frequent and usually self-limiting or easily treated endoscopically. The above-reported definition does not consider as complication the bleeding that occurs while cutting the papilla; it has however been recognized as a risk factor for a further bleeding [2]. Bleeding can usually be controlled endoscopically by inflating a balloon in the papilla, application of pure coagulation current, injection of 1/10,000 diluted epinephrine around the incision, or by placement of one or more hemoclips. Injection of epinephrine and coagulation current could theoretically produce edema in the pancreatic orifice which may determine acute pancreatitis. In a minority of cases, usually when bleeding results from cutting a branch of the retroduodenal artery (usually because of an aberrant branch or a deviated cut), the bleeding can be massive and may require emergency surgery or embolization.

Perforation

Perforation is a rare complication which occurs in less than 1% of cases [11, 17, 18]. The 'conventional' ES is a rare cause of perforation, mainly following a deviated, excessive, or zipper cutting. Perforation is likely to occur more frequently after precut (see the corresponding chapter). Peripapillary diverticula [9, 10], small papilla, narrow bile duct, and Billroth II anatomy are all suspected to be associated to an increased risk of perforation during sphinterotomy. Some perforations develop during the insertion of the endoscope in the duodenum and during its straitening. While ES may result in a retroperitoneal perforation, introduction of the endoscope usually produces a bowel-wall perforation. Perforation can be suspected either during ERCP by demonstrating a leak of air or of contrast in the retroperitoneal space or after the procedure when patients complain of pain. CT scan of abdomen is the technique to be performed to demonstrate retroperitoneal air. Most retroperitoneal perforation can be managed conservatively by the placement of a nasobiliary drainage, systemic antibiotics, nasogastric suction and parenteral nutrition. Development of sign of peritonitis should be an absolute indication to surgery.

References

1 Williams EJ, Green J, Beckingham I, Parks R, Martin D, Lombard M: Guidelines on the management of common bile duct stones. Gut 2008;57;1004–1021.

2 Ferreira LE, Baron TH: Post-sphincterotomy bleeding: who, what, when, and how. Am J Gastroenterol 2007; 102:2850–2858.

3 Kohler A, Maier M, Benz C, et al: A new HF current generator with automatically controlled system (Endocut mode) for endoscopic sphincterotomy: preliminary experience. Endoscopy 1998;30:351–355.

4 Stefanidis G, Karamanolis G, Viazis N, et al: A comparative study of postendoscopic sphincterotomy complications with various types of electrosurgical current in patients with choledocholithiasis. Gastrointest Endosc 2003;57:192–197.

5 Verma D, Kapadia A, Adler DG: Pure versus mixed electrosurgical current for endoscopic biliary sphincterotomy: a meta-analysis of adverse outcomes. Gastrointest Endosc 2007;66:283–290.

6 Gorelick A, Cannon M, Chey W, et al: First cut then blend: an electrocautery technique affecting bleeding at sphincterotomy. Endoscopy 2001;33:976–980.

7 Panteris V, Vezakis A, Filippou G, et al: Influence of juxtapapillary diverticula on the success or difficulty of cannulation and complication rate. Gastrointest Endosc 2008;68:903–910.

8 Zoepf T, Zoepf DS, Arnold JC, et al: The relationship between juxtapapillary duodenal diverticula and disorders of the biliopancreatic system: analysis of 350 patients. Gastrointest Endosc 2001;54:56–61.

9 Boender J, Nix GA, de Ridder MA, et al: Endoscopic papillotomy for common bile duct stones: factors influencing the complication rate. Endoscopy 1994; 26:209–216.

10 Chapman RW: Complications of ERCP. British Society of Gastroenterology Website.

11 Loperfido S, Angelini G, Benedetti G, et al: Major early complications from diagnostic and therapeutic ERCP: a prospective multicenter study. Gastrointest Endosc 1998; 48:1–10.

12 Park DH, Park SH, Kim HJ, et al: A novel method for estimating the safe margin and the adequate direction of endoscopic biliary sphincterotomy in choledocholithiasis with complications. Gastrointest Endosc 2006;64:979–983.

13 Furukawa K, Harada T, Aoyagi Y: Successful endoscopic sphincterotomy using a papillotome tipped with a balloon for cases of choledocholithiasis complicated by duodenal diverticula. Am J Gastroenterol 2001;96:3215–3216.

14 Smithline A, Silverman W, Rogers D, et al: Effect of prophylactic main pancreatic duct stenting on the incidence of biliary endoscopic sphincterotomy-induced pancreatitis in high-risk patients. Gastrointest Endosc 1993;39: 652–657.

15 Singh P, Das A, Isenberg G, et al: Does prophylactic pancreatic stent placement reduce the risk of post-ERCP acute pancreatitis? A meta-analysis of controlled trials. Gastrointest Endosc 2004;60:544–550.

16 Cotton PB, Lehman G, Vennes J, et al: Endoscopic sphincterotomy complications and their management: an attempt at consensus. Gastrointest Endosc 1991;37: 383–393.

17 Freeman ML, Nelson DB, Sherman S: Complication of endoscopic biliary sphincterotomy. N Engl J Med 1996; 335:909–918.

18 Wang P, Li ZS, Liu F: Risk factors for ERCP-related complications: a prospective multicenter study. Am J Gastroenterol 2009;104:31–40.

Gianpiero Manes
Divisione e Cattedra di Gastroenterologia, Ospedale Universitario L. Sacco
Via G.B. Grassi 74, IT–20157 Milano (Italy)
Tel +39 02 39042207, Fax +39 02 39042337, E-Mail gimanes@tin.it

Mönkemüller K, Wilcox CM, Muñoz-Navas M (eds): Interventional and Therapeutic Gastrointestinal Endoscopy.
Front Gastrointest Res. Basel, Karger, 2010, vol 27, pp 328–336

ERCP Cannulation Using Precut Techniques

Nathan J. Shores · John Baillie

Hepatobiliary and Pancreatic Disorders Service, Section on Gastroenterology, Wake Forest University Baptist Medical Center, Winston-Salem, N.C., USA

Abstract

With the emergence of endoscopic ultrasound and magnetic resonance retrograde cholangiopancreatography for the non-invasive diagnosis of hepatobiliary and pancreatic (HBP) disease, ERCP has evolved into a predominantly therapeutic technique. Failed bile duct or pancreatic duct cannulation may result in persistent patient morbidity and the need for more invasive procedures (e.g. biliary surgery and/or percutaneous biliary drainage). So-called needle knife pre-cut (NKP) biliary and pancreatic sphincterotomy has emerged as a useful technique when standard cannulation proves difficult. Multiple small retrospective studies – and handful of prospective reports – suggest that in expert hands, NKP is a safe and effective means of achieving therapeutic cannulation. NKP should only be performed by skilled endoscopists with supervised training in the procedure, a detailed knowledge of HBP anatomy, a thorough understanding of the physics of electrosurgery and the ability to place protective (prophylactic) pancreatic duct stents. Various techniques of 'free-hand' NKP are described, as well as trans-sphincteric papillotomy (the Goff technique). Pre-NKP preparation requires careful attention to coagulation issues, and post-NKP patients need to be monitored for complications including pancreatitis, bleeding, perforation and sepsis. After failed NKP in the setting of biliary obstruction, the patient must remain on broad-spectrum antibiotic coverage and a decision made regarding the urgency of biliary drainage. If this cannot wait at least 2—3 days for the NKP site to mature, the patient should be referred for urgent percutaneous biliary drainage or surgery.

Precutting is the term given to electrocautery-based techniques for accessing the bile duct and pancreatic duct when standard papillotomy ('sphincterotomy') fails or is undesirable. This review will focus mainly on so-called 'free-hand' needle-knife papillotomy (NKP), whereby a bare wire exiting from a plastic catheter is used to apply electrical energy of high intensity in short increments to cut open the duodenal papilla. A number of specialized papillotomes to perform papillotomy when deep access to the desired duct is unavailable have been tried and largely abandoned over the years. Perhaps the best known is the 'shark-fin' device, whose tip is inserted into the orifice of the papilla and the cutting wire – shaped like a shark's dorsal fin – pressed against the suprapapillary fold and electrocautery applied. Precutting 'free hand' has traditionally been associated with increased risk of post-ERCP complications, including bleeding, perforation and pancreatitis. In a large, prospective, multicenter study of ERCP complications, precutting was associated with a 15% post-ERCP pancreatitis (PEP) rate, which was 50% greater than seen for standard sphincterotomy (9.8%) [1]. However, other experts have reported no increase in complication rate using NKP compared to standard sphinctertomy technique [2, 3]. Experience is an important determinant of success when using a needle knife (NK); it also has a bearing on the complication rate. In inexperienced hands, the NK can be a dangerous weapon. An understanding of the ductal anatomy as it relates to the duodenal papilla, and the electrical properties of the NK, are essential for safe application of precutting techniques. In the current era of excellent cross-sectional abdominal imaging (e.g. computed tomography, magnetic resonance imaging), the vast majority of ERCPs are done for therapy: the only truly 'diagnostic' ERCP procedure left is sphincter of Oddi manometry, and even that is often followed by prophylactic pancreatic duct stenting, whether or not sphincterotomy is being performed [4]. Precut papillotomy for biliary access should not be used for purely diagnostic reasons when a less invasive test (e.g. endoscopic ultrasound (EUS)) can provide the same information with less or no morbidity. Precutting into a non-dilated bile duct is technically difficult and prone to failure and complications. Precutting can be justified for therapeutic access to remove bile duct sludge or stones, 'open' a choledochocele, and provide access for stenting of benign and malignant strictures, especially when they are causing obstructive jaundice ± cholangitis. Precutting over a previously placed pancreatic stent is a good (safe) way to perform both major and minor pancreatic sphincterotomy. Free-hand NK techniques can also be used for accessing pancreatic pseudocysts and even necrotic debris in necrotizing pancreatitis, but these techniques are for experts only and beyond the scope of this review. The authors strongly recommend structured, supervised experience of NKP under an experienced mentor before it is attempted unsupervised.

Procedural Aspects

The patient is prepared for ERCP in the usual fashion. If precutting is being considered, attention should be paid to the patient's coagulation status. As precutting is typically all – or mostly – 'cut' and very little 'coag(ulation)', regardless of the electrical generator setting, bleeding is more likely if the patient is therapeutically anticoagulated with Coumadin (warfarin) or receiving antiplatelet therapy with clopridogel (Plavix™). Updated guidelines in preparation by the American Society for Gastrointestinal Endoscopy (ASGE) suggest that aspirin (ASA) and non-steroidal anti-inflammatory drugs (NSAIDs) need not be discontinued for electrocautery procedures, as they are not associated with increased risk of hemodynamically significant bleeding. A variety of NK papillotomes are available from the major equipment manufacturers. Typically, the authors connect these catheters to the ERBE™ generator (ERBE USA, Marietta, Ga., USA) and use standard electrocautery settings for NKP. Due to the rapidity of cut that occurs with this technique, using blended current with the ERBE™ generator does not guarantee the application of significant cautery. That being the case, we typically use the NK papillotome on the pure 'cutting' current setting. As with all electrocautery, the patient must have a grounding pad placed, preferably some distance anatomically from where current will be applied. Patients with cardiac pacemakers and automated implantable cardiac defibrillators need to have the settings of these devices altered if electocautery is used. Typically, these setting changes are made using a magnet held over the implanted device.

Current Density

It is important for the endoscopist to understand the concept of current density as it applies to the NK papillotome. The amount of energy applied to the tissue is inversely proportional to the square of the length of the wire in contact, and the cube of the area. So, the smaller the area of contact, the greater the energy applied. This renders the NK a very powerful weapon! Literally, it cuts like a hot knife through butter. Pressure should *never* be applied when using a NK. One of the great exponents of NKP, Prof. Kees Huibregtse of the University of Amsterdam, compared NK technique to using a paint brush: applying the NK with light strokes is an excellent strategy for avoiding complications.

Techniques

The commonest use for the NK is deroofing the papillary fold to expose the bile duct when standard cannulation techniques fail. There is ongoing debate regarding the 'best' approach: the three principal techniques are cutting cephalad (upward) from the papillary orifice, cutting caudad (downward) from a more proximal incision, and direct puncture of the duct ('fistulotomy'). Although fistulotomy is most direct approach to the bile duct, it is potentially the most risky, especially if the bile duct is not dilated. In general, the more dilated the bile duct, the easier it is to access by direct puncture. However, fistulotomy is a technique that requires considerable experience to ensure safety. The margin for error is measured in millimeters. Puncture of the posterior wall of the bile duct results in retroperitoneal leakage of bile. The author prefers the technique of cutting cephalad from the papillary orifice after it has been protected by a plastic stent inserted into the pancreatic duct. The cut should be kept within the 11- to 1-o'clock arc that is recommended for standard papillotomy. There is often some bleeding from the incision, this typically settles with a few minutes' observation and gentle washing. Although there are no hard data to support the practice, the author likes to use dilute epinephrine solution for washing; this seems to contain capillary oozing. With practice, the cylindrical bile duct can be dissected out and exposed through the papillotomy incision (fig. 1, 2a, b). This structure has a reflective, silvery 'mother-of-pearl' appearance. A small incision in the anterior wall of the bile duct will usually be rewarded with a drop or two of bile. This orifice can then be cannulated with a standard papillotome and guidewire, and the opening extended using normal sphincterotomy technique (fig. 3). If the bile duct is not exposed by this approach, it is tempting to dig deeper to find it. This is almost always a mistake. If the bile duct cannot be safely accessed by initial efforts, the safe response is to abort the procedure and come back another day. Three to seven days later the papillotomy site will have matured, and not infrequently the endoscopist is greeted by an obvious opening with bile exiting from it. If not, the post-papillotomy anatomy is usually easier to 'read' than immediately after the procedure. Second (and rarely subsequent) procedures to complete NKP are frequently successful. If the clinical situation requires it (e.g. acute cholangitis), failed biliary access by NKP may need to be followed quickly by percutaneous transhepatic cholangiography and drain placement. When available, EUS may be very useful for identifying favorable sites for bile duct puncture. The EUS endoscopist can mark a site for NK puncture, or proceed to directly puncture the bile duct using a standard EUS needle (e.g. 19-Fr gauge), through which a guidewire can be advanced. Special care must be taken when using the NK to incise an ampullary tumor, or pancreatic cancer fungating through the duodenal wall, as these are typically quite vascular. Tumors often distort the ductal anatomy, and targeting the bile duct often relies more on experience than visual cues. Using the NK in the vicinity of a periampullary diverticulum (fig. 4) also requires special care, as extension of the cut into the diverticulum will cause a free perforation.

Pancreatic sphincterotomy can be performed easily and safely by cutting down on to a previously placed pancreatic stent (fig. 5). The stent should be left in place after the procedure to

1
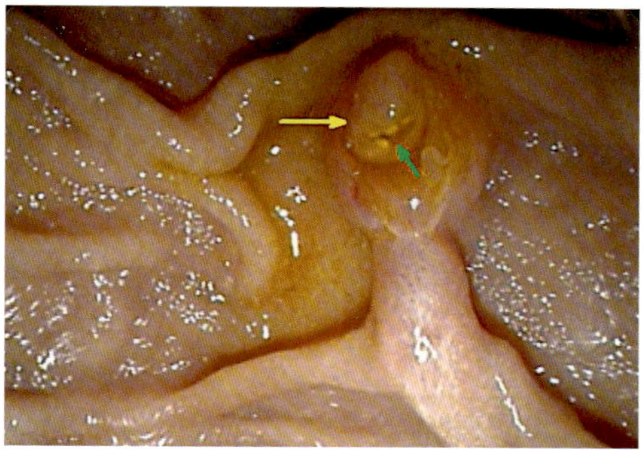

2
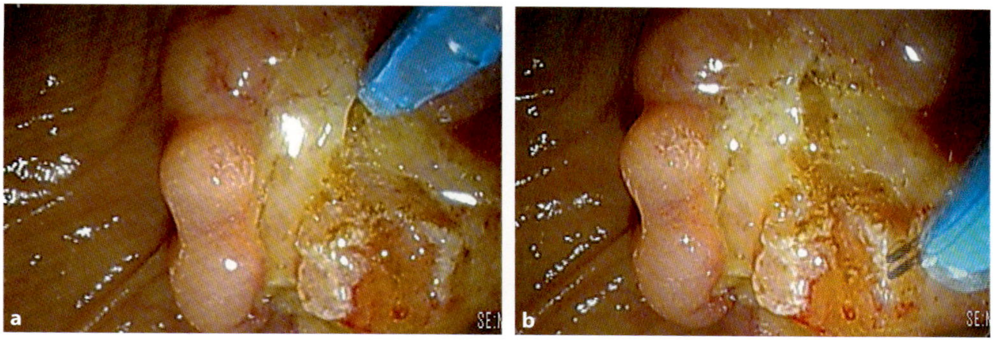

3
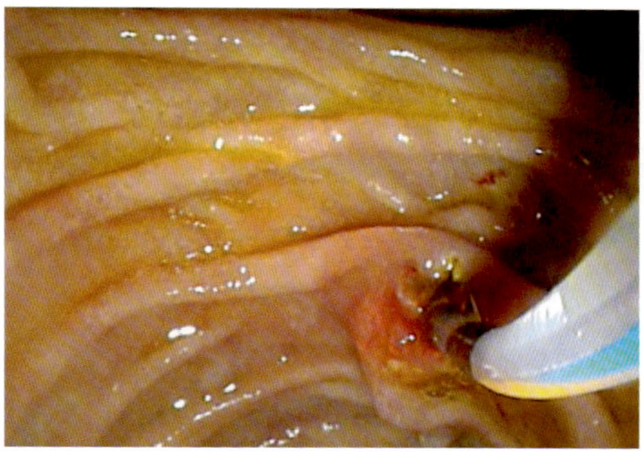

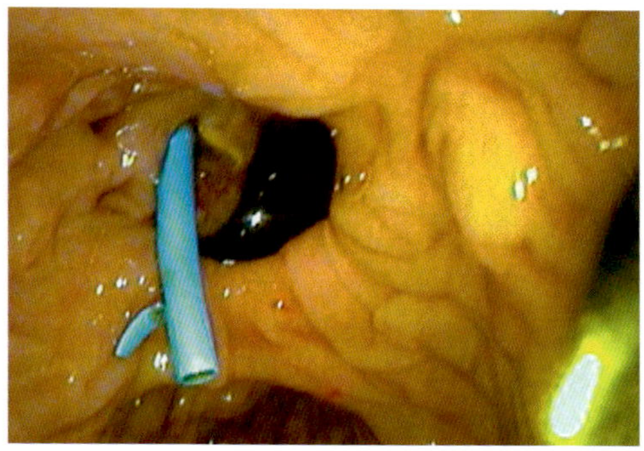
4

Fig. 1. Duodenal papilla after precut. Yellow arrow indicates bulging cystic structure (bile duct). A tiny incision (green arrow) has been made in its wall, which can be accessed using a guidewire and extended with a standard papillotome. **Fig. 2. a, b** NKP of an ampullary tumor. The glistening, mother-of-pearl bile duct wall has been exposed by a superficial incision, then a vertical cut made into the anterior bile duct wall for access. **Fig. 3.** Extension of a NKP using a standard (pull) papillotome. **Fig. 4.** NKP performed over a stent within a periampullary diverticulum.

minimize the risk of PEP. The author likes to use a single-pigtail, single-flanged, 5-Fr pancreatic stent, which will typically migrate spontaneously within a few days. Cutting up though the septum from within the pancreatic duct to achieve both biliary and pancreatic sphincterotomy (the so-called Goff technique) [5] can be done with a NK (fig. 6), but in the author's experience this is achieved in a more controlled fashion with a standard papillotome, after which the pancreatic stent can be placed over a guidewire (see PTS technique, below).

5

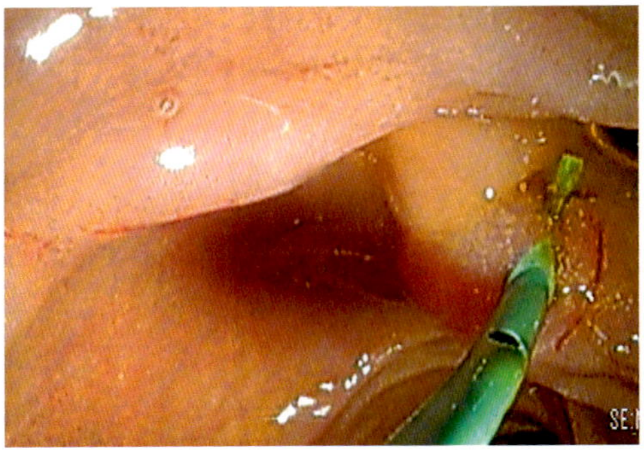

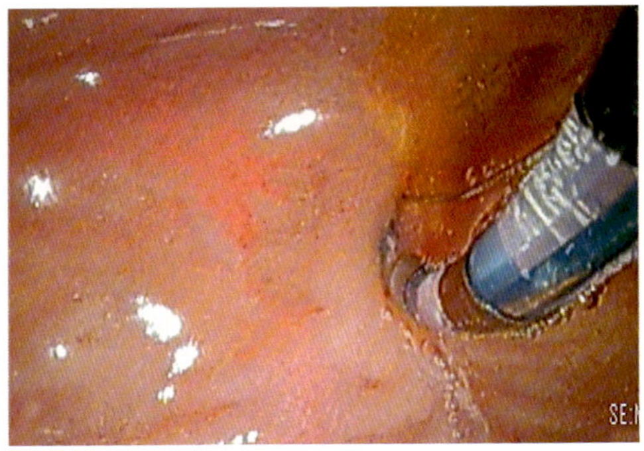

6

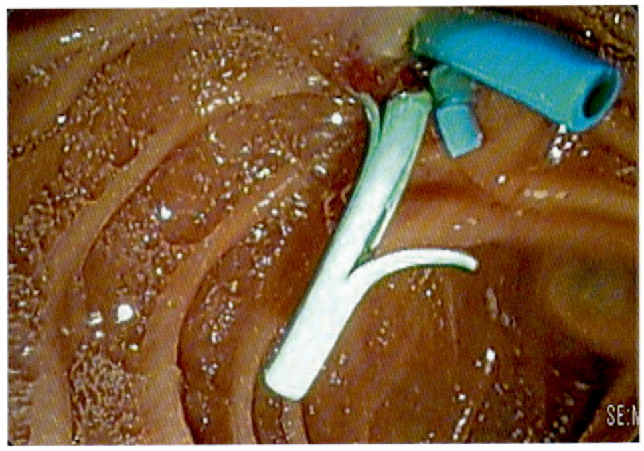

7

Fig. 5. Pancreatic sphincterotomy accomplished by NK cut-down on to a previously placed 5-Fr gauge straight pancreatic stent.

Fig. 6. PTS performed using a standard pull papillotome. The tip of the papillotome is in the pancreatic duct, and the cut proceeds cephalad. The authors recommend that this be done after placing a pancreatic stent for prophylaxis against PEP.

Fig. 7. Biliary and pancreatic stents left at the end of a NKP.

Post-Procedure Care

Successful NKP results in access to the desired duct without perforation or more than minimal bleeding. Special precautions or post-procedural care are not required. It is the author's practice to delay reinstitution of therapeutic anticoagulation for at least 24 h, unless the patient is at high risk for thrombotic complications. Complex anticoagulation issues should be reviewed by a coagulation expert. Patients whose biliary obstruction has not been relieved by the procedure need to remain on broad-spectrum antibiotics, and a decision made regarding the safety or otherwise of delaying biliary drainage by a few days pending another attempt. If there is any concern about the adequacy of biliary drainage after NKP when a stricture is not present (e.g. done for stones or papillary stenosis), it is a wise precaution to place a biliary stent before finishing the procedure (fig. 7). PEP should be uncommon after NKP, as typically the pancreatic duct is protected by a stent. Severe pain following NKP may be due to pancreatitis, but free duodenal or retroperitoneal perforation is in the differential diagnosis. Greatly elevated serum amylase and/or lipase point towards procedure-related pancreatitis, while pain in an ERCP patient with normal pancreatic enzymes should raise concern for perforation, especially if the white cell count is significantly elevated. A contrast-enhanced abdominal computed tomography scan is the investigation of choice to separate pancreatitis from perforation. EUS-guided bile duct puncture through the duodenal bulb wall is particularly prone to cause free retroperitoneal air and/or fluid (bile). This is a particular problem if a stent or other drain is not placed through the fistula. EUS-guided bile duct and pancreatic duct puncture remains an experimental technique and should be used by experts only [6]. Some centers have placed a moratorium on this technique pending more reliable accessories for creating a secure fistula through the duodenal wall into the bile duct or pancreatic duct.

Table 1. Published work on precut techniques for biliary, pancreatic and combined access

Reference (first author)	Techniques
Halttunen, 2009 [10] Retrospective	n = 178. Biliary cannulation succeeded less frequently following NK precutting than following the pancreatic sphincterotomy technique (71.3 vs. 97.3%, $p < 0.001$).
Misra, 2008 [11] Retrospective	n = 169, CBD access in 159 (94%) patients. Complications in 14 (8.2%) patients (mild pancreatitis in 6, moderate pancreatitis in 2, bleeding requiring endoscopic therapy in 5, and perforation in 1).
Fukatsu, 2008 [12] Retrospective	n = 80. CBD access in 95% of 76 difficult cannulation cases (95%). Multivariate analysis indicated that female gender (odds ratio (OR) 2.25), left lobe hypertrophy after hepatectomy (OR 6.25), history of Billroth I gastrectomy (OR 7.49), and malignant biliary stricture (OR 2.31) were significant risk factors for failed standard procedures for biliary cannulation. Complications after NKP were observed in 9 patients (11%): all had pancreatitis.
Fukatsu, 2008 [13] Retrospective	n = 104 were treated in two training periods, A and B. 41 (41/267, 15%) trained in period A, and 63 (63/322, 20%) in period B. No significant difference in success rates was seen between periods A (90%) and B (98%) ($p = 0.08$). However, the initial success rate was higher in period B (95%) than in period A (80%) ($p < 0.05$). Complications were not significantly different between groups (10 vs. 16%; $p = 0.56$). All complications were mild pancreatitis.
Palm, 2007 [14] Retrospective	n = 121. Erlangen type papillotome was used for precutting. Success in 98%. Complication rates similar in the two groups (non-precut 7.1% vs. precut 8.3%, $p =$ 0.7). Hyperamylasemia more common in the precut group (13.3 vs. 31.3%, $p < 0.001$).
Zhou, 2006 [7] Retrospective	n = 91 with difficult biliary cannulation: 43 patients had NKP: success rate 91%, mean cannulation time 5.6 min, complication rate was 9%. 48 patients had persistent cannulation by standard techniques: cannulation success rate 75%, mean cannulation time was 10.2 min, the complication rate 15%.
Tang, 2005 [8] Randomized	n = 62, randomized to 'precut' arm (n = 32) or 'persistence' arm (n = 30). Success rates and complication rates were similar in the two arms (75 and 4%, respectively, for the precut arm vs. 73 and 9% for the persistence arm).
Ahmad, 2005 [15] Retrospective	n = 79, 45 women, 34 men. Precut led to CBD cannulation at first try in 67 patients, and in a further 5 at second attempt, for overall success rate of 91%. Complications in 8 patients (10%): hemorrhage in 5 (6%) and pancreatitis in 3 (4%).
Katsinelos, 2004 [16] Retrospective	n = 64. CBD access was successful immediately after NKP in 44 patients (66%), during a second ERCP in 18 (26%), and during a third ERCP in 2 (3%), for a total cannulation rate of 94%. No related deaths. Complications included bleeding in 5 patients (7%) and pancreatitis in 3 (4%).
Catalano, 2004 [9] Randomized	n = 63. Bile duct access in 29/29 (100%) of patients randomized to TPS, and 26 of 34 (77%) patients who underwent NKP ($p = 0.01$). 7 complications, including bleeding (n = 2) and acute pancreatitis (n = 5). Complications were less frequent in the TPS group (1/29; 3.5%) compared with NKP (6/34; 18%).
Heiss, 2002 [17] Pilot study	(Heiss-Device Flexible Endoscopic Scissors (Telemed™): 8 of 12 could be cannulated.
Rollhauser, 1998 [18] Retrospective	n = 68. Immediate free cannulation in group 1 (non-NKP), 14/22 patients (64%), vs. 34/46 (74%) in group 2 (NKP). The delayed cannulation rate was 5/8 in group 1 (62.5%) vs. 11 of 12 in group 2 (92%). The success rate was 19/22 patients in group 1 (86%) vs. 45/46 in group 2 (98%). The overall success rate was 64/68 (94%). Complication rate 6%, no mortality.

Table 1. Continued

Reference (first author)	Techniques
Rabenstein, 1997 [3] Retrospective	n = 86. In precut NKP. CBD opacification was achieved in 81% (70/86) and pathologic findings were noted in 69% (59/86). Complications not significantly increased by NKP.
Dhir, 1997 [19] Retrospective	n = 100. Patients with malignant obstructive jaundice. 65% success with NKP; 6 complications.
Gholson, 1996 [20] Retrospective	Assessed traction vs. NK papillotomes. Biliary access was immediate in 68 patients (97%). Complications were lower in the precut group. Complications in 5 NKP patients (7%), compared to 11 (4%) of a concurrent 261 patients who underwent standard ES (without NKP).
Foutch, 1995 [21] Prospective, non-randomized cohort study	NKP successful in 47/52 patients (90%). Three complications (6%): 2 (4%) were serious. Morbidity rates for NKP and ES were not significantly different. No procedure-related mortality. NKP increased the overall success rate from 87% (success rate for ES alone) to 97% (success rate for ES and NKP combined).
Tweedle, 1991 [22] Retrospective	24/24 NKP success for cannulation. 12% NKP complication rate (higher than non-NKP group).
Dowsett, 1990 [23] Retrospective	n = 103. Overall success rate of 77% (immediate vs. 2–5 days repeat). The procedure-related morbidity and mortality in the therapeutic group were 5 and 2%, respectively.
Weber, 2008 Retrospective	n = 108. Bile duct cannulation successful in 103 (95%) of 108 patients. 5% required a percutaneous biliary drainage. 12 (11%) complications: acute pancreatitis (n = 6), bleeding (n = 6). 2 severe pancreatitis; 4 required blood transfusion.
Pancreatic sphincterotomy	
Halttunen, 2009 [10] Retrospective	n = 147. Biliary cannulation succeeded less frequently following NKP than after pancreatic sphincterotomy technique (71.3 vs. 97.3%, $p < 0.001$); 25% in PSC patients.
Lawrence, 2009 [2] Retrospective	n = 510 ERCPs. NKP was used for 395/510 (77.5%) cases vs. 115/510 (22.5%) in which PTS was used. PEP was no different between NKS (25/395, 6.4%) and PTS (9/115, 7.8%). 1 severe pancreatitis case in each.
Wilcox, 2001 [24] Retrospective (pilot)	n = 11. 11/11 patients had minor papilla NKP over a wire. 1/11 got pancreatitis.
Both biliary and pancreatic precut papillotomy	
Goff, 2009 [5] Retrospective	n = 143 (biliary sphinterotomy), n = 51 (pancreatic sphincterotomy). Complication rates for standard sphincterotomy and transpancreatic approach were 2.1 and 1.96% respectively. No cases of PEP after transpancreatic precut sphincterotomy. In 2 patients there was failure to enter the bile duct despite the precut.
Siddiqui, 2008 [25] Retrospective	n = 59. 59/515 ERCPs using NKP with success of 95% (56 patients); complications 3% PEP, 5% bleed.

Outcomes

Most of the published data on NKP represent observational experience (table 1). It is difficult to determine the significance of numerous large case series. First, as they lack control subjects, we cannot know if another approach, such as persistence, may have been as safe and as effective.

Second, there is no consensus about the definition of a 'difficult' ERCP case. 'Success' in these studies is similarly ill-defined, and clinically intuitive. What is considered a 'difficult (ERCP) case' varies widely from study to study; the commonest definition is 'failure to cannulate the desired duct without a precut papillotomy'. Frequently, the thorny issue of definition is avoided altogether in published papers. However, certain patterns do emerge. Generally, the available data suggest that successful cannulation of the common bile duct follows precut papillotomy in the majority of cases, with success rates ranging from 77 to 98%. However, in published series, 'success' often was not achieved until the second or even third procedure after initial failure. Experience likely influences success and safety, but there are scant data regarding this. Most centers that report a large and long experience of precut papillotomy fail to stratify the results over time.

If we accept from the published literature that precutting techniques are effective, it is less clear when, or in whom, they are most effective. Zhou et al. [7] randomized patients to NKP or persistence with standard techniques if cannulation took >10 min, or a guidewire entered the pancreatic duct three times. Of 91 patients with difficult biliary cannulation, 43 underwent NKP, with a cannulation success rate of 91%, the mean cannulation time was 5.6 min after the cut was made, with a complication rate of 9%. The remaining 48 patients underwent persistent cannulation by standard techniques with a significantly lower success rate of 75%; the average time to successful cannulation was >10 min. The complication rate was 15%, which was not significantly higher than in the NKP group. Another randomized trial, by Tang et al. [8], supports these findings. Much of the evidence suggests that precut papillotomy can result in successful cannulation in difficult ERCP cases where standard techniques fail after 10–20 min of sustained effort. It may take more than one further ERCP before successful cannulation, even after NKP. Precut papillotomy complications are not significantly increased above controls in most studies.

Precut transpancreatic septotomy (PTS) is an alternative to NKP as a way to facilitate successful bile duct cannulation during ERCP. During difficult cases, the pancreatic duct is often unintentionally cannulated with a guidewire multiple times. In PTS, the pancreatic duct is first stented over a guidewire, then septotomy is performed over the stent. The stent helps guide the cut, and limits PEP related to repeated pancreatic duct instrumentation and the local application of heat. Retrospective observational studies suggest that PTS may be as successful as NKP. The only randomized data available, from Catalano et al. [9], found a higher deep cannulation success rate and fewer complications with PTS than with NKP (100 and 3.5% vs. 77 and 18%, respectively).

Conclusion

Precutting techniques are used to gain access to the bile duct, pancreatic duct and related cystically dilated structures when standard cannulation techniques have failed. Free-hand NKP is a relative 'uncontrolled' procedure compared to standard sphincterotomy, with risks that depend on the indication and the experience of the operator. Supervised experience of NKP is essential before any ERCP endoscopist sets out to do this procedure on his or her own. A thorough understanding of bile duct and pancreatic duct anatomy and the principles of electrosurgery are key if complications of NKP, including bleeding, perforation and pancreatitis are to be avoided. Protecting the pancreas with a plastic transpapillary stent before NKP is an important and effective tool for minimizing the risk of severe necrotizing pancreatitis. NKP increases the success rate of biliary cannulation, but should only be used for therapeutic access. Sometimes a second or subsequent ERCP must be performed before deep access to the desired duct is achieved.

Patients with an urgent need for biliary decompression whose NKP fails to gain deep access to the bile duct should not be kept waiting for another attempt. These patients should proceed to percutaneous transhepatic cholangiography for biliary drainage. PTS is an alternative to free-hand NKP that is reportedly safe and effective. However, the authors recommend that the pancreatic duct always be protected with a transpapillary stent *before* TPS is performed.

References

1 Freeman ML, Nelson DB, Sherman S, et al: Complications of endoscopic biliary sphincterotomy. N Engl J Med 1996;335:909–918.
2 Lawrence C, Romagnuolo J, Cotton PB, et al: Post-ERCP pancreatitis rates do not differ between needle-knife and pull-type pancreatic sphincterotomy techniques: a multiendoscopist 13-year experience. Gastrointest Endosc 2009;69:1271–1275.
3 Rabenstein T, Ruppert T, Schneider HT, et al: Benefits and risks of needle-knife papillotomy. Gastrointest Endosc 1997;46:207–211.
4 Baillie J: Is ERCP headed for extinction? Am J Gastroenterol 2008;103:1888–1890.
5 Goff JS: Long-term experience with the transpancreatic sphincter pre-cut approach to biliary sphincterotomy. Gastrointest Endosc 1999;50:642–645.
6 Brauer B, Chen Y, Fukami N: Single-operator EUS-guided cholangiopancreatography for difficult pancreatobiliary access. Gastrointest Endosc 2009;70: 471–479.
7 Zhou PH, Yao LQ, Xu MD, et al: Application of needle-knife in difficult biliary cannulation for endoscopic retrograde cholangiopancreatography. Hepatobiliary Pancreat Dis Int 2006;5:590–594.
8 Tang SJ, Haber GB, Kortan P, et al: Precut papillotomy versus persistence in difficult biliary cannulation: a prospective randomized trial. Endoscopy 2005;37: 58–65.
9 Catalano MF, Linder JD, Geenen JE. Endoscopic transpancreatic papillary septotomy for inaccessible obstructed bile ducts: comparison with standard pre-cut papillotomy. Gastrointest Endosc 2004;60: 557–561.
10 Halttunen J, Keranen I, Udd M, et al: Pancreatic sphincterotomy versus needle knife precut in difficult biliary cannulation. Surg Endosc 2009;23:745–749.
11 Misra SP, Dwivedi M: Intramural incision technique: a useful and safe procedure for obtaining ductal access during ERCP. Gastrointest Endosc 2008;67: 629–633.
12 Fukatsu H, Kawamoto H, Kato H, et al: Evaluation of needle-knife precut papillotomy after unsuccessful biliary cannulation, especially with regard to postoperative anatomic factors. Surg Endosc 2008; 22:717–723.
13 Fukatsu H, Kawamoto H, Harada R, et al: Quantitative assessment of technical proficiency in performing needle-knife precut papillotomy. Surg Endosc 2009;23:2066–2072.
14 Palm J, Saarela A, Makela J: Safety of Erlangen precut papillotomy: an analysis of 1,044 consecutive ERCP examinations in a single institution. J Clin Gastroenterol 2007;41:528–533.
15 Ahmad I, Khan AA, Alam A, et al: Precut papillotomy outcome. J Coll Physicians Surg Pak 2005;15:701–703.
16 Katsinelos P, Mimidis K, Paroutoglou G, et al: Needle-knife papillotomy: a safe and effective technique in experienced hands. Hepatogastroenterology 2004;51:349–352.
17 Heiss FW, Cimis RS Jr, MacMillan FP Jr: Biliary sphincter scissor for pre-cut access: preliminary experience. Gastrointest Endosc 2002;55:719–722.
18 Rollhauser C, Johnson M, Al-Kawas FH: Needle-knife papillotomy: a helpful and safe adjunct to endoscopic retrograde cholangiopancreatography in a selected population. Endoscopy 1998;30:691–696.
19 Dhir V, Swaroop VS, Mohandas KM, et al: Precut papillotomy using a needle knife: experience in 100 patients with malignant obstructive jaundice. Indian J Gastroenterol 1997;16:52–53.
20 Gholson CF, Favrot D. Needle knife papillotomy in a university referral practice. Safety and efficacy of a modified technique. J Clin Gastroenterol 1996;23: 177–180.
21 Foutch PG: A prospective assessment of results for needle-knife papillotomy and standard endoscopic sphincterotomy. Gastrointest Endosc 1995;41:25–32.
22 Tweedle DE, Martin DF: Needle knife papillotomy for endoscopic sphincterotomy and cholangiography. Gastrointest Endosc 1991;37:518–521.
23 Dowsett JF, Polydorou AA, Vaira D, et al: Needle knife papillotomy: how safe and how effective? Gut 1990;31: 905–908.
24 Wilcox CM, Mönkemüller KF: Wire-assisted minor papilla precut papillotomy. Gastrointest Endosc 2001;54: 83–86.
25 Siddiqui AR, Niaz SK. Needle knife papillotomy for cannulating difficult papilla: two years' experience. J Pak Med Assoc 2008;58:195–197.

John Baillie, MBChB, FRCP
Section of Gastroenterology
Wake Forest University Baptist Medical Center
Winston-Salem, NC 27157 (USA)
Tel. +1 919 713 7311, Fax +1 919 713 7322, E-Mail jbaillie@wfubmc.edu

Mönkemüller K, Wilcox CM, Muñoz-Navas M (eds): Interventional and Therapeutic Gastrointestinal Endoscopy.
Front Gastrointest Res. Basel, Karger, 2010, vol 27, pp 337–344

Biliary Stone Extraction

C. Mel Wilcox

Division of Gastroenterology and Hepatology, University of Alabama at Birmingham, Birmingham, Ala., USA

Abstract

Bile duct stones are a common clinical scenario and their frequency may increase in the future given the rise in gallstones linked to the obesity epidemic. Over the last decade, improved therapeutic tools have been developed which have enhanced the overall success and safety of stone extraction. In some situations, mechanical lithotripsy may be required. Rarely will surgery be required for stone removal.

Common bile duct (CBD) stone disease is one of the more common disorders managed by the therapeutic biliary endoscopist. With the worldwide rise in the obesity epidemic and its associated impact on cholelithiasis, this problem will only further amplify in magnitude. Most patients with CBD stones are managed electively; however, in patients with severe cholangitis, the procedure may require urgent intervention underscoring the importance of effective and safe techniques for management. In this chapter, the methods for successful stone extraction will be reviewed including an update on accessories required for success, and the outcome from such techniques.

Technique

Successful management of CBD stones first requires selective biliary cannulation. When the clinical suspicion for stones is high, cannulation should be initiated using a sphincterotome. In addition, if one cannot achieve an en face view of the papilla, the ability to bow a sphincterotome and change the angulation assists in selective cannulation (fig. 1). In the setting of CBD stones when the papilla is generous in size, selective cannulation can often be achieved. If not, wire-guided access may be necessary. Use of a 'slippery' angled-tip wire (Terumo glidewire®, Boston Scientific) is often times essential for cannulation of the ampulla with extruding biliary epithelium or for those cases where cannulation is difficult. Such wire-guided cannulation requires coordination between a skilled nurse and the endoscopist. A standard wire for cannulation is too stiff and will be traumatic to use. Slow injection of a small amount of contrast is important initially so that the biliary system is not overfilled thereby potentially missing a small stone. Some would use half strength contrast when stones are suspected although it is not necessary when contrast is carefully

1 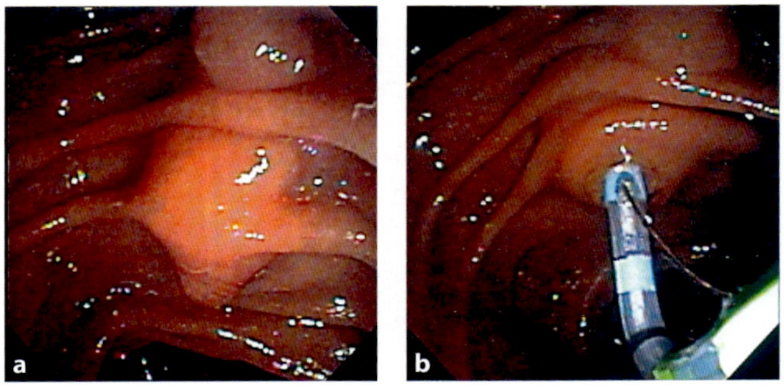 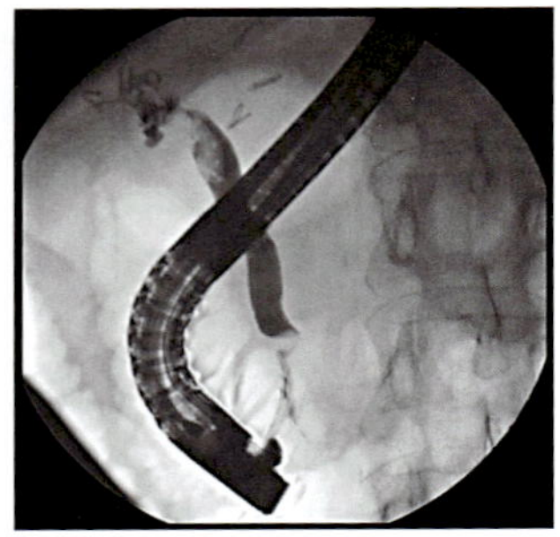 2

Fig. 1. Location of papilla (**a**) and utility of using a sphincterotome for cannulation when the angulation is acute (**b**) to achieve an upwards orientation for the bile duct. **Fig. 2.** Pseudocalculus sign. There appears to be a stone in the distal duct but this represents extrinsic compression on the ampulla.

injected. Excess pressure on the ampulla with the catheter may suggest a stone (pseudocalculus sign; fig. 2). Following slow injection and filling of the distal bile duct to confirm and characterize any abnormalities, further opacification of the more proximal biliary tree is performed.

Biliary sphincterotomy should be performed prior to stone extraction (fig. 3). Balloon dilation alone has been used although it is associated with pancreatitis [1]. The length of the biliary sphincterotomy will be dependent on the size of the papilla and characteristics of the stone(s). For example, if the major papilla is small and the stone is large, additional techniques (see below) for extraction may be required. In contrast, the bulbous papilla provides the opportunity for a generous incision at which point most stones can be extracted. It is important to gauge the size of the sphincterotomy by pulling a balloon through the incision as this confirms the likelihood of removing the identified stone(s) (fig. 3e). Generally stones should be removed separately to avoid impaction especially when large. Once all stones are removed, balloon cholangiography to fully opacify the proximal biliary tree should be done to confirm the absence of other stones and the more proximal biliary anatomy, as well as the location of the cystic duct which would be important for those with a gallbladder in situ when cholecystectomy is anticipated (fig. 3h).

Precut fistulotomy may be needed for those in whom free cannulation cannot be achieved but in whom endoscopic therapy is anticipated or when there is stone impaction (fig. 4). As noted above, selective cannulation can often be achieved using standard techniques when the papilla is generous in size; however, if the papilla is small, initial placement of a pancreatic stent may be necessary before precut incision to assist in identifying the biliary system as well as reducing complications of pancreatitis. Fistulotomy is generally straightforward when the papilla is bulbous, while, in contrast, others may elect precut using a sphincterotome angled toward the biliary orifice or a precut sphincterotome (fig. 4b) [2]. The type of precut incision should be dictated by prior experience.

Accessories

The full complement of biliary tools is mandatory prior to consideration of any stone extraction (table 1). Several sphincterotomes should be available in case of failure. A glidewire may be necessary for selective cannulation as well as a needle knife if precut fistulotomy is required (as noted above). Precut incision carries a higher risk of complications so it should only be performed by

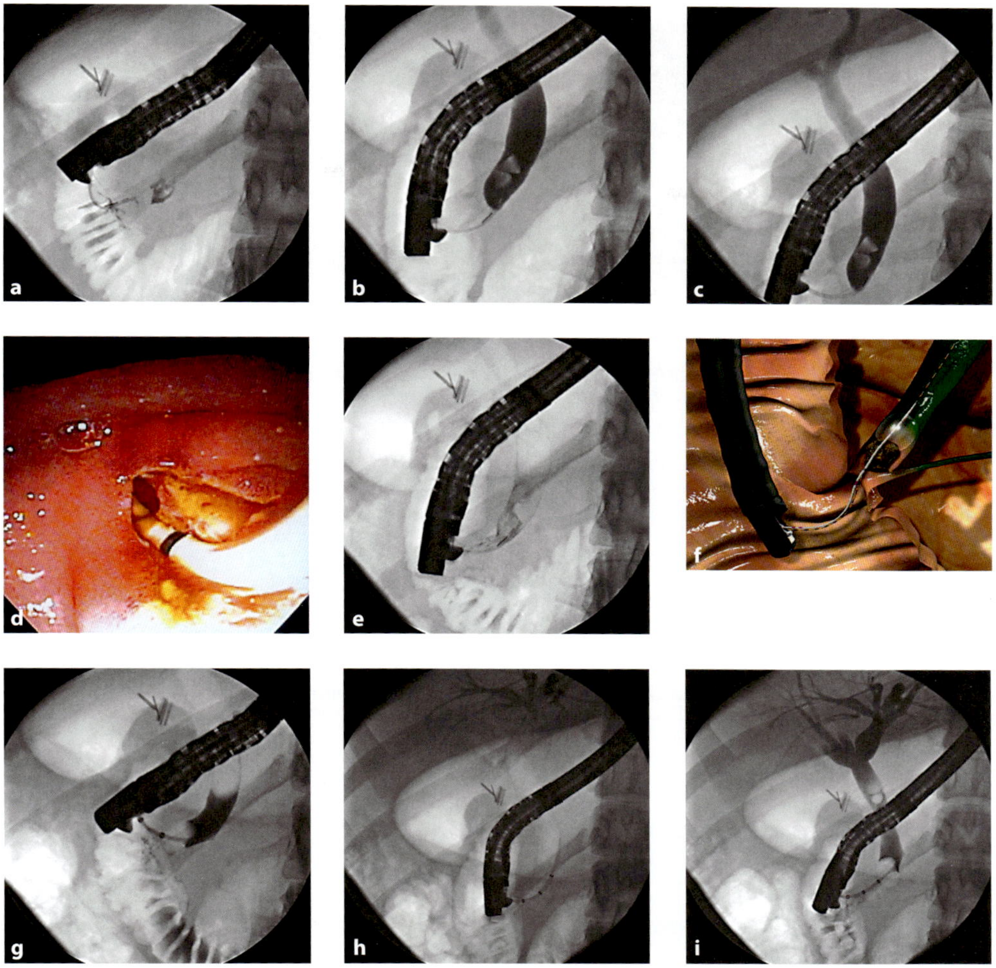

Fig. 3. Removal of several stones. **a** A small amount of contrast is injected showing a filling defect. **b** Further contrast injection confirms 2 stones in a minimally dilated duct. Cholecystectomy clips are seen. **c** Filling of the proximal biliary system shows no additional abnormalities. **d** Biliary sphincterotomy performed to the duodenal wall. **e** Following sphincterotomy air is now seen in the duct somewhat obscuring visualization of the calculi. **f** The balloon can be advanced into the biliary tree alone or over a wire. The use of the wire is generally helpful as it will allow for easier 'return' into the common bile duct. Occasionally, when the papilla becomes swollen and partially destroyed by the sphincterotomy and balloon extraction maneuvers, it may become difficult to regain access into the CBD again. (Permission for use granted by Cook Medical Incorporated, Bloomington, Ind.). **g** The 15-mm balloon is initially placed below the stones and withdrawn through the sphincterotomy to determine the size of the opening and thus gauge the ability to remove the stones. This is important prior to removal of any large stone to rule out the likelihood of impaction. **h** Air fills the duct which suggests complete biliary sphincterotomy. **i** Balloon cholangiogram at completion.

the experienced biliary endoscopist [3]. Most would use a 15-mm balloon with a large sphincterotomy and small stone; wire placement prior to stone extraction may not be necessary (fig. 5). Selective placement of a guidewire proximal to the stone and deep in the left or right intrahepatic ductal system ensures access is maintained if the stone is large or the endoscopic position is

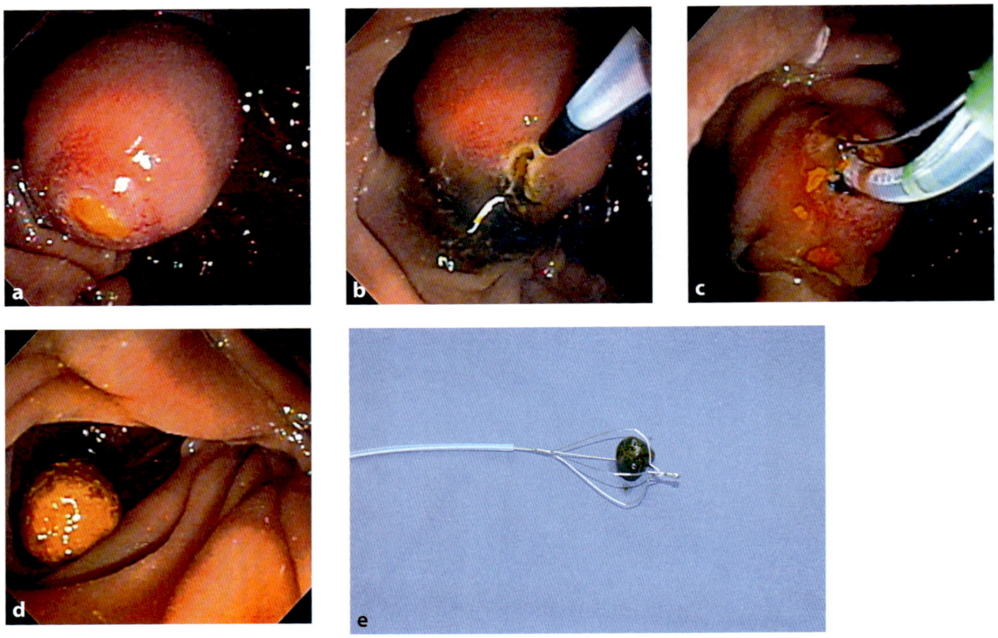

Fig. 4. Precut fistulotomy for impacted stone. **a** Impacted stone in bulbous papilla. **b** Needle knife used to incise papilla over the stone. **c** A standard sphincterotome is used to complete the incision. **d** Stone in the duodenum. **e** Stone captured in basket.

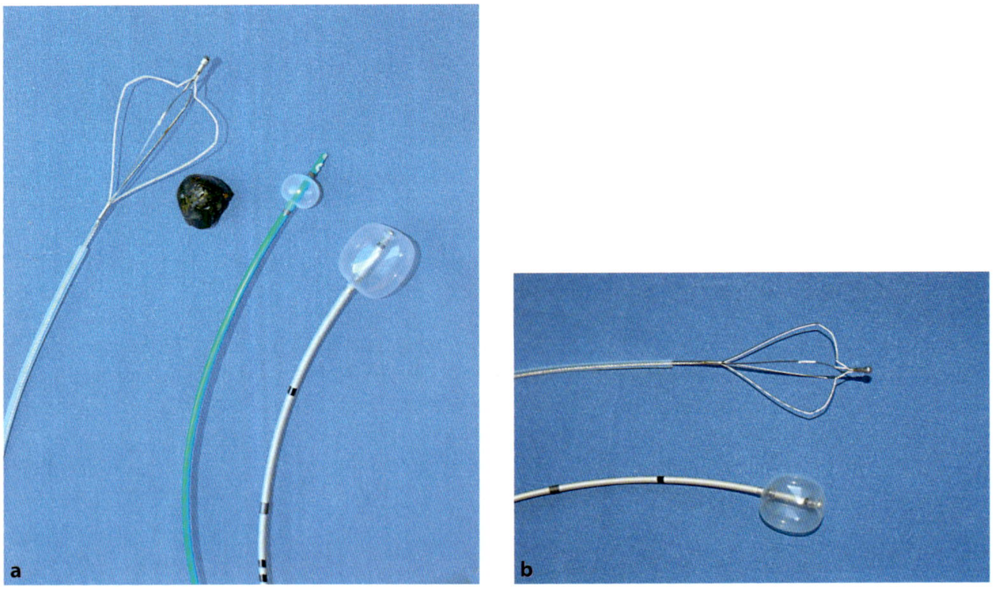

Fig. 5. Balloons and baskets to remove bile duct stones. **a** Note the different sizes of balloons. For slender bile ducts we prefer to use small diameter balloons. **b** Baskets have the advantage of allowing the retrieval of larger stones.

Table 1. Accessories required for extraction of common bile duct stones

Sphincterotomes
Balloons
10 and 15 mm
Basket
Mechanical lithotripter
Crank handle mechanical lithotripter
Sclerotherapy needle

Table 2. Summary of approach to common bile duct stone extraction

Adequate preparation to insure all accessories are available and functioning
For ill patients, assessment of platelet count and prothrombin time
Deep selective cannulation with minimal contrast injection to exclude stone(s)
Opacification of proximal biliary system to evaluate the location and entry of the cystic duct and anatomy of the proximal biliary system
Length of sphincterotomy performed depends on the size and characteristic of the stones
Availability of multiple baskets including mechanical lithotripter for large stones
Placement of a 10-Fr stent proximal to the stone if the stone(s) cannot be removed

tenuous. One must not pull to hard on the balloon above the stone if the stone cannot be easily removed to avoid the wire slipping out or impacting the stone. A mechanical lithotripter may be necessary and should be available. A crank lithotripter is essential to rescue a basket impaction and must be on hand. Laser lithotripsy is relegated to specialized centers given its cost [4]. SpyGlass® or a cholangioscope may occasionally be beneficial to exclude a tumor which may mimic stone disease. Intraductal ultrasound has been used to enhance detection of stones or even microlithiasis [5], but is not widely used.

Outcomes

Using the above techniques, selective biliary cannulation as well as stone extraction can be anticipated in more than 90% of patients (fig. 6). Multiple small stones are relatively easy to remove but if not, stent placement will be required. The stents should be of sufficient size and length to remain in the duct and proximal to all stones and of sufficient length that proximal migration will not occur especially if the sphincterotomy is generous.

Large stones are notoriously difficult to remove especially in those with a slender distal CBD. Thus, the initial cholangiogram is important to evaluate proximal anatomy. Recently ampullary dilatation varying from 12 to 15 mm or larger has been proposed as the method for removing large bile duct stones [6, 7]. Caution must be exercised in choosing the appropriate size for dilatation to avoid perforation. Using such dilatation, larger stones can be removed although giant stones (>2 cm) generally require a mechanical approach which is successful in most but not all patients [8, 9].

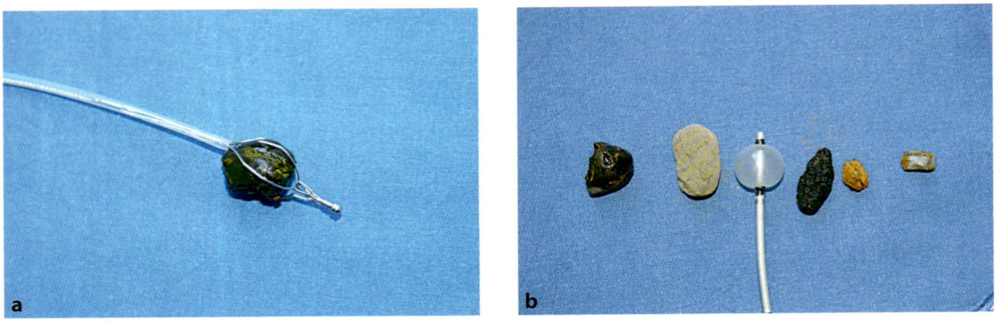

Fig. 6. Removal of stones with basket or balloon. **a** Baskets allow for a tight gripping of the stone. **b** The diameter of the balloon is useful to determine the approximate size of the stones.

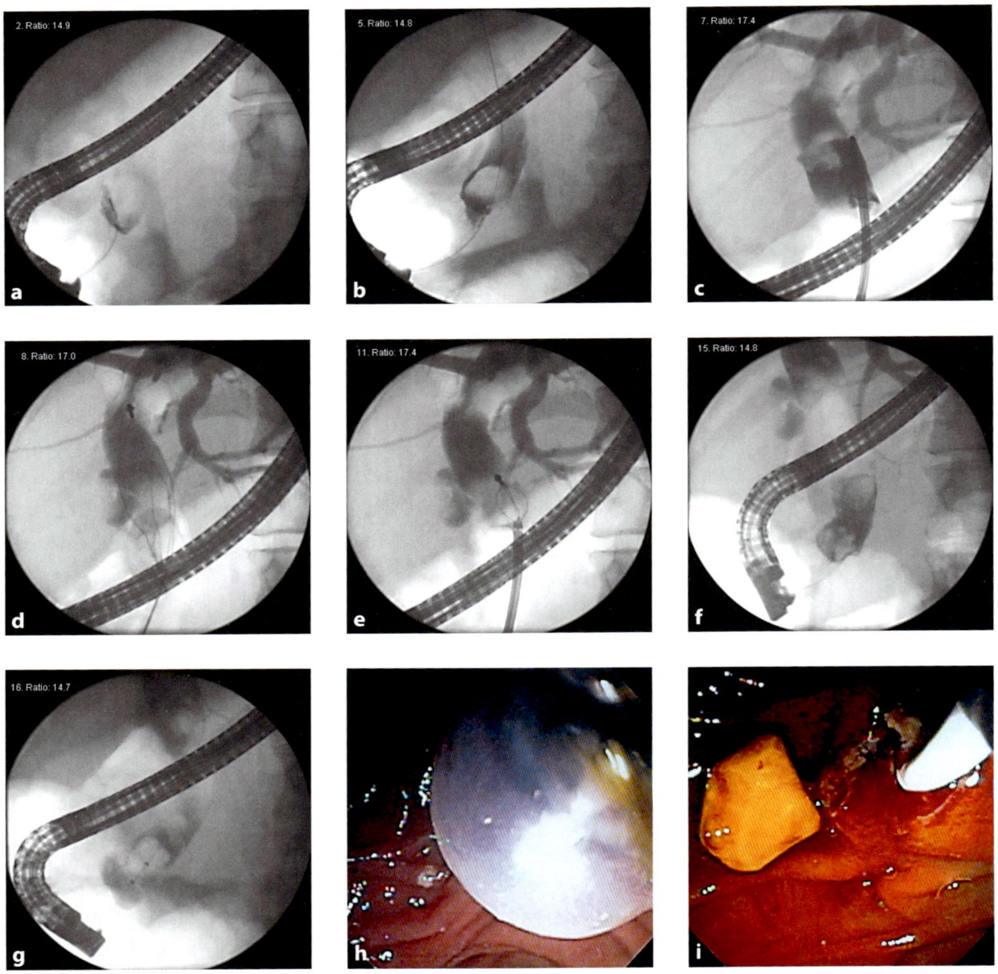

Fig. 7. Removal of large stones with basket lithotripsy. **a, b** Injection shows a large filling defect confirmed with further injection. ERC shows a solitary 11-mm stone. **c** The lithotripter is passed to the level of the stone. **d** The basket is opened and placed around the stone. **e** The stone is captured and lithotripsy begun. **f** Large fragments in the distal duct. **g** Balloon withdrawn through sphincterotomy to gauge size. **h** Balloon withdrawn at 15 mm. **i** Large cholesterol stone removed by the balloon.

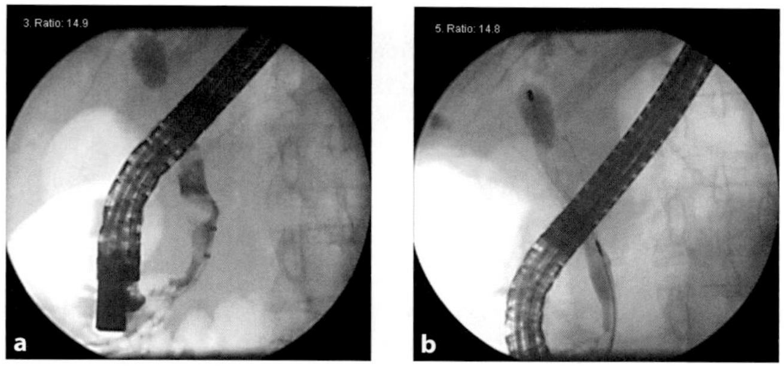

Fig. 8. Bile duct stone and a tapered distal bile duct may require lithotripsy for removal. **a** Stone with tapered distal duct. **b** The basket of the mechanical lithotripter is used to grasp the stone.

When performing mechanical lithotripsy, it is important that the stone is engaged in a dilated portion of the duct (fig. 7). Otherwise, if the stone is in the distal duct and not free floating, it may be difficult for a basket to surround the stone. It is also imperative to maintain adequate position when using the mechanical lithotripter given the difficulty in selective cannulation. In this setting, cannulation with the basket portion alone enhances cannulation. Lithotripsy may also be required when the stone is of modest size but there is tapering of the distal duct (fig. 8).

Post-Procedure Care

Depending on the difficulty of the procedure, the majority of patients can be discharged home following successful stone extraction. High-risk patients may be those in whom the procedure was prolonged, and those at greatest risk of pancreatitis. Bleeding may occur after sphincterotomy in approximately 1–2% of patients but is usually not life-threatening; epinephrine injection of the ampulla delivered via a sclerotherapy needle is generally effective for hemostasis [10–12]. As noted above, balloon dilatation following sphincterotomy also may heighten the risk of bleeding. For patients with large stones that cannot be extracted and in whom a stent is placed, a follow-up procedure in 4–6 months is appropriate. At that time, stones are often times softer and easier to remove. The use of Actigal® is common in this setting although there is very little literature supporting its use.

Conclusions

CBD stones can be removed in most patients. The techniques for extraction are well recognized. Nuances occur in those with altered anatomy and with large calculi. Knowledge of the required equipment or accessories is essential not only for success, but to prevent complications (table 2).

References

1 Weinberg BM, Shindy W, Lo S: Endoscopic balloon sphincter dilation (sphincteroplasty) versus sphincterotomy for common bile duct stones. Cochrane Database Syst Rev 2006;4:CD0004890.

2 Horiuchi A, Nakayama Y, Kajiyama M, Tanaka N: Effect of precut sphincterotomy on biliary cannulation based on the characteristics of the major duodenal papilla. Clin Gastroenterol Hepatol 2007;5: 1113–1118.

3 Robison LS, Varadarajulu S, Wilcox CM: Safety and success of precut biliary sphincterotomy: Is it linked to experience or expertise? World J Gastroenterol 2007;13: 2183–2186.
4 Arya N, Nelles SE, Haber GB, Kim YI, Kortan PK: Electrohydraulic lithotripsy in 111 patients: a safe and effective therapy for difficult bile duct stones. Am J Gastroenterol 2004;99:2330–2334.
5 Varadarajulu S, Eloubeidi MA, Wilcox CM: Prospective evaluation of indeterminate ERCP findings by intraductal ultrasound. J Gastroenterol Hepatol 2007;22:2086–2092.
6 Draganov PV, Evans W, Fazel A, Forsmark CE: Large size balloon dilation of the ampulla after biliary sphincterotomy can facilitate endoscopic extraction of difficult bile duct stones. J Clin Gastroenterol 2009 [Epub ahead of print]
7 Attasaranya S, Cheon YK, Vittal H, Howell DA, Wakelin DE, Cunningham JT, Ajmere N, Ste Marie RW Jr, Bhattacharya K, Gupta K, Freeman ML, Sherman S, McHenry L, Watkins JL, Fogel EL, Schmidt S, Lehman GA: Large-diameter biliary orifice balloon dilation to aid in endoscopic bile duct stone removal: a multicenter series. Gastrointest Endosc 2008;67:1046–1052.
8 Thomas M, Howell DA, Carr-Locke D, Wilcox CM, Chak A, Raijman I, Watkins JL, Schmalz MJ, Geenen JE, Catalano MF: Mechanical lithotripsy of pancreatic and biliary stones: complications and available treatment options collected from expert centers. Am J Gastroenterol 2007;102:1896–1902.
9 Shaw MJ, Mackie RD, Moore JP, Dorsher PJ, Freeman ML, Meier PB, Potter T, Hutton SW, Vennes JA: Results of a multicenter trial using a mechanical lithotripter for the treatment of large bile duct stones. Am J Gastroenterol 1993;88:730–733.
10 Cotton PB, Garrow DA, Gallagher J, Romagnuolo J: Risk factors for complications after ERCP: a multivariate analysis of 11,497 procedures over 12 years. Gastrointest Endosc 2009;70:80–88.
11 Wilcox CM, Canakis J, Mönkemüller KE, Bondora AW, Geels W: Patterns of bleeding after endoscopic sphincterotomy, the subsequent risk of bleeding, and the role of epinephrine injection. Am J Gastroenterol 2004;99:244–248.
12 Leung JW, Chan FK, Sung JJ, Chung S: Endoscopic sphincterotomy-induced hemorrhage: a study of risk factors and the role of epinephrine injection. Gastrointest Endosc 1995;42:550–554.

C. Mel Wilcox, MD, MSPH
Division of Gastroenterology and Hepatology, University of Alabama at Birmingham
703 19th Street, South ZRB 633
Birmingham, AL 35294–0007 (USA)
Tel. +1 205 975 4958, Fax +1 205 934 1546, E-Mail melw@uab.edu

Mönkemüller K, Wilcox CM, Muñoz-Navas M (eds): Interventional and Therapeutic Gastrointestinal Endoscopy.
Front Gastrointest Res. Basel, Karger, 2010, vol 27, pp 345–355

Balloon Sphincteroplasty and Post-Sphincterotomy Balloon Dilation

Jason N. Rogart · David E. Loren

Division of Gastroenterology and Hepatology, Thomas Jefferson University, Philadelphia, Pa., USA

Abstract
Endoscopic dilation of the ampulla of Vater, or endoscopic balloon sphincteroplasty, has been practiced by endoscopists for over 25 years. After initial widespread application of the technique, its use has decreased, largely due to concerns of a high incidence of pancreatitis resulting from the dilation. More recently, balloon sphincteroplasty following biliary sphincterotomy has been demonstrated to be safe and effective for management of complex choledocholithiasis. Additionally, there remains a role for endoscopic balloon sphincteroplasty without prior sphincterotomy for select individuals with coagulopathy or anatomy that may preclude endoscopic sphincterotomy.

Introduction

Endoscopic balloon sphincteroplasty, or 'ampullary balloon dilation' (ABD), was initially described by Staritz et al. [1] in 1983 for the treatment of common bile duct stones and papillary stenosis. Since then, many endoscopists have used this technique as an alternative to endoscopic sphincterotomy (ES). Advocates of the technique argue that ABD may provide advantages including sphincter preservation [2–4], avoiding long-term sequelae of sphincterotomy such as sphincter stenosis and cholangitis [5–6], and a decreased risk of bleeding [7–9] compared to ES. In 2004, however, a randomized controlled multicenter study was published reporting a significant increase in morbidity and mortality of ABD compared with ES [10]. As a result, the routine use of the technique was largely abandoned until later reports demonstrated that ABD in *combination with* ES was effective, with acceptable complication rates compared with ABD alone.

Over recent years, enthusiasm for post-sphincterotomy, transampullary balloon dilation (PSBD) has increased, particularly as an adjunctive therapeutic tool for the extraction of difficult bile duct stones. A list of indications for ABD and PSBD are presented in table 1. In this chapter we will describe the technique for performing PSBD safely, as well as discuss the current literature supporting its use.

Table 1. Indications for ABD and post-sphincterotomy balloon dilation

Extraction of difficult bile duct stones
Alternative to ES in coagulopathic patients
Alternative to ES in high-risk anatomy: Roux-en-Y, periampullary diverticula, intradiverticular ampulla, choledochoenteric anastomosis
Papillary stenosis
Removal of biliary parasites (e.g. *Ascaris*)

Table 2. Equipment suggested for post-sphincterotomy balloon dilation

Therapeutic duodenoscope
Pull-type sphincterotome
Electrocautery generator
Guidewire(s): short (260 cm) and/or long (450 cm)
8 and 10 mm × 4 cm biliary dilation balloons
Controlled radial expansion esophageal balloons, sizes 10–12, 12–15, 15–18 mm
Extraction balloon(s)
Extraction basket(s)
Mechanical lithotripter

Patient Preparation

Patients are instructed to consume nothing by mouth for at least 6 h prior to endoscopic retrograde chloangiopancreatography (ERCP). As with any ERCP, a complete list of medications and allergies are ascertained. It is preferred that patients discontinue anti-platelet (e.g., aspirin, clopidogrel) therapy 1 week prior to the procedure unless the risk-benefit ration favors continuing such medications (e.g. recent drug eluting coronary stent placement). Oral anticoagulant therapy is discontinued days prior to the procedure and 'bridged' with heparin if indicated. Written informed consent is obtained as per institution policy.

Intravenous access should be established, and appropriate sedation determined. There is no modification in sedation requirements when ABD is planned. Any non-fixed dental prosthetics should be removed prior to inserting the bite block and beginning sedation. We prefer the patient be prone on the fluoroscopy table with the head turned to the right.

Accessories

A list of suggested instruments and accessories are presented in table 2. A standard therapeutic duodenoscope is used along with any pull-type sphincterotome and guidewire. For ampullary dilation we use variety of balloon diameters ranging from 8 mm × 4 cm biliary dilation balloons (Hurricane Rx, Boston Scientific, Natick, Mass., USA) to the larger controlled radial expansion esophageal dilation balloons up to 18 mm (Boston Scientific). When a wire-guided device is desired for dilation in excess of 10 mm, the wire-guided controlled radial expansion balloons may be used over a 450-cm long 0.035-in diameter guidewire. The wire that comes prepackaged with the balloon is removed and the balloon is then backloaded over the biliary wire and advanced into the duct. For stone extraction following ABD, any extraction balloon or basket can be employed. A mechanical lithotripter should also be available.

Technique

After preparing and sedating the patient, the major ampulla is identified in the second portion of the duodenum, and the bile duct is deeply cannulated with a sphincterotome and a 0.035-in guidewire (fig. 1). Cholangiography is performed to determine the goals of therapy.

Endoscopic Sphincterotomy and Post-Sphincterotomy Balloon Dilation
We prefer this technique over ABD alone for the extraction of difficult bile duct stones and treatment of ampullary stenosis. We have found that PSBD can also facilitate stone extraction even for small stones (<10 mm) when the distal bile duct is strictured, has a small diameter, or is poorly compliant.

A complete biliary sphincterotomy is performed to the level of the transverse fold overlying the ampulla (fig. 2). We set the electrosurgical unit to the 'endocut' setting to optimize the amount of pure-cut and coagulation currents. Following sphincterotomy, the sphincterotome is exchanged over the wire for a dilation balloon (fig. 3). The initial balloon diameter is selected based primarily on the diameter of the bile duct and secondarily with consideration of the size of the stone. We most often start with a 10-mm (diameter) × 40-mm (length) balloon and perform a single inflation for 60 s. The balloon is positioned across the ampulla such that approximately one-half to two-thirds of the balloon is inside the common bile duct (fig. 4, 5), and the remainder endoscopically visible in the duodenum (fig. 6). After balloon dilation the papilla remains wide open (fig. 7). Stone extraction is then performed using either extraction balloons (which we prefer) or wire baskets (fig. 8). If unsuccessful, larger diameter balloon may be inflated and/or mechanical or electrohydraulic lithotripsy can be performed. Caution should be exercised against the routine use of larger sized balloons (>15 mm) given reports of severe complications and deaths with balloon sizes of 18–20 mm (see below).

In patients with coaguloapthy or altered or unfavorable anatomy, a limited sphincterotomy followed by PSBD can balance the risks of bleeding and pancreatitis with the effectiveness of the procedure (e.g. stone extraction).

Ampullary Balloon Dilation without Sphincterotomy
In situations where sphincterotomy is either contraindicated or technically difficult, ABD can be performed without sphincterotomy. The principles and technique are similar to PSBD described above, though we start with a smaller balloon diameter (6 or 8 mm). Some authors advocate placement of a prophylactic pancreatic stent at the conclusion of the procedure to decrease the risk of post-dilation/post-ERCP pancreatitis; when pancreatic cannulation is readily obtained it is our practice to do so.

Complications
The most common early complications of ampullary dilation are pancreatitis and bleeding. In a recent Cochrane review of 14 randomized controlled trials, pancreatitis occurred twice as often in patients treated with ABD compared with ES (8.6 vs. 4.3%) [11]. The same review showed that

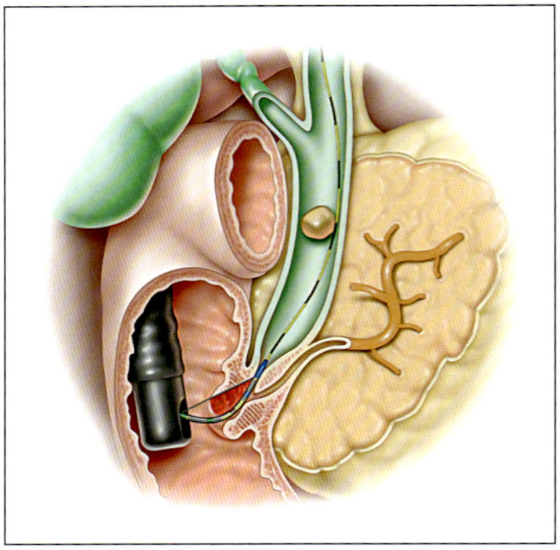
1

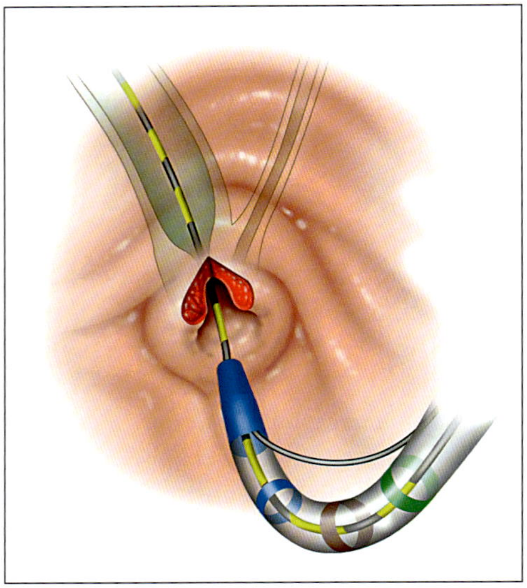
2

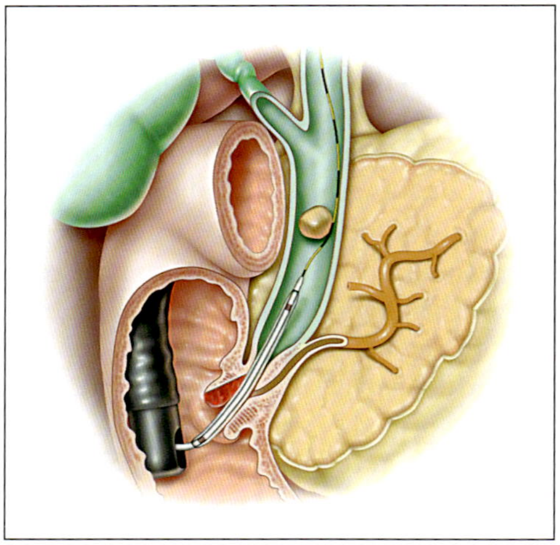
3

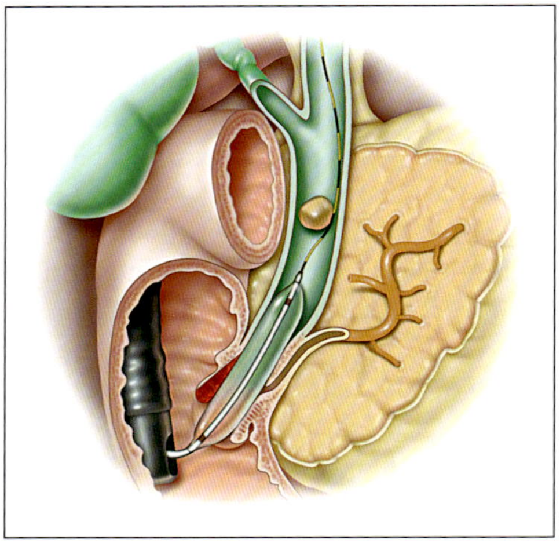
4

Fig. 1. The bile duct is deeply cannulated with a sphincterotome and a 0.035-in guidewire.

Fig. 2. A complete biliary sphincterotomy is performed to the level of the transverse fold overlying the ampulla.

Fig. 3. The sphincterotome is exchanged an over-the-wire for a dilation balloon.

Fig. 4. The balloon is positioned across the ampulla such that approximately one-half to two-thirds of the balloon is inside the common bile duct.

bleeding and infection were significantly less common in ABD than ES (0.1 vs. 4.8% and 2.5 vs. 5.0%, respectively). Perforation is rare (0.3–0.5%). Late 'complications' include recurrent choledocholithiasis (5.5%) and cholecystitis (1.3%), neither of which are likely to be directly related to ABD itself (most of these cases occurred in patients in whom the gallbladder was left in situ) [11]. There is less data available regarding complications after PSBD, with rates of pancreatitis and bleeding ranging from 0 to 8%.

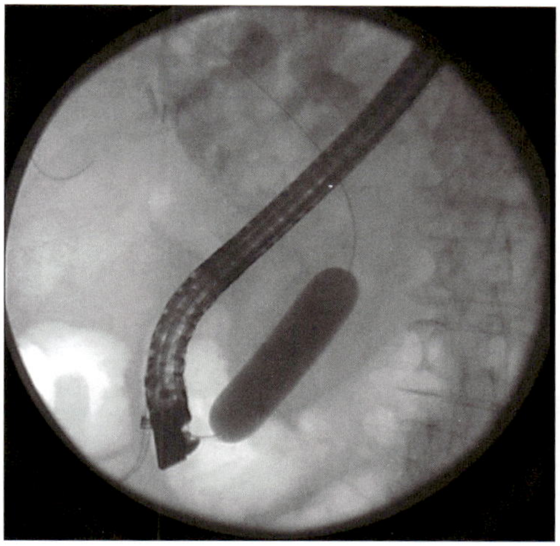

5

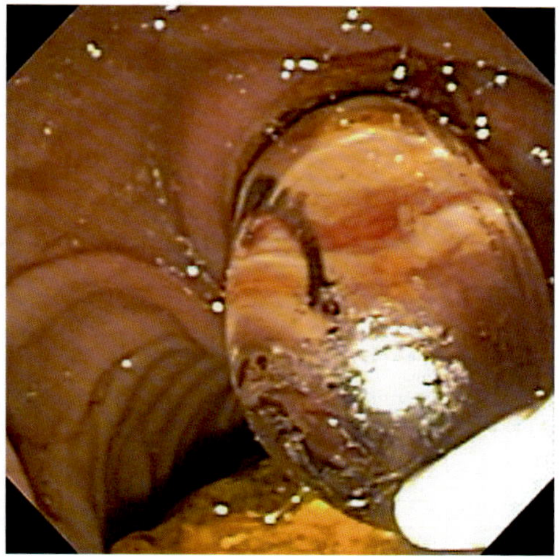

6

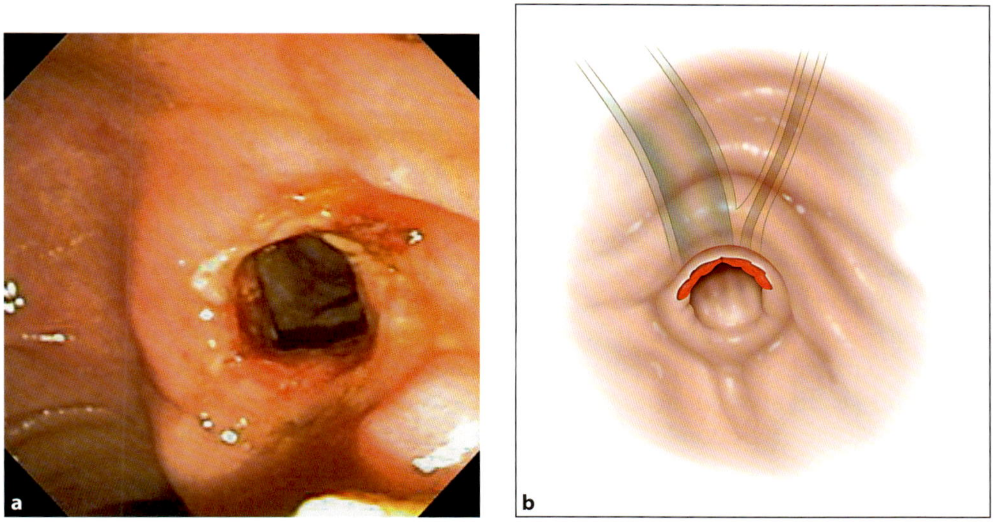

7 a b

Fig. 5. Fluoroscopic image of a completely inflated biliary dilation balloon is seen within the distal bile duct. Inflation of balloon with contrast agent allows for a nice determination of the dilation 'waist'.

Fig. 6. The balloon is positioned across the ampulla such that approximately one-half to two-thirds of the balloon is inside the common bile duct and the remainder endoscopically visible in the duodenum. Each inflation is held for 60 s.

Fig. 7. **a** Endoscopic view of PSBD. After PSBD, the enlarged opening of the biliary os is appreciated. Biliary epithelium of the distal CBD can be seen. We prefer this technique over ABD alone for the extraction of difficult bile duct stones and treatment of ampullary stenosis. We have found that PSBD can also facilitate stone extraction even for small stones (<10 mm) when the distal bile duct is strictured, has a small diameter, or is poorly compliant. **b** Schematic view of PSBD. The objective of balloon dilation after sphincterotomy is to have 'permanent' sphincterotomy, which facilitates the removal of large stones. In the absence of prior sphincteromy, endoscopic removal of stones can result in more damage to the papillary region or even distal impaction.

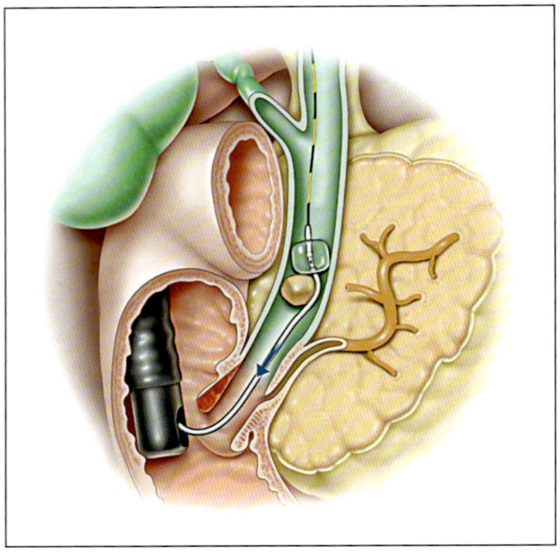

Fig. 8. Stone extraction is then performed using either extraction balloons (which we prefer) or wire baskets.

Outcomes

Preservation of Sphincter of Oddi Function

Long-term manometric studies have shown that ES destroys physiologic sphincter function [12] and may therefore predispose the biliary tract to reflux of gastroduodenal contents and bacterial colonization, which theoretically could lead to higher rates of cholangitis, recurrent bile duct stones due to deconjugation of bilirubin by bacteria, and malignancy from chronic inflammation. At least three studies have demonstrated preservation of sphincter morphology or function following ABD compared with ES [2–4]. Though sphincter function is still present, basal and peak pressures as well as contraction frequency are lower following ABD in both the short- and long-term when compared with pre-procedure manometry.

Despite preservation of sphincter function and a relatively preserved barrier between the biliary system and the gastroduodenal environment, a Cochrane review found no differences in cholangitis, recurrent bile duct stones, or malignancy in long-term follow-up of patients randomized to either ABD or ES [11].

Extraction of Bile Duct Stones

There were numerous randomized controlled studies reported between 1995 and 2005 comparing ABD with ES for the extraction of bile duct stones (table 3). The majority of these used a maximal balloon diameter of 8 mm. A recent Cochrane review demonstrated a lower likelihood of stone extraction during the first attempt with ABD, though a 2004 meta-analysis showed that overall success rates were equivalent [11, 13]. Additionally, mechanical lithotripsy was required more often in the ABD group than the ES group. Though ABD has been shown to have a significantly lower risk of bleeding than ES, the rate of pancreatitis is significantly increased. This higher risk of pancreatitis was highlighted in a well-publicized randomized, controlled multicenter study published in 2004 by DiSario et al. [10]. In this study, there was a significant increase in morbidity (18 vs. 3%) of ABD compared with ES, which was mainly accounted for by an increased incidence of mild to moderate pancreaitits (10 vs. 1%) and severe pancreatitis (5 vs. 0%). There were also 2 deaths in the ABD group, both due to complications of severe pancreatitis. Based on this study and the other available literature, the authors

Table 3. ABD compared with ES for bile duct stone extraction

Reference (first author)	Study design	n	Maximal balloon diameter mm	Success %		Complications %		Comments
				ABD	ES	ABD	ES	
May 1993 [24]	Retro	9	8	100	n/a	22	n/a	stones <8 mm
Mac Mathuna 1995 [25]	Retro	100	8	78	n/a	5	n/a	stones <12 mm
Minami 1995 [4]	RCT	40	8	100	100	10	10	stones <12 mm
Bergman 1997 [9]	RCT	202	8	89	91	17	24	1 death in ABD
Ochi 1999 [26]	RCT	110	8	93	98	2	6	stones <15 mm
Arnold 2001 [27]	RCT	60	8	77	100	30	17	ABD: 2 severe pancreatitis
Bergman 2001 [16]	RCT	34	8	88	78	19	39	all Billroth II patients
Yasuda 2001 [3]	RCT	70	8	100	100	6	9	
Fujita 2003 [28]	RCT	282	8	99	100	15	12	ABD: increased risk of pancreatitis
Vlavianos 2003 [29]	RCT	202	10	87	87	7	3	ABD: 1 severe pancreatitis
DiSario 2004 [10]	RCT	237	8	97	93	18	3	ABD: 2 deaths
Tanaka 2004 [30]	RCT	32	8	100	100	22	22	
Mugica 2007 [15]	Retro	53	10	98	n/a	13	n/a	high-risk anatomy
Tsujino 2007 [31]	Retro	1,000	8	96	n/a	9	n/a	

Retro = Retrospective cohort; RCT = randomized controlled trial.

concluded that balloon dilation of the sphincter of Oddi for stone extraction 'should be avoided in routine practice'.

Because of these 2004 reports, endoscopists were reluctant to adopt balloon sphincteroplasty as a standard technique. There are a number of unique circumstances in which ABD without sphincterotomy should still be considered an appropriate option. In patients with coagulopathy, such as those with cirrhosis, ABD significantly decreases the risk of hemorrhage [7, 8, 14].

Table 4. PSBD compared with ES for bile duct stone extraction

Report	Study design	n	Maximal balloon mm	Success %		Complications %		Comments
				PSBD	ES	PSBD	ES	
Ersoz 2003 [18]	Retro	58	20	88	n/a	16	n/a	all ES failures
Heo 2007 [19]	RCT	200	20	97	98	5	7	
Maydeo 2007 [32]	Prosp	60	10	95	n/a	8	n/a	all ES failures
Minami 2007 [33]	Prosp	88	20	99	n/a	5	n/a	limited ES
Yoo 2007 [20][1]	Prosp	166	20	83	n/a	7	n/a	2 deaths
Attasaranya 2008 [21]	Retro	103	18	95	n/a	5.4	n/a	1 cystic duct perforation
Misra 2008 [34]	Retro	50	20	100	n/a	14	n/a	all ES failures
Kowalski 2009 [17]	Retro	69	15	86	n/a	5.8	n/a	1 perforation in Roux-en-Y

Retro = Retrospective cohort; Prosp = prospective, uncontrolled; RCT = randomized controlled trial.
[1] Abstract only.

In the most recent study of 21 coagulopathic patients with cirrhosis (mean INR 1.9, platelets 65,000/mm^3), the incidence of procedure-related hemorrhage was 0% compared with 30% in a historical control group [8]. Another group of patients in whom ABD may have an acceptable risk-benefit ratio are those with anatomy that makes sphincterotomy either dangerous or technically difficult, e.g. Billroth II gastrectomy, periampullary diverticula, intradiverticular ampulla, or small ampulla [15, 16]. When possible, a limited sphincterotomy prior to dilation is preferred, however it is not always feasible.

The mechanisms leading to the high rates of pancreatitis following ABD, including severe and lethal cases, are not well understood. It has been hypothesized that an expanding balloon against an intact sphincter may cause transmural inflammation and edema which transiently obstructs the pancreatic os and flow of pancreatic secretions [2]. It has subsequently been postulated that performing either a limited or a full biliary sphincterotomy, directed away from the pancreas os, may limit the pressures transmitted toward the pancreatic duct, as the expanding balloon will track along the path of least resistance (i.e., toward the apex of the sphincterotomy) [17]. This technique of PSBD was first reported by Ersoz et al. [18] in 2003 in a group of 58 patients who had failed conventional ES for stone extraction. Esophageal dilating balloons were used up to a size of 20 mm. Success was achieved in 88% of patients, though an overall complication rate of 16% was reported. The majority of complications were due to bleeding; only 3% of patients developed pancreatitis.

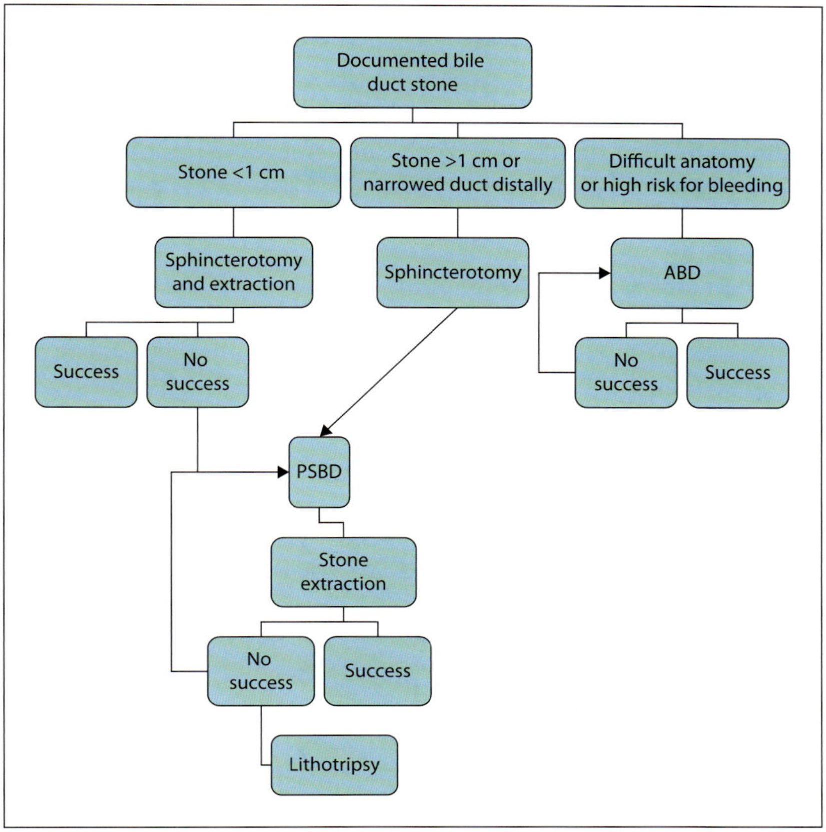

Fig. 9. Algorithm for deciding when to employ PSBD for extraction of bile duct stones.

Over the past few years, enthusiasm for post-sphincterotomy balloon dilation has increased, with several additional reports demonstrating high success rates and a low incidence of complications in patients who fail initial standard ES and stone extraction (table 4). There has, however, been only one randomized controlled trial comparing PSBD with ES alone, which demonstrated equivalent efficacy and complication rates [19]. Caution is advised when using larger balloon sizes (18–20 mm), as 2 deaths and 1 cystic duct perforation were reported in two of the studies [20, 21]. Overall, the risk of hemorrhage following PSBD in recent reports has been variable, ranging from 0 to 8%.

Less Common Indications

There are few published reports describing ABD or PSBD for other indications. Limited data suggest PSBD may be useful for the treatment of papillary stenosis [17, 22]. There is a single case report describing ABD for the extraction of *Ascaris lumbricoides*; the author suggests ABD be used instead of ES for this purpose because of data suggesting ES as a risk factor for new or recurrent biliary ascariasis [23].

Conclusion

Endoscopic sphincteroplasty via ABD should be considered as an alternative to ES in patients with difficult or high-risk anatomy, and in those who are at high risk for post-sphincterotomy hemorrhage. For the routine extraction of bile duct stones, however, we do not recommend ABD alone given the preponderance of data demonstrating an increased risk of pancreatitis in addition to several deaths. We advocate that ES with standard stone extraction technique be attempted first for stones <1 cm. If stone removal is unsuccessful, or for stones >1 cm, or in the relatively common scenario of narrowing or stricture of the distal CBD, ES followed by post-sphincterotomy balloon dilation should be considered as a safe and appropriate alternative (for suggested algorithm, see fig. 9). PSBD uses techniques that are familiar to the endoscopist and are easily applied. The growing body of evidence suggests that PSBD is both safe and effective, and we expect that more endoscopists will adopt PSBD as a useful technique for therapeutic interventions during ERCP.

References

1 Staritz M, Ewe K, Meyer zum Buschenfelde KH: Endoscopic papillary dilation for the treatment of common bile duct stones and papillary stenosis. Endoscopy 1983;15:197–198.

2 Mac Mathuna P, Siegenberg D, Gibbons D, et al: The acute and long-term effect of balloon sphincteroplasty on papillary structure in pigs. Gastrointest Endosc 1996; 44:650–655.

3 Yasuda I, Tomita E, Enya M, et al: Can endoscopic papillary balloon dilation really preserve sphincter of Oddi function? Gut 2001;49:686–691.

4 Minami A, Nakatsu T, Uchida N, et al: Papillary dilation vs. sphincterotomy in endoscopic removal of bile duct stones: a randomized trial with manometric function. Dig Dis Sci 1995;40:2250–2254.

5 Bergman JJ, van der Mey S, Rauws EA, et al: Long-term follow-up after endoscopic sphincterotomy for bile duct stones in patients younger than 60 years of age. Gastrointest Endosc 1996;44:643–649.

6 Hawes RH, Cotton PB, Vallon AG: Follow-up 6–11 years after duodenoscopic sphincterotomy for stones in patients with prior cholecystectomy. Gastroenterology 1990;98: 1008–1012.

7 Kawabe T, Komatsu Y, Tada M, et al: Endoscopic papillary balloon dilation in cirrhotic patients: removal of common bile duct stones without sphincterotomy. Endoscopy 1996;28:694–698.

8 Park DH, Kim MH, Lee SK, et al: Endoscopic sphincterotomy vs. endoscopic papillary balloon dilation for choledocholithiasis in patients with liver cirrhosis and coagulopathy. Gastrointest Endosc 2004; 60:180–185.

9 Bergman J, Rauws EA, Fockens P, et al: Randomised trial of endoscopic balloon dilation versus endoscopic sphincterotomy for removal of bile duct stones. Lancet 1997;349:1124–1129.

10 DiSario JA, Freeman ML, Bjorkman DJ, et al: Endoscopic balloon dilation compared with sphincterotomy for extraction of bile duct stones. Gastroenterology 2004; 127:1291–1299.

11 Weinberg BM, Shindy W, Lo S: Endoscopic balloon sphincter dilation (sphinteroplasty) versus sphincterotomy for common bile duct stones. Cochrane Database of Systematic Reviews 2006;4:CD004890.

12 Bergman JJ, van Berkel AM, Groen AK, et al: Biliary manometry, bacterial characteristics, bile composition and histologic changes 15–17 years after endoscopic sphincterotomy. Gastrointest Endosc 1997;45: 400–405.

13 Baron TH, Harewood GC: Endoscopic balloon dilation of the biliary sphincter compared to endoscopic biliary sphincterotomy for removal of common bile duct stones during ERCP: a meta-analysis of randomized, controlled trials. Am J Gastroenterol 2004; 99:1455–1460.

14 Komatsu Y, Kawabe T, Toda N: Endoscopic papillary balloon dilation for the management of common bile duct stones: experience of 226 cases. Endoscopy 1998;30:12–17.

15 Mugica F, Urdapilleta G, Castiella A, et al: Selective sphincteroplasty of the papilla in cases at risk due to atypical anatomy. World J Gastroenterol 2007;13: 3106–3111.

16 Bergman J, van Berkel AM, Bruno MJ, et al: A randomized trial of endoscopic balloon dilation and endoscopic sphincterotomy for removal of bile duct stones in patients with a prior Billroth II gastrectomy. Gastrointest Endosc 2001;53:19–26.

17 Kowalski T, Nathwani RA, Assis D, et al: Post-sphincterotomy transampullary balloon dilation is a safe and effective technique. Dig Dis Sci 2009;54: 670–674.

18 Ersoz G, Tekesin O, Ozutemiz AO, et al: Biliary sphincterotomy plus dilation with a large balloon for bile duct stones that are difficult to extract. Gastrointest Endosc 2003;57:156–159.
19 Heo JH, Kang DH, Jung J, et al: Endoscopic sphincterotomy plus large-balloon dilation versus endoscopic sphincterotomy for removal of bile-duct stones. Gastrointest Endosc 2007;66:720–726.
20 Yoo B, Kim J, Jung J, et al: Large-balloon sphincteroplasty along with or without sphincterotomy in patients with large extrahepatic bile duct stones: a multicenter study (abstract). Gastrointest Endosc 2007;65:AB97.
21 Attasaranya S, Cheon YK, Vittal H, et al: Large-diameter biliary orifice balloon dilation to aid in endoscopic bile duct stone removal: a multicenter series. Gastrointest Endosc 2008;67:1046–1052.
22 Veldkamp MC, Rauws EA, Dijkgraaf MG, et al: Iatrogenic ampullary stenosis: history, endoscopic management, and outcome in a series of 49 patients. Gastrointest Endosc 2007;66:708–716.
23 Misra SP, Dwivedi M: Removal of *Ascaris lumbricoides* from the bile duct using balloon sphincteroplasty. Endoscopy 1998;30:S6–S7.
24 May GR, Cotton PB, Edmunds SE, Chong W: Removal of stones from the bile duct at ERCP without sphincterotomy. Gastrointest Endosc 1993;39: 749–754.
25 Mac Mathuna P, White P, Clarke E, et al: Endoscopic balloon sphincteroplasty (papillary dilation) for bile duct stones: efficacy, safety, and follow-up in 100 patients. Gastrointest Endosc 1995;42:468–474.
26 Ochi Y, Mukawa K, Kiyosawa K, Akamatsu T: Comparing the treatment outcomes of endoscopic papillary dilation and endoscopic sphincterotomy for removal of bile duct stones. J Gastroenterol Hepatol 1999;14:90–96.
27 Arnold JC, Benz C, Martin WR, et al: Endoscopic papillary balloon dilation vs. sphincterotomy for removal of common bile duct stones: a prospective randomized pilot study. Endoscopy 2001;33:563–567.
28 Fujita N, Maguchi H, Komatsu Y, et al: Endoscopic sphincterotomy and endoscopic papillary balloon dilation for bile duct stones: a prospective randomized controlled multicenter trial. Gastrointest Endosc 2003;57: 151–155.
29 Vlavianos P, Chopra K, Mandalia S, et al: Endoscopic balloon dilation versus endoscopic sphincterotomy for the removal of bile duct stones: a prospective randomized trial. Gut 2003;52:1165–1169.
30 Tanaka S, Sawayama T, Yoshioka T: Endoscopic papillary balloon dilation and endoscopic sphincterotomy for bile duct stones: long-term outcomes in a prospective randomized controlled trial. Gastrointest Endosc 2004;59: 614–618.
31 Tsujino T, Kawabe T, Komatsu Y, et al: Endoscopic papillary balloon dilation for bile duct stone: immediate and long-term outcomes in 1000 patients. Clin Gastroenterol Hepatol 2007;5:130–137.
32 Maydeo A, Bhandari S: Balloon sphincteroplasty for removing difficult bile duct stones. Endoscopy 2007; 39:958–961.
33 Minami A, Hirose S, Monoto T, et al: Small sphincterotomy combined with papillary dilation with large balloon permits retrieval of large stones without mechanical lithotripsy. World J Gastroenterol 2007;13:2179–2182.
34 Misra SP, Dwivedi M: Large-diameter balloon dilation after endoscopic sphincterotomy for removal of difficult bile duct stones. Endoscopy 2008;40:209–213.

David E. Loren, MD
Division of Gastroenterology and Hepatology, Thomas Jefferson University
132 S. 10th Street, Philadelphia, PA 19107 (USA)
Tel. +1 215 955 8900, Fax +1 215 503 2527, E-Mail david.loren@jefferson.edu

Mönkemüller K, Wilcox CM, Muñoz-Navas M (eds): Interventional and Therapeutic Gastrointestinal Endoscopy.
Front Gastrointest Res. Basel, Karger, 2010, vol 27, pp 356–362

Management of Benign Biliary Strictures

Todd H. Baron

Division of Gastroenterology and Hepatology, Mayo Clinic, Rochester, Minn., USA

Abstract

There are a variety of causes of benign biliary strictures including chronic pancreatitis, surgery, and primary sclerosing cholangitis, amongst others. The general treatment of these strictures is dilation followed by stent placement. For postoperative strictures the data shows that placement of multiple, large bore (10-Fr) stents over the course of several procedures is better than placement of fewer stents. Care must be taken to exclude malignancy in cases where benignity is not certain. The use of temporary placement of covered, removable expandable metal stents for the treatment of benign biliary strictures appears promising.

Benign strictures of the biliary tree are encountered commonly in a busy therapeutic ERCP practice. The etiologies of these strictures and their underlying histopathology are highly variable and thus each has a different natural history and response to therapy. This chapter will review the types of benign biliary strictures and the approach to therapy. Benign extrinsic processes that cause biliary obstruction (e.g., pancreatic pseudocyst) will not be considered.

Etiologies of Benign Biliary Strictures

Table 1 shows the etiologies of benign biliary strictures. When approaching the patient with a presumed benign biliary stricture, one must take a careful history of underlying diseases (underlying autoimmune pancreatitis, chronic pancreatitis, and inflammatory bowel disease) and prior pancreaticobiliary surgery. Before assuming a stricture is benign, especially when the clinical history does not suggest an obvious benign process, imaging studies should be obtained to evaluate underlying malignancy. Such imaging studies include CT and MRI, although even after extensive evaluation the strictures may remain indeterminate (discussed later). The other entities will be discussed as if the diagnosis is certain.

Overview of Endoscopic Treatment of Benign Biliary Strictures

Endoscopic therapy consists of rigid or, more commonly, balloon dilation followed by placement of plastic biliary stents (fig. 1a–d). The most recent data suggests that for most causes of benign

Table 1. Causes of benign biliary strictures

Postoperative
Laparoscopic cholecystectomy
Biliary resection
Liver transplantation
Chronic pancreatitis
Primary sclerosing cholangitis
Autoimmune cholangiopathy
Ischemia
Post-endoscopic biliary sphincterotomy

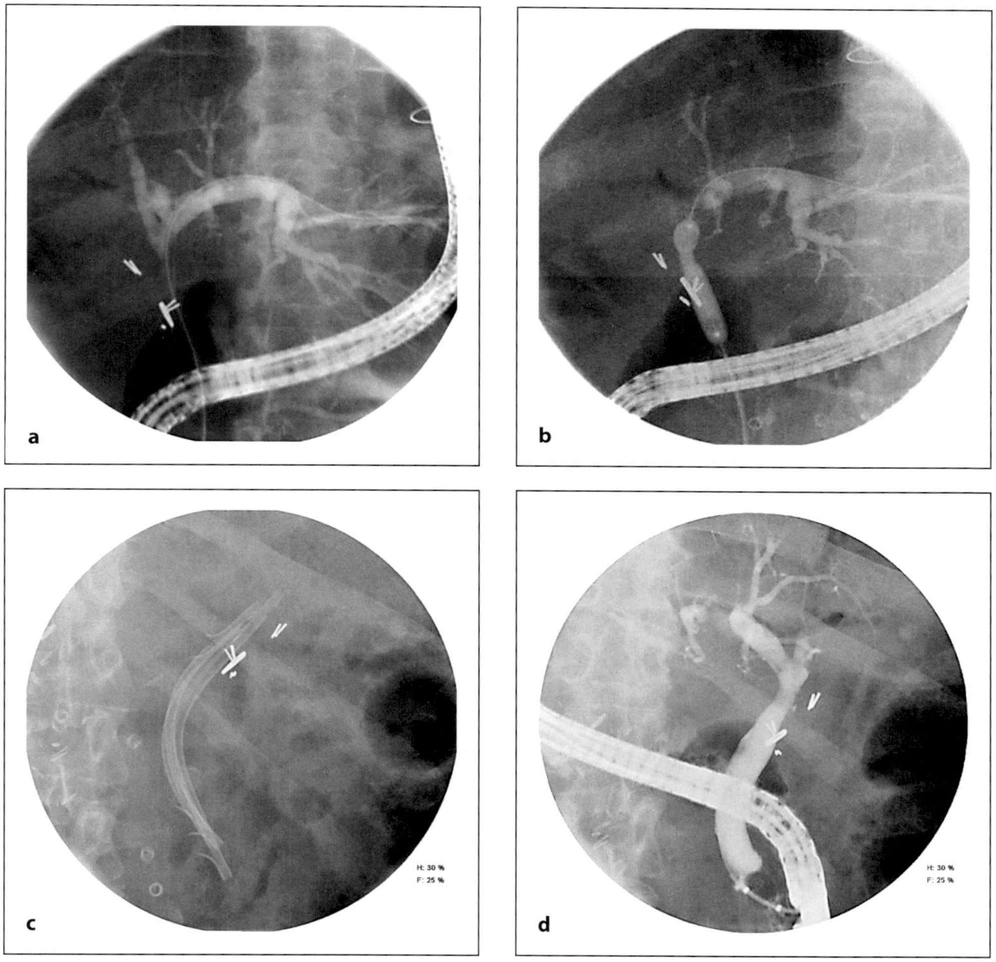

Fig. 1. Endoscopic treatment of post-cholecystectomy biliary stricture using plastic biliary stents. **a** Initial cholangiogram reveals stricture in the common hepatic duct near the previous surgical clips. **b** Balloon dilation of stricture. **c** Placement of multiple stents over two procedures. **d** Cholangiogram after stent removal showing stricture resolution.

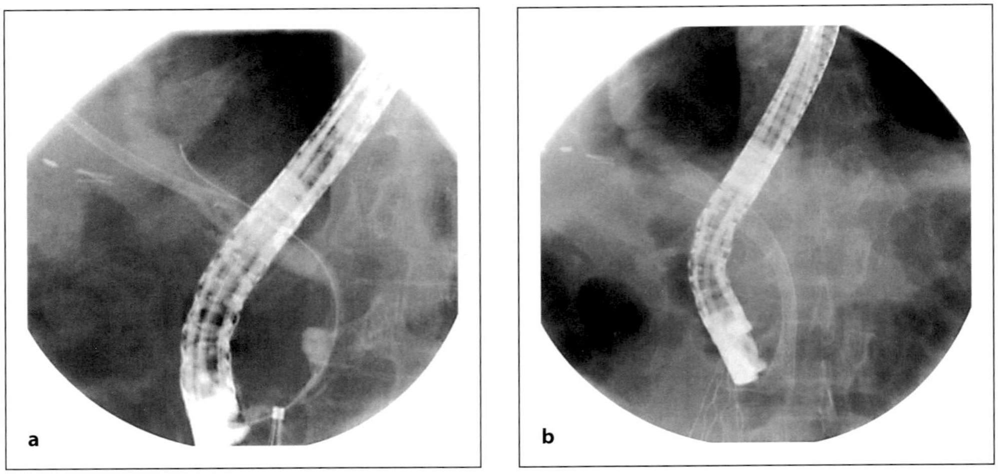

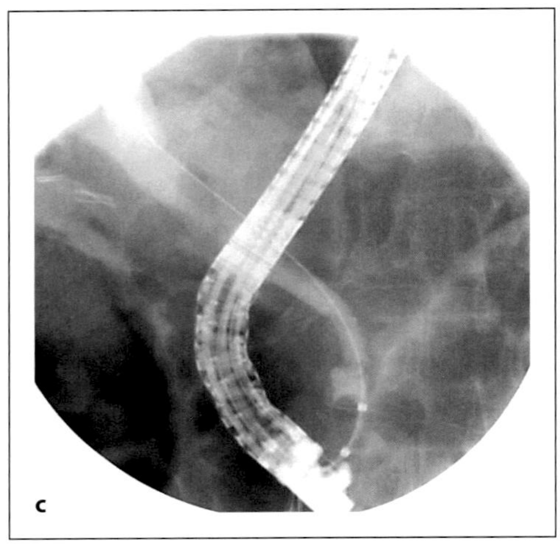

Fig. 2. Endoscopic treatment of distal bile duct stricture from chronic pancreatitis stricture using a plastic-covered metal biliary stent. **a** Initial cholangiogram reveals stricture in the distal common bile duct. **b** Image taken immediately after placement of a 10-mm self-expandable covered stent. **c** Cholangiogram after stent removal showing improvement in stricture.

strictures placement of multiple side-by-side large bore plastic stents over the course of several endoscopic sessions, exchanging periodically (every 3–4 months) for up to 1 year allows a higher rate of successful stricture resolution than when only one or two stents are placed [1, 2].

Self-expandable metal stents (SEMS) placement for management of benign strictures has evolved. Initial studies using uncovered SEMS showed that although the early clinical outcome (relief of biliary obstruction) was favorable, reobstruction occurred from tissue hyperplasia [3]. Moreover, since uncovered SEMS imbed into the bile duct wall, they are non-removable. Thus, the use of uncovered stents for benign biliary strictures has been abandoned. More recently, partially covered and fully covered SEMS have been used since little (partially covered) to no embedding (fully covered) occurs. The stents expand to a diameter of 10 mm and remain in place for a variable period of time to allow dilation and remodeling of the stricture. Then stents are subsequently removed by snare or grasping using a forceps (fig. 2a–c). It is important that these stents be left across the papilla and that enough length remains in the duodenum to allow effective grasping. There is emerging data on the use of covered metal stents for a variety of benign biliary strictures [4].

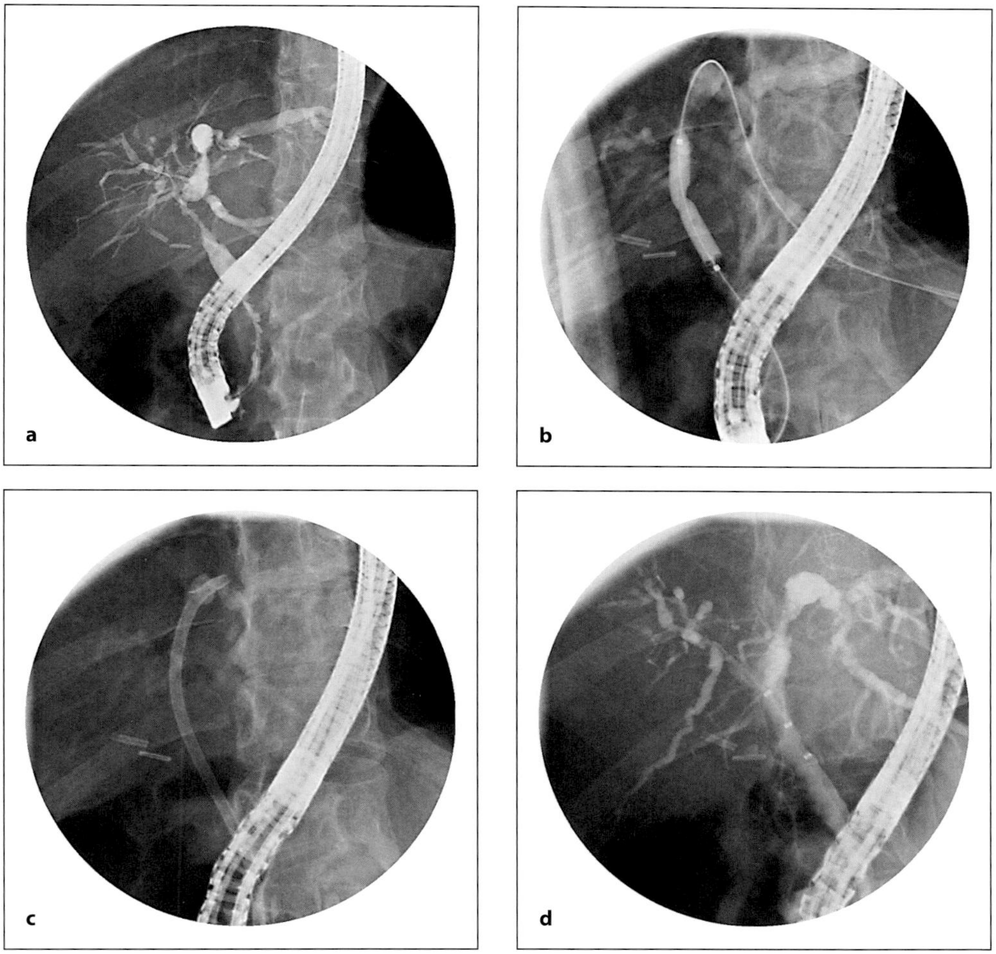

Fig. 3. Endoscopic treatment of dominant biliary stricture in PSC using single plastic biliary stents. **a** Initial cholangiogram reveals stricture in the common hepatic duct extending to the left hepatic duct. **b** Balloon dilation of stricture. **c** Placement of a single 10-Fr plastic biliary stent. **d** Cholangiogram after stent removal showing marked improvement in stricture.

Specific Etiologies

Postoperative Strictures

Cholecystectomy, open or more commonly laparoscopic, can result in injury to the bile duct. These injuries can be recognized early in the postoperative period where there is commonly an associated bile leak, or late. Later presentation may respond less favorably because of the established fibrosis. Other postoperative strictures include post-liver resection (hepatectomy). Post-liver transplant strictures can occur at the anastomosis following either a duct-to-duct (DDA or choledochocholedochal) or hepaticojejunal anastomosis. Living related donor transplantation with DDA anastomosis can be particularly challenging since the arrangement of the anastomoses are variable and can include the cystic duct remnant. There is a large body of literature to support endoscopic therapy for all of these postoperative strictures. With aggressive dilation and placement of multiple stents, the long-term success rate for endoscopic intervention is high [5, 6].

Whether patients who relapse after stent removal respond to additional or more prolonged plastic stent therapy or to removable, metal stents, is unknown.

Chronic Pancreatitis

Chronic pancreatitis produces distal bile duct strictures that are usually refractory to endoscopic therapy with single plastic stents, particularly in those patients with calcific chronic pancreatitis. Multiple plastic stents can be used as a treatment modality for biliary strictures in the setting of chronic pancreatitis [7]. Recently, covered SEMS have been used for the treatment of chronic pancreatitis-induced bile duct strictures [4, 8–10]. The large diameter (10 mm) dilates the stricture over time. The stent is removed after an interval of 3–6 months. Results using this approach have been encouraging, though these devices are not yet approved in the USA for benign disease.

Primary Sclerosing Cholangitis (PSC)

PSC develops in patients with underlying inflammatory bowel disease. Such patients may benefit from endoscopic intervention for treatment of dominant strictures and/or biliary lithiasis [11]. Patients with dominant strictures usually present with worsening biliary obstruction. Underlying cholangiocarcinoma must be considered in these patients. Routine brush cytology has a low sensitivity for detecting cancer in this population. Recently, fluorescence in-situ hybridization has been shown to have a high sensitivity for the detection of underlying cholangiocarcinoma in the setting of PSC [12]. Cholangioscopy has recently been shown to enhance the detection of malignancy in these patients [13].

Endoscopic treatment of dominant strictures involves balloon dilation, often in combination with short-term (≤8 weeks) large bore (10-Fr) stent placement (fig. 3a–d). Endpoints following endoscopic therapy have included clinical, biochemical, and radiological improvement and range from 65 to 100% [14]. Generally, because the bile ducts are small throughout the biliary tree, the use of multiple stents, which has been shown to be effective for the treatment of other strictures, is not an option. There is a small amount of data on the use of removable SEMS for PSC strictures [4].

Autoimmune Cholangiopathy

Autoimmune cholangiopathy is usually seen as an extrapancreatic manifestation of autoimmune pancreatitis (AIP). Biliary obstruction can be caused by an inflammatory mass within the pancreatic head (similar to chronic pancreatitis of other etiologies) or by coexisting sclerosing cholangitis. Biliary tract involvement occurs in 17% of patients with AIP. Pancreatic and extrapancreatic manifestations of AIP respond to corticosteroid therapy. Elevated levels of serum IgG_4 are characteristic of AIP though normal IgG_4 serology does not exclude a diagnosis of AIP. IgG_4-associated cholangitis (IAC) refers to the manifestation of IgG_4-related systemic disease in the biliary tree and can occur with AIP or as an isolated biliary disease.

IAC can cause intrahepatic, proximal extrahepatic, or intrapancreatic biliary strictures. Establishing a diagnosis of IAC relies on histologic analysis or response to a corticosteroid trial. Endoscopic biopsy specimens often do not provide sufficient tissue to diagnose IAC. Intrahepatic strictures in patients with IAC can mimic those of PSC, but IAC strictures are more segmental, longer, with prestenotic dilatation and more commonly affected the distal common bile duct.

Stent placement is used to temporarily relieve biliary obstruction while patients are being diagnosed and treated with corticosteroids.

Ischemic Strictures

Ischemic strictures usually involve the bifurcation and intrahepatics. They are often seen in post-liver transplant patients and are associated with multiple factors but often seen as a result of poor hepatic arterial flow. Similar strictures have been reported after other causes of localized or systemic ischemia in non-transplant patients. Such strictures can be treated endoscopically with placement of multiple stents [15], though they respond less well to dilation and stent therapy than anastomotic strictures and require more endoscopic procedures [16].

Post-Endoscopic Biliary Sphincterotomy Strictures

Endoscopic biliary sphincterotomy can occasionally be complicated by the development of a cautery-induced stricture. Similar to other biliary strictures, dilation and multiple plastic stents can be placed to allow resolution of the stricture [17].

Indeterminate Biliary Obstruction

Some patients with biliary strictures cannot be readily classified into benign or malignant based upon imaging studies and tissue sampling. Tissue-sampling techniques at ERCP consist of wire-guided biliary brush cytology and intraductal forceps biopsy [18]. Adjuvant techniques to assess strictures include intraductal ultrasonography [19] and direct cholangioscopy with or without directed biopsy [20]. In a small percentage of patients the diagnosis remains unclear. In some patients the final diagnosis can only be established during long-term follow-up or at surgical exploration and resection.

References

1 Matlock J, Freeman ML: Endoscopic therapy of benign biliary strictures. Rev Gastroenterol Disord 2005;5:206–214.

2 Draganov P, Hoffman B, Marsh W, Cotton P, Cunningham J: Long-term outcome in patients with benign biliary strictures treated endoscopically with multiple stents Gastrointest Endosc 2002;55:680–686.

3 Dumonceau JM, Devière J, Delhaye M, Baize M, Cremer M: Plastic and metal stents for postoperative benign bile duct strictures: the best and the worst. Gastrointest Endosc 1998;47:8–17.

4 Kahaleh M, Behm B, Clarke BW, Brock A, Shami VM, De La Rue SA, Sundaram V, Tokar J, Adams RB, Yeaton P: Temporary placement of covered self-expandable metal stents in benign biliary strictures: a new paradigm? Gastrointest Endosc 2008;67:446–454.

5 Costamagna G, Pandolfi M, Mutignani M, Spada C, Perri V: Long-term results of endoscopic management of postoperative bile duct strictures with increasing numbers of stents. Gastrointest Endosc 2001;54:162–168.

6 Morelli G, Fazel A, Judah J, Pan JJ, Forsmark C, Draganov P: Rapid-sequence endoscopic management of post-transplant anastomotic biliary strictures. Gastrointest Endosc 2008;67:879–885.

7 Catalano MF, Linder JD, George S, Alcocer E, Geenen JE: Treatment of symptomatic distal common bile duct stenosis secondary to chronic pancreatitis: comparison of single vs. multiple simultaneous stents. Gastrointest Endosc 2004;60:945–952.

8 Cantù P, Hookey LC, Morales A, Le Moine O, Devière J: The treatment of patients with symptomatic common bile duct stenosis secondary to chronic pancreatitis using partially covered metal stents: a pilot study. Endoscopy 2005;37:735–739.

9 Cahen DL, Rauws EA, Gouma DJ, Fockens P, Bruno MJ: Removable fully covered self-expandable metal stents in the treatment of common bile duct strictures due to chronic pancreatitis: a case series. Endoscopy 2008;40: 697–700.
10 Mahajan A, Ho H, Sauer B, Phillips MS, Shami VM, Ellen K, Rehan M, Schmitt TM, Kahaleh M: Temporary placement of fully covered self-expandable metal stents in benign biliary strictures: midterm evaluation (with video). Gastrointest Endosc 2009;70:303–309.
11 Gluck M, Cantone NR, Brandabur JJ, Patterson DJ, Bredfeldt JE, Kozarek RA: A twenty-year experience with endoscopic therapy for symptomatic primary sclerosing cholangitis. J Clin Gastroenterol 2008;42: 1032–1039.
12 Charatcharoenwitthaya P, Enders FB, Halling KC, Lindor KD: Utility of serum tumor markers, imaging, and biliary cytology for detecting cholangiocarcinoma in primary sclerosing cholangitis. Hepatology 2008;48:1106–1017.
13 Tischendorf JJ, Krüger M, Trautwein C, Duckstein N, Schneider A, Manns MP, Meier PN: Cholangioscopic characterization of dominant bile duct stenoses in patients with primary sclerosing cholangitis. Endoscopy 2006;38:665–669.
14 McLoughlin M, Enns R: Endoscopy in the management of primary sclerosing cholangitis. Curr Gastroenterol Rep 2008;10:177–185.
15 Tabibian JH, Asham EH, Goldstein L, Han SH, Saab S, Tong MJ, Busuttil RW, Durazo FA: Endoscopic treatment with multiple stents for post-liver transplantation non-anastomotic biliary strictures. Gastrointest Endosc 2009;69:1236–1243.
16 Barriga J, Thompson R, Shokouh-Amiri H, Davila R, Ismail MK, Waters B, Tombazzi CR: Biliary strictures after liver transplantation. Predictive factors for response to endoscopic management and long-term outcome. Am J Med Sci 2008;335:439–443.
17 Pozsár J, Sahin P, László F, Topa L: Endoscopic treatment of sphincterotomy-associated distal common bile duct strictures by using sequential insertion of multiple plastic stents. Gastrointest Endosc 2005;62: 85–91.
18 Papachristou GI, Smyrk TC, Baron TH: Endoscopic retrograde cholangiopancreatography tissue sampling: when and how? Clin Gastroenterol Hepatol 2007;5:783–790.
19 Varadarajulu S, Eloubeidi MA, Wilcox CM: Prospective evaluation of indeterminate ERCP findings by intraductal ultrasound. J Gastroenterol Hepatol 2007;22:2086–2092.
20 Shah RJ, Langer DA, Antillon MR, Chen YK: Cholangioscopy and cholangioscopic forceps biopsy in patients with indeterminate pancreaticobiliary pathology. Clin Gastroenterol Hepatol 2006;4:219–225.

Todd H. Baron, MD
200 First Street S.W., Charlton 8A
Rochester, MN 55905 (USA)
Tel. +1 507 266 6931, Fax +1 507 266 3939, E-Mail baron.todd@mayo.edu

Mönkemüller K, Wilcox CM, Muñoz-Navas M (eds): Interventional and Therapeutic Gastrointestinal Endoscopy.
Front Gastrointest Res. Basel, Karger, 2010, vol 27, pp 363–374

Endoscopic Management of Malignant Biliary Obstruction

Dalton Marques Chaves

University of São Paulo Medical School Clinics Hospital, São Paulo, Brazil

Abstract

Distal and proximal biliary obstructions have distinct etiologies and anatomic characteristics which are reflected in the differential diagnosis and therapeutic management. Cholangiocarcinoma is the most frequent malignant neoplasia of the biliary tract and the Klatskin tumor accounts for 60–80% of the cases. Biliary decompression increases survival and improves the patient's quality of life. Endoscopic drainage has been the technique most employed because of its high rate of success, fewer complications and best cost. The use of stents for biliary decompression is the most common form of endoscopic treatment of malignant biliary obstruction. There are 2 basics types of stents: plastic and metallic. Both have their advantages and disadvantages, and the choice between the 2 stents should take the patient's health, life expectancy and quality of life into consideration.

Biliary obstruction has always been a diagnostic and therapeutic challenge. It is very important for those who perform endoscopic retrograde cholangiopancreatography (ERCP) to be familiarized with the management techniques of malignant biliary obstruction in order to improve the success rate of the procedure and avoiding serious complications for the patient.

The causes of malignant biliary obstructions arise from the biliary tract or from infiltration or compression from extrinsic tumors. The most common causes are: cholangiocarcinoma, pancreatic tumor, gallbladder tumor, ampullary tumor, hepatocellular carcinoma and metastasis.

Cholangiocarcinoma is the most frequent malignant neoplasm of the biliary tract and its incidence varies in different geographic locations, being highest in some Asiatic countries. Considering the location of the tumor it may be classified into 3 groups: intrahepatic, perihilar and distal extrahepatic.

For unknown reasons, the incidence of and mortality from intrahepatic cholangiocarcinoma have been increasing in recent years in relation to the extrahepatic location [1]. The Klatskin tumor or perihilar tumor is the most common cholangiocarcinoma, accounting for 60–80% of the cases [2].

Endoscopic Treatment

The prognosis for cholangiocarcinoma is usually poor, ranging between 5 and 10% in 5 years. The only curative possibility for these patients is surgery; however most of these cases are inoperable when diagnosis is made. At the time of diagnosis only 10–20% of the patients have indications for surgical treatment secondary to advanced disease or poor medical health. The prognosis for inoperable patients is poor with a median survival time of 6.7–11.6 months [3].

Biliary decompression to increase survival and improve the patient's quality of life may be accomplished surgically, radiologically or endoscopically. The endoscopic techniques are the most employed of because of their high rate of success, fewer complications and lower cost [4–6].

The use of stents for biliary decompression was first described in 1980 and still being the most common form of endoscopic treatment of malignant biliary obstruction.

Indications

Malignant biliary obstruction is the most frequent indication for endoscopic decompression. Endoscopic drainage may be employed as a definitive or temporary method.

Definitive endoscopic biliary drainage is indicated in cases with advanced and unresectable tumors or for non-surgical candidates with poor health. Resectability may be ascertained by surgical exploration or by radiographic findings, such as vascular encasement, involvement of adjacent organs, retropancreatic and paraceliac nodal metastases, non-regional liver metastases or distant metastases.

Temporary biliary decompression is indicated before surgery in the following situations: patients with acute cholangitis; for the prevention of cholangitis after endoscopic biliary contrasting, or if surgery is to be delayed due to unfavorable clinical conditions. Excluding these situations, endoscopic biliary drainage is controversial if done before surgery since it may increase the risk of postoperative infection [2, 7].

Technical Aspects

In most institutions, ERCP is performed with anesthesia or deep sedation. For deep sedation, the anesthetics that have been most used are propofol associated with fentanyl. However, the procedure can be performed with moderate sedation using midazolam combined with a narcotic, such as fentanyl.

After deep cannulation of the biliary tract, enough contrast should be injected to identify the stricture and to define the management strategy. It is important to avoid over injection of contrast to prevent acute cholangitis in cases where adequate local drainage has not been achieved and to prevent cholecystitis as this is more frequent after the employment of metallic stents.

After the stricture has been identified and analyzed, it must be traversed with a guidewire for endoscopic drainage. In case of accentuated stenosis, traversing may be difficult and for the success of the procedure it is important that some maneuvers be performed with the wire. The movement of pushing and pulling back associated with rotation is the proper way to manipulate the guidewire. In some situations the sphincterotome may help to achieve selective cannulation.

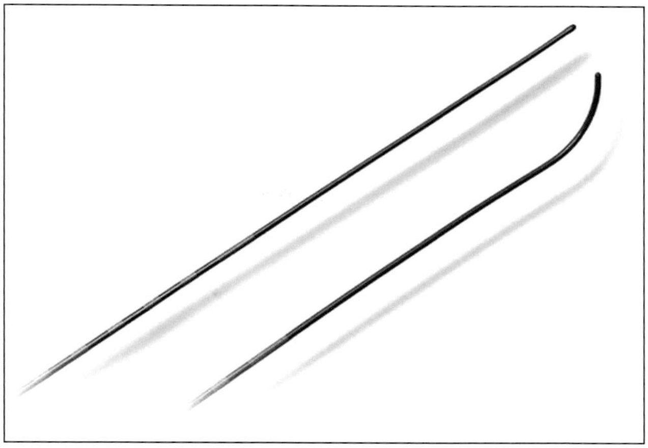

Fig. 1. The two shapes of guidewire: straight and angled.

If it is angled in the required direction the guidewire may be properly placed. The 0.09-cm guidewire is preferable if the introduction of a stent is intended; however, in certain cases it may be necessary to employ a thinner guidewire such as one measuring 0.06 cm to pass through the stenosis.

There are two basics types of guidewire defined by tip shape: straight or angled (fig. 1). The angulated tip is better for selective cannulation of the hepatic ducts.

Regarding the nature of the guidewire, it can be fully hydrophilic, non-hydrophilic or only have a hydrophilic tip. Guidewires with hydrophilic tips are preferred by most because they improve the cannulation capacity without compromising the stability for passing stents.

It is important to pass the wire well above the stricture to prevent misplacing the cannula during the procedure.

Choosing the right length of stent is important for the success of the drainage. One good way to do this is by withdrawing the initial cannulating catheter to measure the distance from the proximal end of the stenosis up to the papilla. The length of the catheter exteriorized outside the biopsy port between these two points corresponds to the stent's length. Another method is to measure this distance and comparing it with the thickness of the endoscope using radioscopy.

The long distal end of the stent should be avoided to prevent damaging the opposite duodenal wall as it may lead to perforation.

Bilateral stenting is technically difficult; the left system should be drained first as it is more difficult and usually produces more effective drainage than the right system stent. This is due to the longer length of the main left duct before branching, leading to larger volumes of the liver being drained. However, this is questioned by many others.

Dilatation

Dilation before placement of a 10-Fr plastic stent for distal biliary stenosis is not usually necessary. In case resistance is felt during cannulation, or there is uncertainty during the procedure, the dilation should be done with a 10-Fr dilating catheter (Soehendra dilator, Cook Endoscopy) or hydrostatic balloon dilation (Wilson-Cook, Boston Scientific).

2 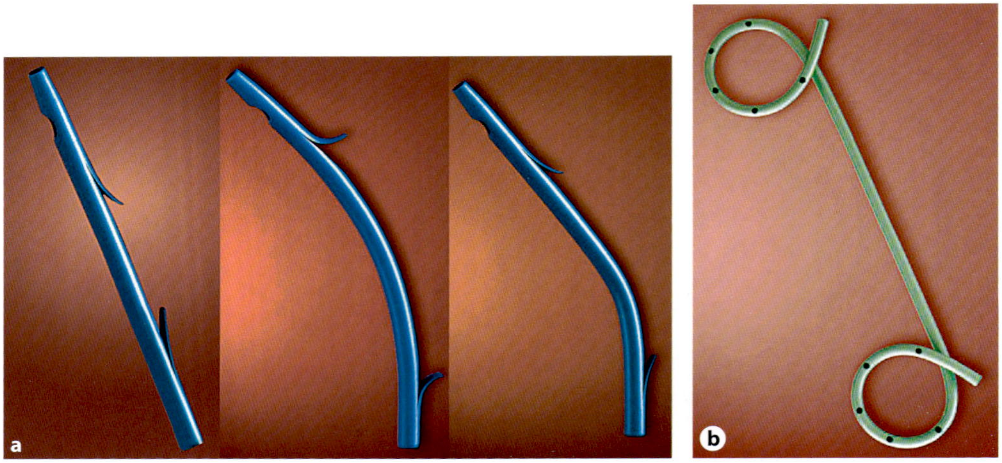

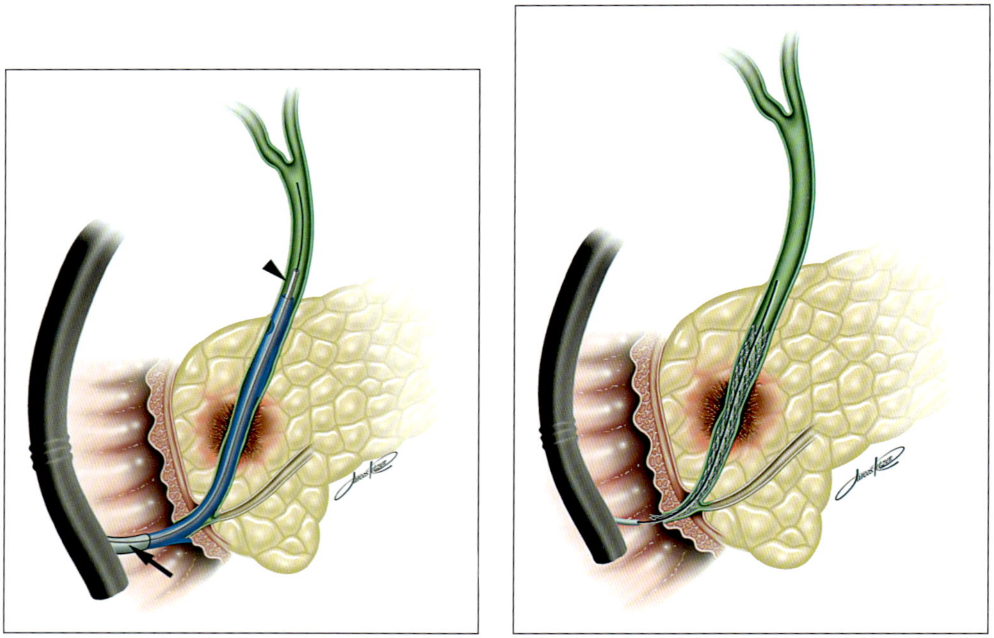

3 4

Fig. 2. Plastic stents. **a** Straight, curved, angled. **b** Double pigtail. **Fig. 3.** Illustration of the plastic stent being placed through of distal stenosis caused by pancreatic cancer. Inner guiding catheter (arrowhead), stent (blue) and pusher tube (arrow). **Fig. 4.** Illustration of the metallic stent being placed through a distal stenosis caused by pancreatic cancer.

For hilar obstruction, stricture dilation is frequently required. The longer distance from the tumor to the tip of the endoscope determines the loss mechanical force transmission to the stent during its insertion making its placement more difficult. The frequent necessity of 2 stents is another important factor that demands dilation.

For placement of metallic stents, routine stricture dilation is not required.

Sphincterotomy

The real need for biliary sphincterotomy before insertion of the 10-Fr plastic stent has not been proven [8, 9], but most prefer to perform it to facilitate stent insertion and to prevent obstruction of pancreatic drainage or acute pancreatitis. In a retrospective study, it was observed that the rate of pancreatitis following transpapillary plastic stenting without sphincterotomy was higher in patients with proximal biliary stenosis. The supposed cause was because this type of lesion worked as a fulcrum causing a distal deflection of the stent and the consequent compression of the pancreatic orifice [9]. For patients with coagulation disorders sphincterotomy is contraindicated. In addition, for the metallic stent, transpapillary stent placement without previous sphincterotomy is unfounded.

If sphincterotomy was decided before stent insertion, an economic sphincterotomy may avoid complications.

When the insertion of more than one stent is intended, sphincterotomy is required.

Plastic Stents

Plastic stents are composed of polyethylene or polytetrafluoroethylene (Teflon).

There are a variety of plastic stents available with different shapes, calibers, lengths and materials. Most are made of polyethylene, Teflon, and polyurethane. More recently a 2-layer stent composed of an inner perfluorinated water-repellent layer and an outer structural layer composed of a stainless steel mesh coated with a polyamide elastomer has been designed to enhance deployment (Olympus).

As to the shape, the plastic stent can be straight, angled, curved or pigtailed (fig. 2). The straight stents have 1 or more side flaps on each end to anchor them, whereas pigtail stents have a 360° curved section at 1 or both ends for anchoring. Straight biliary stents may or may not have side holes located at the barb flaps at each end, whereas pigtail stents have numerous side holes at each end.

More recently, a stent with an antireflux valve (Cook) has become available to prevent occlusion due to food.

The diameters of these stents vary from 5 to 12 Fr in caliber and from 1 to 15 cm in length. As the capacity of drainage is directly related to the diameter of the stent, it is important to choose a stent with the maximum caliber that each case can accommodate.

Stents of 8.5 Fr or more usually come with an inner guiding catheter that should be used to promote stability when passing through the strictures. The setup kit has been commercialized by different companies (fig. 3).

Metallic Stents

The metallic stent was developed in an attempt to resolve premature obstruction by plastic stents.

This stent has a delivery system of no more than 12 Fr, mostly between 7.5 and 8.0 Fr. It can be easily deployed in the biliary tree and self-expand up to 10 mm (fig. 4, 5).

There are 2 categories of metallic stents: uncovered and covered.

The most acknowledged types of uncovered stents are: Wallstent, Diamond Ultraflex, Zilver and Flexxus.

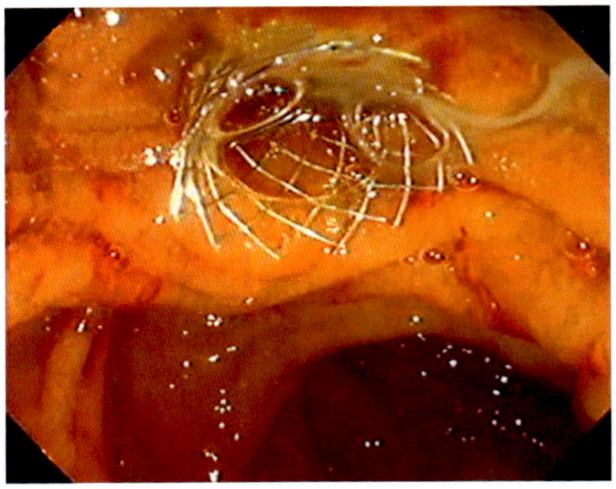

5

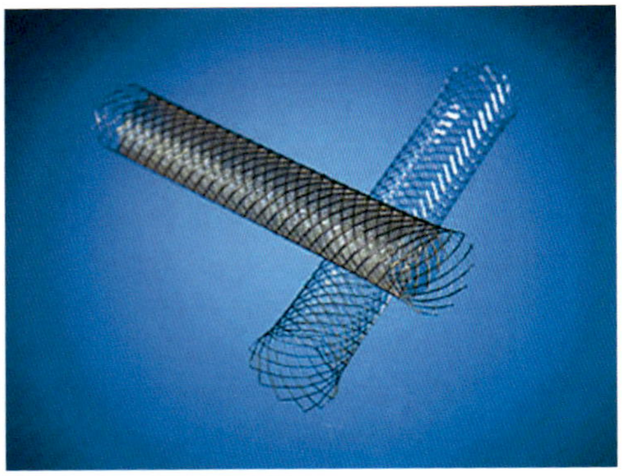

6

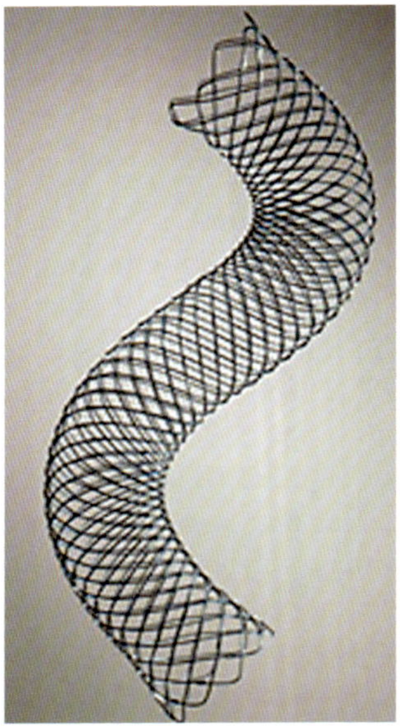

7

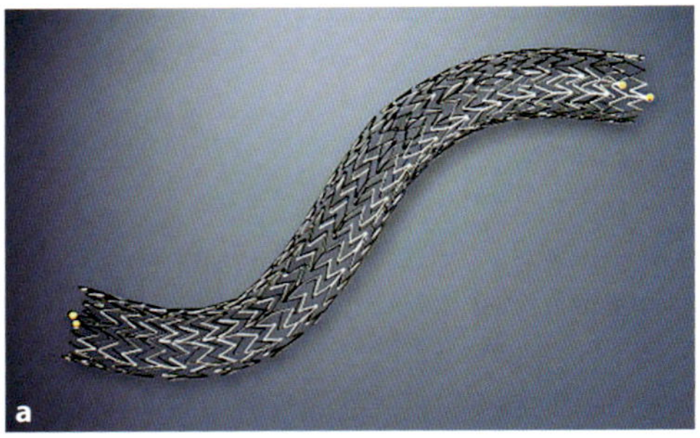

a

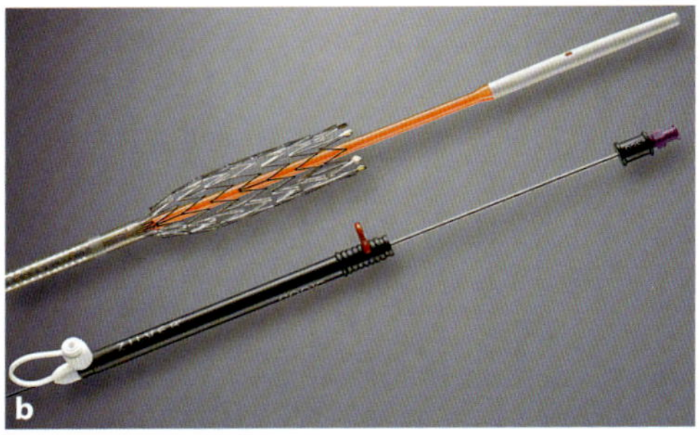

b

8

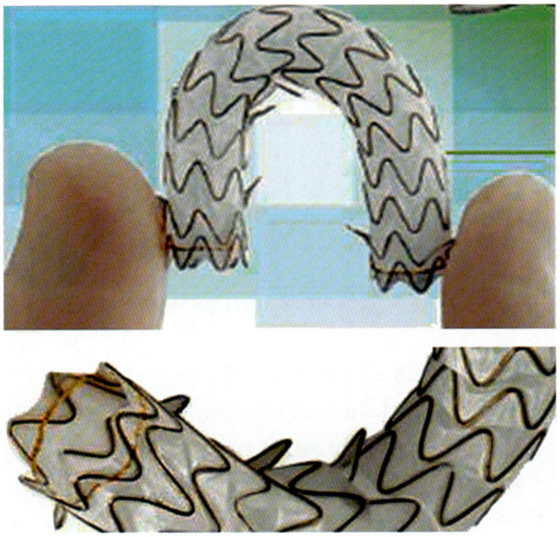

9

Fig. 5. Transpapillary metallic stent draining purulent bile.

Fig. 6. Wall stent covered and uncovered (Boston Scientific).

Fig. 7. WallFlex Stent – platinum-cored nitinol construction (Boston Scientific).

Fig. 8. **a**, **b** Zilver stent (Wilson Cook). Permission for use granted by Cook Medical Inc. (Bloomington, Ind.).

Fig. 9. Viabil® stent.

The Wallstent stent is considered the first metallic stent, and is composed of braided stainless steel mesh (fig. 6). The Ultraflex stent is made of nitinol which provides high flexibility (fig. 7). The Zilver stent is known as the spiral Z stent because it is a modification of the original Gianturco-Rösch Z stent made of stainless steel wire bent in a continuous Z-shaped pattern (fig. 8). The Flexxus stent is made of highly flexible nitinol.

The covered stents include: Wallstent and Viabil® Stent.

The Wallstent has a polyurethane covering. The Viabil® stent is a nitinol stent with expanded polytetrafluoroethylene (ePTFE) and fluoroethylenepropylene (FEP) lining, which is a more bio-inert material. It has anchoring fins to prevent migrations (fig. 9).

Plastic versus Metallic Stents

The most common form of endoscopic treatment for malignant biliary obstruction is insertion of plastic or metallic stents in the biliary tract. Both have their advantages and disadvantages.

Plastic stents have the important advantage of being relatively more affordable and can be changed several times. However, they are associated with a high rate of obstruction in a short time, 30–70% in a period of 3–6 months, and should be replaced every 3 months to prevent complications due to obstruction [10, 11]. The obstruction occurs due to a bio-film formed by bacterial colonization and duodenal reflux [12, 13].

Self-expanding metal stents have the advantage of a higher diameter and consequent higher patency, with fewer interventions being needed because of obstruction. However, when in place they are very difficult to remove or mobilize. Their higher costs are compensated by their higher patency time of approximately 12 months. Some studies have compared plastic versus metallic stents with regard to cost, complication rates and survival. In 1 recent meta-analysis [14] involving 7 randomized controlled trials, 724 participants were randomized to either metal (Wallstent) or plastic endoscopic stents. No significant difference was seen between the two stent types in terms of technical success, therapeutic success, 30-day mortality or complications. The median plastic stent patency ranged from 62 to 165 days, and metal stent patency from 111 to 273 days. Metal stents were associated with a significantly lower relative risk of occlusion after 4 months than plastic stents. The overall risk of recurrent biliary obstruction was also significantly lower in patients treated with metal stents.

For patients with a life expectancy of more than 6 months, the lower cost of the plastic stent does not make a difference, because its shorter patency time makes frequent replacements necessary.

The choice between the 2 stents should take in consideration the patient's health, life expectancy and quality of life. If the patient has a life expectancy of more than 6 months, the metallic stent is preferred because its higher patency decreases the need to repeat the procedure and consequently the risk of complications.

Covered Metallic Stent

One of the major causes of uncovered stent occlusion is tumor or hyperplastic tissue ingrowth. The covered stent was developed to impede tissue growth into the stent through the mesh using a silicone polymer coat. It may be removed in the case of obstruction but has a higher tendency to migrate than the uncovered stents. Another important observation about the covered stent is that it cannot be used in the intrahepatic biliary tract because the covering prevents draining of the bile ducts.

In a retrospective study [15] a higher incidence of stent migration was observed in the covered stent group (3/36) compared to the uncovered (1/41), but without being statistically significant. The overall patency time did not differ significantly, although there was a trend in favor of the covered stent.

A prospective randomized controlled study [14] comparing these 2 stent types showed longer patency of the covered stent with a significantly lower mean cost of treatment. In the covered stent group, stent obstruction occurred in 8 (14%) patients after a mean period of 304 days, and in the uncovered group in 21 (38%) patients after a mean period of 166 days. The cumulative patency of the covered stent was significantly higher in pancreatic cancer and metastatic lymph node subgroups, but not in the subgroup with gallbladder cancer and cholangiocarcinoma. Tumor ingrowth was observed in 15 patients in the uncovered stent group and was not observed in the covered group. The difference in survival time between the 2 groups was not significant, and acute cholecystitis was observed in 2 patients in the covered stent group and was not observed in the uncovered group. Mild pancreatitis occurred in 5 patients in the covered stent group and in 1 of the uncovered group.

One important advantage of the covered stent is that it can be removed with a snare or alligator forceps with relative ease and safety, which permits the immediate introduction of a new stent [16].

Distal Malignant Obstruction

Distal and proximal biliary obstructions have distinct etiologies and anatomic characteristics which are reflected in the differential diagnosis and therapeutic management.

The most common cause of medium and distal biliary malignant obstruction is pancreatic cancer, responsible for more than 90% of the cases [17], followed by gallbladder cancer, cholangiocarcinoma, malignant lymphadenopathy and ampullary tumors.

Due to their anatomical characteristics, distal tumors have a better chance of curative or palliative surgical treatment than hilar tumors.

Studies comparing surgical bypass versus endoscopic plastic stent placement for palliative treatment of biliary distal neoplastic obstruction have not shown differences in efficacy for relief of jaundice, improvement in quality of life and survival time [18] (fig. 10).

A recent meta-analysis [19] analyzed 3 randomized controlled studies comparing plastic stent versus surgery. Between 64 and 80% of the patients had pancreatic cancer and there was no difference in the rates of technical and therapeutic success. Endoscopic stenting appears to be associated with a reduced risk of complications, but with a higher risk of recurrent biliary obstruction prior to death when compared with surgery.

There were no significant differences in survival or quality of life between the 2 treatment groups in any of the studies. The median survival of participants was 84–152 days in these trials. Two of the trials demonstrated shorter total hospital stay for those in the stent group.

An evidence-based review suggests that endoscopic palliative treatment is better than surgical bypass (same efficacy but lower morbidity, mortality, and hospital stay) in mid-lower strictures, but at the present time this issue must be considered unsettled. Surgical or endoscopic palliative

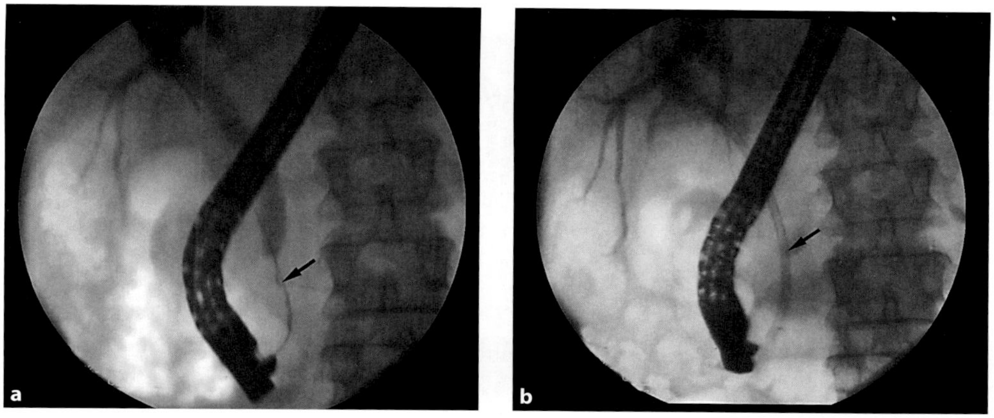

Fig. 10. Malignant biliary distal obstruction. **a** Malignant stricture (arrow). **b** Plastic stent placed (arrow).

care should be selected on an individual basis: older patients and patients with advanced or metastatic disease should undergo endoscopic stent placement, while younger patients or those with locally advanced tumor may be best treated with surgery [20].

There are very few studies about metallic versus surgical drainage of biliary obstruction. In a prospective, randomized controlled trial Artifon et al. [4] conclude that endoscopic biliary drainage with metallic stents is cheaper and provides better quality of life for patients with biliary obstruction and metastatic pancreatic cancer. There was no difference between the 2 groups in relation to complication rate, readmissions due to complications, and survival time.

Hilar Malignant Obstruction

Biliary hilar obstruction represents a significantly greater challenge than distal obstruction. The vast majority of patients with hilar cancer die within the first year and less than 10% of patients survive 5 years after diagnosis. Few cases of hilar cancer are resectable, ranging from 5 to 20%. Palliative surgery is usually difficult or impossible and operative mortality is high, approximately 20% [21].

The most common malignant etiology of proximal biliary obstruction is cholangiocarcinoma, gallbladder carcinoma, nodal metastases, hepatocellular carcinoma, and hepatic metastases.

The Bismuth classification is frequently used for hilar tumors. This classification has important prognostic significance both for surgical resectability and for palliative drainage. In Bismuth type I, the stenosis is at the level of the common hepatic duct, within 2 cm of the bifurcation, but with communication between left and right hepatic ducts. Bismuth type II, the lesions separately obstruct the left and right hepatic ducts. Bismuth type III, the lesions involve either the right (type IIIA) or left (type IIIB) secondary intrahepatic ducts with the contralateral ductal system intact. Bismuth type IV, the lesions involve bilateral secondary or tertiary branch obstruction or may be multifocal [20] (fig. 11).

Considering the reserved prognosis of primary hilar cancer or Klatskin tumor and the technical difficulties of surgical drainage, endoscopic stent placement is accepted as the first option for palliative treatment of these patients.

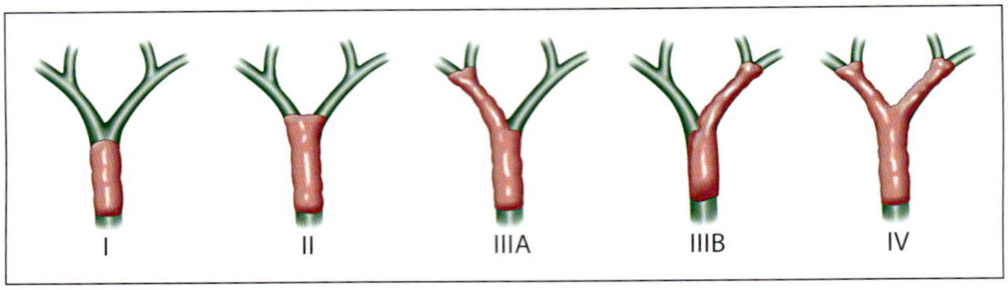

Fig. 11. Illustration of the Bismuth classification.

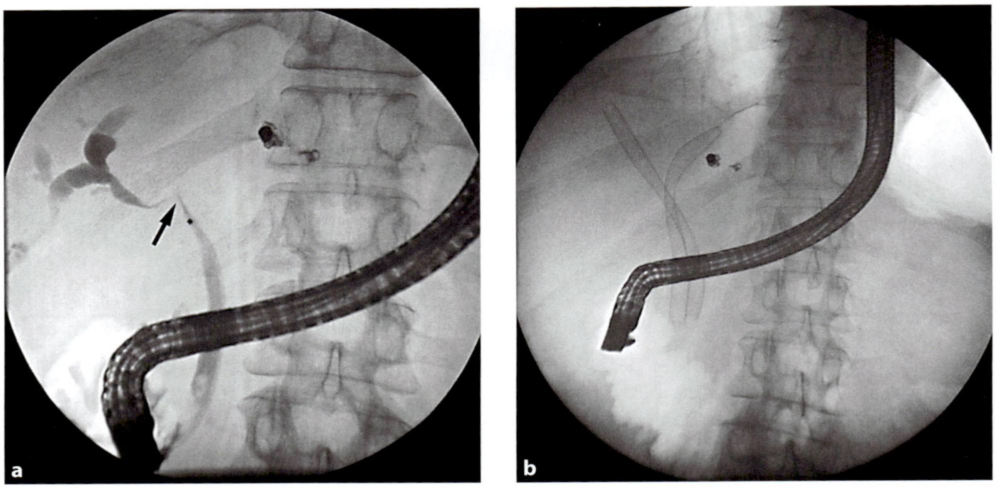

Fig. 12. Bilateral drainage of a Klatskin tumor with metallic stents. **a** Hilar stenosis (arrow). **b** Bilateral metallic stents placed.

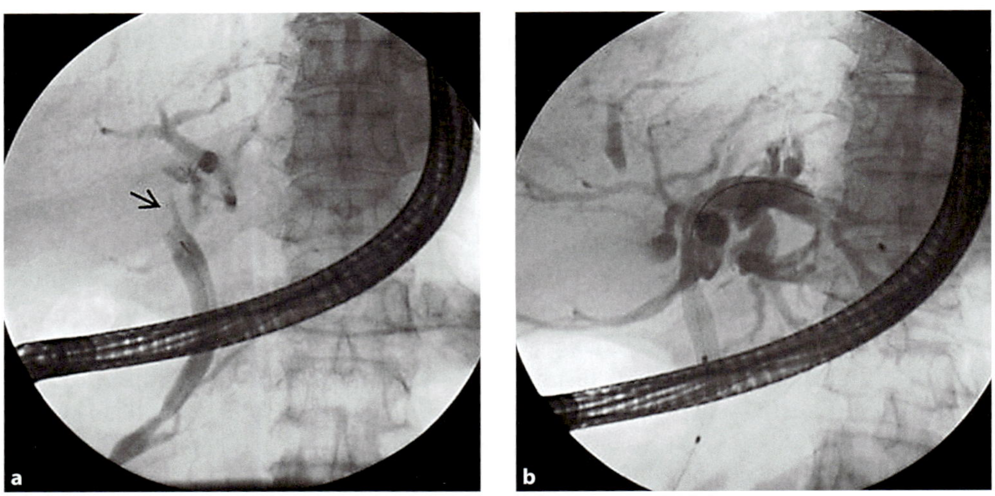

Fig. 13. Unilateral drainage of a Klatskin tumor with metallic stent. **a** Hilar stricture (arrow) and left hepatic duct opacified. **b** Stent placed in left hepatic duct.

Bilateral versus Unilateral Drainage

The necessity to drain the bilateral lobes for Bismuth II and III is considered controversial, but the literature is clear that failure to drain an opacified lobe will worsen the patient's prognosis. Drainage of only one side does not completely relieve jaundice and can induce acute cholangitis. However, drainage of both liver lobes is technically more difficult and may require a longer time or multiple procedures, with an increased risk of complications and mortality. Some studies have concluded that insertion of more than one stent does not appear justified as a routine procedure in patients with biliary bifurcation tumors [21, 22].

Dowsett et al. [23] have shown that drainage of 25% of the liver volume can achieve adequate palliative treatment with improvement in the biochemical parameters and in the patient's quality of life. However, Deviere et al. [24] showed that mean survival, 30-day mortality, and deaths from sepsis were all significantly less with bilateral versus unilateral drainage. In a prospective, randomized and controlled study, comparing unilateral versus bilateral hepatic duct drainage, Giovanni et al. [21] observed a higher rate of early cholangitis in the bilateral drainage group (16.6 vs. 8.8%) with no statistical differences for the success rate of drainage, median survival time and late complications. However, the survival time varied significantly for the subgroup of patients with cholangiocarcinoma, gallbladder cancer and metastatic tumor: 179, 104 and 89 days, respectively. They concluded that single stent insertion is effective and avoids the risk of further procedure-related complications and mortality.

In a retrospective study, Chang et al. [25] evaluated patients with Bismuth type II and III strictures. They were classified into 3 groups: group A, one lobe opacified with the same lobe drained; group B, both lobes opacified and both lobes drained, and group C, both lobes opacified with one lobe drained. Group C patients had a significantly higher rate of early cholangitis (32%) than either group A (6.3%, $p < 0.01$) and group B (0%, $p < 0.001$). The median survival of groups A, B, and C was 145, 225, and 46 days, respectively. Survival was significantly longer in group A versus group C ($p < 0.001$) and in group B versus group C.

An evidence-based review by Cipolletta et al. [20] concluded that unilateral endoscopic stenting is safe and effective in most cases, and bilateral stenting may be appropriate in selected patients with Bismuth type II cancer and those in whom bilateral ducts have been contaminated (fig. 12, 13).

References

1 Patel T: Cholangiocarcinoma. Nat Clin Pract Gastroenterol Hepatol 2006;3:33–42.

2 Freeman ML, Sielaff TD: A modern approach to malignant hilarbiliary obstruction. Rev Gastroenterol Disord 2003;3:187–201.

3 Weber SM, Jarnagin WR, Klimstra D, DeMatteo RP, Fong Y,Blumgart LH: Intrahepatic cholangiocarcinoma: resectability, recurrence pattern, and outcomes. J Am Coll Surg 2001;193:384–391.

4 Artifon EL, Sakai P, Cunha JE, Dupont A, Filho FM, Hondo FY, Ishioka S, Raju GS: Surgery or endoscopy for palliation of biliary obstruction due to metastatic pancreatic cancer. Am J Gastroenterol 2006;101:2031–2037.

5 Smith AC, Dowsett JF, Russell RC, et al: Randomized trial of endoscopic stenting versus surgical bypass in malignant low bile duct obstruction. Lancet 1994; 344:1655–1660.

6 Knyrim K, Wagner HJ, Pausch J, et al: A prospective, randomized, controlled trial of metal stents for malignant obstruction of the common bile duct. Endoscopy 1993;25:207–212.

7 Strasberg SM: ERCP and surgical intervention in pancreatic and biliary malignancies. Gastrointest Endosc 2002;56:S213–S217.

8 Giorgio PD, Luca LD: Comparison of treatment outcomes between biliary plastic stent placement with and without endoscopic sphincterotomy for inoperable malignant common bile duct obstruction. World J Gastroenterol 2004;10:1212–1214.
9 Tarnasky PR, Cunningham JT, Hawes RH, Hoffman BJ, Uflacker R, Vujic I, Cotton PB: Transpapillary stenting of proximal biliary strictures: does biliary sphincterotomy reduce the risk of postprocedure pancreatitis? Gastrointest Endosc 1997;45:46–51.
10 Huibregtse K: Plastic or expandable biliary endoprostheses? Scand J Gastroenterol Suppl 1993;200:3–7.
11 Prat F, Chapat O, Ducot B, Ponchon T, Pelletier G, Fritsch J, Choury AD, Buffet C: A randomized trial of endoscopic drainage methods for inoperable malignant strictures of the common bile duct. Gastrointest Endosc 1998;47:1–7.
12 Sung JY, Leung JW, Shaffer EA, Lam K, Costerton JW: Bacterial biofilm, brown pigment stone and blockage of biliary stents. J Gastroenterol Hepatol 1993;8:28–34.
13 Van Berkel AM, Van MJ, Groen AK, Bruno MJ: Mechanisms of biliary stent clogging: confocal laser scanning and scanning electron microscopy. Endoscopy 2005;37:729–734.
14 Isayama H, Komatsu Y, Tsujino T, et al: A prospective randomised study of 'covered' versus 'uncovered' diamond stents for the management of distal malignant biliary obstruction. Gut 2004;53:729–734.
15 Yoon WJ, Lee JK, Lee KH, Lee WJ, Ryu JK, Kim YT, et al: A comparison of covered and uncovered Wallstents for the management of distal malignant biliary obstruction. Gastrointest Endosc 2006;63: 996–1000.
16 Familiari P, Bulajic M, Mutignani M, Lee LS, Spera G, Spada C, et al: Endoscopic removal of malfunctioning biliary self-expandable metallic stents. Gastrointest Endosc 2005;62:903–910.
17 Jemal A, Tiwari RC, Murray T, et al: Cancer statistics, 2004. CA Cancer J Clin 2004;54:8.
18 Andersen JR, Sorensen SM, Kruse A, Rokkjaer M, Matzen P: Randomised trial of endoscopic endoprosthesis versus operative bypass in malignant obstructive jaundice. Gut 1989;30:1132–1135.
19 Moss AC, Morris E, Mac Mathuna P: Palliative biliary stents for obstructing pancreatic carcinoma. Cochrane Database Syst Rev 2006;2:CD004200.
20 Cipolletta L, Rotondano G, Marmo R, Bianco MA: Endoscopic palliation of malignant obstructive jaundice: an evidence-based review. Dig Liver Dis 2007; 39:375–388.
21 De Palma GD, Galloro G, Siciliano S, Iovino P, Catanzano C: Unilateral versus bilateral endoscopic hepatic duct drainage in patients with malignant hilar biliary obstruction: results of a prospective, randomized, and controlled study. Gastrointest Endosc 2001;53:547–553.
22 Polydorou AA, Chislom EM, Romanos AA, Dowsett SF, Cotton PB, Hatelfied AK, et al: A comparison or right versus left hepatic endoprosthesis insertion in malignant hilar biliary obstruction. Endoscopy 1989;21:266–271.
23 Dowsett JF, Vaira D, Hatfield ARW, Cairns SR, Polydorou AA, Frost R, et al: Endoscopic biliary therapy using the combined percutaneous and endoscopic technique. Gastroenterology 1989;96:1180–1186.
24 Deviere J, Baize M, de Toeuf J, Cremer M: Long-term follow-up of patients with hilar malignant stricture treated by endoscopic internal biliary drainage. Gastrointest Endosc 1988;34:95–101.
25 Chang WH, Kortan P, Haber GB: Outcome in patients with bifurcation tumors who undergo unilateral versus bilateral hepatic duct drainage. Gastrointest Endosc 1998; 47:354–362.

Dalton Marques Chaves, MD, PhD
University of São Paulo Medical School Clinics Hospital
São Paulo (Brazil)
Tel./Fax +55 11 3069 6221, Fax +55 11 3069 7579, E-Mail dalton.chaves@fleury.com.br

Mönkemüller K, Wilcox CM, Muñoz-Navas M (eds): Interventional and Therapeutic Gastrointestinal Endoscopy.
Front Gastrointest Res. Basel, Karger, 2010, vol 27, pp 375–383

Stents for Benign and Malignant Biliary Tract Diseases

Júlio C. Pereira-Lima · César Vivian Lopes

Department of Gastroenterology and Endoscopy Unit of the Santa Casa University Hospital/University of Health Sciences of Porto Alegre, UFCSPA, Medical School, Porto Alegre, Brazil

Abstract

Biliary endoscopy has had a great impact on therapeutic strategy for biliary diseases, especially with the insertion of plastic or auto-expandable metallic stents, Endoscopic biliary stent insertion is the definitive therapy for the majority of unresectable malignant biliary strictures, relieving pruritis and increasing quality of life. Indications for benign diseases include dilation of benign strictures (post-cholecystectomy or liver transplantation), bridging of leakages and prevention of stone impaction when all calculi cannot be retrieved. In this scenario, an endoscopic approach is successful in 60–90% of these case at mid-term, and this less invasive therapy does not preclude further surgery.

During the past three decades the development of therapeutic biliary endoscopy has provided a profound impact on treatment regimens for biliary diseases. Although deep cannulation, papillotomy, stone extraction and prosthesis insertion remain the cornerstone of therapeutic endoscopic retrograde cholangiopancreatography (ERCP), some fine adjustments have been developed in recent years. Endoprostheses insertion and balloon dilatation is successful, at least on mid term, in 60–90% of benign strictures, according to its type and etiology [1]. Endoscopic biliary stent insertion is the treatment of choice for unresectable malignant jaundice [2, 3] and should be preferred over the percutaneous approach, except for cases of complex intrahepatic biliary strictures, unapproachableness to the papilla with the duodenoscope due to prior surgery, or in hospitals endowed with expert interventional radiologists and average endoscopists [1].

Technique

Biliary endoprostheses are placed as definitive therapy for malignant obstruction in order to relieve pruritus, occasionally to allow chemotherapy, which may be precluded by jaundice, and mainly, to increase quality of life and survival [2, 4]. Indications in benign diseases include dilation of benign strictures, bridging of leakages and preventing stone impaction when all calculi are not retrieved. There is no difference among the several plastic endoprostheses types [1]. We begin every ERCP with a Jumbo duodenoscope of 4.2 mm working channel and employ straight

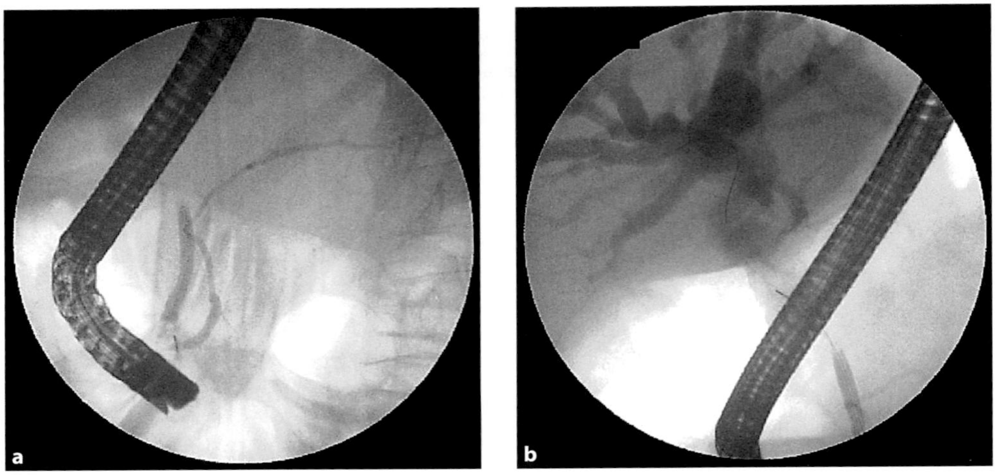

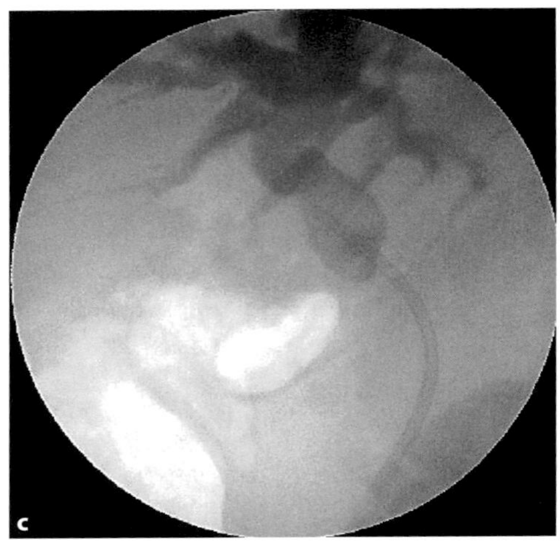

Fig. 1. a Patient with cholangiocarcinoma. The main pancreatic duct was normal and there was a choledochal stricture. **b** No contrast was injected beyond the stenosis. The papillotome was inserted along the guidewire, through the stenosis, and a dilated biliary tree proximal to the stricture was demonstrated. **c** A plastic stent was introduced.

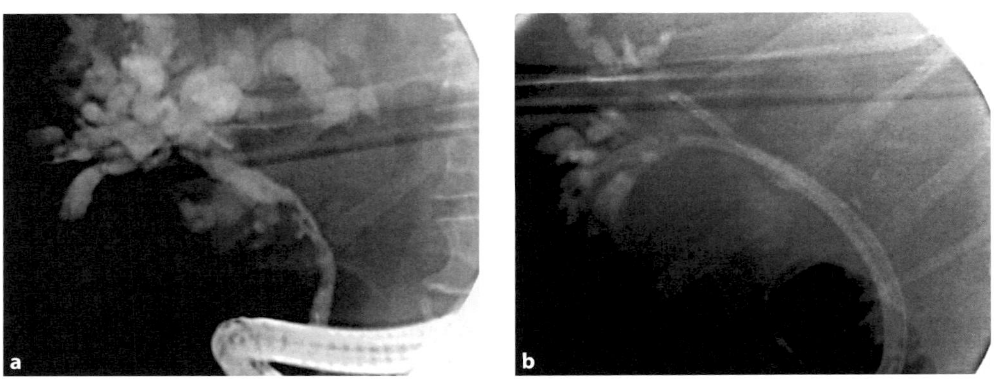

Fig. 2. a Gallbladder tumor invading the common hepatic duct and liver hilum. Note severe bilateral intrahepatic dilation. **b** Two plastic stents were inserted.

Amsterdam-type stents of 10 Fr [they are easier to place than an 11.5-Fr stent and the latter does not offer advantage in terms of patency [2]] from 5 to 15 cm in length according to stricture's extension and location.

In cases of low bile duct obstruction, after deep biliary cannulation, contrast is injected in order to perform a full cholangiography. This is essential in order to evaluate whether there is metastatic disease at the liver hilum. Then a flexible tip guidewire is negotiated through the stricture and the stent is introduced across the stenosis with a pre-mounted stent set (inner catheter and a pusher). Pre-dilatation of the stricture is never performed in case of malignancy. The insertion of metal stents follows the same rules. Since most complications of stent insertion (bleeding, perforation and a percentage of cases of pancreatitis) are due to sphincterotomy, the latter is not routinely performed, although it facilitates stent positioning.

In clinical practice, we do not recommend pre-scheduled stents changes or revisions for distal malignant strictures. In cases of stent dysfunction, a new plastic stent or a metal one is inserted according to life expectancy and 'clogging tendency of the patient'. Patients who have their stent clogged early (<2 months), tend to have the next stent clogged even earlier [1].

The approach to proximal duct obstruction is somewhat different. After selective biliary cannulation, contrast is injected to recognize, but not to trespass the stricture (fig. 1). Then the guidewire is introduced across the stricture into one of the hepatic ducts. Afterwards, the catheter is placed through the stenosis along the guidewire and contrast is injected. We usually place one stent into the 'easiest' trespassed duct. The endoscopist should have in mind that every hepatic segment that is contrasted must be drained. Thus, if contrast is injected in both hepatic ducts, they must be drained in order to avoid cholangitis (fig. 2). Since cholangiocarcinoma patients live longer than pancreatic cancer ones, we prefer to insert metal stents in these cases. Covered metal stents should never be placed in Klatskin tumors, because the stent will obstruct small intrahepatic ducts. Moreover, metal stents (7 Fr) are easier to place in Klatskin tumors than plastic stents (10 Fr), not only due to their diameter, but also because the former stents are stiffer, and consequently, proportionate a better torque.

If two prostheses are placed (one in each hepatic duct), it is less difficult to insert firstly the guidewires in both ducts, and then to introduce the stents. If one stent is inserted first, the introduction of another guidewire will tend strongly to come along the stent into the same duct.

Stenting benign biliary strictures (post-cholecystectomy or liver transplantation) is more cumbersome. The insertion of the guidewire across the stricture is more difficult, because these stenoses are tighter, have more irregular (sometimes even S-shaped) shapes or are longer than malignant ones (especially in comparison to distal bile duct strictures).

In case of benign strictures, we recommend to inject contrast (as with distal bile duct obstruction) to 'draw' the stenosis. Afterwards, the guidewire is negotiated through the stricture and a balloon for dilation (EBD) up to about 30 Fr, which is performed at 4–8 atm (according to the balloon's manufacturer instructions), is inserted. With inflation the waist of the balloon disappears and the dilation is considered complete. Following the dilation, 2–3 stents are left in place to cast the stenosis. We repeat this procedure every 4 months for 1 year and papillotomy is always performed to make possible the insertion of multiple stents. In patients with bile duct fistulas, we routinely perform endoscopic papillotomy (even in the absence of stones) and insert a plastic stent bridging the leakage point.

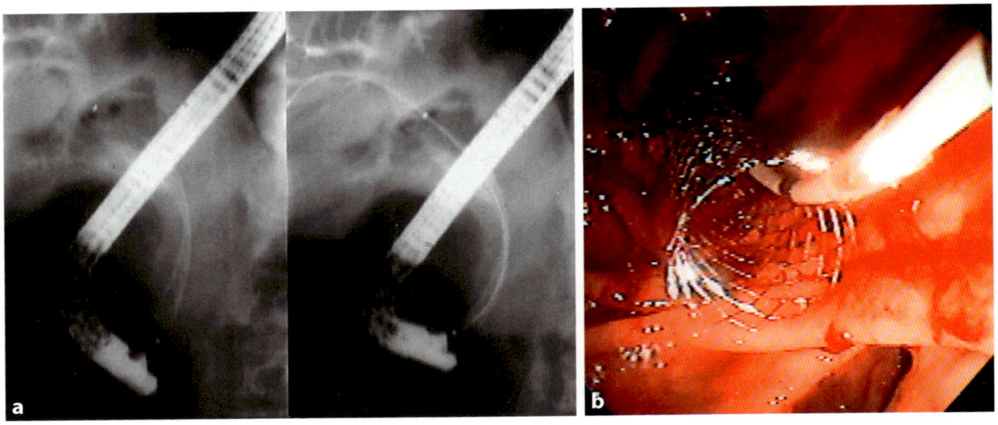

Fig. 3. **a** Pancreatic cancer with a metal stent inserted in the bile duct. **b** Metal stent viewed from the duodenum.

Accessories

As for the majority of ERCP procedures, the following devices are needed: papillotomes, cannulas, balloons, dilation balloons, guidewires and stents.

Outcomes

Distal Malignant Bile Duct Obstruction

Patients should be carefully staged prior to therapy (either surgical or not) in terms of disease extension before curative intent pancreatoduodenectomy by means of endoscopic ultrasound (EUS) with biopsy, computed tomography (CT), CT or magnetic resonance (MR) angiography and clinical evaluation. Curative intent surgery was feasible in less than 15% of the cases in a US population-based study evaluating 32,348 cases of pancreatic cancer [5]. Most cases of choledochal or ampullary cancers (<20% of the cases of distal obstruction) are resectable and hence these patients should be operated, unless they are unfit for surgery or have distant metastasis [6]. ERCP with stent insertion should not be performed prior to pancreatoduodenectomy, except in patients with cholangitis. Stenting before surgery does not affect surgical mortality (neither positively nor negatively) according to a Cochrane review [7].

ERCP with stent placement is the preferable treatment for three quarters of the patients with malignant low bile duct obstruction. In a Cochrane review of 21 trials involving 1,454 subjects, endoscopic stenting with plastic endoprostheses was associated with fewer complications and 30-day mortality when compared to surgical bypass. There was no difference in technical or therapeutic success. However, with endoscopic treatment there is a higher risk of recurrent biliary obstruction prior to death [3]. Prosthesis occlusion can be easily resolved with stent changing. In a series of 103 pancreatic cancer patients treated by biliary stenting, about half of the patients died with a functioning stent in situ and stent patency had a mean of 3–4 months. There was no difference when comparing 11.5- and 10-Fr stents in terms of patency [2]. There is also no difference in stent patency when comparing stent materials (teflon vs. polyethylene, polyurethane;

hydrophilic coated, etc.) or shape (straight, tannenbaum, etc.). Neither the use of antibiotics nor ursodeoxycholic acid can prevent clogging, although obstruction is caused by deposition of a brownstone-like material formed by the aggregation of bacteria, bile glycoproteins and bile salts [1]. The only way to enhance stent patency is to increase stent diameter. Self-expanding metal stents can reach a 30-Fr diameter after insertion (fig. 3). In randomized controlled trials, their permeability was longer in comparison to 10- and 11.5-Fr plastic stents with consequent less reinterventions and better quality of life during patient's survival [1, 3]. Nevertheless, this was not translated into a statistically significant better survival in these studies.

Prognostic factors have been used to determine in which cases a plastic or a metal stent should be inserted. Liver metastases, tumor size >3 cm, anemia, pain and CEA/CA19-9 levels are prognostic factors associated with shorter survival and should be used to select which patients should receive metal or plastic stents [6] from an economical point of view. In terms of economics, the most expensive procedure everywhere is surgery [8]. In general, as a whole, plastic stents should be inserted in patients with a survival expectancy of <4 months and metal prostheses in those with a better prognosis [1, 3].

The occlusion of metal stents is usually caused by tumor in-growth through the stent meshes and typically happens from 5 to 9 months after insertion. In case of obstruction, a plastic stent should be placed across the stricture. In specific cases, the metal stents could be removed, another metal stent might be inserted or the tumor in-growth may be ablated with APC [9–11]. Covered metal stents solves the problem of tumor in-growth, but they also cover the cystic and the pancreatic ducts. They confer higher patency rates, but also a higher risk of complications [9, 11], namely cholecystitis and pancreatitis. Patients who have already undergone cholecystectomy are the ideal candidates for covered metal stents. It should be kept in mind that this population has a short life expectancy and all efforts should be made to give them a better quality of life for their remaining survival time, with as few days in hospital as possible.

Proximal Malignant Bile Duct Obstruction

Malignant proximal duct strictures are mostly caused by hilar tumors. About a quarter of these cases are caused by hilar metastases (e.g. from colon cancer) or in-growth of gallbladder neoplasms [1, 4]. Primary hilar tumors have a better prognosis than pancreatic cancer, but at diagnosis, most patients are unresectable due to vessel invasion, hepatic metastases or spreading through the biliary tree. EUS is usually not useful in tumor staging and is replaced by intraductal EUS in these cases. MR or CT angiography and cholangiography (preferable with MRCP) are essential for staging.

The introduction of one (draining just one lobe) or two stents (draining both liver lobes) produces similar clinical results in comparative trials [12]. Moreover, the placement of two stents is associated with a higher risk of early complications, due to failure in the insertion of the second stent and a longer procedure time [12]. Some authors [13, 14] advocate selective drainage with one stent placed in the dominant duct, determined by MRCP. On the other hand, De Palma et al. [15] demonstrated that draining the easiest duct reached by the guidewire provides the same clinical results. This approach is more feasible because it is not always possible to reach the desired duct with the guidewire.

It would seem logical, at first sight, to drain the right lobe in cases of placement of just one stent, since this lobe drains about 60% of the liver volume. However, 25% of volume drainage

Table 1. Etiology of benign biliary strictures

Postoperative
Cholecystectomy
Common bile duct exploration
Hepatic resection or transplantation
Bilioenteric anastomosis
Post-sphincterotomy
Rarely from other surgeries such as pancreatic resections
Inflammatory
Acute and chronic pancreatitis and related complications
Primary sclerosing cholangitis
Biliary lithiasis/Mirizzi's syndrome
Post-radiation and chemotherapy
Infections (viral, tuberculosis, parasites, fungal)
Other causes
Abdominal trauma
Recurrent pyogenic cholangitis
Retroperitoneal fibrosis
Vascular indentations
Idiopathic

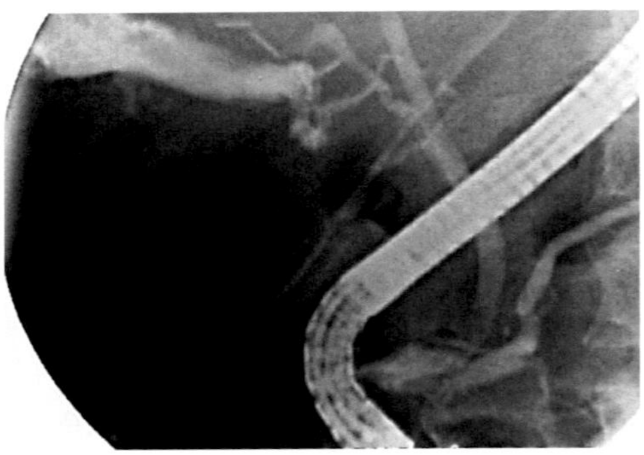

4

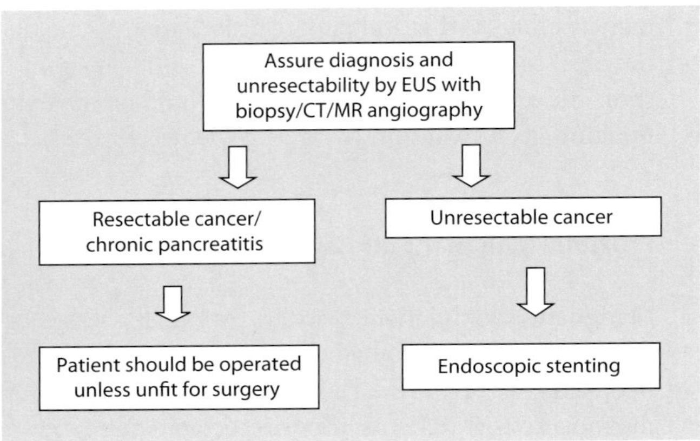

5

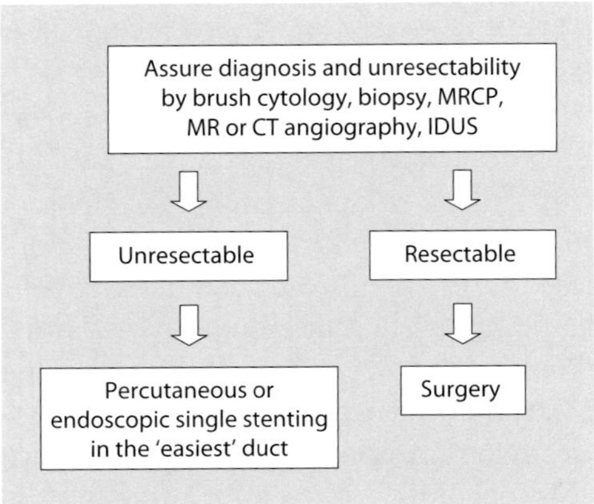

6

Fig. 4. Cholangiopancreatography demonstrating bile duct leakage from the cystic duct near to the surgical clips. There was a stone in the distal bile duct. This patient was treated by papillotomy with stone removal and stent insertion.

Fig. 5. Distal bile duct obstruction.

Fig. 6. Proximal bile duct obstruction.

is needed to normalize liver function and the right hepatic duct is divided nearer the bifurcation in comparison to the left duct (0.9 vs. 3.2 cm), what makes tumor infiltration spread more in the right duct, making the results of draining in the left or right lobe clinically similar [16]. What is essential in stenting hilar cancers is to drain the ducts in which contrast was injected. Nondraining opacified ducts are associated with higher morbidity and mortality [17]. New techniques for treating cholangiocarcinoma such as endoscopic intraluminal brachytherapy with metal stent [18] and a combination of metal stents and photodynamic therapy are considered promising by some groups [1]. However, these techniques have existed for more than a decade and are not widely used.

Benign Biliary Strictures

Postoperative biliary lesions occur after 0.4% of cholecystectomies and after 10–30% of liver transplantations [19]. These lesions are seldom caused by other surgical procedures (table 1). Success rates of endoscopic therapy are variable and largely dependent on the underlying etiology of the stricture, as well as a wide variation in location, shape and severity of these strictures. Since endoscopy by itself may be unsuccessful, a combined approach with a percutaneous radiological intervention may warrant entrance to intrahepatic ducts that are otherwise inaccessible. In addition, minimal invasive therapy by endoscopic or radiological means does not preclude further surgery.

The differential diagnosis of benign and malignant strictures is determined most of the time by a combination of clinical history, radiographic appearance, brush cytology/biopsy and serum CEA/CA19-9. It can be extremely difficult to settle if a dominant stricture in a patient with primary sclerosing cholangitis is benign or not. The combination of multiple techniques such as biopsy/cytology and CEA/CA19-9 do not reach 80% in diagnostic certainty [20]. On the other hand, beyond the clinical setting of primary sclerosing cholangitis, post-liver transplantation or post-cholecystectomy strictures are easily and correctly diagnosed by cholangiographic aspect and the clinical history. The same is true for malignant strictures due to pancreatic cancer or Klatskin's tumors.

Complete bile duct transection must be treated surgically, but bile duct strictures with or without leakage can be effectively treated by endoscopy. Initial success is reported to be at least 90% of the cases [20–24]. However, even after dilation and insertion of multiple stents, stenosis recur in about a fifth of the cases in a 3- to 5-year follow-up [21–24]. These results are similar to the ones obtained with surgery [24]. The placement of temporary covered self-expandable metal stents has been described by some authors, especially in strictures secondary to chronic pancreatitis and liver transplantation [19]. Endoscopic stricture dilatation with stent insertion is indisputably the therapy of choice for biliary stenoses after orthotopic liver transplantation [20]. Bile duct leakages are easily treated endoscopically by endoscopic papillotomy with stent insertion and duct healing approaches 98–100% [25], endoscopy being considered the treatment of choice (fig. 4).

Endoscopy obtains disappointing results in obstructive jaundice due to chronic pancreatitis [1, 20] with a long-term success rate of 10–30%. Balloon dilation and stenting can also be used in some patients with primary sclerosing cholangitis, mainly those with dominant strictures in the extrahepatic bile ducts or near the hilum [1, 20]. Finally, the results of the present study are summarized in the algorithms shown in figures 5–8.

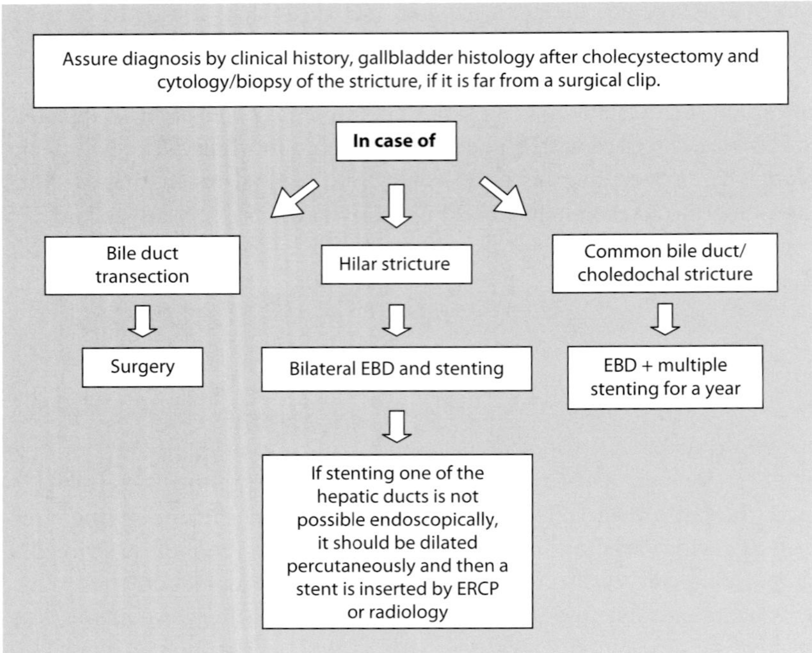

Fig. 7. Post-surgical strictures.

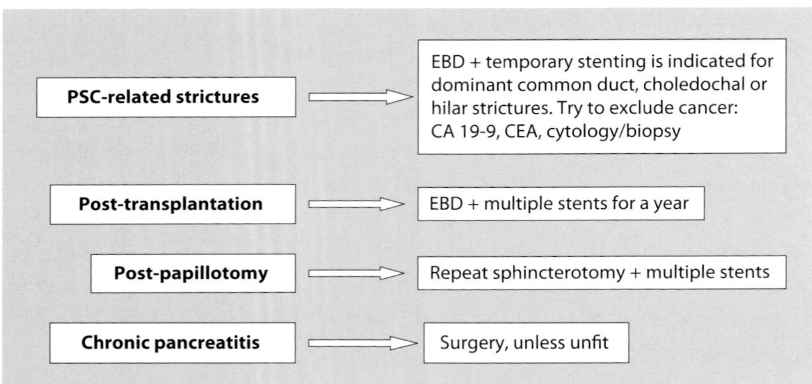

Fig. 8. Treatment for other common reasons for benign strictures.

References

1 Jakobs R, Weickert U, Hartmann D, et al: Interventional endoscopy for benign and malignant bile duct strictures. Z Gastroenterol 2005;43:295–303.

2 Pereira-Lima JC, Jakobs R, Maier M, et al: Endoscopic biliary stenting for the palliation of pancreatic cancer: results, survival predictive factors, and comparison of 10-french with 11.5-french gauge stents. Am J Gastroenterol 1996;91:2179–2184.

3 Moss AC, Morris E, Mac Mathuna P: Palliative biliary stents for obstructing pancreatic carcinoma. Cochrane Databse Syst Rev 2006;19:CD004200.

4 Pereira-Lima JC, Jakobs R, Maier M, et al: Endoscopic stenting in obstructive jaundice due to liver metastases: does it have a benefit for the patient? Hepatogastroenterology 1996;43:944–948.

5 Shaib Y, Davila J, Naumann C, et al: The impact of curative intent surgery on the survival of pancreatic cancer patients: a US population-based study. Am J Gastroenterol 2007;102:1377–1382.
6 Müller MW, Friess H, Köninger J, et al: Factors influencing survival after bypass procedures in patients with advanced pancreatic adenocarcinomas. Am J Surg 2008; 195:221–228.
7 Mumtaz K, Hamid S, Jafri W: Endoscopic retrograde cholangiopancreaticography with or without stenting in patients with pancreaticobiliary malignancy, prior to surgery. Cochrane Database Syst Rev 2007;18: CD006001.
8 Artifon EL, Sakai P, Cunha JE, et al: Surgery or endoscopy for palliation of biliary obstruction due to metaplastic pancreatic cancer. Am J Gastroenterol 2006; 101:2031–2037.
9 Yoon WJ, Lee JK, Lee KH, et al: A comparison of covered and uncovered Wallstents for the management of distal malignant biliary obstruction. Gastrointest Endosc 2006;63:996–1000.
10 Bueno JT, Gerdes H, Kurtz RC: Endoscopic management of occluded biliary Wallstents: a cancer center experience. Gastrointest Endosc 2003;58:879–884.
11 Isayama H, Komatsu Y, Tsujino T, et al: A prospective randomised study of covered versus uncovered diamond stents for the management of distal malignant biliary obstruction. Gut 2004;53:729–734.
12 De Palma GD, Galloro G, Siciliano S, et al: Unilateral versus bilateral endoscopic hepatic duct drainage in patients with malignant hilar biliary obstruction: results of a prospective, randomized, and controlled study. Gastrointest Endosc 2001;53:681–684.
13 Freeman ML, Overby C: Selective MRCP and CT-target drainage of malignant hilar biliary obstruction with self-expanding metallic stents. Gastrointest Endosc 2003; 58:41–49.
14 Hintze RE, Abou-Rebyeh H, Adler A, et al: Magnetic resonance cholangiopancreaticography-guided unilateral endoscopic stent placement for Klatskin tumors. Gastrointest Endosc 2001;53:40–46.
15 De Palma GD, Pezzullo A, Rega M, et al: Unilateral placement of metallic stents for malignant hilar obstruction: a prospective study. Gastrointest Endosc 2003;58:50–53.
16 Polydorou AA, Chisholm EM, Romanos AA, et al: A comparison of right versus left hepatic duct endoprosthesis insertion in malignant hilar biliary obstruction. Endoscopy 1989;21:266–271.
17 Chang WH, Kortan P, Haber GB: Outcomes in patients with bifurcation tumors who undergo unilateral versus bilateral hepatic duct drainage. Gastrointest Endosc 1998;47:354–362.
18 Singh V, Kapoor R, Solanki KK, et al: Endoscopic intraluminal brachytherapy and metal stent in malignant hilar biliary obstruction: a pilot study. Liver Int 2007;27:347–352.
19 Kahaleh M, Behm B, Clarke BW, et al: Temporary placement of covered self-expandable metal stents in benign biliary strictures: a new paradigm? Gastrointest Endosc 2008;67:446–454.
20 Farah M, McLoughlin M, Byrne MF, et al: Endoscopic retrograde cholangiopancreatography in the management of benign biliary strictures. Curr Gastroenterol Rep 2008;10:150–156.
21 Bergman JJ, Burgemeister L, Bruno MJ, et al: Long-term follow-up after biliary stent placement for postoperative bile duct stenosis. Gastrointest Endosc 2001;54:154–161.
22 Costamagna C, Pandolfi M, Mutignani M, et al: Long-term results of endoscopic management of postoperative bile duct strictures with increasing number of stents. Gastrointest Endosc 2001;54:162–168.
23 Draganov P, Hoffman B, Marsh W, et al: Long-term outcome in patients with benign biliary strictures treated endoscopically with multiple stents. Gastrointest Endosc 2002;55:680–686.
24 Davids H, Tanka AK, Rau EA, et al: Benign biliary strictures – surgery or endoscopy? Ann Surg 1993; 217:237–243.
25 Huang CS, Lichtenstein DR. Postcholecystectomy bile leak: what is the optimal treatment? Gastrointest Endosc 2005;61:276–278.

Júlio C. Pereira-Lima
Rua Com. Rheingantz 910/801
90450-020 Porto Alegre (Brazil)
Tel. +55 51 3022 5794, Fax +55 51 3022 5791
E-Mail jpereiralima@terra.com.br

Mönkemüller K, Wilcox CM, Muñoz-Navas M (eds): Interventional and Therapeutic Gastrointestinal Endoscopy.
Front Gastrointest Res. Basel, Karger, 2010, vol 27, pp 384–389

Endoscopic Management of Bile Leaks

Jennifer Chennat · Irving Waxman

Center for Endoscopic Research and Therapeutics, University of Chicago Medical Center, Chicago, Ill., USA

Abstract

Bile duct injuries resulting in leaks are often the result of iatrogenic causes. They can be associated with significant morbidity and mortality, particularly if not effectively diagnosed and treated. The treatment of bile leaks has evolved from traditional surgical approaches to innovative minimally invasive endoscopic techniques. We focus on the technical aspects of endoscopic bile leak management.

Bile leaks occur most commonly as a surgical complication, particularly following laparoscopic cholecystectomy or liver transplantation. In larger series this procedural complication has a reported incidence of 0.5% or less following open cholecystectomy and up to 1% after a laparoscopic approach (fig. 1–4). It also occurs in approximately 26% of orthotopic liver transplantations, 53% of living donor transplantations, and in 6% of donors (often in the early postoperative 1- to 3-month period) [1–9].

Those bile leakages associated with liver transplantation can be further subdivided into biliary anastomosis-related and non-anastomosis leakage (from T-tube-related injury or from the cut surface of reduced grafts; fig. 5, 6). Additionally, iatrogenic nonsurgical biliary injury can occur during liver biopsy, intrahepatic portosystemic shunting or hepatic tumor ablations. Penetrating or blunt trauma remains the primary cause of non-iatrogenic biliary leaks.

Four types of postoperative bile duct injuries have been described by Bergman et al. [10]: type A = cystic duct leaks or leakage from aberrant or peripheral hepatic radicles; type B = major bile duct leaks with or without concomitant biliary strictures; type C = bile duct strictures without bile leakage, and type D = complete transection of the duct with or without excision of some portion of the biliary tree.

A more recently reported classification subdivides bile leaks into low grade (leak identified only after intrahepatic contrast opacification) or high grade (leak observed before intrahepatic opacification) for purposes of guiding endoscopic therapy [11].

Technical Aspects

Diagnostic Workup

Early clinical suspicion and diagnosis of bile leak is imperative, as unrecognized disruptions can result in peritonitis and worsening sepsis. Diffuse abdominal pain may be associated with leaks

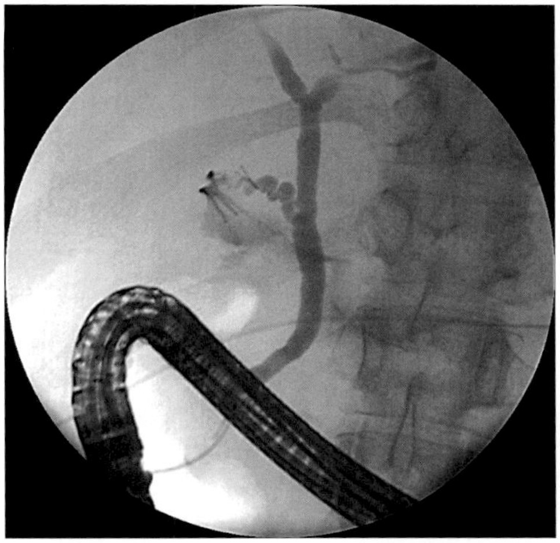

1

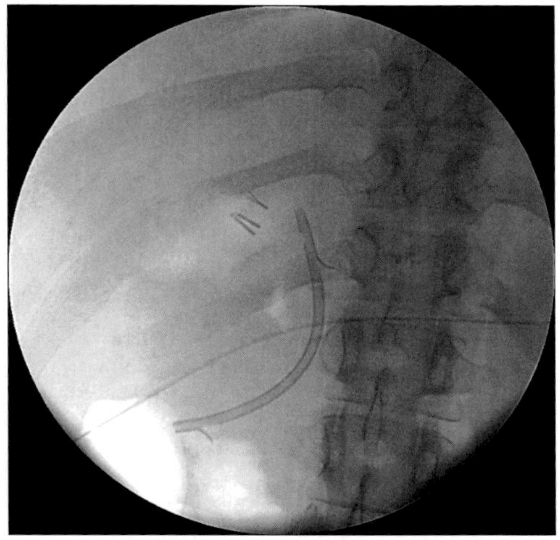

2

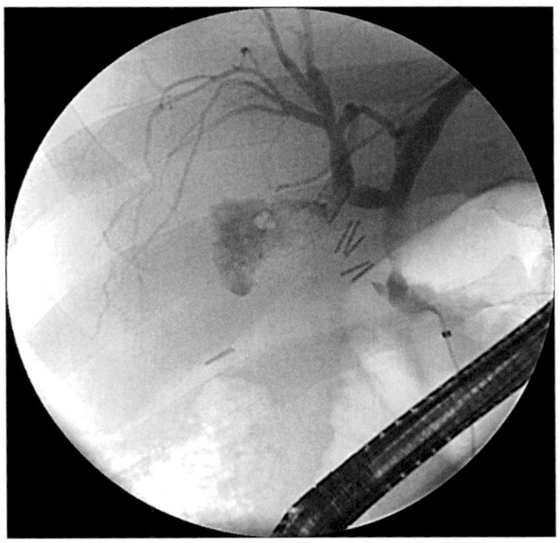

3

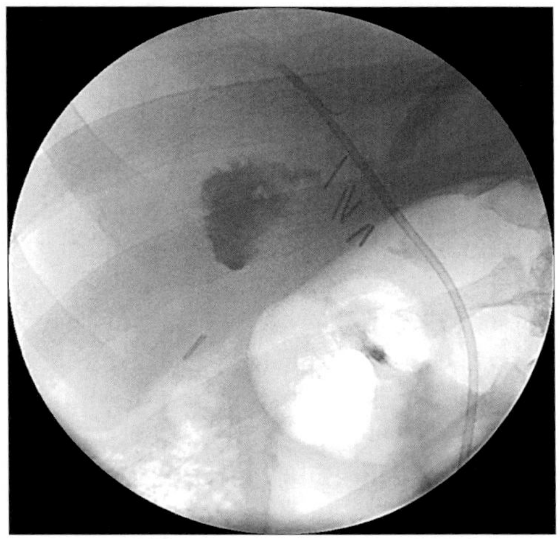

4

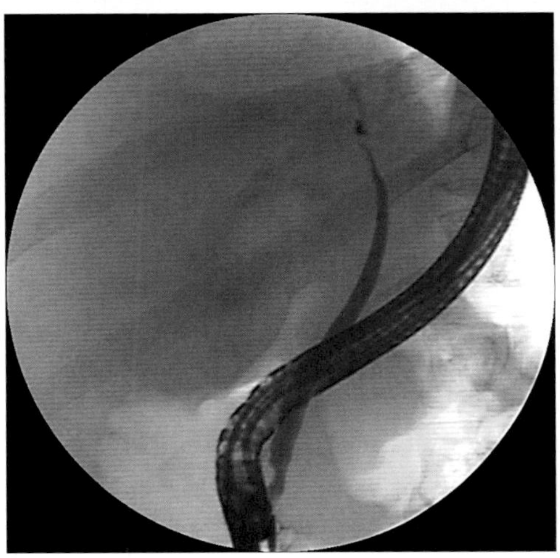

5

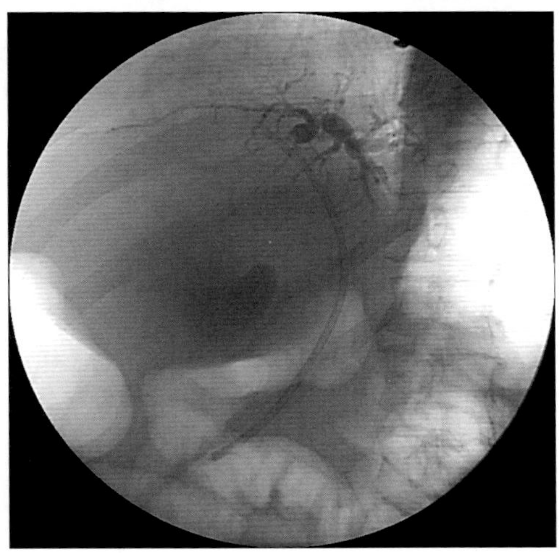

6

Fig. 1. Post-cholecystectomy cystic duct stump leak. **Fig. 2.** Post-cholecystectomy cystic duct stump leak stent placement. **Fig. 3.** Post-cholecystectomy right intrahepatic duct leak. **Fig. 4.** Post-cholecystectomy right intrahepatic duct leak stent. **Fig. 5.** Orthotopic liver transplant biliary duct to duct anastomosis leak. **Fig. 6.** Orthotopic liver transplant biliary duct to duct anastomosis leak stent.

that freely communicate with the peritoneal cavity. More focal tenderness may occur with localized bilious fluid collections (bilomas). These abdominal findings may be attenuated or masked by concomitant immunosuppressive or steroid therapy [12]. Transient elevations in liver chemistries with or without associated leukocytosis can occur [13].

Due to its lack of adequate sensitivity in detecting smaller yet clinically significant leaks, transabdominal ultrasound is reserved in our practice for patients who are critically ill and unable to be transported for more detailed imaging [14]. Hepatobiliary scintigraphy carries a sensitivity of >85% in detecting bile leaks, but cannot provide detailed knowledge about anatomic location with respect to ductal anatomy. Computed tomography with contrast enhancement is superior to ultrasound for detecting smaller bilomas [15, 16]. Therefore, when the clinical suspicion of bile leak arises, our practice is to obtain a computed tomogram with intravenous contrast as the initial diagnostic imaging of choice, with placement of a percutaneous drain into significant and accessible bilomas for quantitative assessment of the fluid collection. This percutaneous drainage provides a controlled outflow for the leakage contents which yields diagnostic fluid bilirubin sampling and cultures to tailor potential antimicrobial therapy. In the post-endoscopic healing period, drain output is carefully recorded, and it is removed if the total external drainage is <50 ml/day.

Endoscopic retrograde cholangiography provides the dual ability to diagnose and treat biliary leaks. Prior to commencing with the procedure, a detailed review of all abdominal operative reports is done to fully understand the postoperative biliary anatomy. Pre-procedural broad-spectrum antibiotics are administered intravenously and continued in cases of suspected bile peritonitis. Endoscopic management includes biliary sphincterotomy with or without drainage via a stent or nasobiliary tube insertion. All of these alternatives share the common intention of reducing the transpapillary pressure gradient between the bile duct and duodenum, thus preferentially facilitating bile flow into the duodenum, instead of out through the ductal disruption, thus promoting healing of the defect site [17]. An algorithm is shown in figure 7 for proposed bile leak management.

Technique

A balloon occlusion cholangiogram is obtained, and transpapillary 10-Fr biliary stenting is preferred after biliary sphincterotomy. The rationale for larger diameter (10 Fr or larger) stent placement is to enhance bile flow compared with smaller caliber stents. We prefer to use longer stents that bridge the disruption and cover the leak site. Repeat endoscopic stent removal and cholangiogram are performed in 4–8 weeks, with re-stenting with larger or multiple stents as deemed necessary by cholangiographic and clinical findings. Nasobiliary catheters are reserved for surveillance cholangiography of critically ill patients who cannot medically tolerate repetitive endoscopic procedures. These drains are frequently uncomfortable for conscious patients, and are prone to spontaneous or intentional dislodgement.

If guidewire access across the disruption site into the proximal biliary tree proves to be challenging, we typically utilize a stone extraction balloon or bowed sphincterotome for alteration of the wire trajectory. The use of hydrophilic or smaller caliber (0.025 or 0.018 mm) guidewires is sometimes necessary to traverse stenotic biliary regions or angulated post-surgical anatomy. For post-surgical anatomy that is not amenable to standard duodenoscope access of the biliary tree, we utilize double balloon enteroscopy with or without laparoscopic assistance (fig. 8, 9). Percutaneous cholangiography is reserved for patients who have significant adhesions and bowel angulations that obviate endoscopic advancement to the biliary tree.

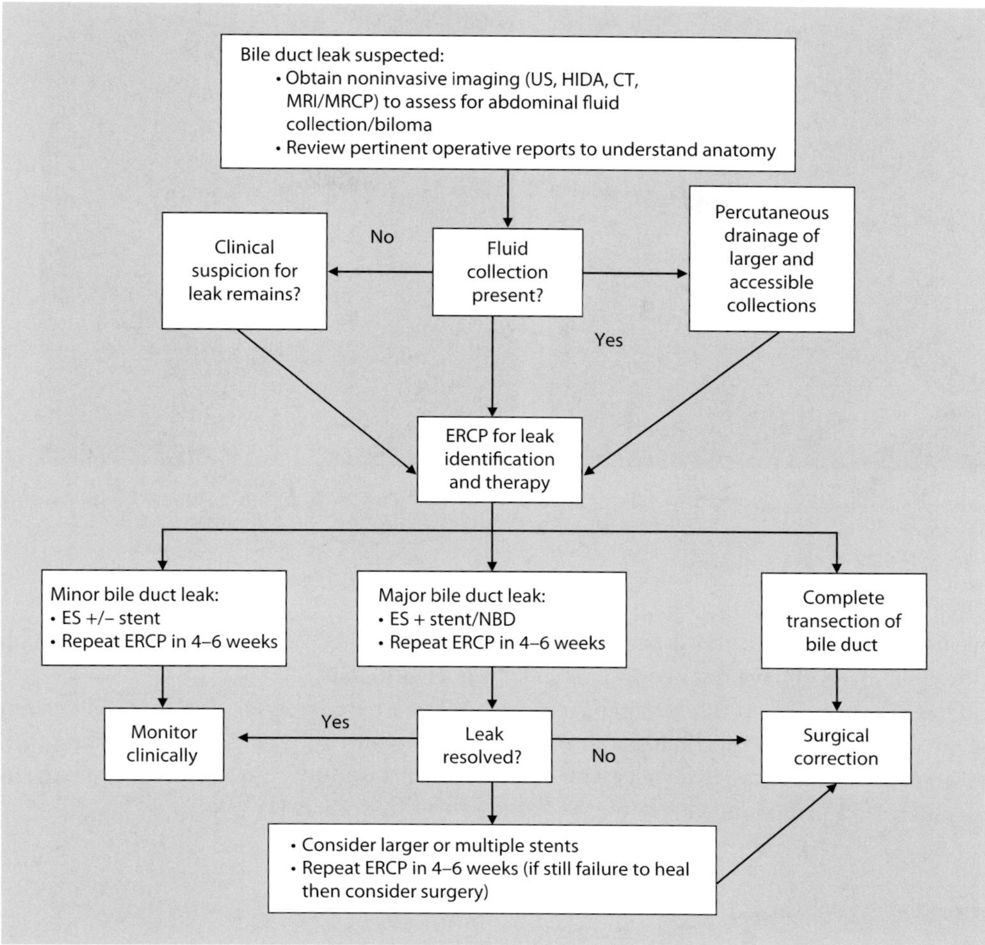

Fig. 7. Algorithm for management of suspected bile leak.

Outcomes

The success rate for endoscopic bile leak therapy has been reported to be 88–100%, largely replacing surgical approaches [18]. Endoscopic biliary sphincterotomy as sole therapy for bile leak was effective in 88% of 25 patients treated in one study [19]. This offers the potential advantage of a single endoscopic session for bile leak therapy. However, a canine model study found significant healing delay for biliary injury in the group that received only sphincterotomy as compared to the sphincterotomy with stenting group [20]. Another disadvantage to sole endoscopic sphincterotomy therapy is the associated need for repeat procedures, as noted in a report of 100 patients undergoing endoscopic treatment for post-cholecystectomy bile leak [21]. Plastic biliary stents and nasobiliary drains effectively treat leaks in >85% of cases. However, indwelling biliary stents have a reported higher success rate compared to nasobiliary tubes for post-cholecystectomy leaks [7, 8, 17, 22, 23]. For surgically altered anatomy that precludes usage of a standard duodenoscope for endoscopic access, double balloon enteroscopy assistance, if available,

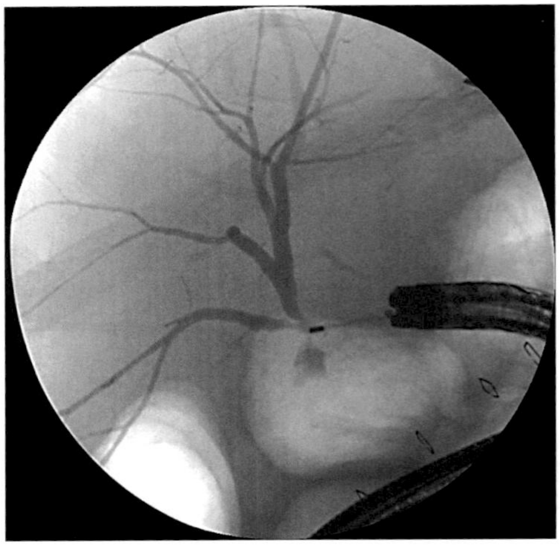

8

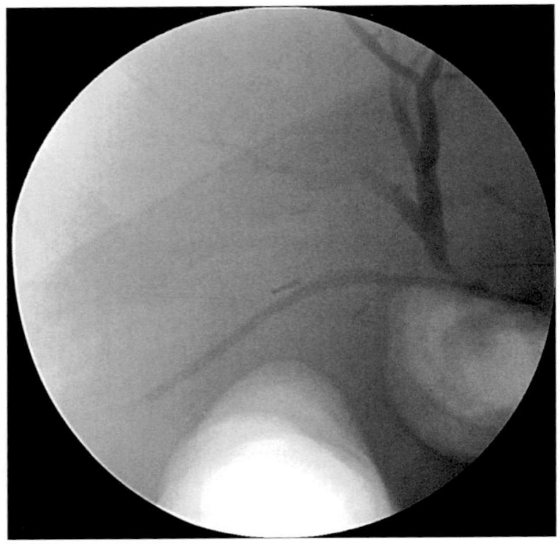

9

Fig. 8. Roux-en-Y hepaticojejunostomy biliary anastomosis leak. **Fig. 9.** Roux-en-Y hepaticojejunostomy biliary leak stent.

can prove useful in this setting. However long-term data on management of biliary leaks through this endoscopic method have not been specifically reported to date.

The standard approach to biloma management has been percutaneous drainage, which can often be uncomfortable. Surgical biloma drainage is reserved for refractory and complex cases. A recent small case series reported successful endoscopic ultrasound-guided biloma drainage in 5 patients, offering a promising alternative to both of these options [24].

Conclusions

This brief report describes the clinical technical approach to the endoscopic management of biliary leaks. The majority of cases managed at our institution have been successfully handled through the above-mentioned algorithmic approach (fig. 7). As endoscopic ancillary devices and imaging continue to improve, we believe the therapeutic efficiency of endoscopic biliary injury treatment will also improve.

References

1 Larson GM, Vitale GC, Casey J, et al: Multipractice analysis of laparoscopic cholecystectomy in 1,983 patients. Am J Surg 1992;163:221–226.

2 Scott TR, Zucker KA, Bailey RW: Laparoscopic cholecystectomy: a review of 12,397 patients. Surg Laparosc Endosc 1992;2:191–198.

3 Greif F, Bronsther OL, Van Thiel DH, et al: The incidence, timing, and management of biliary tract complications after orthotopic liver transplantation. Ann Surg 1994;219:40–45.

4 O'Connor TP, Lewis WD, Jenkins RL: Biliary tract complications after liver transplantation. Arch Surg 1995;130: 312–317.

5 Mehta SN, Pavone E, Barkun JS, et al: A review of the management of post-cholecystectomy biliary leaks during the laparoscopic era. Am J Gastroenterol 1997;92: 1262–1267.

6 MacFadyen BV Jr, Vecchio R, Ricardo AE, et al: Bile duct injury after laparoscopic cholecystectomy. The United States experience. Surg Endosc 1998;12:315–321.

7 Pfau PR, Kochman ML, Lewis JD, et al: Endoscopic management of postoperative biliary complications in orthotopic liver transplantation. Gastrointest Endosc 2000;52: 55–63.
8 Rerknimitr R, Sherman S, Fogel EL, et al: Biliary tract complications after orthotopic liver transplantation with choledochocholedochostomy anastomosis: endoscopic findings and results of therapy. Gastrointest Endosc 2002;55:224–231.
9 Shah JN, Ahmad NA, Shetty K, et al: Endoscopic management of biliary complications after adult living donor liver transplantation. Am J Gastroenterol 2004;99:1291–1295.
10 Bergman JJ, van den Brink GR, Rauws EA, et al: Treatment of bile duct lesions after laparoscopic cholecystectomy. Gut 1996;38:141–147.
11 Sandha GS, Bourke MJ, Haber GB, et al: Endoscopic therapy for bile leak based on a new classification: results in 207 patients. Gastrointest Endosc 2004;60: 567–574.
12 Tung BY, Kimmey MB: Biliary complications of orthotopic liver transplantation. Dig Dis 1999;17: 133–144.
13 Mutignani M, Shah SK, Tringali A, et al: Endoscopic therapy for biliary leaks from aberrant right hepatic ducts severed during cholecystectomy. Gastrointest Endosc 2002;55:932–936.
14 Kok T, Van der Sluis A, Klein JP, et al: Ultrasound and cholangiography for the diagnosis of biliary complications after orthotopic liver transplantation: a comparative study. J Clin Ultrasound 1996;24:103–115.
15 Brooks DC, Becker JM, Connors PJ, et al: Management of bile leaks following laparoscopic cholecystectomy. Surg Endosc 1993;7:292–295.
16 Brugge WR, Rosenberg DJ, Alavi A: Diagnosis of postoperative bile leaks. Am J Gastroenterol 1994; 89:2178–2183.
17 Bjorkman DJ, Carr-Locke DL, Lichtenstein DR, et al: Postsurgical bile leaks: endoscopic obliteration of the transpapillary pressure gradient is enough. Am J Gastroenterol 1995;90:2128–233.
18 Costamagna G, Shah SK, Tringali A: Current management of postoperative complications and benign biliary strictures. Gastrointest Endosc Clin N Am 2003;13:635–648, ix.
19 Llach J, Bordas JM, Elizalde JI, et al: Sphincterotomy in the treatment of biliary leakage. Hepatogastroenterology 2002;49:1496–1498.
20 Marks JM, Ponsky JL, Shillingstad RB, et al: Biliary stenting is more effective than sphincterotomy in the resolution of biliary leaks. Surg Endosc 1998;12: 327–330.
21 Kaffes AJ, Hourigan L, De Luca N, et al: Impact of endoscopic intervention in 100 patients with suspected postcholecystectomy bile leak. Gastrointest Endosc 2005;61:269–275.
22 Morelli J, Mulcahy HE, Willner IR, et al: Endoscopic treatment of post-liver transplantation biliary leaks with stent placement across the leak site. Gastrointest Endosc 2001;54:471–475.
23 Neidich R, Soper N, Edmundowicz S, et al: Endoscopic management of bile duct leaks after attempted laparoscopic cholecystectomy. Surg Laparosc Endosc 1996;6: 348–354.
24 Shami VM, Talreja JP, Mahajan A, et al: EUS-guided drainage of bilomas: a new alternative? Gastrointest Endosc 2008;67:136–140.

Irving Waxman, MD
Center for Endoscopic Research and Therapeutics,
University of Chicago Medical Center
5758 S. Maryland Ave., MC 9028, Chicago, IL 60637 (USA)
Tel. +1 773 702 5997, Fax +1 773 834 8891, E-Mail iwaxman@medicine.bsd.uchicago.edu

Mönkemüller K, Wilcox CM, Muñoz-Navas M (eds): Interventional and Therapeutic Gastrointestinal Endoscopy.
Front Gastrointest Res. Basel, Karger, 2010, vol 27, pp 390–402

Endoscopic Treatment of Biliary Complications after Liver Transplantation

Julius Spicak

Institute of Clinical and Experimental Medicine, Prague, Czech Republic

Abstract

Biliary complications remain a frequent and significant issue occurring in up to 30% of patients after liver transplantation. Their development and presentation are associated with specific transplant issues such as surgery technique, immunosuppression, rejection, damage of vascular supply, infections and disease recurrence. With the expanding and demanding surgical techniques in reduced, living related and splitting donors, the technical factors play a crucial role. Biliary complications comprise a long list of varied events corresponding to biliary problems in non-transplant conditions. The most frequent are anastomotic strictures and leaks followed by hilar (ischemic-like) and intrahepatic strictures, sphincter Oddi dysfunction, stones and stenoses due the extraluminal pressure. The diagnostic work-up and treatment involve usual modalities. The treatment of biliary complications requires a multidisciplinary approach, in which all three main options – endoscopic, radiologic and surgical – play a role. Endoscopic management is usually preferred due its comprehensiveness, efficacy and safety. Alternatively, the radiologic approach can be used particularly if there is not a comfortable transluminal access to the biliary tree. Both approaches can be combined and the success can be expected in up to 80% of patients. As in non-transplant conditions, sphincterotomy, multiple stent insertion with or without dilatation, and extraction of stones are used. The specific issues of endoscopic procedures after liver transplantation include postprocedural cholangitis prevention, consideration of coagulation disorders and sedation of patients with various mental impairments. Surgery, usually Roux-en-Y hepaticojejunostomy, is a demanding procedure potentially solving the obstruction for ever. Nevertheless, stenosis of the anastomosis and the episodes of reflux cholangitis can compromise long-term outcomes in up to 20% of patients. A universally acceptable therapeutic approach to biliary complications has not been defined, and local expertise, usually inevitably uneven, plays an important role.

Biliary complications continue to be a significant cause of morbidity and even mortality after orthotopic liver transplantation (OLT) [1–8] (table 1). Given the generally increased patients' vulnerability after OLT, it is necessary to manage these complications promptly and effectively to prevent an irreversible liver damage and a threat to the recipient's life. Biliary complications cannot be considered as a separate issue. They often develop as a consequence of the underlying problems specifically associated with liver transplantation in patients with immunosuppression modulating clinical manifestations and laboratory findings. Not exceptionally, they can occur together with other complications such as primary disease recurrence, rejection, vascular problems or cytomegalovirus (CMV) infection. To assess the problem comprehensively and to correctly organize the management of such a complicated patient is the masterpiece of medical skill.

Table 1. Biliary complications in various surgical anastomosis techniques

Reference (first author)	Center	Year	n	Total %	Leaks %	Strictures %
Duct-to-duct anastomosis						
Lebeau [1]	Pittsburgh	1990	193	20	2	18
Davidson [2]	Royal Free	1999	100	31	17	14
Graziadei [3]	Innsbruck	2006	515	16	NA	16
Roux-en-Y hepaticojejunostomy						
Ringe [4]	Hannover	1989	84	24	12	2
Lebeau [1]	Pittsburgh	1990	187	12	9	3
Living donor liver transplantation						
Giacomoni [5]	Milano	2006	23	48	22	26
Wojcicki [6]	Birmingham	2006	70	26	20	4
Cardiac death donors						
Suarez [7]	Coruna	2008	27	42	4	
De Vera [8]	Pittsburgh	2008	141	25	NA	NA

NA = Not analyzed.

Biliary Reconstruction of Liver Transplantation

To achieve high technical success of endoscopic treatment of biliary complications, a detailed knowledge of the anatomy of biliary reconstruction as well as knowledge of specific issues of post-transplant pathophysiology is essential. Biliary reconstruction is created as the final step of OLT after vascular anastomoses. The gallbladder interposition technique was used in the pioneering years utilizing the gallbladder as the graft conduit between the donor and recipient bile ducts. In early reports by Starzl and Calne, the association of bile stasis with stone formation and cholangitis resulted in morbidity of up to 50% and mortality up to 30%, fully deserving the reference of being the 'Achilles heel' of this demanding surgical technique.

Nowadays, end-to-end duct-to-duct anastomosis in recipients with healthy native bile ducts of compatible caliber is the preferred technique in most centers. The resulting continuity of bile ducts most corresponding to original structure allows access to and efficient treatment of complications by standard endoscopic techniques. Similarly good results were obtained by other centers using a side-to-side variant. Occasionally and more often in the past, the reconstruction was complemented by temporary T-tube biliary drainage with two presumed aims: to visualize the bile ducts whenever needed, and to prevent anastomotic stricture. The results of several comparative studies differ but the second premise was never reliably met, and leaks prevailing in T-tube groups caused that the use of preventive drainage has been mostly abandoned [9–12].

Roux-en-Y hepaticojejunostomy is utilized in patients with bile ducts altered by the pre-existing disease such as sclerosing cholangitis. It can be also used in the presence of major disparity in size of ducts, and it is often preferred in the case of retransplantation because of inadequate recipient duct length. Roux-en-Y was also the routine reconstruction technique in the first series of living-related, reduced graft and split liver transplantation. With the growing body of knowledge of the blood supply around the biliary ducts and experience, duct-to-duct anastomosis has been increasingly constructed even if multiple anastomoses are needed [13].

Table 2. Classification of biliary complications

Intrinsic	Extrinsic
Strictures	False aneurysm
Intrahepatic	Cystic duct mucocele
PSC recurrence	Lymphoproliferative disease
Secondary cholangitis	Cystic duct mucocele
Perihilar	Chronic pancreatitis
Ischemic	Recurrent/de novo cancer
Idiopathic (ischemic-like)	
Anastomotic	
Distal	
Papillary dysfunction	
Leaks	
Anastomotic duct-to-duct	
Anastomotic HJA	
T-tube location	
Cut surface	
Missed segmental duct	
Stones, cast, T-tube remnant	
Hemobilia	
Recurrent sclerosing cholangitis	

Cadaveric Death Brain Donors, Living Donors, and Non-Heart Beating Donors

A liver transplantation program provides full recovery from various otherwise inevitably lethal conditions (chronic end-stage liver disease, acute liver failure, selected tumors and others) in a large majority of transplanted patients. With an expansion of indications and technical progress the shortage of organs has arisen as a critical issue. Various ways have been explored to enlarge and optimally utilize the pool of donors. There are three different donor sources with specific biliary consequences: cadaveric brain donors are utilized in Europe and the USA in a large majority of cases. The advantage of the living donor technique prevailing in some Asian countries is the optimal timing of the elective procedure with a minimal time loss, which could be, on the other hand, compromised by more complicated biliary anastomoses of a reduced donor organ. Using donation after cardiac death, the relative risk of graft failure in several series was increased with the higher rate of biliary complications being one of the reasons [7, 8].

Classification and Etiology of Biliary Complications

The complex pathogenesis of biliary complications is attributable to various factors including technical reasons, ischemic damage mostly due to hepatic artery thrombosis and ischemia-reperfusion injury, immunological factors such as ABO incompatibility, CMV infection, disease recurrence in primary sclerosing cholangitis, and others [14]. The consequent cholestasis contributes to the generally increased vulnerability after liver transplantation, heavily affecting particularly the outcome of patients with recurrent hepatitis C virus (HCV) [15]. Technical reasons for biliary complications include imperfect suture with early T-tube-related leak or anastomotic stricture, leaks from the liver surface or inadvertent bile duct injuries. Biliary complications comprise a long and varied list of events with different frequency involving both the ductal and extraluminal causes. In fact, the scale of complications corresponds to biliary problems appearing in non-transplant conditions. The difference consists in the proportions and several specific aspects [13] (table 2).

Clinical Manifestations and Diagnosis

Symptoms indicating biliary complications include fever, right upper quadrant pain, non-specific abdominal discomfort, and elevation of liver particularly cholestatic enzymes. They can rapidly proceed to the development of biliary peritonitis in large leaks, but more often they remain mild and undistinguishable from other causes of cholestasis such as HCV recurrence, and acute rejection to mention at least two other common complications. The diagnosis is based on a detailed analysis of the clinical picture, laboratory examinations, liver biopsy and imaging methods. Typically, there is absence of intrahepatic bile ducts dilatation on ultrasound particularly early after liver transplantation even above tight obstruction. The direct imaging by endoscopic retrograde cholangiopancreatography (ERCP) or percutaneous transhepatic cholangiography is the final step of the diagnostic work-up, which should be preceded by magnetic resonance cholangiopancreatography (MRCP).

Specific Measurements before the Scope Is Inserted

Infection Prevention

Infection is one of major complications of ERCP occurring in about 1% of procedures overall. Several reasons can play a role. Similarly to other invasive procedures, ERCP, even though poorly documented, may cause endocarditis in high-risk patients. Infection transmitted by the contaminated scope should be completely preventable by proper use of disposable accessories and utilization of the standard technique of disinfection. Thanks to universally adopted measures, cases of endocarditis and nosocomial infection including HCV, hepatitis B, and human immunodeficiency virus related to endoscopy have been exceptional in recent series. The American Heart Association recently revised their guidelines for prophylaxis of infective endocarditis, and a crucial change regarding endoscopic procedures is that antibiotic prophylaxis solely to prevent infective endocarditis is not recommended. The exceptions are the high-risk cardiac conditions including: a prosthetic cardiac valve, history of previous infective endocarditis, cardiac transplant recipients who develop valvulopathy, patients with congenital heart disease with either unrepaired cyanosis or those repaired by prosthetic material within 6 months after the procedure, or those with a residual defect. Since the enterococci, which make part of the common bile duct flora in cholangitis, are the invading agents in endocarditis, either amoxicillin or ampicillin should be included for the antibiotic protocol for enterococcal coverage in these patients.

The most frequent cause of cholangitis after ERCP is the flare-up of infection being already present in the bile ducts. The common pathogens include *Pseudomonas aeruginosa, Klebsiella* spp., *E. coli, Bacteroides* spp., and *Enterococci.* Precipitation of the infection is caused by the elevated intraductal pressure when complete bile drainage is not achieved. To eliminate these factors, it is highly recommended to aspirate bile before contrast injection and to complete endoscopic treatment (removal of stones, drainage of all relevant visualized strictures) within one session. Risk factors to be considered also involve jaundice, previous cholangitis, previous endoscopic treatment, combined endoscopic-percutaneous procedures, hilar tumors and primary sclerosing cholangitis because the bile duct obstruction is difficult to be relieved completely, and transplant patients on immunosuppressive regimens.

The role of antibiotic prophylaxis is controversial and a variety of practices exist. Several randomized clinical trials (RCTs) have been published showing reduction of bacteremia, but their relevance was inevitably limited due to the small number of clinical infections. No RCT has been conducted exclusively with transplant patients. For all these reasons, the general attitude to antibiotic prophylaxis is becoming more and more selective with their application in highly suspected risk-related conditions only, with transplant patients being exactly the case. ERCP should only be employed in transplant patients with highly suspected biliary obstruction and after MRCP. In fact, most of these patients are already on an antibiotic regimen due to clinical/laboratory manifestation of infection. If not, we recommend 400 mg of ciprofloxacin to be given intravenously (peroral administration is probably similarly effective) 2 h before the procedure and to continue with the administration until complete drainage is achieved. Other options involve gentamicin, cephalosporins and ureidopenicillins [16, 17].

Coagulopathy – Bleeding Disorders

ERCP and subsequent endoscopic treatment are commonly undertaken in transplant recipients with abnormal coagulation due to liver dysfunction or anticoagulation therapy. Other risk factors include thrombocytopenia (including hemodialysis-caused coagulation disorder) and initiation of anticoagulation therapy within 3 days after the invasive procedure; on the other hand, enlarging of previous sphincterotomy and the use of aspirin or non-steroidal anti-inflammatory drugs do not seem to raise the risk. Data dealing specifically with sphincterotomy in patients with liver disorders are unavailable and a commonly shared view is that coagulopathy should be managed according to rules applied to liver biopsy. Generally, there are widely divergent opinions about the values at which abnormal coagulation indexes signal a significant risk for any kind of invasive procedures including endoscopic sphincterotomy. The patient's platelet count as a part of complete blood count, and prothrombin time or international normalized ratio should be checked at a suitable juncture prior sphincterotomy. However, the utility of these tests (which are not equal) in predicting bleeding risk is uncertain and generally not sufficiently supported by scientific evidence. Probably more important than any laboratory parameters is taking a detailed medical history as to whether any bleeding episode had followed an invasive procedure in the past, and to search for any possible signs of recent bleeding. Whether the prophylactic use of blood products alters the risk of bleeding is currently unknown. Nevertheless, it is commonly assumed that platelet transfusion should be considered when the thrombocyte count is <50,000–60,000/ml and, if the prothrombin time is >4 s longer (or international normalized ratio >1.6), then a transfusion of fresh-frozen plasma may bring the bleeding risk into the desired range [18]. The mixture of factors concentrates could be considered in severe coagulation disorder. The appropriate practice of endoscopic procedures on patients on anticoagulation or antiplatelet therapy is specified in detail in the guidelines of the endoscopic societies and the conditions of post-transplant care do not possess any specificity. Adoption of all these measures cannot completely eliminate the increased risk of hemorrhage in the complex bleeding disorder accompanying the liver dysfunction in the post-transplant patient. The endoscopist should avoid the use of pure cutting current and to stop actively, using local endoscopic techniques, any bleeding that may occur immediately after sphincterotomy.

Sedation and Anesthesia
During the thorough pre-transplant evaluation and post-transplant follow-up, patients are often exposed to many endoscopic procedures which could make them more anxious and less tolerant. The procedures early after transplantations or in impaired condition (ASA class IV-V-E) have to be performed with the assistance of an anesthesiologist, often under general anesthesia. The therapeutic procedures due to an abnormal anatomy of reconstructed bile ducts are often prolonged. A considerable proportion of transplant procedures are performed in alcohol abusers. Chronic alcohol use increases the dose requirements for anesthetic, sedative or analgesic agents. This is thought to be because in part of enzyme (particularly cytochrome P450 2E1) induction, or through the development of cross-tolerance. The effective doses of propofol, opioids and other drugs are increased, the patients may become paradoxically agitated, uneasily controlled and less tolerant to any disturbing procedures. The increased requirements for anesthetics may exacerbate the risk of cardiovascular instability in patients suffering from cardiomyopathy, and increase the risk of adverse effects of all kinds. All these consequences make the endoscopic procedures particularly demanding. The administered drugs have to be precisely titrated and the patient adequately monitored. The participation of an anesthesiologist on presumably risk-associated procedures is highly recommended [19].

Biliary Complications after Liver Transplantation – Specific Issues and Their Management

Basically, treatment of biliary complications does not differ from the treatment of the identical structural entities and its techniques have been repeatedly described in detail and are more or less standardized. Nevertheless, there are several specific features which have to be considered to avoid an unexpected surprise and to achieve optimal results. Since few data from well-designed prospective trials are available, the specific techniques and tricks described below are based besides a search of the literature on the continuous experience with more then 700 liver transplantations and management of approximately 200 biliary complications being followed in the single department. This has made it possible to follow the results of treatment from both immediately and in the long run and to discuss all individual aspects with representatives of other specialties participating on the transplantation program such as invasive radiologists, surgeons and transplant hepatologists. A retrospective analysis of the first 500 consecutive primary transplant procedures revealed biliary complications in 147 (29.4%) patients. Choledochocholedochal anastomotic stricture was found in 90 patients, and leak in 38 patients. The scale of other less frequent complications included non-anastomotic hilar (ischemic-like) strictures, strictures due to post-transplant lymphoproliferative disorder, choledocholithiasis and papillary stenosis. Endoscopic treatment was fully successful in 88 out of the 117 (75.2%) patients with anastomotic strictures or leaks. Retransplantation rate was higher in patients with than in those without biliary complications (10.9 vs. 5%). The occurrence of biliary strictures did not have any effect on mortality. We have learnt that, in transplantology more than in non-transplant medicine, every patient is a unique complex entity, and that clinical decision-making should be, as a rule, preceded by a detailed analysis of the patient's condition and a careful evaluation of all available, usually unequally established techniques, skill and experience.

Endoscopic Sphincterotomy
The technique itself does not differ from the sphincterotomy performed in other patients. Nevertheless, the spontaneous motility of the bile duct is abolished due to the surgical

reconstruction resulting in the denervation of the biliary tree. Therefore, evacuation of the contrast material cannot serve as a reliable parameter of bile duct function, and cholestasis tends to occur after sphincterotomy of a standard size which would be otherwise fully sufficient for what it is aimed – stent insertion or bile duct stones extraction in a non-transplant condition. As a result, we always recommend to perform the sphincterotomy to the maximum possible (safe) extent.

Anastomotic Strictures
Anastomotic strictures, being, together with leaks, the most common post-transplant biliary complication, are highly specific and almost unparalleled to non-transplant conditions. They are often asymmetrical with the shape which can be difficult to precisely project on x-ray due to overlap with one or two cysticus stumps. The shape of a prolonged reconstructed bile duct in the anastomotic area may resemble letter 'S'. For the irregular lumen of the anastomosis with cysticus stumps, it may be exceptionally quite difficult to pass the guidewire through the stricture. Often, several types of wire with different properties concerning the diameter, flexibility/rigidity and slipperiness have to be tried. The direction of the tip of the wire can be enhanced by the use of an angled tip, sphincterotome or balloon catheter. The stricture can be dilated by balloon before stenting, but we do not find it necessary if planning to insert a single stent. The strategic principle is that a benign anastomotic stricture unlike a malignant stenosis does not need to be bridged only, but the lumen of the bile duct has to be fully reconstituted to respond to normal anatomy, and therefore, multiple stents according to the size of the bile ducts below and above the stricture have to be inserted. Both basic techniques of multiple stent insertion can be used: two wires prior to inserting either stent, or to insert the wire along and after the first stent insertion. The optimal number and position of multiple stents is usually achieved in several sessions separated by short 1- or 2-week intervals. Even if, in our opinion, stenting should be the preferred technique, there are several studies showing that simple balloon dilation without stenting relieves the stricture with similar success, and even with reduced complication rates. It seems that the chance for the optimal remodeling of the anastomosis and the stricture is higher early after transplantation and lower later on, if a firm fibrotic stricture has already developed. If the reconstructed bile duct after liver transplantation is prolonged with the S shape, we select a longer stent that can be estimated from the distance between the stricture and duodenum. The reason is that the stent passing through the S-shaped bile duct creates friction making the insertion more difficult. If the stent is not long enough, its end may become impacted in the orifice of the stricture, which makes it impossible to go through. On the other hand, when a curved stricture is overcome, the shape straightens and this can expel the proximal end of the stent far above the stricture, possibly above the hilar junction. This unfavorable position of the proximal end can hardly be prevented. One stent alone inserted into S-shaped bile duct with anastomotic stricture may adopt the curvature of the duct, while multiple stents straighten it, which is the optimal outcome. If the first one or two inserted stents are located with their proximal ends far above the stricture, the length of the third stent should be shorter to drain the bile from various levels of the bile ducts to avoid cholestasis and debris accumulation above the stricture. A firm S-shaped bile duct can expel the stent back to the duodenum with the risk of duodenal perforation by the stent on the opposite side to the orifice. More stents inserted in parallel make the expulsion less probable. The stents should be exchanged regularly at 3-month intervals as recommended elsewhere, and are usually removed after an interval of 6 months to 1 year. If there is a failure of endoscopic access, the transhepatic approach follows. The first plastic stent can be inserted either transhepatically or using the rendezvous technique transpapillarily [20–22] (fig. 1–3).

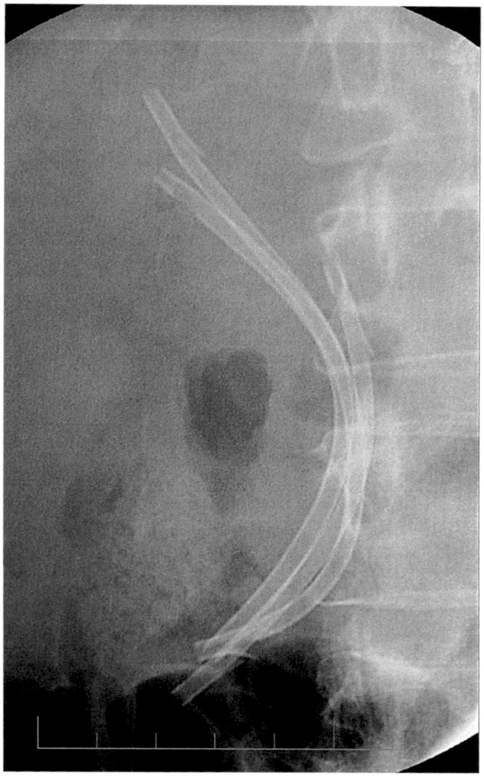

1

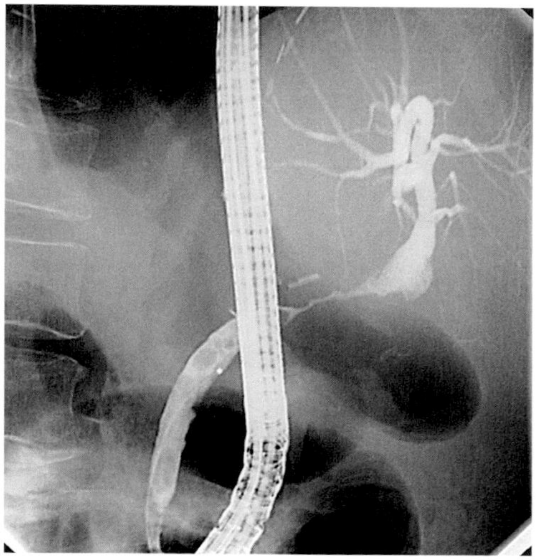

2

Fig. 1. Multiple plastic stents.
Fig. 2. Hilar ischemic-like stricture.
Fig. 3. Anastomotic stricture on MRCP.
Fig. 4. S-shaped reconstructed bile duct.

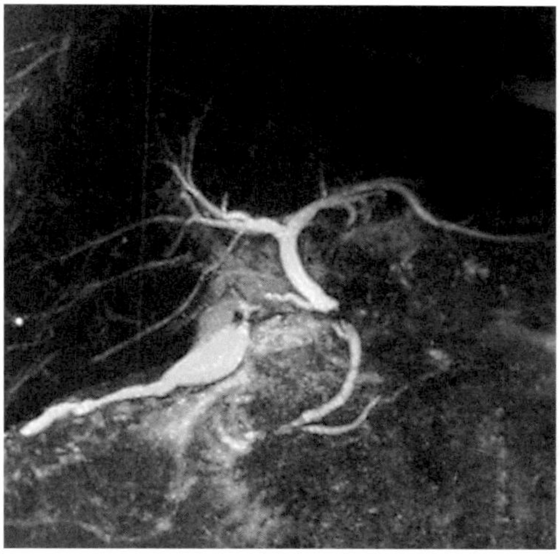

3

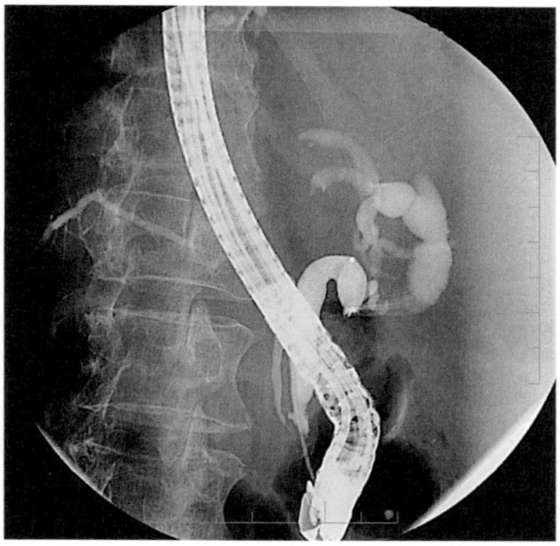

4

Non-Anastomotic Hilar Strictures (Ischemic-Type Biliary Lesions)
With an incidence ranging between 5 and 15%, these biliary complications remain, more than anastomotic strictures, a substantial source of morbidity, graft loss and even mortality after liver transplantation. Their multifactorial origin embraces a variety of events (risk factors) including ischemia due to hepatic artery thrombosis or prolonged cold and warm ischemia, use of

University of Wisconsin solution vs. histidine tryptophan ketoglutarate, ABO incompatibility, extramural pressure by lymph nodes or tumor, original disease recurrence, or it remains obscure. The altered bile composition with the significantly lower phospholipids/bile salts ratio after liver transplantation and graft steatosis may likewise contribute to their pathogenesis [23, 24]. Endoscopic treatment consists of stent insertion similar to that in non-transplant patients, but detailed exploration and management of underlining conditions is essential. If the stricture involves segmental branches, multiple stent bridging the strictures of all ducts are necessary. In specific conditions of malignant stricture, metallic stent insertion according to commonly shared rules is the choice. Full success of the endoscopic treatment is less probable due to the location distant to the papilla making the endoscopic manipulation less effective, and due to various underlying conditions, with different outcomes. The endoscopic treatment can be combined with the transhepatic approach, if necessary [25] (fig. 4).

Intrahepatic Strictures
They are not unequivocally classified against non-anastomotic hilar ischemic-type biliary lesions, and the pathogenesis involves identical principles. Lee et al. [26] classified intrahepatic stenoses into four groups: unilateral focal, confluence, bilateral multifocal, and diffuse. The success of either non-surgical endoscopic or transhepatic interventions is inversely related to the extent of the duct involvement with the frequent need of early retransplantation [26].

Distal Strictures
The strictures below the anastomosis are usually caused by chronic pancreatitis. Surprisingly, pancreatitis is often asymptomatic and cholestasis is the only manifestation of advanced pancreatic disease. Other causes involve extramural pressure by malignancies, mucocele, and biloma. They can be managed similarly to non-transplant conditions [13, 25].

Papillary Stenosis (Sphincter of Oddi Dysfunction – SOD)
Data concerning the occurrence of papillary stenosis/dysfunction after liver transplantation are less consistent compared to other specific and well-defined biliary complications (anastomotic strictures, leaks). Cholestasis was observed in 3–7% of patients following T-tube clamping early after liver transplantation but, according to some authorities, it seems to be transient and self-limited. Papillary stenosis can be facilitated or unmasked by liver transplantation since the abolished bile duct spontaneous motility by ducts reconstruction and denervation. On the other hand, the fact that some patients develop SOD and others do not while undergoing the same surgical technique, is intriguing [13, 25, 27]. The embarrassment and inevitable diversity of approaches can be demonstrated on a model case: A patient developed significant cholestasis several months after liver transplantation. Liver biopsy excluded other causes, sonography and MRCP have shown dilatation of the recipient choledochus, which was confirmed by ERCP. Multiple acceptable choices included: either to perform manometry or sphincterotomy immediately without manometry, or to wait for possible spontaneous resolution or, perhaps, to insert a stent and wait – if the cholestasis has resolved, the patient can be either followed only and, if reappearing, it would pose a strong argument for sphincterotomy. If sphincterotomy is the choice, the cut of maximal safe extent is recommended.

Bile Duct Stones
Bile duct stones are less frequent compared to leaks and anastomotic strictures, but still relatively common complication after liver transplantation. Two basic categories of choledocholithiasis

can be classified: Sludge or small stones usually develop as a late complication. Soft pigmented composition prevails suggesting that cholestasis and infection play a decisive role. Cholesterol supersaturation and related changes in lithogenicity are probably less important. The occurrence of stones is often associated with biliary strictures. More rarely, extensive casts completely filling the biliary tree have been described. Casts usually appear relatively early after liver transplantation due to prolonged ischemia resulting in severe diffuse biliary mucosal damage and defoliation. Endoscopic treatment responding to non-transplant conditions should be preferred to be followed alternatively by the transhepatic approach or surgery in the event of failure. Nevertheless, the long-term outcome reflecting the underlying conditions can be limited when multiple stones or cast with diffuse bile duct damage occur [13, 25, 28, 29].

Port-Transplant Lymphoproliferative Disorder

Port-transplant lymphoproliferative disorder is a serious and complex clinicopathologic disorder that has been related to several specific factors, particularly overimmunosuppression and viral infection. The rate of post-transplant lymphoproliferative disorder is close to 3.0%. The early cases are located in the liver hilum causing biliary stenosis with cholestasis. The treatment is based on several principles. The degree of immunosuppression should be reduced. Antiviral drugs have been used mostly in children. Chemotherapy has been used in the presence Epstein-Barr Virus-negative monoclonal lymphomas developing with delay after transplantation. Other options involve rituximab, a chimeric anti-CD20 antibody, radiotherapy and interferon-α. The local biliary involvement can be relieved by stent insertion from either the endoscopic or transhepatic approach or, exceptionally, by surgery. Endoscopic treatment is consistent with the endoscopic approach to hilar strictures of other causes with commonly required transhepatic assistance. Survival is determined by the pathobiology of the PTDL with a worse prognosis in early disease similar to the prognosis of other post-transplant malignancies [30].

Bile Leaks

Bile leaks have been reported in 1–25% of OLTs performed. They can be dividend into early, defined by a time period of 1–3 months after OLT, and late leaks. Anastomotic leaks are related to technically insufficient suture, or to ischemic damage, usually to the donor bile duct. Other risk factors considered include recipient and donors age and the MELD score [31]. They seem to be unrelated to the type of biliary duct-to-duct reconstruction. According to a recent RCT, end-to-end versus side-to side choledochocholedochostomy did not reveal a significant difference in terms of the occurrence of biliary complications [29]. Early leakage may develop at the T-tube insertion site any time but typically after T-tube removal, in up to 30% of procedures [32, 33]. Other sites of leak comprise surface leaks and leaks from inadvertent bile ducts usually after graft reduction. The leaks can be treated either by stent or nasobiliary drainage insertion (after sphincterotomy). In small leaks, sphincterotomy alone may be sufficient (fig. 5).

Roux-en-Y Anastomosis

Several small studies were focused on endoscopic management of patients with Roux-en-Y anastomosis, which in the past could be managed with either a standard duodenoscope, gastroscope or pediatric colonoscope with limited success only. Both with double- or single-balloon enteroscope, ERCP is a feasible option with a high success rate. Limitations of this technique include the time requirements (1–2 h), and the relatively narrow scale of accessories [34].

5

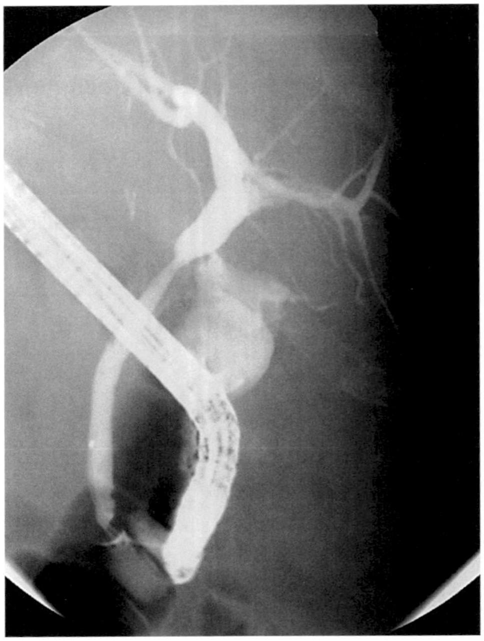

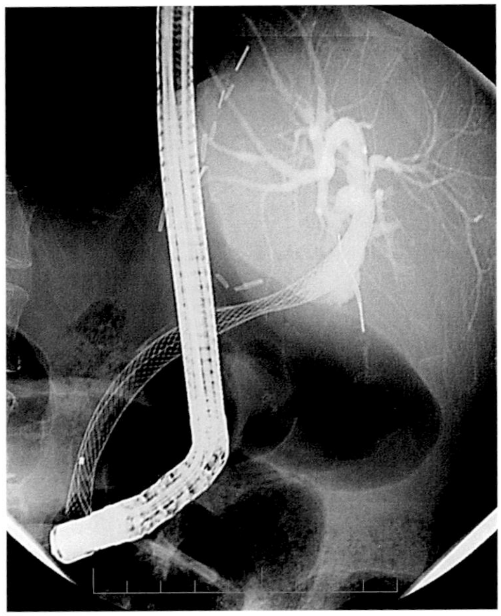

6

Fig. 5. Anastomotic leak. **Fig. 6.** Covered metallic stent.

Metallic Stents

The first bare self-expanding metallic stents have been shown to maintain patency longer than plastic ones in malignant strictures. Nevertheless, in benign strictures, they were mostly rejected due to failure related to mucosal hyperplasia and the fact they could not be removed. The mostly welcome feature of the metallic stents is the single-session treatment, with an additional advantage of (semi)covered metallic stents in benign strictures being they prevent tissue ingrowth and thus ensure removability using the snare or rat-tooth technique [35, 36]. Several studies have shown the potential of (semi)covered metallic stents to offer high efficacy and recurrence while keeping complication rates on an acceptable level. Comparative studies with conventional plastic stents are warranted to evaluate also the various radial forces, traumatic ends and, perhaps, also resorbable material (fig. 6).

Conclusion

The high rate and wide range of biliary complications after liver transplantation remain a challenging issue. The advent of new strategies and techniques, such as split- or reduced-size liver, living related liver transplantation, and non-heart beating donors comprising new technical and pathogenetical principles will maintain the rate of complications on a significant level. Management has to arise from individual assessment of the patient with their unique complexity comprising the morphology of the lesion, presumed pathogenesis, comorbidity, prior surgery and the patient's own preferences. Analyses that consider all these factors should determine the strategy that may offer optimal benefit for the patient. The management of biliary complications requires a multidisciplinary approach, in which all three main options – endoscopic, radiologic and surgical – have to be weighed up one against each other. Generally, endoscopic management has to be considered in the majority of patients as the first therapeutic option due its comprehensiveness, efficacy and safety. Alternatively, the radiologic approach can be used in the majority of complications, preferably if there is not a comfortable transluminal access to the biliary tree. Proper stent placement using x-ray alone is more difficult to control, and multiple stents usually cannot be inserted [37]. Both approaches can be combined. The disadvantage of these methods is the need for multiple sessions annoying the patient and increasing the risk of complications. Surgery, usually Roux-en-Y anastomosis, is a demanding technique potentially solving the obstruction for ever. Nevertheless, obstruction of the anastomosis and the episodes of reflux cholangitis can compromise long-term outcomes in up to 20% of patients [38]. A standard therapeutic approach to biliary complications has not been uniformly defined, and local expertise, usually inevitably uneven, plays an important role. The same biliary complication, e.g. extrahepatic stricture, can be (and used to be) treated by either endoscopy, or interventional radiology, or surgery, without a significant difference in the outcome among the studies. Direct comparative studies are scanty and it is not realistic to expect a well-designed prospective trial, even in the future [39]. The diverse nature of the complications requires usual endoscopic techniques of treatment and, the same as in non-transplant conditions, sphincterotomy, stent insertion with or without dilatation, and extraction of stones are the principal steps. With the advent of new technologies, such as metallic (semi)covered stents and balloon enteroscopes, the range of options will expand. The specific issues of endoscopic procedures after liver transplantation include post-procedural cholangitis prevention, consideration of coagulation disorders and sedation of patients with various mental impairments.

References

1 Lebeau G, Yanaga K, Marsch JW, et al: Analysis of surgical complications after 397 hepatic transplantations. Surg Gynecol Obstet 1990;170:317–322.

2 Davidson BR, Rai R, Kurzawinski TR, et al: Prospective randomized trial of end-to-end versus side-to-side biliary reconstruction after orthotopic liver transplantation. Br J Surg 1999;86:447–452.

3 Graziadei IW, Schwaighofer H, Koch R, et al: Long-term outcome of endoscopic treatment of biliary strictures after liver transplantation. Liver Transplant 2006;12:718–725.

4 Ringe B, Oldhafer K, Bunzendahl H, et al: Analysis of biliary complications following orthotopic liver transplantation. Transplant Proc 1989;21:2472–2476.

5 Giacomoni A, Lauterio A, Slim AO, et al: Biliary complications after living donor adult liver transplantation. Transplant Int 2006;19:466–473.

6 Wojcicki M, Silva MA, Jethwa P, et al: Biliary complications following adult right lobe ex vivo split liver transplantation. Liver Transpl 2006;12:839–844.

7 Suarez F, Otero A, Solla M, et al: Biliary complications after liver transplantation from Maastricht category-2 non-heart beating donors. Transplantation 2008;85:9–14.

8 De Vera ME, Solis-Lopez R, Dvorchik I, et al: Liver transplantation using donation after cardiac death donors: long-term follow-up from a single center. Am J Transplant 2009;9:773–781.

9 Alsharabi A, Zieniewicz K, Michalowicz B, et al: Biliary complications to relation to the technique of biliary reconstruction in adult liver transplant recipients. Transplant Proc 2007;39:2785–2787.

10 Grande L, Pérez-Castilla A, Matus D, et al: Routine use of the T-tube in the biliary reconstruction of liver transplantation: is it worthwhile? Transplant Proc 1999;31:2396.

11 Kobayashi T, Sato Y, Yamamooto S, et al: Long-term follow-up study of biliary reconstruction and complications after adult donor liver transplantation: feasibility of duct-to-duct reconstruction with a T-tube stent. Transplant Proc 2009;41:265–267.

12 Vougas V, Rela M, Gane E, et al: A prospective randomised trial of bile duct reconstruction at liver transplantation: T tube or no T tube? Transpl Int 1996;9:392–395.

13 Wojcicki M, Milkiewicz P, Silva M: Biliary complications after liver transplantation. A review. Dig Surg 2008;25:245–257.

14 Sanni A, Asher J, Wilson C, et al: Predisposing factors for biliary complications following liver transplantation. Transplant Proc 2006;38:2677–2678.
15 Katz LH, Mor E, Brown M, et al: Recurrent hepatitis C virus disease after liver transplantation and concurrent biliary tract complications: poor outcome. Clin Transplant 2006;20:465–470.
16 Cotton PB, Conner P, Eawls E, et al: Infection after ERCP, and antibiotic prophylaxis: a sequential duality-improvement approach over 11 years. Gastrointest Endosc 2008; 67:471–475.
17 ASGE guideline: Antibiotic prophylaxis for GI endoscopy. Gastrointest Endosc 2008;67:781–798.
18 Rockey DC, Caldwell SH, Goodman ZD, et al: Liver biopsy. Hepatology 2009;49:1017–1043.
19 Chapman R, Plaat F: Alcohol and anaesthesia. Cont Edu Anaesth Crit Care Pain 2009;9:10–13.
20 Holt AP, Thorburn D, Mizra D, et al: A prospective study of standardized nonsurgical therapy in the management of biliary anastomotic strictures complicating liver transplantation. Transplantation 2007;84: 857–863.
21 Pasha SF, Harrison ME, Das A, et al: Endoscopic treatment of anastomotic biliary strictures after deceased donor liver transplantation. Outcomes after maximal stent therapy. Gastrointest Endosc 2007;66:44–51.
22 Kulaksiz H, Weiss KH, Gotthardt D, et al: Is stenting necessary after balloon dilation of post-transplantation biliary strictures? Results of a prospective comparative study. Endoscopy 2008;40:746–751.
23 Buis CI, Geuken E, Visser DS, et al: Altered bile composition after liver transplantation is associated with the development of non-anastomotic biliary strictures. J Hepatol 2009;2009:69–79.
24 Buis CI, Hoekstra H, Verdonk RC, et al: Causes and consequences of ischemic-type biliary lesions after liver transplantation. J Hepatobil Pancreat Surg 2006;13:517–524.
25 Pascher A, Neuhaus P: Bile duct complications after liver transplantation. Transplant Int 2005;18:627–642.
26 Lee HW, Suh KS, Shin WY, et al: Classification and prognosis of intrahepatic biliary stricture after liver transplantation. Liver Transpl 2007;13:1736–1742.
27 Douzdjian V, Abecassis MM, Johlin FC, et al: Sphincter of Oddi dysfunction following liver transplantation. Screening by bedside manometric evaluation. Dig Dis Sci 1994;39:253–256.
28 Sheng R, Ramirez CB, Zajko AB, et al: Biliary stones and sludge in liver transplant patients: a 13-year experience. Radiology 1996;198:243–247.
29 Spier BJ, Pfau PR, Lorenze KR, et al: Risk factors and outcomes in post-liver transplantation bile duct stones and casts: a case-control study. Liver Transpl 2008;14: 1461–1465.
30 Aucejo F, Rofaiel G, Miller C: Who is at risk for post-transplant lymphoproliferative disorders after liver transplantation? J Hepatol 2006;44:19–23.
31 Weiling TH, Heidt DG, Englesbe MJ, et al: Biliary complications following liver transplantation in the model for end-stage liver disease era: effect of donor, recipient, and technical factors. Liver Transpl 2008; 14:73–80.
32 Skuhart MC, Kowdley KV, McVicar JP, et al: Predictors of bile leaks after T-tube removal in orthotopic liver transplant recipients. Liver Transpl Surg 1998;4:62.
33 Hwang S, Lee SG, Sung KB, et al: Long-term incidence, risk factors, and management of biliary complications after adult living donor liver transplantation. Liver Transpl 2006;12:831–838.
34 Mönkemüller K, Belluti M, Neumann H, et al: Therapeutic ERCP with the double-balloon enteroscope in patients with Roux-en-Y anastomosis. Gastrointest Endosc 2008;67:992–996.
35 Kahaleh M, Behm B, Clarke BW, et al: Temporary placement of covered self-expandable metal stents in benign biliary strictures: a new paradigm? Gastrointest Endosc 2008;67:446–454.
36 Costamagna G: Covered self-expanding metal stents in benign biliary strictures: not yet a 'new paradigm' but a promising alternative. Gastrointest Endosc 2008;67:455–457.
37 Aytekin C, Boyvat F, Harman A, et al: Percutaneous management of anastomotic bile leaks following liver transplantation. Diagn Interv Radiol 2007;13: 101–104.
38 Langer FB, Györi GP, Pokorny H, et al: Outcome of hepaticojejunostomy for biliary obstruction following liver transplantation. Clin Transplant 2009;23: 361–367.
39 Kuo PC, Lewis DW, Stokes K, et al: A comparison of operation, endoscopic retrograde cholangiopancreatography, and percutaneous transhepaptic cholangiography in biliary complications. J Am Coll Surg 1994;179:177–181.

Julius Spicak
Institute of Clinical and Experimental Medicine
Videnska 1958/9, CZ–140 21 Prague 4 (Czech Republic)
Tel. +420 261 364016, Fax +420 602 103284,
E-Mail julius.spicak@medicon.cz

Mönkemüller K, Wilcox CM, Muñoz-Navas M (eds): Interventional and Therapeutic Gastrointestinal Endoscopy.
Front Gastrointest Res. Basel, Karger, 2010, vol 27, pp 403–411

Peroral Cholangioscopy

Rinse K. Weersma

Department of Gastroenterology and Hepatology, University Medical Centre Groningen, University of Groningen, Groningen, The Netherlands

Abstract

Peroral cholangioscopy using the mother-baby technique allows the direct visualization of the bile ducts and enables the performance of targeted biopsies and the intraductal treatment of stones. Although the technique has long been available, there is very little evidence-based literature. Due to the limited number of indications and the time-consuming technique, it has only been available in tertiary referral centers. The addition of peroral cholangioscopy to regular endoscopic retrograde cholangiopancreatography with brush cytology is highly accurate in determining the origin of bile duct strictures or filling defects of unknown origin. A second indication is the evaluation of cholangiocarcinoma in patients with dominant bile duct strictures in primary sclerosing cholangitis. Furthermore, the intraductal treatment of complex biliary stones, either with electrohydraulic or laser lithotripsy, is an established therapeutic application of peroral cholangioscopy.

Cholangioscopy is the direct endoscopic visualization of the intra- and extrahepatic bile ducts. This can be achieved using either a percutaneous transhepatic approach or a peroral approach [1]. The first technique is performed by creating a bilio-cutaneous tract which is dilated stepwise until the appropriate diameter for the cholangioscope is achieved. The latter technique is achieved using the so-called 'mother-baby technique'. A 'mother' scope, usually a regular duodenoscope is placed in the duodenum and a second 'baby' scope is advanced through the working channel of the duodenoscope into the common bile duct (CBD). The focus of this chapter will be the peroral approach.

The first reports of direct peroral cholangioscopy already date back to the early years of endoscopy [2]. Since then, the technique has not been widely adopted and has only been employed in specialized centers. There are several reasons for this. First of all the technique is difficult, time-consuming and, until recently, required 2 endoscopists trained in advanced endoscopic retrograde cholangiopancreatography (ERCP). Second, the choledochoscopes used are fragile, expensive and need frequent repairs. Third, the proper visualization of the bile ducts and performing intraductal biopsies are cumbersome. Due to these limitations the range of indications for the procedure have been limited.

The main diagnostic indications for performing cholangioscopy have been the evaluation of biliary strictures of unknown origin and the evaluation of dominant bile duct strictures in patients with primary sclerosing cholangitis (PSC). Furthermore, for therapeutic reasons, cholangioscopy is being used to apply intraductal laser or electrohydraulic lithotripsy (EHL) of complex intra- or extrahepatic bile duct stones [1].

Procedural Aspects

Patient Preparation

As for conventional ERCP procedures, patients should be kept on overnight fasting before the procedure. Prophylactic antibiotics should be considered, given the chance of post-procedural cholangitis due to extensive manipulation within the bile ducts. Since most of the procedures are extensive and will include additional techniques next to the actual cholangioscopy, the procedure can be scheduled under general anesthesia. However, it can usually be performed under conscious sedation using propofol, or a combination of midazolam with pethidine or fentanyl. In the latter situation, a topical fluid anesthetic is usually administered in the throat. Patients are placed in the supine position.

Instruments and Accessories

There are several dedicated choledochoscopes available (table 1). Most of these endoscopes can be advanced through the working channel of a regular duodenoscope and have a small working channel (usually 1.2 mm in diameter). Most of them are steerable in two directions with a limited angle. The endoscopic images of the video endoscopes are superior to the choledochoscopes with fiber optics, but these video endoscopes tend to be more fragile and need frequent repairs. Recently Boston Scientific introduced the Spyglass cholangioscopy system (fig. 1) [3]. This system consists of a four-way steerable endoscope through which an optical fiber can be advanced. The advantage of this system is the fact that it is disposable. The endoscope is for single-use only, while the optical fiber can be used up to 20 times. Another advantage of the Spyglass system is the fact that it can be performed by a single operator, while for the other choledochoscopes, 2 skilled endoscopists are needed. However, the quality of the images is inferior to that of the video choledochoscopes.

Three monitors are needed: one for the fluoroscopic images, one for the regular ERCP images, and one for the actual cholangioscopy. We use an automatic irrigation pump with a footswitch which can be attached to the working channel of the cholangioscope to flush the bile ducts with sterile saline to ensure good visibility. Since there is no possibility of suction, we use a 10-ml vial for vacuum suction on the working channel when debris is perturbing visibility. Before we start we preferably go through all the steps of the procedure with the assisting endoscopy nurses and make sure that all equipment that is expected to be necessary is available within the endoscopy suite.

Technique

The procedure starts as a regular ERCP with selective cannulation of the CBD. Cholangiography is then performed. Although it is not absolutely necessary, a sphincterotomy is usually performed, which facilitates the introduction of the choledochoscope and subsequent therapeutic accessories. If the indication for the procedure is the analysis of bile duct strictures of unknown origin or strictures in PSC, one should try to avoid the passage of catheters or sphincterotomes through the stenosis before the introduction of the choledochoscope, because this can cause damage to the epithelium and severely hamper the endoscopic evaluation of the origin of the lesion. A long guidewire (e.g. 450-cm Jagwire) is left in the biliary tree. The cholangioscope is then advanced over the guidewire through the working channel of the duodenoscope. One of the most difficult

Table 1. Commercially available peroral cholangioscopes

Manufacturer	Type	Diameter mm	Working channel mm	Type
Olympus	CHF-B20	4.5	1.7	Fiber
	CHF-B30	3.4	1.2	Fiber
	CHF-B160	3.1	1.2	Video
	CHF-B260	3.1	1.2	Video
Pentax	FCP-8P	2.8	0.75	Fiber
	FCP-9P	3.1	1.2	Fiber
Boston Scientific	Spyglass	3.3	1.2	Fiber
Clinical Supply Ltd	Optiscope	2.1	–	Fiber
Polydiagnost	ERCP-Scope	3.0	1.2/1.6	Fiber
Medisecur	3D-Microendoscope	3.0	1.2	Fiber

parts of the procedure is the introduction of the choledochoscope into the CBD. One should try to avoid the use of the elevator at the distal end of the duodenoscope, since too much flexion can cause severe damage to the choledochoscope or break the optical fibers. It is usually best to align the choledochoscope as much as possible with the CBD and advance the scope slowly into the CBD under fluoroscopic control. Once the choledochoscope is within the CBD the guidewire can be removed and the flushing catheter can be attached to the working channel of the cholangioscope. The guidewire can later be reintroduced to cannulate specific segments of the liver and to advance the cholangioscope into the intrahepatic ducts. One should try to avoid flushing when the cholangioscope is in a 'wedge' position in the intrahepatic bile ducts.

Evaluation of Biliary Strictures

One of the most important indications for cholangioscopy is the evaluation of biliary strictures of unknown origin or dominant bile duct strictures in PSC with suspicion of a developing cholangiocarcinoma [4, 5]. Most patients will be referred from other centers where a previous ERCP has usually been performed and a biliary stent is already inserted. After removal the endoprosthesis should be sent for cytological examination. Following insertion of the cholangioscope one could additionally obtain bile for cytology, although the diagnostic yield is limited. We start with the endoscopic evaluation of the stricture and get an impression whether the stenosis has a benign, fibrotic appearance (fig. 2) or an irregular vulnerable malignant appearance (fig. 3). One of the best endoscopic discriminating features for malignancy is the presence of neovascularization [6]. One has to bear in mind that endoscopic evaluation of a stricture can be difficult after stent removal or scope passage as the epithelium is usually damaged and can mimic an exophytically growing cholangiocarcinoma. Small caliber biopsy forceps are available that can be advanced through the working channel of the cholangioscope. Biopsies can therefore be obtained under direct visual control. Due to the acute angulation of the cholangioscope at the tip of the duodenoscope it is sometimes difficult or impossible to advance the biopsy forceps. A maneuver to overcome this is to withdraw the cholangioscope several centimeters, advance the biopsy forceps until it cannot be advanced any further due to the angulation, and

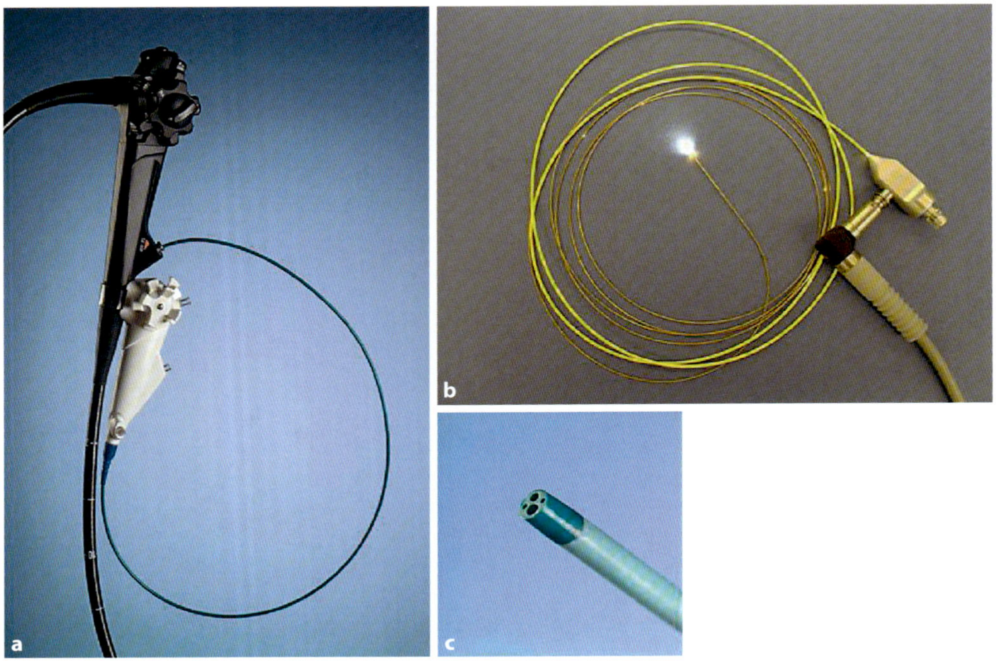

Fig. 1. The disposable Spyglass® peroral cholangioscopy system consisting of a disposable four-way steerable endoscope which can be attached to a regular duodenoscope (**a**) and a multi-usable fiber optic (**b**) which is advanced through a dedicated channel of the endoscope. Separate working channels are available for flushing and the introduction of instruments (**c**). Reproduced with permission from Boston Scientific, Natick, Mass., USA.

then readvance the cholangioscope again with the biopsy forceps in situ. Usually, it is then possible to advance the biopsy forceps easily into the bile duct. We perform 4–6 biopsies of suspected biliary strictures. After removal of the cholangioscope we also perform brush cytology. It is important to discuss the clinical background, origin of the biopsies and brush cytology with the pathologist to ensure optimal interpretation. Afterwards the ERCP with, e.g., dilation of the stricture and/or the placement of an endoprothesis if necessary should be finished in a regular manner.

Intraductal Lithotripsy of Complex Biliary Stones

The intraductal treatment of complex biliary stones is an established therapeutic application of peroral cholangioscopy [7]. The most often used techniques are lithotripsy through EHL or laser lithotripsy. Additionally, in order to prevent accidental tissue damage of the bile duct, a stone-detection system was developed, allowing 'blind' laser fragmentation under fluoroscopic control [8].

EHL is established through the underwater discharge of 18,000 V leading to a spark gap and subsequent plasma formation. Plasma expansion induces a shockwave which can be used for stone disintegration [9]. In urology EHL has been used for the fragmentation of urinary stones, but due to the potentially severe complications, it has mostly been replaced by laser lithotripsy. Bile duct perforations have also been described during treatment of biliary stones [10].

2
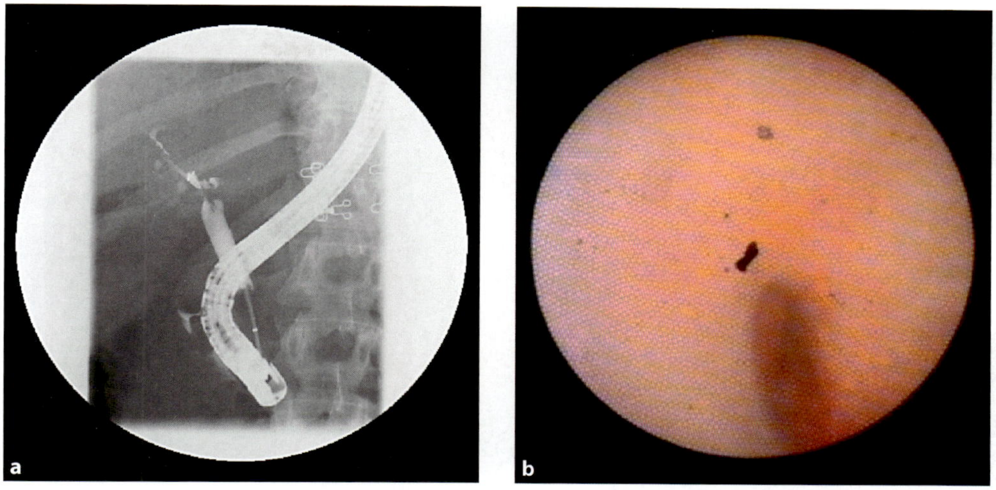

3
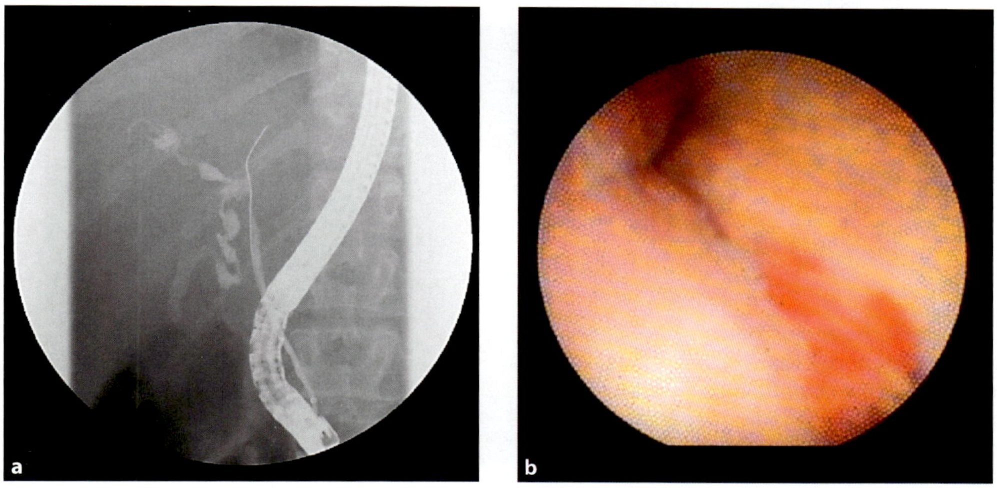

Fig. 2. Benign stricture of the common bile duct in a patient with primary sclerosing cholangitis. Fluoroscopic image (**a**) and cholangioscopic image (**b**) revealing a stricture with a fibrotic non-malignant endoscopic appearance. **Fig. 3.** Malignant stricture of the common bile duct in a patient with primary sclerosing cholangitis. Fluoroscopic image (**a**) and cholangioscopic image (**b**) revealing a stricture with an irregular, vulnerable surface with neovascularization.

We use a holmium:yttrium aluminum garnet (Ho:YAG laser) Versapulse Power Suite (Lumenis Inc. Santa Clara, Calif., USA) which is extensively used by urologists to treat urinary stones, urethral strictures or even enucleation of the prostate [11]. The Ho:YAG laser has been proven to be an effective and safe treatment modality for all types of urinary calculi and has also been used to treat biliary calculi. The laser delivers pulsed energy through a small quartz fiber, which is introduced in the bile duct through the working channel of the cholangioscope allowing direct visual control (fig. 4). It is capable of fragmenting stones of mixed cholesterol and calcium bilirubinate composition and mixed bile pigments [12, 13]. The laser can be applied through fibers of various diameters. We use a 250- or 365-μm fiber allowing sufficient flexibility to move the endoscope.

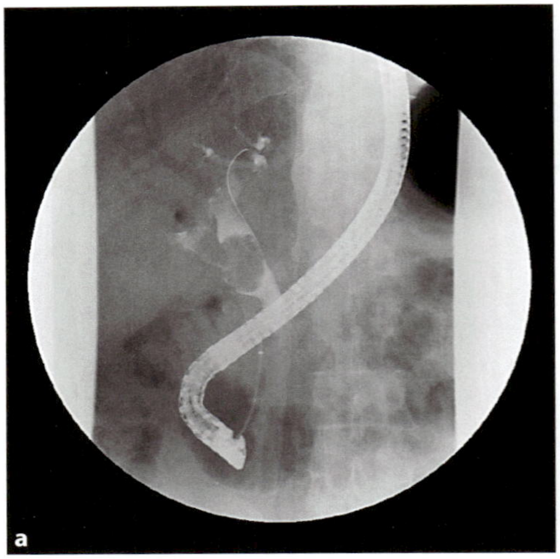

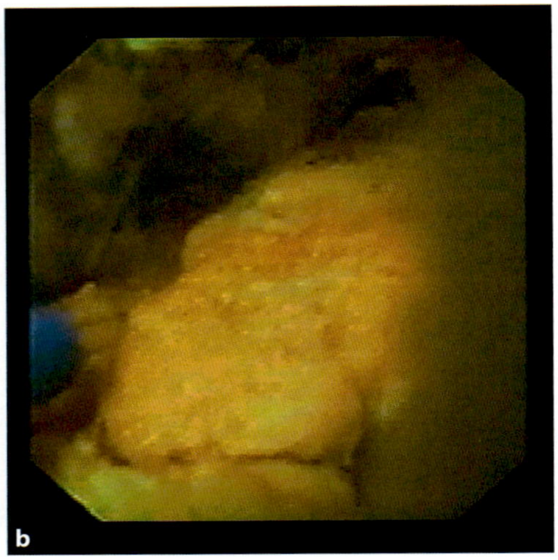

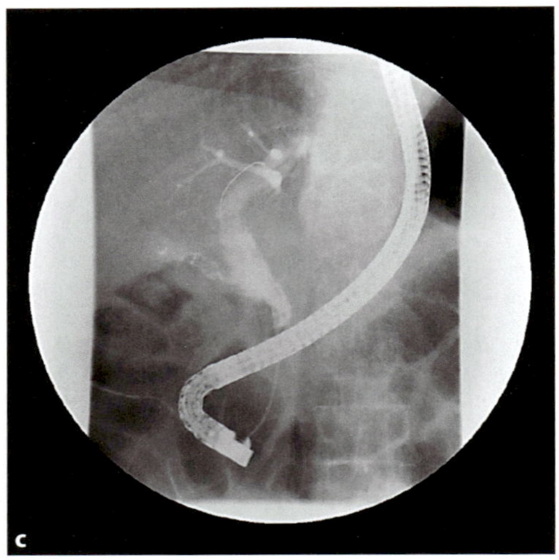

Fig. 4. Peroral cholangioscopic-guided intraductal laser lithotripsy. Fluoroscopic image with a large stone in the common bile duct (**a**). Cholangioscopic image showing the stone and the laser fiber (**b**). Fluoroscopic image after successful treatment (**c**).

Lithotripsy is established by the laser which creates a vaporization bubble in the surrounding water. Due to the difference in impedance, this vaporization bubble generates a shockwave at the boundary between the water and stone leading to stone fragmentation. The laser beam should be applied in close range to the stone (0.5 mm) and at a straight angle in order to be effective. This can be quite difficult to achieve, not only because of poor vision but also because of poor maneuverability of the cholangioscope once inside the bile duct. The required irrigation of the bile duct, necessary for clearance of debris and to provide a medium to transfer laser energy to the stone, is established by infusion of a saline solution through a 3-way lock attached to the proximal end of the cholangioscope working channel or through the flushing channel of the Spyglass endoscope. The calculi are fragmented with a laser frequency of 5–10 Hz and energy of 0.5–1.0 J. Fragments are then removed by conventional endoscopic methods, i.e. with a basket or extraction balloon. At the end of the procedure a nasobiliary drain can be inserted for additional irrigation of retained debris.

Limitations and Complications

There are several limitations to the use of peroral cholangioscopy, which have already been described at the start of the chapter, namely the difficult and time-consuming technique, the fragility of the choledochoscopes and the still cumbersome proper visualization of the bile ducts. In combination with the limited indications, the procedure is available only in a few specialized tertiary referral centers. Furthermore the quality of the biopsies obtained cholangioscopically is poor and remains a challenge for the pathologist.

The complications of the procedure are similar to that of regular ERCPs. Although there is no evidence in the literature, transient bacteremia with fever might be observed after the procedure more often than after regular ERCP due to extensive irrigation and manipulation of the bile ducts. This is usually successfully treated with prolonged administration of antibiotics. Epithelial damage and even perforation of the bile duct is a severe complication of intraductal laser lithotripsy or EHL. Further post-procedural care is similar to that of conventional ERCP.

Outcomes

Although the technique of peroral cholangioscopy has been available for some time, there is very little evidence-based literature and most data are presented as case reports or case series. Therefore when the diagnostic and therapeutic accuracy of peroral cholangioscopy is presented, one should consider the small number of cases, the lack of control groups, and the limited data on clinical outcome.

Peroral cholangioscopy can aid in determining the origin of bile duct strictures or filling defects. The two largest series from Japan and the USA that have been published show that the addition of peroral cholangioscopy to regular ERCP with brush cytology improves diagnostic ability and is highly accurate in diagnosing pancreaticobiliary malignancy [4, 14]. The first study evaluated 97 patients with indeterminate biliary strictures (n = 76) and filling defects (n = 21). The final diagnosis was obtained from the surgical resection specimens or clinical follow-up. In the group with indeterminate strictures, peroral cholangioscopy correctly identified all 38 malignant strictures and 35 of the 38 benign strictures. For the 21 patients with filling defects of the bile ducts, cholangioscopy diagnosed all 8 malignant lesions and 13 benign lesions [14]. In the second study 72 examinations were performed in 62 patients with pancreaticobiliary pathology suspicious for malignancy with inconclusive previous studies. Cholangioscopy with and without biopsies detected 16 of 18 patients with a final diagnosis of malignancy. Both missed cancers were intrahepatic cholangiocarcinomas. The positive predictive value in this study was 89% and the negative predictive value 96% [4]. The administration of methylene blue has been reported to be helpful in distinguishing malignant or benign lesions in the bile duct [15].

Another indication for peroral cholangioscopy is the evaluation of dominant bile strictures in patients with PSC. The incidence of cholangiocarcinoma is increased in PSC and this is frequently difficult to diagnose. ERCP with brush cytology and/or fluoroscopic-guided biopsies in combination with tumor markers such as CA19–9 and carcinoembryonic antigen yield variable results [16, 17]. Cholangioscopy might have two advantages in the setting of PSC. First, it enables performing targeted biopsies under direct visual control and direct endoscopic evaluation of the stricture (fig. 2, 3). One study showed that cholangioscopy was significantly superior to ERCP in detecting malignant bile duct strictures in 12 of 53 PSC patients [18]. A second case series showed that cholangioscopic tissue sampling yielded adequate biopsies but the diagnosis of cholangiocarcinoma remained challenging [5]. Second, it detected biliary stones and casts that were not seen in up to one third of patients on regular cholangiography and the subsequent treatment of these stones resulted in clinical improvement [5].

The management of complex biliary tract calculi when standard endoscopic therapy fails, is challenging. Endoscopic procedures with mechanical lithotripsy fail in 5–10% because of the large size or the number of calculi [19]. For these patients different treatment modalities are available, such as laparotomic and laparoscopic choledochotomy with stone extraction, extracorporeal shockwave lithotripsy (ESWL) or percutaneous or peroral cholangioscopy with intraductal lithotripsy [9].

The intraductal treatment of complex biliary stones either with electrohydraulic or laser lithotripsy is an established therapeutic application of peroral cholangioscopy [7]. There have been 2 randomized studies comparing intraductal laser lithotripsy with ESWL for complex bile duct stones. Both studies used laser systems with an integrated stone detection system that can be used under fluoroscopic control and does not need direct cholangioscopic visualization of the stone. Both studies showed that the intraductal laser lithotripsy was more effective than ESWL regarding bile duct clearance and treatment duration [20, 21]. Case series have shown good results for the intraductal treatment of complex bile duct stones with both the Ho:YAG laser and EHL [22, 23].

Conclusions

Peroral cholangioscopy using the mother-baby technique allows direct visualization of the bile ducts and enables the performance of targeted biopsies and the intraductal treatment of stones. Although the technique has been available for some time, there is very little evidence-based literature. Due to the limited number of indications and the time-consuming technique, it is only available in tertiary referral centers. With the availability of new single-operator cholangioscopy systems, it is becoming more widespread. The addition of peroral cholangioscopy to regular ERCP with brush cytology is highly accurate in determining the origin of bile duct strictures or filling defects of unknown origin. A second indication is the evaluation of cholangiocarcinoma in patients with dominant bile duct strictures in PSC. Furthermore, the intraductal treatment of complex biliary stones either with electrohydraulic or laser lithotripsy is an established therapeutic application of peroral cholangioscopy.

References

1 Shim CS, Neuhaus H, Tamada K: Direct cholangioscopy. Endoscopy 2003;35:752–758.

2 Kawai K, Nakajima M, Akasaka Y, Shimamotu K, Murakami K: A new endoscopic method: the peroral choledocho-pancreatoscopy. Leber Magen Darm 1976;6:121–124.

3 Chen YK, Pleskow DK: SpyGlass single-operator peroral cholangio-pancreatoscopy system for the diagnosis and therapy of bile-duct disorders: a clinical feasibility study. Gastrointest Endosc 2007;65: 832–841.

4 Shah RJ, Langer DA, Antillon MR, Chen YK: Cholangioscopy and cholangioscopic forceps biopsy in patients with indeterminate pancreaticobiliary pathology. Clin Gastroenterol Hepatol 2006;4:219–225.

5 Awadallah NS, Chen YK, Piraka C, Antillon MR, Shah RJ: Is there a role for cholangioscopy in patients with primary sclerosing cholangitis? Am J Gastroenterol 2006; 101:284–291.

6 Kim HJ, Kim MH, Lee SK, Yoo KS, Seo DW, Min YI: Tumor vessel: a valuable cholangioscopic clue of malignant biliary stricture. Gastrointest Endosc 2000;52:635–638.

7 Williams EJ, Green J, Beckingham I, Parks R, Martin D, Lombard M; British Society of Gastroenterology: Guidelines on the management of common bile duct stones (CBDS). Gut 2008;57:1004–1021.
8 Ell C, Hochberger J, May A: Laser lithotripsy of difficult bile duct stones by means of a rhodamine-6G laser and an integrated automatic stone-tissue detection system. Gastrointest Endosc 1993;39:755–762.
9 Hochberger J, Tex S, Maiss J, Hahn EG: Management of difficult common bile duct stones. Gastrointest Endosc Clin N Am 2003;13:623–634.
10 Josephs LG, Birkett DH: Electrohydraulic lithotripsy (EHL) for the treatment of large retained common duct stones. Am Surg 1990;56:232–234.
11 Delvecchio FC, Preminger GM: Endoscopic management of urologic disease with the holmium laser. Curr Opin Urol 2000;10:233–237.
12 Shamamian P, Grasso MJ: Management of complex biliary tract calculi with a holmium laser. Gastrointest Surg 2004;8:191–199.
13 Blomley MJ, Nicholson DA, Bartal G: Holmium-YAG laser for gall stone fragmentation: an endoscopic tool. Gut 1995 ;36:442–445.
14 Fukuda Y, Tsuyuguchi T, Sakai Y, Tsuchiya S, Saisyo H: Diagnostic utility of peroral cholangioscopy for various bile-duct lesions. Gastrointest Endosc 2005; 62:374–382.
15 Hoffman A, Kiesslich R, Bittinger F, Galle PR, Neurath MF: Methylene blue-aided cholangioscopy in patients with biliary strictures: feasibility and outcome analysis. Endoscopy 2008;40:563–571.
16 Wiesner RH, Grambsch PM, Dickson ER, Ludwig J, MacCarty RL, Hunter EB, Fleming TR, Fisher LD, Beaver SJ, LaRusso NF: Primary sclerosing cholangitis: natural history, prognostic factors and survival analysis. Hepatology 1989;10:430–436.
17 Björnsson E, Kilander A, Olsson R: CA 19–9 and CEA are unreliable markers for cholangiocarcinoma in patients with primary sclerosing cholangitis. Liver 1999; 19:501–508.
18 Tischendorf JJ, Krüger M, Trautwein C, Duckstein N, Schneider A, Manns MP, Meier PN: Cholangioscopic characterization of dominant bile duct stenoses in patients with primary sclerosing cholangitis. Endoscopy 2006;38:665–669.
19 Classen M, Hagenmuller F, Knyrim K, Frimberger E: Giant bile duct stones – non-surgical treatment. Endoscopy 1988;20:21–26.
20 Neuhaus H, Zillinger C, Born P, Ott R, Allescher H, Rösch T, Classen M: Randomized study of intracorporeal laser lithotripsy versus extracorporeal shock-wave lithotripsy for difficult bile duct stones. Gastrointest Endosc 1998;47:327–334.
21 Jakobs R, Adamek HE, Maier M, Krömer M, Benz C, Martin WR, Riemann JF: Fluoroscopically guided laser lithotripsy versus extracorporeal shock wave lithotripsy for retained bile duct stones: a prospective randomised study. Gut 1997;40:678–682.
22 Das AK, Chiura A, Conlin MJ: Treatment of biliary calculi using holmium: yttrium aluminum garnet laser. Gastrointest Endosc 1998;48:207–209.
23 Hixson LJ, Fennerty MB, Jaffee PE: Peroral cholangioscopy with intracorporeal electrohydraulic lithotripsy for choledocholithiasis. Am J Gastroenterol 1992;87:296–299.

Rinse K. Weersma, MD, PhD
Department of Gastroenterology and Hepatology
University Medical Centre Groningen, University of Groningen
Hanzeplein 1, NL–9700RB Groningen (The Netherlands)
Tel. +31 503612406, Fax +31 503619306, E-Mail r.k.weersma@int.umcg.nl

Mönkemüller K, Wilcox CM, Muñoz-Navas M (eds): Interventional and Therapeutic Gastrointestinal Endoscopy.
Front Gastrointest Res. Basel, Karger, 2010, vol 27, pp 412–422

Endoscopic Papillectomy

Jaume Boix · Vicente Lorenzo-Zúñiga · Vicente Moreno de Vega

Endoscopy Unit, University Hospital Germans Trias i Pujol Badalona, Barcelona, Spain

Abstract

Tumors of the ampulla of Vater are called ampullary tumors and can arise from any of the three epithelia (duodenal, pancreatic and biliary) that delimit the papilla. These tumors are clinically important and early identification, appropriate staging and proper treatment are essential. The symptoms of these tumors are non-specific and not always evident. Ampullary tumors at an early stage must be resected, but opinions differ on the optimal method of excision. Currently, controlled trials are lacking and consequently the treatment chosen must be individually tailored according to the characteristics of the patient and the tumor. Curative treatment may be endoscopic or surgical. In patients who are not candidates for curative treatment, palliative treatment through drainage can be performed. Endoscopic papillectomy is a safe procedure that can be used as an alternative first-line therapy in the hands of an experienced endoscopist. Endoscopic benign features cannot predict complete removal of ampullary tumors. Because of the high risk for endoscopic failure, it is necessary to perform endoscopic ultrasound before papillectomy to assess tumor extension. Patients undergoing endoscopic removal of ampullary and duodenal neoplasms should undergo postprocedure surveillance to ensure complete tissue removal and lack of disease recurrence.

Overview of Treatment Approach

A wide variety of tumors arise at the major duodenal papilla. They account for 5% of gastrointestinal neoplasms [1] but are being identified more frequently with increasing use of upper endoscopic examination and ERCP. Most of them are adenomas, which can potentially undergo to adenoma-carcinoma sequence [2], making complete removal mandatory for curative therapy. Unfortunately, endoscopic biopsy of ampullary tumors carries an alarming 30% false-negative rate for detecting carcinoma in situ and invasive carcinoma [3]. This means that a preoperative biopsy of an ampullary neoplasm that shows benign histology can be of limited value.

The therapeutic approach to benign tumors of the main duodenal papilla continues to be a challenging issue. Until recently, radical surgery with duodenopancreatectomy has been considered as the standard treatment of papillary tumors. However, for management of a frequently benign condition, this aggressive approach appears to be an 'overtherapy' and, therefore, unsatisfactory, especially because the majority of patients are elderly, with significant comorbidity, and, hence, are poor surgical candidates. As an alternative to radical surgery, surgical ampullectomy and the use of endoscopic methods (snare ampullectomy, with or without thermal ablation) have been performed.

Endoscopic resection of papillary tumors seems to be an interesting alternative to surgery. Its advantage is clearly a less invasive approach, omitting the need for general anesthesia and laparotomy. For adenomas of the major duodenal papilla, the endoscopically resectable area is limited

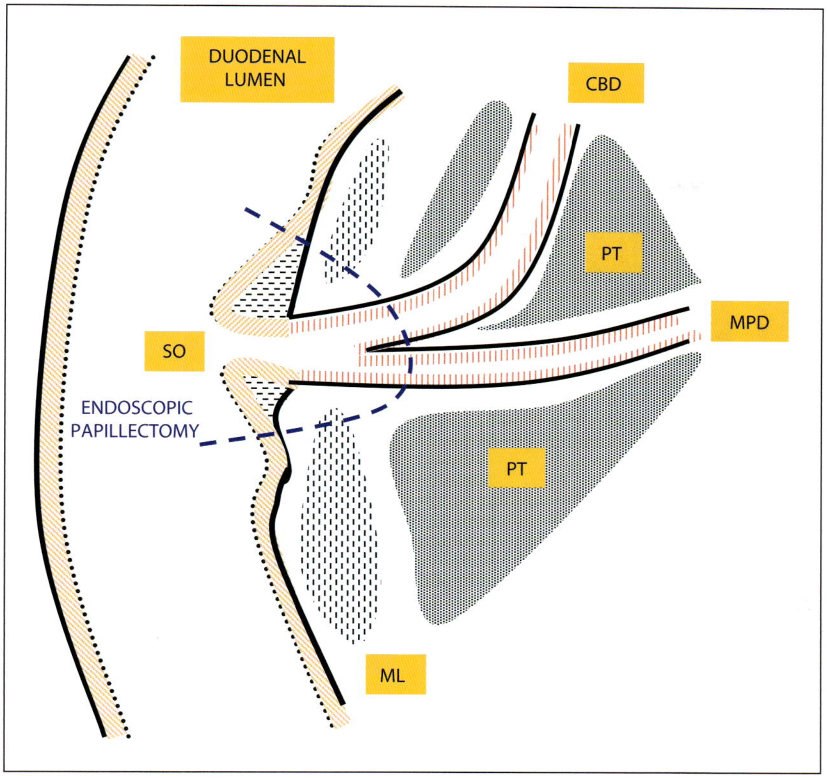

Fig. 1. Schematic presentation of the anatomy of the ampulla of Vater. Line indicates the plane of resection in endoscopic papillectomy. CBD = Common bile duct; MPD = main pancreatic duct; PT = pancreatic tissue; ML = muscular layer; SO = sphincter of Oddi.

only to mucosa and submucosa of the duodenal wall, and the resection of this area is termed endoscopic papillectomy [4] (fig. 1). Tissue around the bile duct and the pancreatic-duct orifices located at the major duodenal papilla almost are always removed along with the tumor. With endoscopic papillectomy, it is impossible to remove tumor tissues that invade into the common bile duct or the main pancreatic duct. In clinical practice, the terms 'endoscopic papillectomy' and 'endoscopic ampullectomy' are used interchangeably. Strictly speaking, however, ampullectomy consists of circumferential resection of the ampulla of Vater, with complete reinsertion of the common bile duct and separate reinsertion of the main pancreatic duct into the duodenal wall. This necessitates surgical duodenotomy and resection of pancreatic-head tissue in the area of the anatomical attachments of the ampulla to the wall of the duodenum. 'Endoscopic papillectomy', therefore, is a more appropriate term than 'endoscopic ampullectomy' in patients who undergo endoscopic resection for papillary adenoma.

Local Staging

Evaluating the major papilla with conventional endoscopy may be not a reliable method of predicting malignancy. Various methods have been adopted to help decide whether a patient is an appropriate

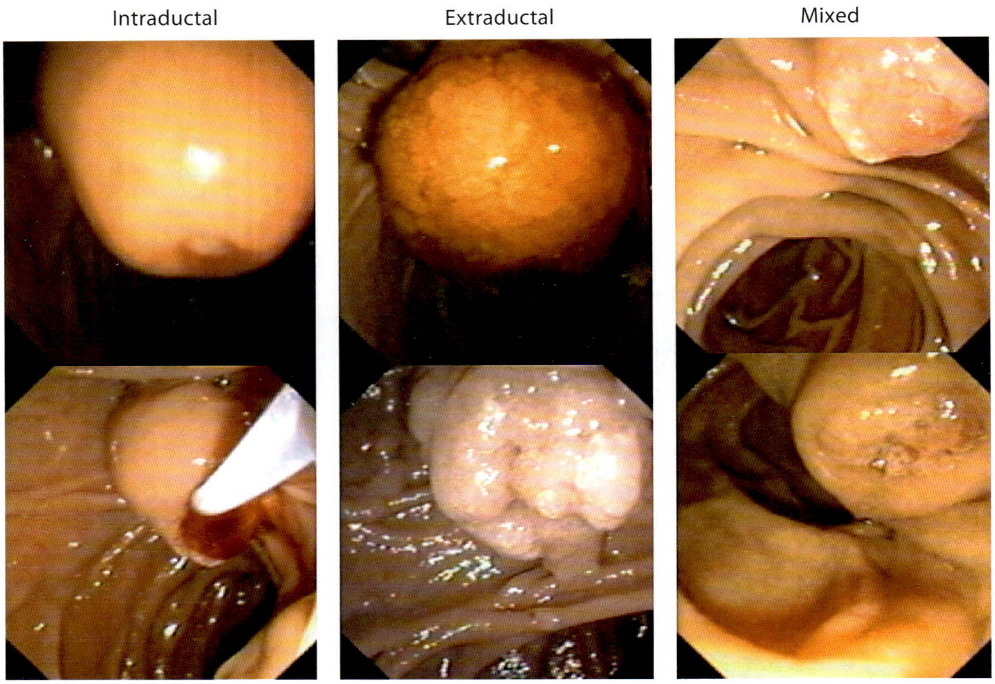

Fig. 2. Growth patterns of ampullary tumors.

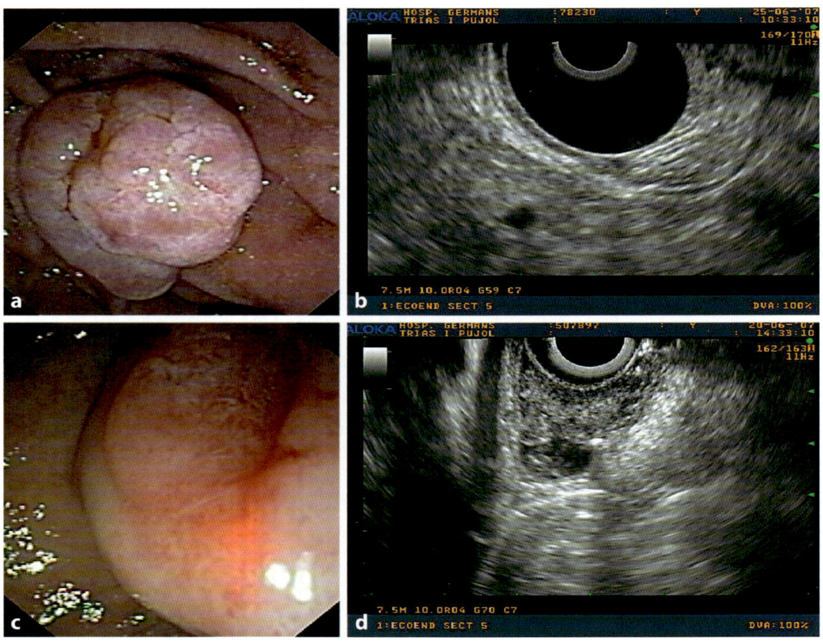

Fig. 3. Endoscopic ultrasonography in papillary tumors. **a** Endoscopic appearance of villous tumor of the papilla. **b** EUS of the previous case without muscular layer invasion. **c** Adenocarcinoma of the papilla. **d** EUS of the previous case with deep penetration of the duodenal wall.

candidate for endoscopic papillectomy, by providing information on lateral extension and tumor depth. The gross appearance of the tumor was classified as the intraductal type, the extraductal type, or the mixed type (fig. 2) [5]. With regard to lateral extension, chromoendoscopy, and more recently, magnifying endoscopy and narrow-band imaging can reasonably predict histology [6].

ERCP is the sine qua non of completing a successful endoscopic papillectomy. Not only can ERCP provide access to the pancreatic and biliary ducts for sphincterotomy and stenting, it can also provide information on the extent of tumor growth. Other complementary local staging modalities include endoscopic ultrasonography (EUS) and transpapillary intraductal ultrasound (IDUS) (fig. 3). EUS and IDUS, using frequencies of 7.5–10 and 20–30 MHz respectively, can give detailed images of the periampullary area and can show the presence of invasion of the duodenal muscularis propia, pancreas, or bile duct. The overall accuracy by EUS and IDUS in T staging was 63 and 78%, respectively [7]. However, we need a randomized controlled trial with long-term follow-up to show that the use of EUS and IDUS as a staging modality prior to endoscopic papillectomy has no negative effect on patient outcome.

Indication

Endoscopic biopsies obtained after sphincterotomy have only reached accuracy rates of approximately 80% [8], therefore a common problem is to achieve a reliable pretreatment distinction between benign and malignant papillary tumors (fig. 4, 5). Snare removal of the entire papilla as a single specimen was advocated as early as 1993 [9]. Endoscopic ampullectomy is being increasingly performed with curative intent for benign papillary tumors [4, 10–16].

Although careful patient selection is a prerequisite to successful endoscopic papillectomy, indications for endoscopic papillectomy are not yet fully established. Indications for endoscopic papillectomy are the collection of features that can predict complete removal of adenomas, while minimizing procedure-related morbidities. Criteria for selecting patients who would benefit the most from endoscopic papillectomy vary from one study to another, but nowadays the more used criteria to select patients for endoscopic papillectomy are [4, 15, 18] (table 1): (a) no endoscopic evidence of malignancy (e.g., absence of ulceration, excessive friability, and spontaneous bleeding); (b) the size of papillary tumor is not a limitation; (c) without invasion of duodenal muscularis; (d) no infiltration into the pancreas or the bile duct demonstrated at ERCP or at EUS; (e) exposed-type adenoma or carcinoma in situ and absence of histologically proven carcinoma, and (f) simple intraductal extension does not seem to be an absolute contraindication for endoscopic papillectomy, because the tumor can be exposed to the luminal side with sphincterotomy and/or balloon sweeping and, thus, resected completely.

Large, prospective studies with long-term follow-up are needed to demonstrate that endoscopic papillectomy provides curative treatment for ampullary adenoma with HGIN/Tis (high-grade intraepithelial neoplasia) and focal T_1 cancer.

Procedural Aspects and Patient Preparation

Eligible patients included were also checked for coagulation abnormalities and use of anticoagulants or antiplatelet drugs. A written informed consent must be obtained from all patients. Due to the length and complexity of the procedure, general anesthesia is our preferred method

Table 1. Indications for endoscopic papillectomy

• No endoscopic evidence of malignancy (e.g., absence of ulceration, excessive friability, and spontaneous bleeding)
• The size of papillary tumor is not a limitation
• Without invasion of duodenal muscularis
• No infiltration into the pancreas or the bile duct demonstrated at ERCP or at EUS
• Exposed-type adenoma or carcinoma in situ and absence of histologically proven carcinoma
• Intraductal growth <1 cm in length

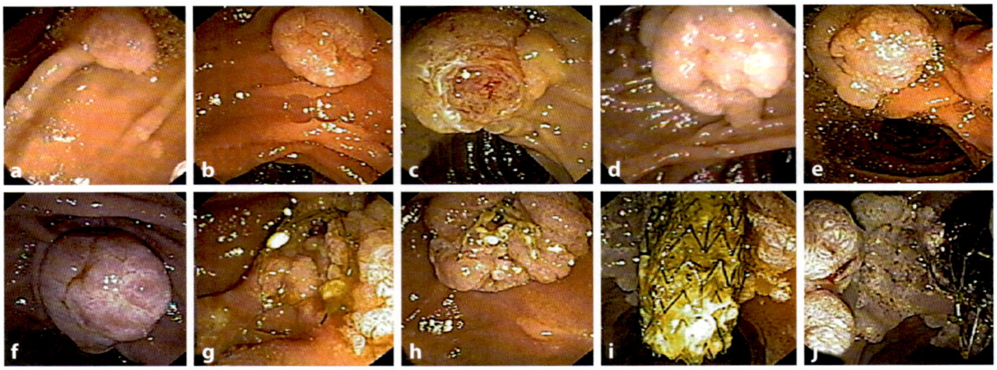

4

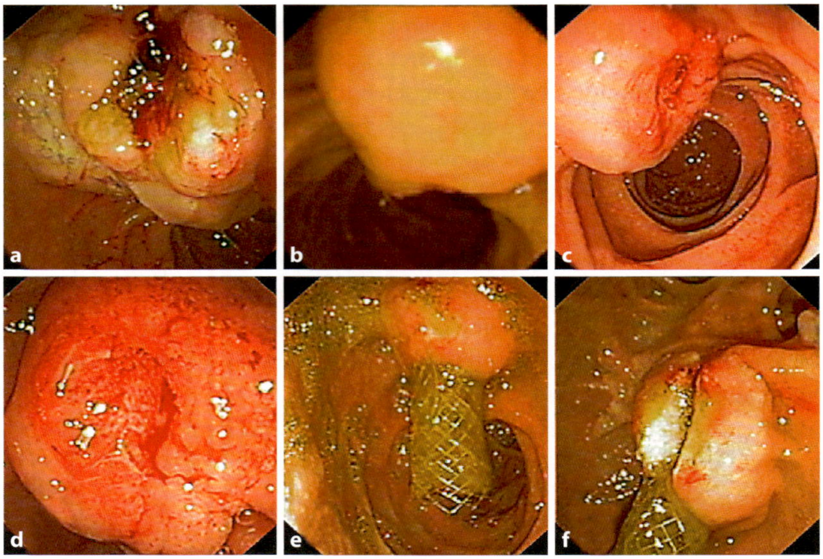

5

Fig. 4. Endoscopic appearance of papillary tumors. **a** Small villous tumor in FAP. **b** Small adenomatous villous tumor. **c** High-grade intraepithelial neoplasia of the papilla. **d**, **e** Villous papillary tumor. **f** Extraductal villous papillary tumor. **g**, **h** Malignant papillary tumor with partially destructed metallic stent. **i**, **j** Biliary metallic stent in malignant ampullary villous tumor. **Fig. 5.** Endoscopic appearance of ampullary tumors (II). **a** Ulcerated ampullary tumor. **b** Intraductal tumor. **c**, **d** Malignant extraductal tumor. **e** Intraductal tumor with metallic stent. **f** Intraductal tumor with metallic stent after sphincterotomy.

of sedation. ERCP is performed to assess intraductal extension and is combined immediately before endoscopic papillectomy as one session. A standard polypectomy snare can be used to grasp the tumor either from the cephalad to the caudal side or from the caudal to the cephalad side on an individual case basis.

There is no established consensus regarding power output and the mode of electrosurgical current used for endoscopic papillectomy. The mode of the current also varies from study to study. Some investigators advocate the use of pure-cutting current to avoid edema caused by the coagulation mode. We use blended electrosurgical monopolar current at a power output of 50 W [16]. It is difficult to compare various power outputs and modes of current used, because there is no randomized controlled trial that compares these settings.

Technique

Preresection Sphincterotomy

A preresection sphincterotomy and pancreatic-duct stent placement prior to endoscopic papillectomy ensures duct access postpapillectomy and permits a more aggressive treatment [11]. However, there are some concerns over its safety and efficacy. Furthermore, mechanical and thermal injury exerted may alter the anatomy of the resected specimen and make precise histopathologic evaluation of the tumor difficult.

A preresection stent placement (a 5-Fr, 5-cm, double-barbed, pancreatic-duct stent) may protect the pancreatic-duct orifice, but may hinder complete excision of the tumor, especially around the stent [11]. This problem can be solved with the use of wire-guided papillectomy that simplifies the procedure and improves the probability of complete resection [17].

Submucosal Injection

The systematic use of submucosal injection of either physiologic saline solution or dilute epinephrine has not been established. Submucosal injection may reduce the risk of bleeding, and may be useful for avoiding inappropriate resection if the tumor does not lift. However, we do not recommend this technique because capturing the lesion with a snare becomes difficult, and may blur the margin of the tumor [4]. Otherwise, studies conducted without submucosal injection have not reported any difficulty in complete resection or an increase in complications [4].

En-Bloc or Piecemeal Resection

En-bloc resection is fundamental to the treatment of neoplastic lesions, and is the preferred technique to guide the pathologist in assessing tumor margins. However, for larger lesions (>2 cm in diameter), piecemeal polypectomy will have to be performed. In most centers, a combination of en-bloc and piecemeal resection is used [10–16]. Aggressive efforts are then made to retrieve all resected tissue in all patients for histolopathologic evaluation.

Thermal Ablation

Thermal ablation is mainly used as a complementary method, to destroy residual tumor in the area of resection and surrounding margin, and to produce hemostasis. Modalities for adjunct thermal ablation include argon plasma coagulation (APC), monopolar/multipolar electrocoagulation, neodymium-yttrium aluminum garnet (Nd:YAG) laser photoablation, and photodynamic therapy. Selection is dependent on availability and preference of individual endoscopists,

Fig. 6. Pancreatic stent after sphincterotomy.

Fig. 7. Endoscopic postpapillectomy surveillance. **a**, **b** Endoscopic appearance 1 month after papillectomy. **c–g** Duodenoscopy after 3–6 months after papillectomy without recurrence. **h** One-year follow-up after papillectomy with a small adenoma (arrow).

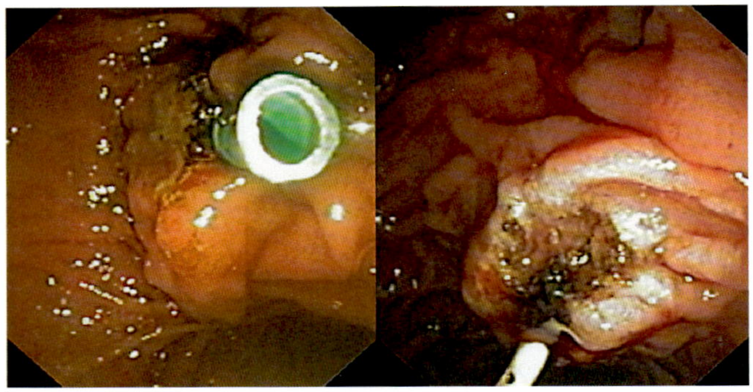

6

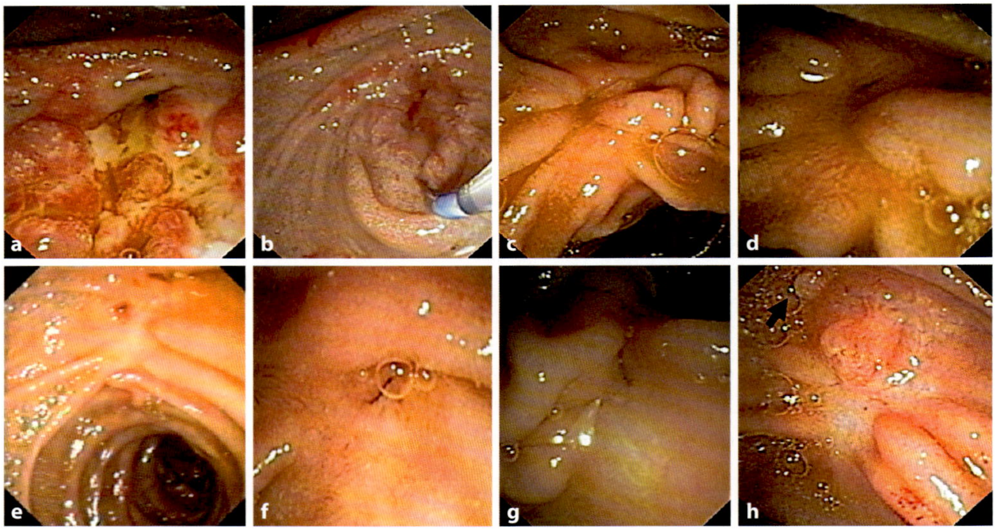

7

and there is no randomized controlled trial that compares individual modality [4]. We always use APC for fulguration of small tissue remnants not amenable to snare resection, and to manage procedural bleeding.

The only retrospective study that evaluated the efficacy of adjunct thermal ablation after endoscopic papillectomy demonstrated that patients who had thermal ablation with APC showed a lower rate of recurrence [13].

Pancreatic-Duct Stents

Experts agree that the use of pancreatic-duct stents is essential to prevent postendoscopic papillectomy pancreatitis. The only prospective, randomized, controlled trial that has evaluated the roles of prophylactic pancreatic duct stenting for the reduction of post-ERCP pancreatitis after endoscopic papillectomy showed a statistically significant decrease in the rate of postprocedure pancreatitis in the stent group [15].

Routine placement of a pancreatic stent may decrease both postpapillectomy pancreatitis and papillary stenosis [4]. Some authors have expressed concerns on the possibility of not identifying the pancreatic duct orifice after endoscopic papillectomy due to edema and electrocautery effect, but this can be lessened by performing a pancreatic duct sphincterotomy [18]. We recommend selective placement use a pancreatic stent only in the setting of delayed pancreatic-duct drainage after pancreatic sphincterotomy or visual evidence of remnant lesion in close approximation to the ductal epithelium requiring additional intervention. Endoscopists prefer to place a stent of small caliber (3- to 5-Fr) without flaps for the shortest duration possible (fig. 6).

Postpapillectomy Surveillance

Neither is there consensus on the appropriate surveillance interval for patients after undergoing endoscopic papillectomy. We arbitrarily perform a follow-up examination using a side-viewing endoscope after 3 months, then every 6–12 months for about 2 years depending on the disease and completeness of excision [19] (fig. 7).

Outcomes

Definition of endoscopic success is not standardized. It is noteworthy that the goal of endoscopic papillectomy is to resect the mucosa and submucosa, unlike surgical transduodenal excision in which the intent is to extend the resection beyond the muscularis propia. We define endoscopic success as complete excision of the lesion without considering the number of sessions required and the absence of recurrence or a recurrence during long-term follow-up that was easily treated endoscopically [16]. On the contrary, endoscopic failure is defined as inability to completely remove the lesion, regardless of the number of sessions, recurrence treated surgically, and discovery of carcinoma beyond the mucosal layer [16].

The results of published studies on endoscopic papillectomy are summarized in table 2. Reported success rates for endoscopic papillectomy range from 46 to 92% [9–14]. Recurrence rates of ampullary adenoma after endoscopic papillectomy range from 0 to 33% [9–14]. Predictors of successful endoscopic papillectomy in the largest multicenter study [13] included age >48 years, lesion size ≤24 mm, and male gender. Indeed, endoscopic papillectomy is a relatively safe and effective therapy and should be established as a first-line therapy for adenomas of the major duodenal papilla (table 3).

Limitations

The final decision on whether endoscopic resection is really curative depends on histopathologic assessment of the entire resected specimen confirming complete removal and absence of malignancy.

Although endoscopic resection of benign papillary tumors is very promising, the lack of long-term results on large study populations has not yet allowed establishment of clear indications and limitations of the technique [20]. The more delicate question is about adenomas harboring T_1 cancer, defined according to the TNM classification as tumor limited to the ampulla or the sphincter of Oddi. Apart from complete resection, lymphovascular invasion seems to be another decisive prognostic criterion in the treatment of T_1 ampullary cancers.

Another limitation of the local excision that applies to both surgical and endoscopic ampullectomy is the presence of intraductal growth [20]. If the intraductal growth is <1 cm in length, an endoscopic resection can be attempted by experienced hands. If the intraductal growth extends beyond 1 cm, surgery should be recommended because complete endoscopic removal becomes technically unfeasible. Maximum endoscopic sphincterotomy followed by balloon extraction should be performed to expose the intraductal part of the tumor, enabling further endoscopic snare resection.

Table 2. Endoscopic success rate and recurrence after endoscopic papillectomy

Reference (first author)	n	Endoscopic success, %	Incomplete resection	Recurrence, %	Malignant foci	Need for surgery
Binmoeller [9]	25	92	2	26	0	3
Fukushima [10]	31	65	1	0	1	2
Desilets [11]	13	92	1	0	0	1
Norton [12]	26	46	14	10	1	1
Catalano [13]	103	81	20	10	6	16
Cheng [14]	55	71	0	33	7	4

Table 3. Comparison of the outcomes among various methods of treating ampullary adenoma [cf. 4]

	Pancreatico-duodenectomy	Surgical ampullectomy	Endoscopic papillectomy
Recurrence rate, %	0	25.8	12.7
Morbidity, %	25–65	27.5	12
Mortality, %	12.9	0.03	0.04
Duration of hospital stay, weeks	2–4	1–3	<1
Need for endoscopic surveillance	No	Yes	Yes

Table 4. Complications related to endoscopic papillectomy

Reference (first author)	n	Bleeding %	Pancreatitis %	Perforation %	Cholangitis	Papillary stricture, %	Mortality
Binmoeller [9]	25	8	12	0	0	0	0
Fukushima [10]	31	13	13	0	0	0	0
Desilets [11]	13	0	8	0	0	0	0
Norton [12]	26	0	15	4	0	8	0
Catalano [13]	103	2	5	0	0	3	0
Cheng [14]	55	7	9	2	0	4	0

Complications Postprocedure Care

The perceived risk of complications is probably still a major barrier to its use in the community. Early experience of endoscopic papillectomy was marred by postprocedure acute pancreatitis, which on occasion had led to death. Fortunately, mortality resulting from endoscopic papillectomy has remained quite rare in the literature [21].

Complications of endoscopic papillectomy can be classified as early (pancreatitis, bleeding, perforation, and cholangitis) and late (papillary stenosis) complications [13]. Acute pancreatitis is one of the complications commonly associated with endoscopic papillectomy. In the literature it is difficult to assess the true rate of postendoscopic papillectomy acute pancreatitis because there are nuances in technique that were not standardized (such as type of current used, timing of ERCP prior to endoscopic papillectomy, and if biliary and/or pancreatic sphincterotomy was performed) [18]. Endoscopic papillectomy-related complications are summarized in table 4. The overall morbidity rate was 18.8% (range 10–27%).

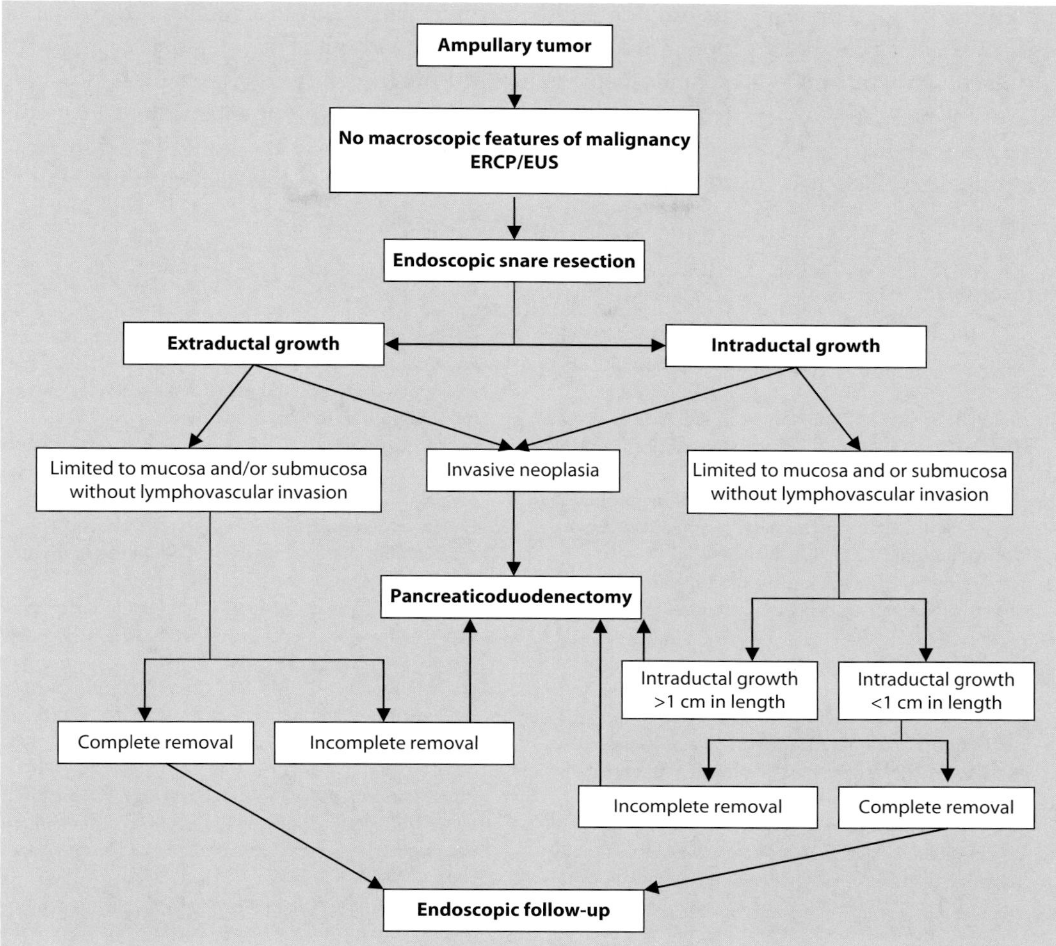

Fig. 8. Algorithm for endoscopic snare resection of tumor of the ampulla of Vater.

Algorithm

Every patient with ampullary tumor should be given a chance of endoscopic resection as long as the tumor appears benign, as we propose in figure 8.

Conclusion

To conclude: (1) Endoscopic papillectomy is a safe procedure that can be used as a alternative first-line therapy, in the hands of experienced endoscopist. (2) Ampullary and duodenal adenomas have the potential for malignant transformation and require appropriate diagnostic evaluation. (3) Both ERCP and EUS are important tools in the evaluation and staging of ampullary adenomas and can assist in selecting candidates for endoscopic or surgical therapy. (4) Endoscopic benign features cannot predict complete removal of ampullary tumors. An increased application of EUS or using magnifying endoscopy and narrow-band imaging (MENBI) can assist in selecting candidates for endoscopic therapy, those without invasive neoplasia and with extraductal growth, and to avoid endoscopic failure. (5) Because of the high risk for endoscopic failure, it is necessary to perform a prepapillectomy EUS to assess tumor extension. (6) Patients undergoing endoscopic removal of ampullary and duodenal neoplasms should undergo post-procedure surveillance to ensure complete tissue removal and lack of disease recurrence.

References

1 Scarpa A, Capelli P, Zamboni G, et al: Neoplasia of the ampulla of Vater. Ki-ras and p53 mutations. Am J Pathol 1993;142:163–172.
2 Stolte M, Pscherer C: Adenoma-carcinoma sequence in the papilla of Vater. Scand J Gastroenterol 1996; 31:376–382.
3 Yamaguchi K, Enjoji M, Kitamura K: Endoscopic biopsy has limited accuracy in diagnosis of ampullary tumors. Gastrointest Endosc 1990;36:588–592.
4 Han J, Kim MH: Endoscopic papillectomy for adenomas of the major duodenal papilla. Gastrointest Endosc 2006; 63:292–301.
5 Lee SY, Jang KT, Lee KT, et al: Can endoscopic resection be applied for early stage ampulla of Vater cancer? Gastrointest Endosc 2006;63:783–788.
6 Uchiyama Y, Imazu H, Kakutani H, et al: New approach to diagnosing ampullary tumors by magnifying endoscopy combined with a narrow-band imaging system. J Gastroenterol 2006;41:483–490.
7 Ito K, Fujita N, Noda Y, et al: Preoperative evaluation of ampullary neoplasm with EUS and transpapillary intraductal US: a prospective and histopathologically controlled study. Gastrointest Endosc 2007;66: 740–747.
8 Menzel J, Poremba D, Dietl KH, et al: Tumors of the papilla of Vater inadequate diagnostic impact of endoscopic forceps biopsies taken prior to and following sphincterotomy. Ann Oncol 1999;10:1227–1231.
9 Binmoeller KF, Boaventura S, Ramsperger K, et al: Endoscopic snare excision of benign adenomas of the papilla of Vater. Gastrointest Endosc 1993;39: 127–131.
10 Fukushima T, Fogel EL, Devereaux BM, et al: Use of ERCP and papillectomy in management of ampullary tumors: seven-year review of 75 cases at Indiana University Medical Center (abstract). Gastrointest Endosc 2001;53: AB88.
11 Desilets DJ, Dy RM, Ku PM, et al: Endoscopic management of tumors of the major papilla: refined techniques to improve outcome and avoid complications. Gastrointest Endosc 2001;54:202–208.
12 Norton ID, Gostout CJ, Baron TH, et al: Safety and outcome of endoscopic snare excision of the major duodenal papilla. Gastrointest Endosc 2002;56:239–243.
13 Catalano MF, Linder JD, Chak A, et al: Endoscopic management of adenoma of the major duodenal papilla. Gastrointest Endosc 2004;59:225–232.
14 Cheng CL, Sherman S, Fogel EL, et al: Endoscopic snare papillectomy for tumors of the duodenal papillae. Gastrointest Endosc 2004;60:757–764.
15 Harewood GC, Prochron NL, Gostout CJ: Prospective, randomized, controlled trial of prophylactic pancreatic stent placement for endoscopic snare excision of the duodenal ampulla. Gastrointest Endosc 2005;62:367–370.
16 Boix J, Lorenzo-Zúñiga V, Moreno de Vega V, Domènech E, Gassull MA: Endoscopic resection of ampullary tumors: twelve-year review of 21 cases. Surg Endosc 2009;23:45–49.
17 Moon JH, Cha SW, Cho YD, et al: Wire-guided endoscopic snare papillectomy for tumors of the major duodenal papilla. Gastrointest Endosc 2005; 61:461–466.
18 Hernández LV, Catalano MF: Endoscopic papillectomy. Curr Opin Gastroenterol 2008;24:617–622.
19 Lorenzo-Zúñiga V, Moreno de Vega V, Domènech E, Boix J: Diagnóstico y tratamiento de los tumores de la papilla de Vater. Gastroenterol Hepatol 2009; 32:101–108.
20 Seewald S, Omar S, Soehendra N: Endoscopic resection of tumors of the ampulla of Vater: how far up and how deep down can we go? Gastrointest Endosc 2006;6:789–791.
21 Adler DG, Qureshi W, Davila R, et al: Standards of Practice Committee. The role of endoscopy in ampullary and duodenal adenomas. Gastrointest Endosc 2006; 64:849–854.

Jaume Boix
Endoscopy Unit, Hospital Universitari Germans Trias i Pujol
Carretera del Canyet s/n, ES–08916 Badalona, Barcelona (Spain)
Tel. +34 934978866, Fax +34 934978946
E-Mail jboix.germanstrias@gencat.cat

Mönkemüller K, Wilcox CM, Muñoz-Navas M (eds): Interventional and Therapeutic Gastrointestinal Endoscopy.
Front Gastrointest Res. Basel, Karger, 2010, vol 27, pp 423–429

Photodynamic Therapy: Palliation and Endoscopic Technique in Cholangiocellular Carcinoma

Tommy Ibrahim · Michel Kahaleh

University of Virginia Health System, Charlottesville, Va., USA

Abstract

Cholangiocarcinoma is the primary malignancy arising from the biliary epithelium. The disease is marked by jaundice, cholestasis, and cholangitis. Over 50% of patients present with advanced stage disease, precluding curative surgical resection as an option of treatment. Typically, prognosis is poor and survival has been measured in months even after biliary decompression. Palliative management has become the standard of care for unresectable disease and has evolved to include the endoscopic approach. Photodynamic therapy (PDT) consists in administration of a photosensitizer followed by local irradiation with laser therapy. It has been used as a means of palliation for bile duct tumors with promising results. Several studies conducted in Europe and the United States have shown a marked improvement in the symptoms of cholestasis, survival, and quality of life. The published experience regarding PDT for cholangiocarcinoma and the steps required to administer this therapy safely are summarized.

Cholangiocarcinoma is the primary malignancy arising from the biliary epithelium of the bile ducts. The incidence rate is 1–2 per 100,000 people per year in the United States [1]. Initially thought to be an uncommon disease, the number of cases being reported annually is climbing [2]. Nearly two thirds of cases of cholangiocarcinoma occur between the ages of 50 and 70, and the tumor appears to have a male predominance [3]. The tumor seems to be the result of an underlying chronic inflammation of the biliary tract. Predisposing conditions include disorders such as primary sclerosing cholangitis, intrahepatic stones and choledocholithiasis, choledochal cysts, liver flukes, and previous exposure to the contrast agent thorium dioxide (Thorotrast) [4].

Complete surgical resection is the only treatment with potential for a cure. Unfortunately, patients usually present with advanced disease, with greater than 50% found to be unresectable at the time of diagnosis [5–7]. The prognosis in advanced disease is dismal, being approximately 3 months without intervention and 4–6 months after palliative biliary decompression [8–13]. Successful palliation of biliary obstruction remains the main goal to reduce morbidity and mortality in these patients with unresectable disease [9, 14].

The approach to biliary decompression has evolved from a surgical approach, to percutaneous drainage, and finally to endoscopic management. Hepaticojejunostomy is associated with a 30-day postoperative mortality rate between 7 and 24% [15–19]. Furthermore, quality of life was only improved in a minority of patients undergoing surgery because of the time needed to recover [12, 20, 21]. Even after biliary stenting, the prognosis remains grim [22–27]. Adding chemotherapeutic agents to biliary decompression has largely been unsuccessful [28]. Radiotherapy is an area of great controversy with regard to improved outcomes [29]. However, concurrent chemoradiotherapy with helical tomotherapy intensity-modulated radiotherapy and capecitabine, in conjunction with photodynamic therapy (PDT) has been shown to be well tolerated in patients with hilar cholangiocarcinoma [30].

PDT has been gaining increased awareness in the palliative management of cholangiocarcinoma. PDT is a two-step process. Initially, a photosensitizer is administered before the photoradiation process can occur [31]. Photofrin (porfimer sodium, Axcan Pharma Inc., Mont-Saint Hilaire, Que., Canada) has a selective nature and is preferentially retained by neoplastic tissue [32]. Laser application at a specific wavelength starts the activation process by transforming the drug from its neutral ground state into its active excited state. In the presence of oxygen, cytotoxic singlet oxygen species are formed, destroying the dysplastic cells to which they are bound. These free radicals then directly induce apoptosis and necrosis of the tumor cells [33]. Synergistically, nearby vascular channels are also affected, indirectly accelerating the process by cutting off the supply of vital nutrients.

PDT was demonstrated to reduce xenografted human cholangiocarcinoma tumor volume by 60% in a mouse model [34]. Recent reports and randomized controlled studies in which PDT was used as an adjuvant therapy, have shown a significant survival benefit in patients with unresectable cholangiocarcinoma, as well as a significant improvement in the quality of life after PDT and stenting [35–37].

Techniques

The technique used to execute the procedure has become standardized. PDT should be offered to all patients with nonresectable cholangiocarcinoma. Staging can be performed with computed tomography and/or magnetic resonance imaging [36]. Resectability is usually defined according to the criteria of Vauthey and Blumgart [38].

Each patient found to be a candidate for PDT undergoes a thorough educational process. Specific education regarding sun exposure and protection is necessary to avoid severe sun-related phototoxicity and should be provided to all patients prior to the procedure [36].

Endoscopic retrograde cholangiopancreatography (ERCP) is performed using a large channel duodenoscope (TJF-140, TJF-160, and TJF-160VF; Olympus America, Center Valley, Pa., USA) permitting 10-Fr stent placement. After cannulation into the biliary tract, a cholangiogram is performed to help define the anatomic distribution of malignant tissue and the extent of disease within the biliary ducts. Careful opacification of the dilated segments should be performed selectively (fig. 1). Next, selective bougie and balloon dilation of the stricture(s) to be treated are performed to facilitate diffuser placement within the malignant stricture.

Photoactivation is performed at 630 nm with a light dose of 180 J/cm^2, fluency of 0.250 W/cm^2 and irradiation time of 750 s (fig. 2). One or more segments can be treated at the discretion of the endoscopist. When the tumor length exceeds the maximal diffuser length, overlap of treated areas should be avoided by a stepwise pull-back of the fiber under radiologic control. Placement of endoprostheses is performed systematically after the photodynamic treatment

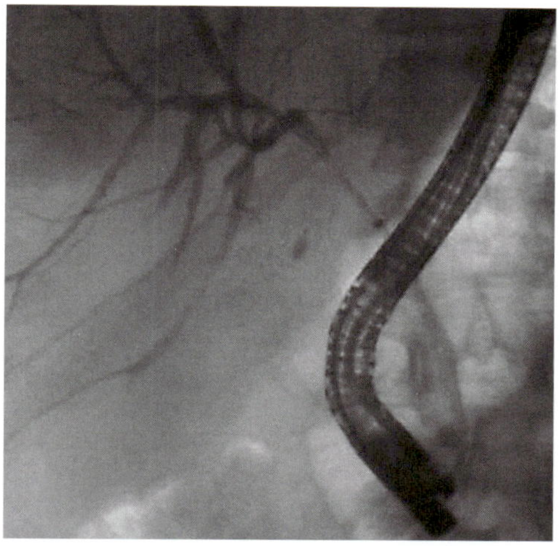

1

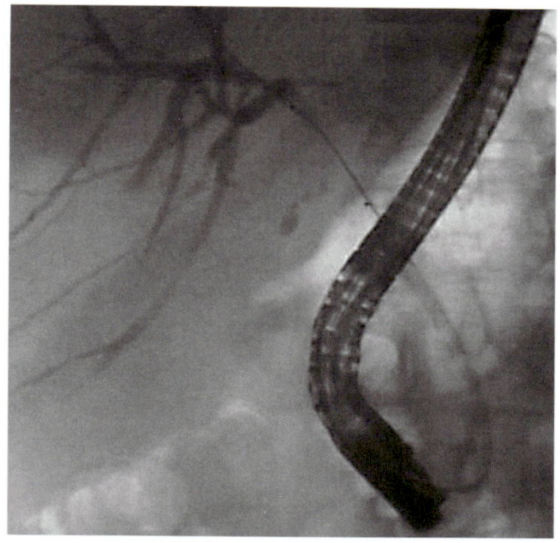

2

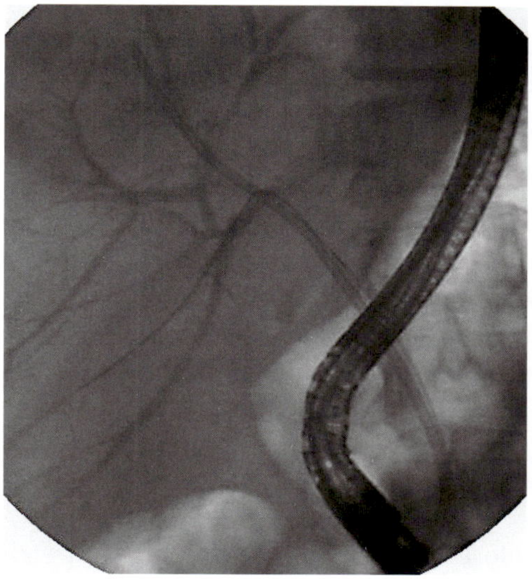

3

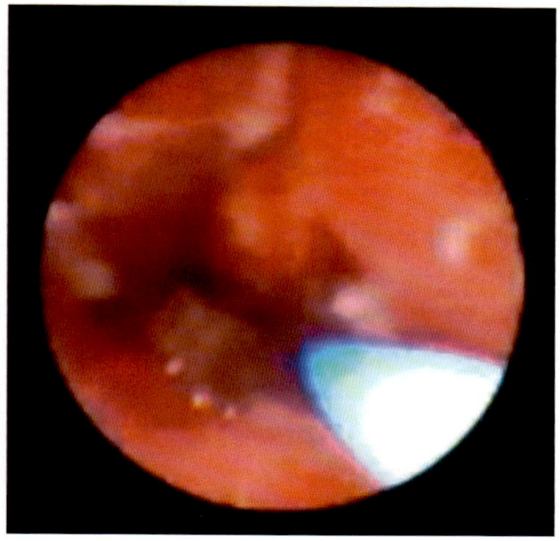

4

Fig. 1. Fluoroscopic image after contrast injection showing a malignant stricture, Bismuth III lesion (patient 1). **Fig. 2.** Fluoroscopic image after advancement of the PDT fiber along side the guidewire through the 10-Fr sheath of a plastic stent delivery system (patient 1). **Fig. 3.** Fluoroscopic images a 8.5-Fr plastic stent across the stricture treated (patient 1). **Fig. 4.** Choledochoscopic images of a malignant stricture at the hilum (patient 2).

to prevent cholangitis (fig. 3). Our group has recently demonstrated the safety and efficacy of choledochoscopy-guided PDT, allowing specific intraductal visualization of the stricture(s) to be treated (fig. 4–6) [37].

Prasad et al. [39] described a technique for PDT using percutaneous biliary access. Patients that failed biliary cannulation or those with preexisting biliary drains were successfully treated using this method [39]. The percutaneous biliary drain was replaced with an 8-Fr vascular sheath over a guidewire. PDT was administered by fluoroscopically guided placement of the cylindrical diffusing fiber. After the treatment was completed, a standard 10-Fr biliary drain was placed to facilitate biliary drainage.

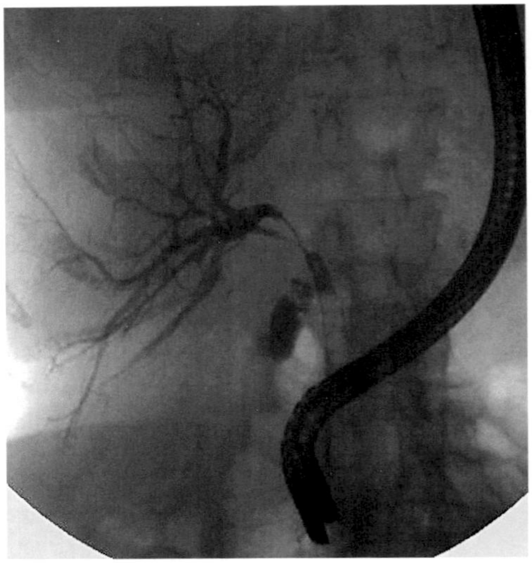

5

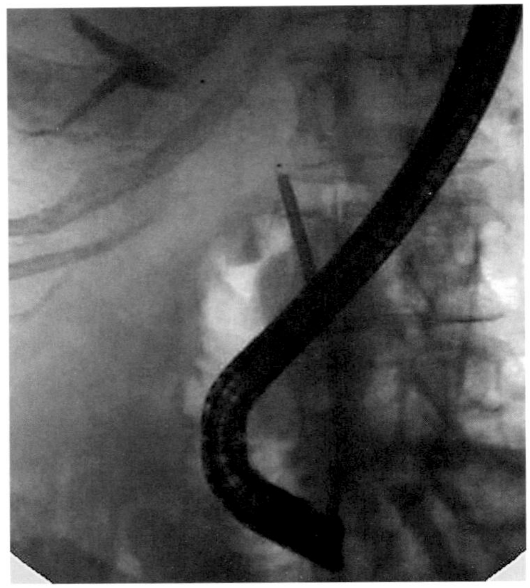

6

Fig. 5. Fluoroscopic image of a malignant stricture at the hilum (patient 2). **Fig. 6.** Fluoroscopic image after advancement of the PDT fiber into the malignant stricture through the choledochoscope (patient 2).

PDT is typically repeated at 3-month intervals at which time all stents should be replaced; stents are exchanged earlier in the case of premature occlusion or migration to maintain optimal decompression. All patients should receive perioperative antibiotic prophylaxis, usually with a fluoroquinolone. Postoperatively, patients treated with PDT are advised to remain out of direct sunlight as porfimer sodium may cause prolonged photosensitivity lasting 30–90 days [39].

Accessories

Porfimer sodium is the most commonly used photosensitizer. It is administered intravenously at a dose of 2 mg/kg body weight 48 h prior to illumination. Though other photosensitizers are now available, porfimer sodium is the most studied and the only photosensitizer approved by the FDA. A diode laser system (InGaAIP Laser Diode; Diomed Inc, Andover, Mass., USA) with a maximum power output of 2,000 mW and a wavelength of 630 nm is used as a light source, delivered through a 3.0-m length fiber having a 2.5-cm-long cylindrical diffuser at its distal end (Pioneer Optics, Windsor Locks, Conn., USA). The diffuser can be inserted into a 10-Fr sheath of a plastic stent delivery system (MAJ-1419; Olympus America) and placed at the level of the stricture being treated. Alternatively, our group has been using the choledochoscope as a platform to administer PDT (Spyglass, Boston Scientific, Natick, Mass., USA) [37].

Outcomes

There have been several uncontrolled reports that suggest that PDT can provide a survival benefit (table 1). In 2003, Ortner et al. [31] conducted the first randomized controlled trial comparing survival between biliary stenting alone vs. biliary decompression combined with PDT. After

Table 1. Studies performed using ERCP with PDT with photofrin sodium for palliation of cholangiocarcinoma

Study	Patients n	Study type	Median TB before and after PDT	Mean PDT sessions (range)	Median survival months	Adverse events phototoxicity, cholangitis
Ortner et al. [40], 1998	9	Single arm	18.6 > 6	1.5 (1–2)	14.6	1 (11%),0 (0%)
Berr et al. [41], 2000	23	Single arm	11.2 > 1.1	3 (1–5)	11.1	3 (13%), 8 (35%)
Rumalia et al. [42], 2001	6	Single arm	2.7 > 1.3	2.3 (1–2)	>6	2 (33%), 2 (33%)
Dumoulin et al. [43], 2003	24	Single arm	13.3 > 2.6	1–2	9.9	2 (8%), 5 (21%)
Ortner et al. [31], 2003	20	Randomized	NA (decreased)	2.4 (1–5)	16.4	2 (10%), 5 (25%)
Ortner et al. [31], 2003	31	Nonrandomized	11.8 > 3.1	1.5 (1–4)	14.2	3 (10%), 6 (19%)
Harewood et al. [44], 2005	8	Single arm	7.7 > 1.1	2 (1–5)	9.2	2(25%), 2(25%)
Witzigmann et al. [45], 2006	68	Single arm	NA (decreased)	2 (1–6)	12	8 (12%), 38 (56%)
Prasad et al. [38], 2007	25	Single arm	6.1 > 3.5	1.6 (1–4)	13.4	1 (4%), 2 (8%)
Kahaleh et al. [36], 2008	19	Comparative	6.3 > 3.5	1.6 (1–3)	16.2	3 (16%), 7 (37%)

TB = Total bilirubin; NA = not available.

carefully examining the initial 39 patients enrolled in the study, improvement in survival and quality of life in the randomized PDT group was found to be very impressive. Patients had a median prolongation of survival of 493 days (n = 20) in the group treated with PDT and stenting vs. a median prolongation of 98 days (n = 19) in the stent-alone group ($p < 0.0001$). The trial was terminated prematurely as continued data collection and randomization was thought to be unnecessary and ethically unacceptable. The PDT arm of the study showed a clear improvement in cholestasis, physical functioning and global quality of life, keeping patients well integrated in their own social lives. This study was criticized as only patients failing conventional ERCP were enrolled in the study, making a repeat ERCP indispensable which might account for the benefit attributed to PDT.

In 2007, Prasad et al. [39] found that patients with unresectable cholangiocarcinoma without a visible mass benefited from early treatment with PDT. In 2008, our group [36] published their findings comparing stenting alone versus combination therapy of stenting and PDT. Kaplan-Meier analysis demonstrated improved survival in the PDT group compared with the stent-alone group (16.2 vs. 7.4 months, $p < 0.004$). Mortality in the PDT group at 3, 6, and 12 months was 0, 16, and 56%, respectively. The corresponding mortality in the stent group was 28, 52, and 82%, respectively. The difference between the 2 groups was statistically significant at 3 and 6 months, but not at 12 months. Although it was not entirely clear whether the benefit was directly related to PDT or the number of ERCP sessions, this key study helped to strengthen the findings published by Ortner et al. [31] in 2003. In that study, not only was there a survival benefit, but overall quality of life was again found to be significantly improved in the PDT group. Furthermore, adverse effects in the PDT group were minor, largely related to phototoxicity, and essentially self-limiting. Other complications occurring included cholangitis, hemobilia, cholecystitis, pancreatitis, duodenal perforation, hepatic abscess and myocardial infarction, were a result of the endoscopic procedure and found in both groups treated [36].

In summary, the majority of patients with cholangiocarcinoma present with advanced and unresectable disease. Treatment needs to be initiated as soon as possible in order to improve survival and quality of life. PDT in conjunction with stenting has shown very promising outcomes. Further multicenter, randomized, prospective controlled trials are needed to confirm the benefit of PDT and stenting compared to stenting alone.

References

1 Callery MR, Meyers WC: Bile duct cancer; in Cameron JL (ed): Current Surgical Therapy, ed 6. Baltimore, Mosby, 1998, p 455.

2 Shahib Y, El-Serag HB: The epidemiology of cholangiocarcinoma. Semin Liver Dis 2004;24:115–125.

3 Burgos San Juan L: Cholangiocarcinoma (in Spanish). Rev Med Chil 2008;136:240–248.

4 Rubel LR, Ishak KG: Thorotrast-associated cholangiocarcinoma. Cancer 1982;50:1408–1415.

5 de Groen PC, Gores GJ, LaRusso NF, et al: Biliary tract cancers. N Engl J Med 1999;341:1368–1378.

6 Jarnagin WR, Fong Y, DeMatteo RP, et al: Staging respectability, and outcome in 225 patients with hilar cholangiocarcinoma. Ann Surg 2001;234:507–519.

7 Reed DN Jr, Vitale GC, Martin R, et al: Bile duct carcinoma: trends in treatment in the nineties. Am Surg 2000;66:711–715.

8 Liu CL, Lo CM,Lai EC, et al: Endoscopic retrograde cholangio-pancreatography and endoscopic endoprosthesis insertion in patients with Klatskin tumors. Arch Surg 1998;133:293–296.

9 Polydorou AA, Cairns SR, Dowsett JF, et al: Palliation of proximal malignant biliary obstruction by endoscopic endoprosthesis insertion. Gut 1991; 32:685–689.

10 Ducreux M, Liguory C, Lefebvre JF, et al: Management of malignant hilar biliary obstruction by endoscopy: results and prognostic factors. Dig Dis Sci 1992;37:778–783.

11 Farley DR, Weaver AL, Nagorney DM. 'Natural history' of unresected cholangiocarcinoma: patient outcome after noncurative intervention. Mayo Clin Proc 1995;70:425–429.

12 Baer HU, Stain SC, Dennison AR, et al: Improvements in survival by aggressive resections of hilar cholangiocarcinoma. Ann Surg 1993;217:20–27.

13 Deviere J, Baize M, de Toeuf J, et al: Long-term follow-up of patients with hilar malignant stricture treated by endoscopic internal biliary drainage. Gastrointest Endosc 1988;34:95–101.

14 Gibson RN, Yeung E, Hadjis N, et al: Percutaneous transhepatic endoprosthesis for hilar cholangiocarcinoma. Am J Surg 1988;156:363–367.

15 Lai EC, Tompkins RK, Mann LL, et al: Proximal bile duct cancer: quality of survival. Ann Surg 1987;205:111–118.

16 Havlik R, Sbisa E, Tullo A, et al: Results of resection for hilar cholangiocarcinoma with analysis of prognostic factors. Hepatogastroenterology 2000;47:927–931.

17 Kapoor VK, Pradeep R, Haribhakti SP, et al: Intrahepatic segment III cholangiojejunostomy in advanced carcinoma of the gallbladder. Br J Surg 1996;83:1709–1711.

18 Chaudhary A, Dhar P, Tomey S, et al: Segment III cholangiojejunostomy for carcinoma of the gallbladder. World J Surg 1997;21:866–871.

19 Guthrie CM, Banting SW, Garden OJ, et al: Segment III cholangiojejunostomy for palliation of malignant hilar obstruction. Br J Surg 1994;81:1639–1641.

20 Figueras J, Llado L, Valls C, et al: Changing strategies in diagnosis and management of hilar cholangiocarcinoma Liver Transpl 2000;6:786–794.

21 Blom D, Schwartz SI: Surgical treatment and outcome in carcinoma of the extrahepatic bile ducts: the University of Rochester experience. Arch Surg 2001;136:209–215.

22 Smith AC, Dowse JF, Russell RC, Hatfield AR, Cotton PB: Randomized trial of endoscopic stenting versus surgical bypass in malignant low bile duct obstruction. Lancet 1994;344:1655–1660.

23 Davids PH, Groen AK, Rauws EA, Tytgat GN, Huibregtse K: Randomized trial of self-expanding metal stents versus polyethylene stents for distal malignant biliary obstruction. Lancet 1992;34:1488–1492.
24 Schmassmann A, von-Gunten E, Knuchel J, Scheurer U, Fehr HF, Halter F: Wall stents versus plastic stents in malignant biliary obstruction: effect of stent patency of the first and second stent on patient compliance and survival. Am J Gastroenterol 1996;91:654–659.
25 Born P, Rosch T, Bruhl K, Sandschin W, Weigert N, Ott R, et al: Long-term outcome in patients with advanced hilar bile duct tumors undergoing palliative endoscopic or percutaneous drainage. Z Gastroenterol 2000;38:483–489.
26 Peters RA, Williams SG, Lombard M, Karani J, Westaby D: The management of high grade hilar strictures by endoscopic insertion of self-expanding metal prostheses. Endoscopy 1997;29:10–16.
27 Prat F, Chapat O, Ducot B, Ponchon T, et al: A randomized trial of endoscopic drainage methods for inoperable malignant strictures of the common bile duct. Gastrointest Endosc 1998;42:76–80.
28 Van Groeningen CJ: Intravenous and intra-arterial chemotherapeutic possibilities in biliopancreatic cancer. Ann Oncol 1999;10:305–307.
29 Bowling TE, Galbraith SM, Hatfield AR, et al: A retrospective comparison of endoscopic stenting alone with stenting and radiotherapy in non-resectable cholangiocarcinoma. Gut 1996;39:852–855.
30 Baisden JM, Kahaleh M, Weiss GR, Sanfey H, Moskaluk CA, Yeaton P, de Lange EE, Rich TA: Multimodality treatment with helical tomotherapy intensity modulated radiotherapy, capecitabine, and photodynamic therapy is feasible and well tolerated in patients with hilar cholangiocarcinoma. Gastrointest Cancer Res 2008;2:219–224.
31 Ortner ME, Caca K, Berr F, et al: Successful photodynamic therapy for nonresectable cholangiocarcinoma: a randomized prospective study. Gastroenterology 2003;125:1355–1363.
32 Giuliano EA, Ota J, Tucker SA: Photodynamic therapy: basic principles and potential uses for the veterinary ophthalmologist. Vet Ophthalmol 2007;10: 337–343.
33 Henderson B, Waldow S, Mang T, et al: Tumor destruction and kinetics of cell death in tow experimental mouse tumors following photodynamic therapy. Cancer Res 1985;45:572–576.
34 Wong Kee Song LM, Wang KK, Zinsmeister AR: Mono-L-aspartyl chlorine e6 (NPe6) and hematoporphyrin derivative (HpD) in photodynamic therapy administered to a human cholangiocarcinoma model. Cancer 1998;82:421–427.
35 Zoepf T, Jakobs R, Arnold JC, et al: Palliation of nonresectablebile duct cancer: Improved survival after photodynamic therapy. Am J Gastroenterol 2005;100:2426–2430.
36 Kahaleh M, Mishra R, Shami V, et al: Unresectable cholangiocarcinoma: comparison of survival in biliary stenting alone versus stenting with photodynamic therapy. Clin Gastroenterol Hepatol 2008;6: 290–297.
37 Talreja JP, Sauer B, Ellen K, Rehan ME, Shami VM, Kahaleh M: Photodynamic therapy for unresectable cholangiocarcinoma: what is the contribution of single operator cholangioscopy for targeted Treatment? Gastrointest Endosc 2009;69:AB146.
38 Vauthey JN, Blumgart LH: Recent advances in the management of cholangiocarcinomas. Semin Liver Dis 1994; 14:109–114.
39 Prasad G, Wang K, Baron TH, et al: Factors associated with increased survival after photodynamic therapy for cholangiocarcinoma. Clin Gastroenterol Hepatol 2007;5:743–748.
40 Ortner MA, Liebetruth J, Schreiber S, et al: Photodynamic therapy of nonresectable cholangiocarcinoma. Gastroenterology 1998;114:536–542.
41 Berr F, Weidmann M, Taanapfel A, et al: Photodynamic therapy for advanced bile duct cancer: evidence for improved palliation and extended survival. Hepatology 2000;31:291–298.
42 Rumalla A, Baron TH, Wang KK, et al: Endoscopic application of photodynamic therapy cholangiocarcinoma. Gastrointest Endosc 2001;53:500–504.
43 Dumoulin FL, Gerhardt T, Fuchs S, et al: Phase II study of photodynamic therapy and metal stent as palliative treatment for nonresectable hilar cholangiocarcinoma. Gastrointest Endosc 2003;57:860–867.
44 Harewood GC, Baron TH, Rumalla A, et al: Pilot study to assess patient outcomes following endoscopic application of photodynamic therapy for advanced cholangiocarcinoma. J Gastroenterol Hepatol 2005;20: 415–420.
45 Witzigmann H, Berr F, Ringel U, et al: Surgical and palliative management and outcome in 184 patients with hilar cholangiocarcinoma: palliative photodynamic therapy plus stenting is comparable to r1/r2 resection. Ann Surg 2006;244:230.

Michel Kahaleh, MD, Director Pancreatico-Biliary Services
Digestive Health Center Box 800708
University of Virginia Health System
Charlottesville, VA 22908–0708 (USA)
Tel. +1 434 243 9259, Fax +1 434 924 0491, E-Mail mk5ke@virginia.edu

Mönkemüller K, Wilcox CM, Muñoz-Navas M (eds): Interventional and Therapeutic Gastrointestinal Endoscopy.
Front Gastrointest Res. Basel, Karger, 2010, vol 27, pp 430–437

ERCP in Patients with Altered Upper Gastrointestinal Tract Anatomy

Jan J. Koornstra

Department of Gastroenterology and Hepatology, University Medical Centre Groningen, University of Groningen, Groningen, The Netherlands

Abstract

Balloon-assisted enteroscopy has allowed endoscopists to access intestinal areas which were until recently inaccessible with conventional endoscopes. Even after surgical reconstruction procedures, diagnostic and therapeutic endoscopic interventions are feasible and safe. In this chapter, the safety and feasibility of balloon-assisted techniques for endoscopic retrograde cholangiopancreaticography in patients with surgically altered anatomy is reviewed. In addition, an overview of currently available accessories is given. Double-balloon endoscopy, as well as single-balloon endoscopy, has been shown to be technically possible for this purpose. Successful interventions described include balloon dilation of stenotic biliodigestive anastomoses, sphincterotomy, extraction of bile stones and stent placement. No serious complications have been reported yet. Overall, balloon-assisted enteroscopy has great diagnostic and therapeutic potential as a technique to obtain biliary or pancreatic access in patients with surgically altered anatomical configurations.

Patients with surgically altered upper gastrointestinal anatomy are a serious challenge to the endoscopist when access to the biliary or pancreatic system is required. Using conventional endoscopes, endoscopic retrograde cholangiopancreaticography (ERCP) in these patients generally has limited success. Until recently, percutaneous transhepatic cholangiography or surgical interventions were the alternative possibilities when conventional endoscopy failed. The introduction of the double-balloon enteroscope (DBE) has contributed considerably to the endoscopists' ability to access the small bowel [1]. DBE has also shown to facilitate ERCP in patients with previously inaccessible areas and anatomical configurations resulting from upper gastrointestinal tract surgery [2]. Indications for a balloon-assisted ERCP include suspected biliary or pancreatic disease in patients with a history of a pylorus-preserving pancreaticoduodenectomy, classical Whipple resection or total gastrectomy with a Roux-en-Y reconstruction, patients with a hepaticojejunostomy with Roux-en-Y reconstruction, gastric bypass surgery and patients with a partial gastrectomy with BII gastrojejunostomy, in whom ERCP with conventional endoscopes failed (fig. 1–3). In this chapter, the safety and feasibility of balloon-assisted techniques for ERCP in patients with surgically altered anatomy is discussed.

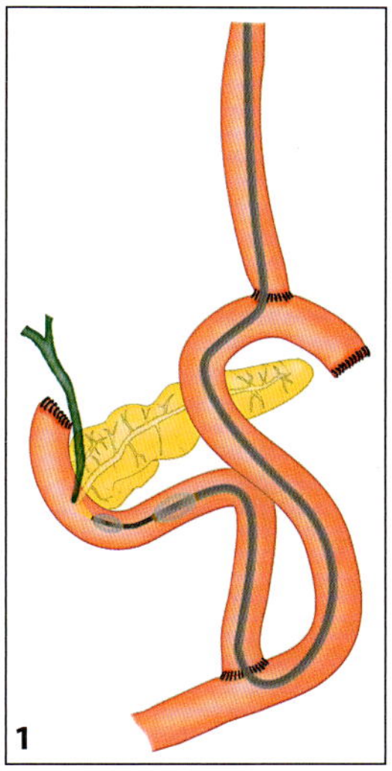

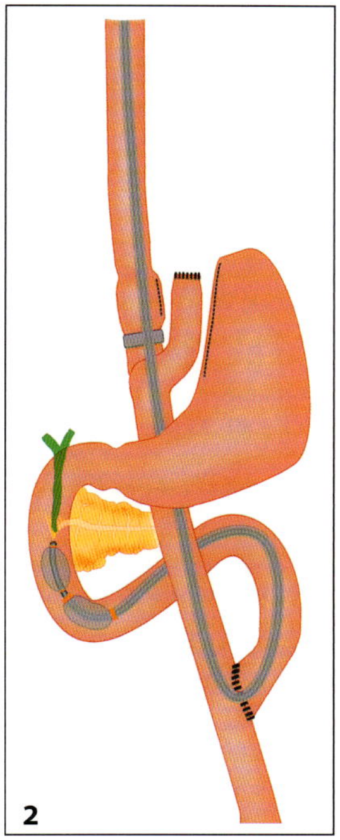

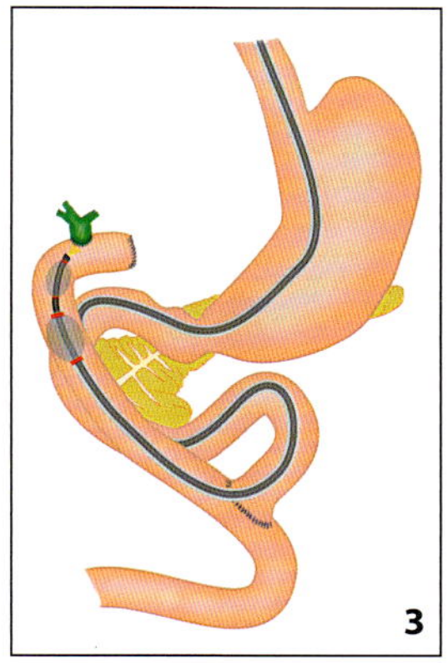

Fig. 1. DBE-ERCP in Roux-en-Y total gastrectomy [reproduced with permission, Karger Publishers; Kuga et al. Dig Dis 2008]. **Fig. 2.** DBE-ERCP in Roux-en-Y vertical banded gastroplasty [reproduced with permission, Karger Publishers; Kuga et al. Dig Dis 2008]. **Fig. 3.** DBE-ERCP in Roux-en-Y hepaticojejunostomy [reproduced with permission, Karger Publishers; Kuga et al. Dig Dis 2008].

Procedural Aspects

Patient Preparation

Before the procedure, the endoscopist should gather as much information as possible with respect to the current patients' anatomy, especially from surgical and radiological reports. As for conventional ERCP procedures, patients should be kept on overnight fasting before the procedure. In patients with biliary obstruction, prophylactic antibiotics can be considered, given the chance of cholangitis due to extensive instrument manipulation. Bowel preparation is generally not necessary. Depending on the local facilities, the procedure can be scheduled under general anesthesia, but can usually also be performed under conscious sedation using propofol, or a combination of midazolam with pethidine or fentanyl. In the latter situation, a topical fluid anesthetic is usually administered in the throat. Patients are best placed in the prone position. As for any ERCP, the procedure is performed under fluoroscopic control.

Accessories

The procedure may be performed with a double-balloon or a single-balloon endoscope. There are a few double-balloon endoscopes available; a diagnostic endoscope (EN-450P5, Fujinon Corp., Saitama, Japan) which has a working channel diameter of 2.0 mm, and a therapeutic endoscope (EN-450T5, Fujinon), with a 2.8-mm diameter working channel. Both endoscopes have a working length of 200 cm and a 12-mm diameter overtube with a length of 140 cm. Both the endoscope

Table 1. Available accessory devices for balloon-assisted ERCP

Material	Length, cm	Manufacturer[1], product code
ERCP catheter	250 260 320	Fujinon, F3CTPK1810250M Medwork, CAN1-B3-18-260-35 Cook, GT-1-TE
Guidewires	650 500 600	Fujinon, F3LQPK 0850650X-S; ø 0.035" Medwork, WIR1-F1-21-500; ø 0.021" Cook, METII-35-600E
Sphincterotome	250 320	Fujinon, F3QTEW1830250-S Cook, CCPT-25 ME
Precut sphincterotome	250	Fujinon, F3QYEW1802250Z-S
Needle knife	320	Cook, PTW-1E
Extraction balloon	275	Cook, TXR-ME (ø 8.5, 12 and 15 mm)
Basket	250 260 260 230 230	Fujinon, F1NSEW1825250Z-S (25 mm) Medwork, BAS1-C1-20-18-260 (20 mm) Medwork, BAS1-C2-25-23-260 (25 mm) Cook, WEB2×4 (2 × 4 cm) Cook, WEB3×6 (3 × 6 cm)
Cytology brush	350	US Endoscopy, 0071 1405
Snares	230 250 350	MTW, S052011212 Fujinon, various snares US Endoscopy, 0071 1101
Plastic stents	320	Cook, OASIS OA-XXE 8.5- or 10-Fr stents
Pusher for 7-Fr stent	270 320	Fujinon, FPU7270 Cook, PC-X-E
Dilation balloons	240 320	Boston Scientific, CRE balloon (ø 6–8 mm; 8–10 mm, etc.) Cook, QBD-XX×3 (ø 6, 8 and 10 mm)
Dilation catheter	275	Cook, SBDC-7E (7-Fr)
Bipolar coag. probe	350	Cook, BCP-XXA/B (7- or 10-Fr)
Injection needle	250 320 230	Fujinon, F2EZTV1805250HP-S Cook, LDVI-XXE US Endoscopy, 00711811

[1] Fujinon, Willich, Germany; Medwork, Höchstadt/Aisch, Germany; Cook, Limerick, Ireland; US Endoscopy, Mentor, Ohio, USA; MTW, Wesel, Germany; Boston Scientific, Natick, Mass., USA.

and the overtube are balloon-loaded. The single-balloon endoscope (XSIF-Q260Y, Olympus Optical Co., Tokyo, Japan) has a working length of 200 cm with a working channel of 2.8 mm, and an overtube with a length of 140 cm. Given the potential chance of performing endoscopic interventions, an endoscope with a 2.8-mm working channel is preferred, as it allows the passage of accessories if required. A shorter version of a double-balloon scope with a working length of 152 cm has become available (EC-450B15, Fujinon) that allows for the use of standard accessories.

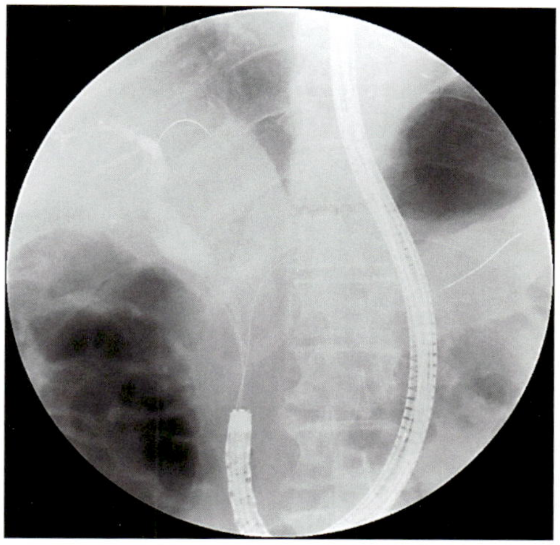

4

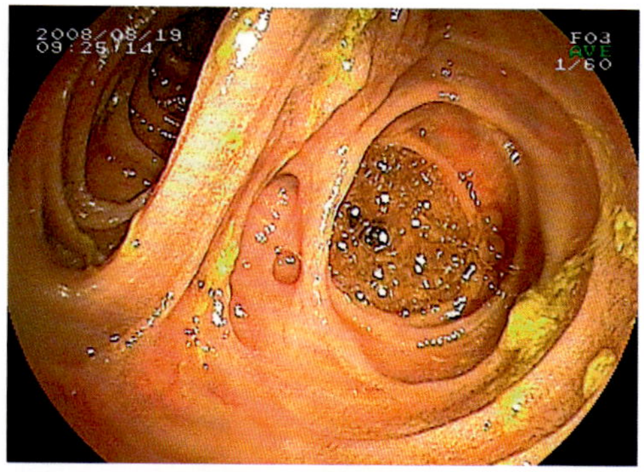

5

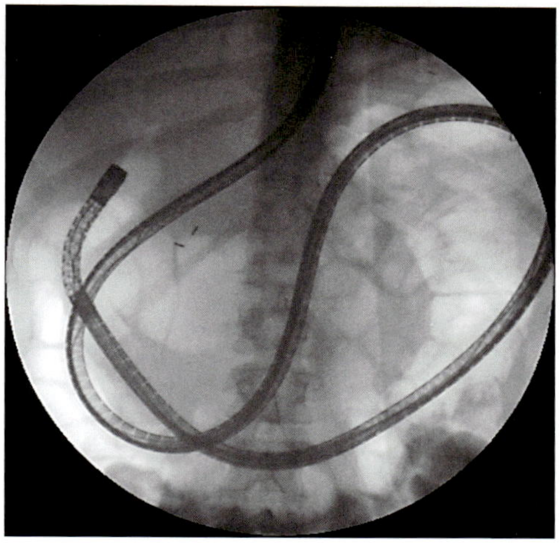

6

Fig. 4. Fluoroscopic image of the endoscope advanced into the afferent limb after BII resection showing a sharp bend between limb and remnant stomach; guidewires are positioned in the pancreatic duct and common bile duct.

Fig. 5. Endoscopic view of the jejunojejunal anastomosis, showing air bubbles and bile coming from the Roux limb on the right.

Fig. 6. Fluoroscopic image of the endoscope and overtube advanced into the Roux limb approaching surgical clips.

With respect to accessories, there was until recently limited availability of suitable equipment, as all accessories have to be of sufficient length. However, the availability of accessories for balloon-assisted ERCP has increased rapidly over the last years. These are summarized in table 1. Currently available accessories include ERCP catheters, guidewires, dilation balloons, sphincterotomes, precut sphincterotomes/needle knifes, extraction balloons, retrieval baskets and stent placement accessories.

Technique

In double-balloon enteroscopy, alternately inflating and deflating the two balloons and straightening the endoscope with the overtube achieve a stepwise progression of the enteroscope throughout the small intestine. In single-balloon enteroscopy, only the tip of the overtube has an inflatable balloon attached. The basic principle of single-balloon endoscopy is similar to that of DBE, with repeated advancement of the endoscope, insertion of the overtube towards the tip of the endoscope, followed by pulling back both endoscope and overtube after inflation of the balloon. Advancement of the endoscope can be hindered by adhesions as a consequence of previous surgery.

In patients with a BII gastrojejunostomy, the target limb usually makes a sharp angle with the stomach remnant, which can make cannulation of the limb difficult (fig. 4). Applying abdominal pressure or changing the patients' position may be helpful. In patients with a Roux-en-Y jejunojejunostomy, the endoscope has to be passed beyond the ligament of Treitz, as the

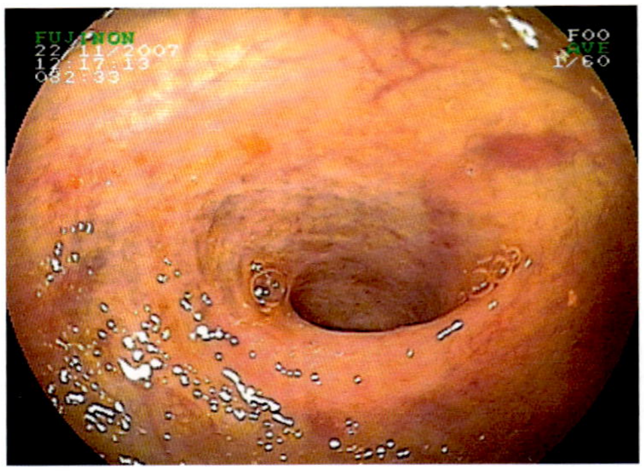
7

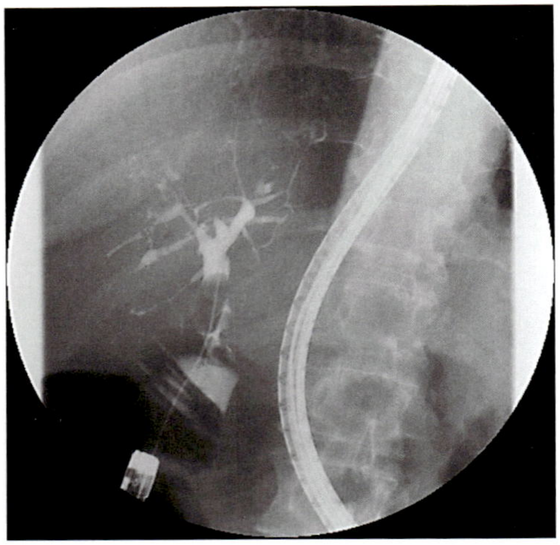
8

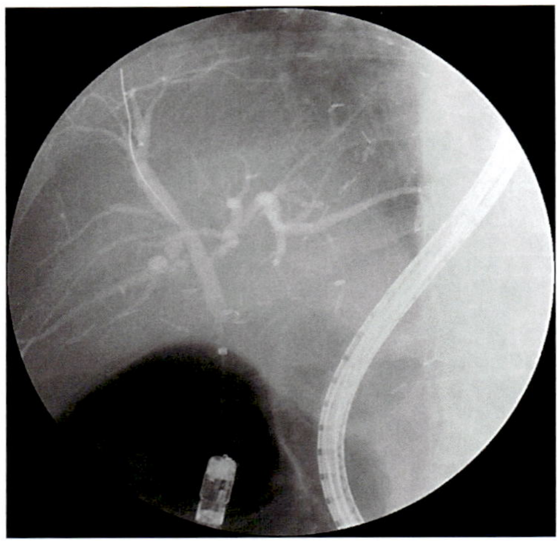
9

Fig. 7. Endoscopic view of the opening of a normal, non-stenotic hepaticojejunostomy.

Fig. 8. Cholangiography with inflated CRE balloon showing diffuse stricturing and dilation of biliary branches consistent with sclerosing cholangitis.

Fig. 9. Fluoroscopic image of balloon dilation of the right hepatic duct using an 8-mm CRE balloon.

anastomosis is usually located another 40–60 cm downstream in the small bowel. At this point, a typical crossroad can be identified (fig. 5) where it is not always readily clear which limb should be accessed. The target limb is usually accessed by taking the 'turn to the left'. Clues pointing to which limb is the appropriate one are the appearance of bile from one of the limbs or air bubbles, resulting from bile saponification (fig. 5). Evidently, fluoroscopy may help indicating the appropriate route. The presence of surgical clips may serve as localizing points (fig. 6). Once the enteroscope is at the desired position in the Roux limb, the overtube should be advanced just behind the enteroscope, to fix the overtube and allow the enteroscope to approach the biliary or pancreatic system as flexible as possible. Beware that the biliodigestive anastomosis or native papilla is usually not located at the far end of the blind small bowel loop, but a few centimeters downstream of this point.

Once positioned, the endoscopist usually is able to get a good impression of the biliodigestive anastomosis (fig. 7). Access to a biliodigestive anastomosis can be difficult given that the biliary tract usually makes an angle with the Roux limb, which can seriously limit the advancement of accessories. Introduction of a native major papilla is relatively easy given the fact that the endoscope is

Table 2. Overview of case series on balloon-assisted ERCP

Patients	Anatomy	Intervention	Ref.
5	Gastric bypass with Roux-en-Y; LT with Roux-en-Y hepaticojejunostomy	Balloon dilation of stenotic anastomosis and sphincterotomy	4
14	Various (mostly gastric bypass with Roux-en-Y; Whipple with pancreaticojejunostomy	Balloon dilation; sphincterotomy; biliary stent placement; pancreatic stent placement and removal	5
13	Various (mostly LT with Roux-en-Y hepaticojejunostomy)	Biliary stent placement and stone extraction	6
2	Roux-en-Y gastrojejunostomy PPPD with Roux-en-Y	Biliary stent placement and removal Balloon dilation of stenotic anastomosis	7
3	LT with Roux-en-Y hepaticojejunostomy	Balloon dilation and stone extraction	8
11	Various (mostly BII gastrojejunostomy and PPPD)	Various (sphincterotomy, balloon dilation, stent placement)	9
4	Various (mostly BII gastrojejunostomy)	Stent placement, sphincterotomy and stone extraction	10
3	BII gastrojejunostomy (2) and PPPD (1)	Sphincterotomy and stone extraction; stent placement	11
38	Various (mostly BII and Roux-en-Y gastrectomies)	Sphincterotomy, stone extraction, balloon dilation, plastic and metal stent placement, bile duct biopsy, pancreatic interventions	12
4	Various (all Roux-en-Y)	None	13
11	Roux-en-Y anastomosis	Biopsies, stent placement and removal, balloon dilation, papillectomy, stone extraction	14
6	Roux-en-Y anastomosis	Sphincterotomy, stone extraction, balloon dilation	15
2	Roux-en-Y anastomosis	Stent removal, sludge removal	16

LT = Liver transplantation; BII = Billroth II; PPPD = pylorus-preserving pancreaticoduodenectomy.

forward-viewing and the angle of the biliary tract relative to the small bowel limb is rather straight. For cannulation of the biliary tract, an ERCP catheter, guidewire or papillotome can be used. When injecting contrast to obtain a cholangiogram, this usually leaks straight into the small bowel. To obtain a cholangiogram effectively, it can be helpful to make an 'occlusion cholangiogram', injecting contrast after inflating a dilatation balloon in the biliodigestive anastomosis (fig. 8). The advancement of accessories can be difficult and is usually due to a curved tip of the endoscope. In these cases it can be helpful to straighten the tip of the endoscope by pulling back slightly.

The purpose of the procedure often is to obtain a cholangiogram, which usually guides further management. Biliary interventions like balloon dilation (fig. 9), crushing and removal of stones, and plastic stent placement are all technically possible. Stent placement is usually performed by pushing a stent over a long guidewire with a pushing catheter or the ERCP catheter. Recently, an all-in-one stent delivery system became available (table 1).

After finishing the procedure, the endoscope is gently pulled back. When it is clear or suspected that a second balloon-assisted procedure is necessary in the future, it can be considered to mark the appropriate small bowel limb with submucosal ink on withdrawal of the endoscope, to facilitate recognition of the target limb.

Outcomes

There are several case series and case reports available reporting on ERCP procedures in patients with altered upper gastrointestinal anatomy [reviewed in 3]. All published case series are summarized in table 2. Balloon-assisted ERCP procedures have been described in patients aged 2–81 years [4–16]. In almost all published cases, the objective of the procedure was to gain biliary access. The experience in pancreatic interventions is scarce. In practically all patients reported, access into the targeted limb was obtained. However, entry into the native papilla, biliodigestive or pancreaticodigestive anastomosis was not always possible. Nevertheless, a diagnosis can be made in the majority of patients, based on findings of either direct visualization of the papilla or biliodigestive anastomosis or cholangiography. Therapeutic interventions like balloon dilation, biliary stent placement, biliary stone extraction and pancreatic duct interventions have been shown to be technically possible. The relatively short endoscope from Fujinon has recently been used successfully in 48 balloon-assisted ERCP procedures in 38 patients [12]. The Olympus single-balloon endoscope has also shown to be useful in the setting of ERCP, although published experience is limited to 6 patients [13, 16]. It is not known which endoscope is best for ERCP in patients with altered upper gastrointestinal anatomy, but the short Fujinon double-balloon endoscope has a great advantage over the other endoscopes in that all conventional accessories can be used. This allows for almost all conventional interventions including metallic stent placement. In selected cases, double-balloon enteroscopy can be combined with percutaneous transhepatic cholangioscopy in a rendezvous approach [17, 18]. It has been suggested to use the unifying term balloon-assisted enteroscopy for all procedures involving the use of a balloon-loaded endoscope or overtube [19].

Importantly, serious complications are rarely encountered during or following balloon-assisted procedures. Sometimes, cholangitis following the procedure occurs, probably due to manipulation in the biliary system. This can usually be treated conservatively. There is one reported case of perforation of the hepaticojejunostomy following balloon dilation, which was managed by surgery [14]. The risk of complications using balloon-assisted enteroscopy for ERCP appears to be considerably lower than that of percutaneous transhepatic biliary interventions, which is estimated to be around 5% [20].

Conclusion

Balloon-assisted enteroscopy has allowed endoscopists to access intestinal areas which were until recently inaccessible with the conventional endoscopes. Even after surgical reconstruction procedures, diagnostic and therapeutic endoscopic interventions are feasible and safe. Double-balloon procedures, as well as single-balloon techniques, have shown to be possible. Successful interventions described include balloon dilation of stenotic biliodigestive anastomoses, sphincterotomy, extraction of bile stones and stent placement. No serious complications have yet been reported.

In conclusion, balloon-assisted enteroscopy is a safe and feasible technique to obtain biliary or pancreatic access in patients with surgically altered anatomical configurations with great diagnostic and therapeutic potential.

References

1 Yamamoto H, Sekine Y, Sato Y, et al: Total enteroscopy with a nonsurgical steerable double-balloon method. Gastrointest Endosc 2001;53:216–220.

2 Haber GB: Double-balloon endoscopy for pancreatic and biliary access in altered anatomy. Gastrointest Endosc 2007;66(suppl):S47–S50.

3 Koornstra JJ, Fry L, Mönkemüller K: ERCP with the balloon-assisted enteroscopy technique: a systematic review. Dig Dis 2008;26:324–329.

4 Mehdizadeh S, Ross A, Gerson L, et al: What is the learning curve associated with double-balloon enteroscopy? Technical details and early experience in 6 US tertiary care centers. Gastrointest Endosc 2006; 64:740–750.

5 Emmett DS, Mallat DB: Double-balloon ERCP in patients who have undergone Roux-en-Y surgery: a case series. Gastrointest Endosc 2007;66:1038–1041.

6 Aabakken L, Bretthauer M, Line PD: Double-balloon enteroscopy for endoscopic retrograde cholangiography in patients with a Roux-en-Y anastomosis. Endoscopy 2007;39:1068–1071.

7 Mönkemüller K, Bellutti M, Neumann H, Malfertheiner P: Therapeutic ERCP with the double-balloon enteroscope in patients with Roux-en-Y anastomosis. Gastrointest Endosc 2008;67:992–996.

8 Koornstra JJ: Double-balloon enteroscopy for endoscopic retrograde cholangiopancreaticography after Roux-en-Y reconstruction: case series and review of the literature. Neth J Med 2008;66:275–279.

9 Maaser C, Lenze F, Bokemeyer M, Ullerich H, Domagk D, Bruewer M, Luegering A, Domschke W, Kucharzik T: Double-balloon enteroscopy: a useful tool for diagnostic and therapeutic procedures in the pancreaticobiliary system. Am J Gastroenterol 2008;103:894–900.

10 Chu YC, Yang CC, Yeh YH, Chen CH, Yueh SK: Double-balloon enteroscopy application in biliary tract disease – its therapeutic and diagnostic functions. Gastrointest Endosc 2008;68;585–591.

11 Fähndrich M, Sandmann M, Heike M: A facilitated method for endoscopic interventions at the bile duct after Roux-en-Y reconstruction using double-balloon enteroscopy. Z Gastroenterol 2008;46:335–338.

12 Matsushita M, Shimatani M, Takaoka M, Okazaki K. 'Short' double-balloon enteroscope for diagnostic and therapeutic ERCP in patients with altered gastrointestinal anatomy. Am J Gastroenterol 2008; 103:3218–3219.

13 Dellon ES, Kohn GP, Morgan DR, Grimm IS: Endoscopic retrograde pancreaticography with single-balloon enteroscopy is feasible in patients with a prior Roux-en-Y anastomosis. Dig Dis Sick 2009;54: 1798-1803.

14 Mönkemüller K, Fry LC, Bellutti M, Neumann H, Malfertheiner P: ERCP with the double-balloon enteroscope in patients with Roux-en-Y anastomosis. Surg Endosc 2009;23:1961–1967.

15 Kuga R, Furuya CK Jr, Hondo FY, Ide E, Ishioka S, Sakai P: ERCP using double-balloon enteroscopy in patients with Roux-en-Y anatomy. Dig Dis 2008;26: 330–335.

16 Mönkemüller K, Fry LC, Bellutti M, Neumann H, Malfertheiner P: ERCP using single-balloon instead of double-balloon enteroscopy in patients with Roux-en-Y anastomosis. Endoscopy 2008;40(suppl 2):E19–E20.

17 Kawano Y, Mizuta K, Hishikawa S, Egami S, Fujiwara T, Hyodo M, Yasuda Y, Yano T, Nakazawa K, Yamamoto H, Kawarasaki H: Rendezvous penetration method using double-balloon endoscopy for complete anastomosis obstruction of hepaticojejunostomy after pediatric living donor liver transplantation. Liver Transpl 2008;14:385–387.

18 Tsukui D, Yano T, Nakazawa K, Osawa H, Kawano Y, Mizuta K, Kawarasaki H, Yamamoto H: Rendezvous technique combining double-balloon endoscopy with percutaneous cholangioscopy is useful for the treatment of biliary anastomotic obstruction after liver transplantation. Gastrointest Endosc 2008;68: 1013–1015.

19 Mönkemüller K, Fry LC, Bellutti M, Malfertheiner P: Balloon-assisted enteroscopy: unifying double-balloon and single-balloon enteroscopy. Endoscopy 2008;40:537.

20 Winick AB, Waybill PN, Venbrux AC: Complications of percutaneous transhepatic biliary interventions. Tech Vasc Interv Radiol 2001;4:200–206.

Jan J. Koornstra, MD, PhD
Department of Gastroenterology and Hepatology
University Medical Centre Groningen, University of Groningen
PO Box 30001, NL–9700 RB Groningen (The Netherlands)
Tel. +31 503613354, Fax +31 503619306, E-Mail j.j.koornstra@int.umcg.nl

Mönkemüller K, Wilcox CM, Muñoz-Navas M (eds): Interventional and Therapeutic Gastrointestinal Endoscopy.
Front Gastrointest Res. Basel, Karger, 2010, vol 27, pp 438–448

Techniques for Minor Papilla Access and Sphincterotomy

John T. Maple

Division of Digestive Diseases and Nutrition, University of Oklahoma Health Sciences Center, Oklahoma City, Okla., USA

Abstract

Endoscopic access to the minor papilla is most commonly sought in cases of symptomatic pancreas divisum. Dorsal duct access can be achieved using a variety of techniques and accessories, with technical success in about 90% cases at experienced centers. Meticulous attention to technique, and occasionally the use of adjunctive measures such as intravenous secretin or local application of methylene blue, will increase cannulation success in challenging cases. The main techniques for minor papillotomy include pull-type sphincterotomy, needle-knife over stent, and needle-knife over wire; all appear to be effective and no method has been shown to yield superior outcomes. Dorsal duct stenting may reduce the risk of post-endoscopic retrograde cholangiopancreatography (ERCP) pancreatitis, but longer durations of stenting may induce ductal strictures. Patients with idiopathic recurrent acute pancreatitis are more likely to benefit from minor papilla endotherapy than those with chronic pancreatitis or pain alone. The incidence of post-ERCP pancreatitis is about three times more frequent with minor papilla cases than with unselected ERCPs, again highlighting the need for appropriate expertise in the endoscopic care of these patients.

The pancreatic body, tail, and anterior aspect of the head arise from the embryonic dorsal pancreatic bud, whereas the posterior portion of the pancreatic head arises from the ventral bud; the origin of the uncinate process is variable. At about 7 weeks' gestation, the ventral bud rotates clockwise around the duodenum and fuses with the dorsal bud; the dorsal and ventral ducts usually join at this time as well. The proximal aspect of the dorsal duct typically regresses to form a petite accessory duct (duct of Santorini), and in dye-injection studies at endoscopic retrograde cholangiopancreatography (ERCP) and in cadavers, the accessory duct is only patent in 40–50% of individuals [1]. The ventral pancreatic duct (duct of Wirsung) drains via the major duodenal papilla along with the common bile duct, whereas the accessory pancreatic duct drains through the minor duodenal papilla (fig. 1). The minor papilla lacks a discrete sphincter musculature per se, but in cases of pancreas divisum or patent accessory duct, muscle fibers from the duodenal muscularis propria surround the duct and appear to perform sphincteric actions [1].

Pancreas divisum is a common congenital anatomic variant referring to non-fusion of the dorsal and ventral pancreatic ducts (fig. 1). The prevalence of pancreas divisum has ranged from 3 to 13% in autopsy, ERCP, and magnetic resonance cholangiopancreatography (MRCP) series in Western patients [1–3]. Although most patients with pancreas divisum are asymptomatic, a subset will present with idiopathic recurrent acute pancreatitis (IRAP), chronic pancreatitis, or pancreatic-type pain. Historically this has been attributed to a relative stenosis posing outflow obstruction in these symptomatic patients, though the mechanisms underlying these associations are not fully understood. Recently an association between IRAP and cystic fibrosis transmembrane conductance regulator *(CFTR)* gene mutation [4] and/or impaired CFTR protein function [4, 5] has been reported. Also, patients with pancreas divisum appear to have more *CFTR* mutations than do healthy controls [6]. Suboptimal CFTR function causes impaired epithelial ion transport, and may result in hyperviscous pancreatic secretions that may encounter difficulty in draining from pancreata with divisum anatomy.

Endoscopic access to the dorsal pancreatic duct, with subsequent interventions including minor papilla sphincterotomy, may be sought in a variety of clinical situations. Most commonly, minor papilla access is desired in patients with pancreas divisum associated with IRAP or chronic pancreatitis. However, minor papilla access may facilitate endoscopic treatment of pancreatic duct strictures, stones, or leaks, even in patients without divisum, when the ventral duct is obstructed or tortuous [7]. Dorsal ductography may also help delineate true pancreas divisum from pseudodivisum due to obstructing pathology (e.g. neoplasm) when the ventral duct does not opacify beyond the pancreatic head.

Techniques and Accessories

Minor Papilla Localization and Endoscopic Approach

Prone or supine patient positioning are optimal for pancreatography and should be employed when approaching the minor papilla. The minor papilla can range from pinpoint in size to quite prominent and nearly the size of the major papilla. However, on average it is 5 mm in diameter [1], and usually located about 10–20 mm proximal/cephalad and 5–10 mm anterior to the major papilla (fig. 2). The minor papilla may be difficult to locate; if it cannot be visualized by withdrawing the duodenoscope from the level of the major papilla, the scope should be withdrawn to the gastric antrum and passed antegradely through the duodenum again, as this may facilitate localization. Intravenous glucagon (0.5 mg) is useful to achieve duodenal aperistalsis, and in patients with multiple bunched or overlapping duodenal mucosal folds, a sphincterotome or catheter can be used to splay the folds apart to aid in minor papilla localization. Spraying dilute methylene blue onto the duodenal mucosa may be useful if the above measures fail to conclusively identify the minor papilla; it may highlight the subtle raised and frond-like papillary mucosa, and clear pancreatic effluent can be seen washing away the blue dye [8]. Intravenous synthetic porcine secretin (0.2 μg/kg, i.v. over 1 min, maximum 16 μg) will stimulate prompt pancreatic secretion and induce dilation of the pancreatic ductal orifices. Secretin may be utilized with or without prior methylene blue application, and is useful both in localization and cannulation efforts, given its effects on the minor papillary os [9]. Lastly, endoscopic ultrasound (EUS)-guided puncture of the pancreatic duct with a 22-gauge needle with subsequent instillation of contrast and methylene blue into the duct has been reported when prior attempts to localize the minor papilla had failed [10].

Following localization, stable positioning of the endoscope with an en-face view of the minor papilla is necessary for successful cannulation. Most commonly, this is achieved via a 'long' scope position (fig. 3), though occasionally a 'very short' scope position may be adequately stable. The first approaches to the minor papilla will have the greatest likelihood of

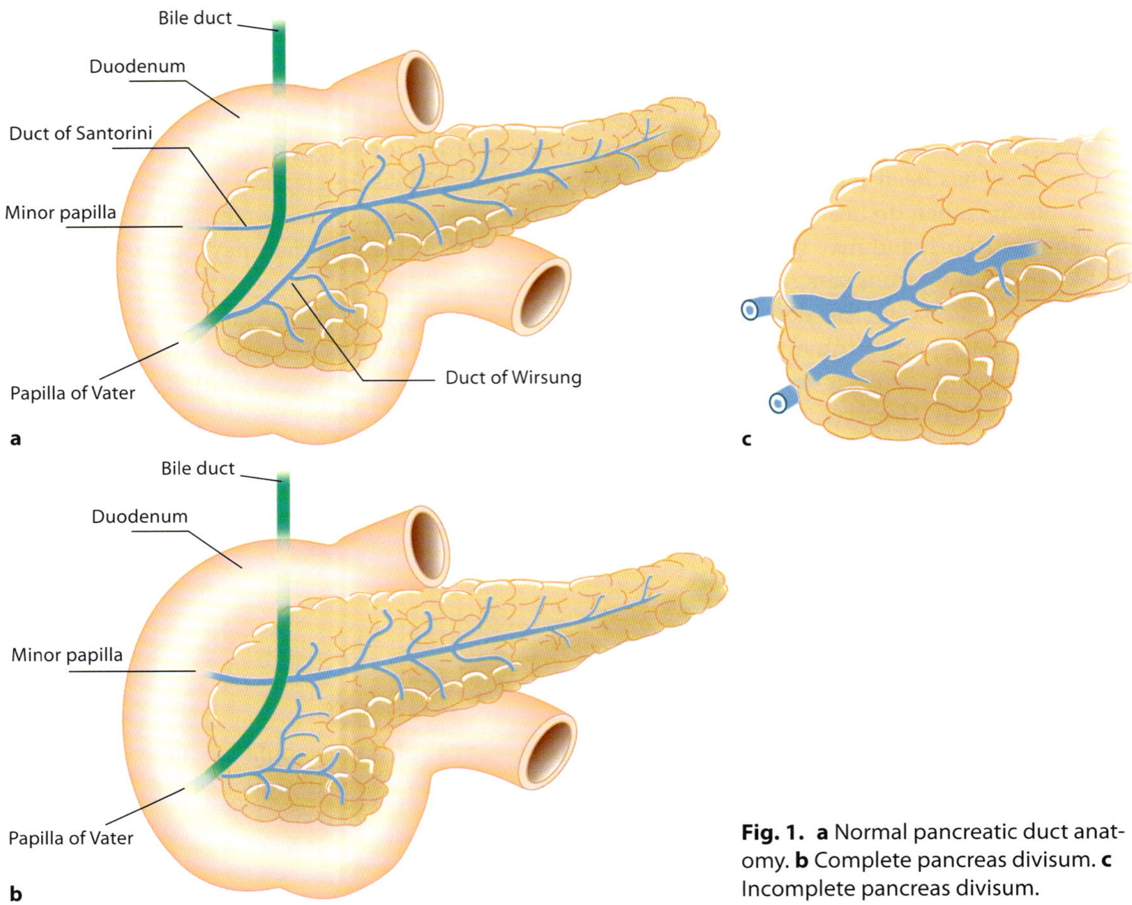

Fig. 1. **a** Normal pancreatic duct anatomy. **b** Complete pancreas divisum. **c** Incomplete pancreas divisum.

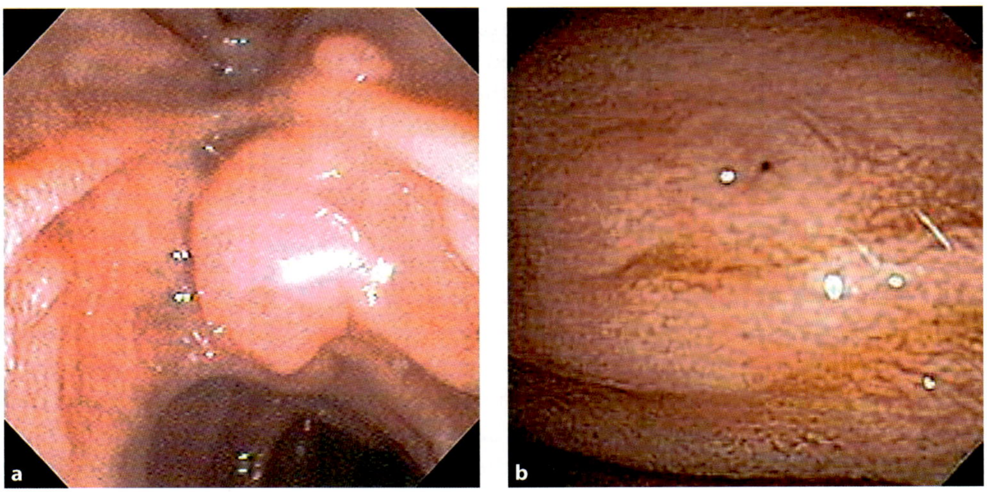

Fig. 2. **a** Endoscopic photograph demonstrating the position of the minor papilla, cephalad and slightly anterior to the major papilla. **b** Endoscopic photograph of the minor papilla, with a tiny central papillary os visible.

successful dorsal ductography or wire cannulation; repeated touches with a device or wire will tend to induce papillary edema, oozing, and spasm of the papillary sphincter musculature – all impeding further cannulation attempts. For this reason, a dedicated effort should me made to clearly visualize the minor papillary os prior to the initial cannulation approach. If the os is not apparent, strong consideration should be given to secretin administration. In two large series of minor papilla cannulation, secretin was utilized in 17–35% of cases [11, 12]. In a randomized, double-blind controlled trial conducted on patients in whom initial minor papilla cannulation was unsuccessful, secretin infusion was associated with an 81% successful cannulation rate, compared with 8% for placebo [13]. In the trial's second phase, patients whose minor papillae were still inaccessible crossed over to the alternate study drug; impressively, an ultimate 89% cannulation success rate was seen after exposure to secretin across the entire study group, which again, was defined by difficulty with initial cannulation. As adequate dorsal ductography may be more challenging in a vigorously secreting gland, the optimal use of secretin remains reserved for cases of non-visualization of the minor papilla or its orifice, or cases of difficult cannulation.

Minor Papilla Access and Dorsal Ductography

When dorsal ductography alone is desired, a blunt needle-tip catheter (e.g. Cremer metal tip cannula, Cook Endoscopy, Inc., Winston-Salem, N.C., USA) is frequently useful. While a variety of other devices may also be used as a platform for initial minor papilla cannulation, including various tapered catheters and sphincterotomes (fig. 4), in the vast majority of cases a guidewire will be needed to achieve deep dorsal duct cannulation. To achieve deep wire access, the selected catheter may be lightly impacted into the papillary os, and subsequently, gentle wire advancement (with or without prior dorsal ductography) can be undertaken. Alternatively, the device can be positioned in the duodenal lumen, 'hovering' over the minor papilla, with subsequent wire advancement into the papillary os without touching the papilla with the device. Ideally these maneuvers are undertaken with either control of the guidewire by the endoscopist or a highly skilled assistant. If dorsal ductography is not performed prior to attaining superficial wire entry (10–20 mm) into the dorsal duct, contrast injection generally should be performed prior to attempting wire passage deeply to the pancreatic tail. This will help avoid potentially traumatic wire passage into a side branch, as well as define any anatomic obstructions (e.g. strictures, stones) that may impede wire advancement.

As traditional pull-type sphincterotomy (PTS) is frequently possible when minor papillotomy is warranted, a standard short-nose pull-type sphincterotome is a reasonable choice as a cannulation device. Most conventional sphincterotomes have a 4- to 5-Fr tip and accommodate either 0.025- or 0.035-inch guidewires. While smaller caliber wires (e.g. 0.018- or 0.021-inch) for use in highly tapered catheters (e.g. Glo-Tip 5-4-3 catheter, Cook Endoscopy, Inc.) and sphincterotomes (e.g. MiniTome or UTS sphincterotomes, Cook Endoscopy, Inc.) are available and advocated by some when the need for minor papilla access is anticipated, it is unknown whether these specialty accessories improve cannulation success. In some cases, a smaller device and wire system may succeed in cannulation where standard accessories and a 0.035-inch wire have failed. However, some small caliber wires are not electrically insulated to allow for sphincterotomy (e.g. Roadrunner, Cook Endoscopy, Inc.), and in general small wire platforms provide less stability during stent placement, with some risk of loss of cannulation. It should also be noted that pancreas divisum is frequently an unanticipated finding (at ventral ductography) during an ERCP in which standard accessories and a 0.035-inch wire may

3

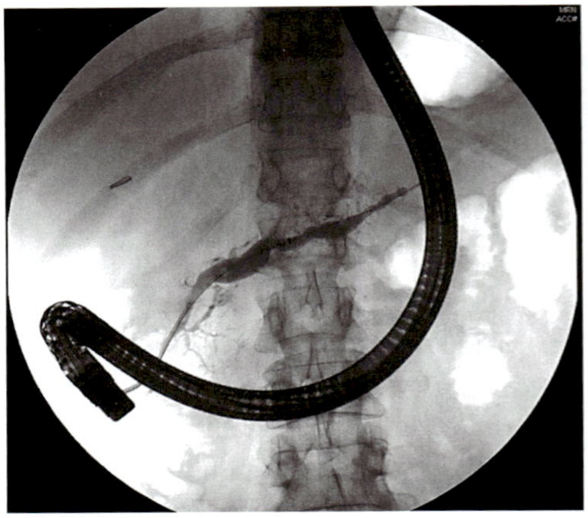

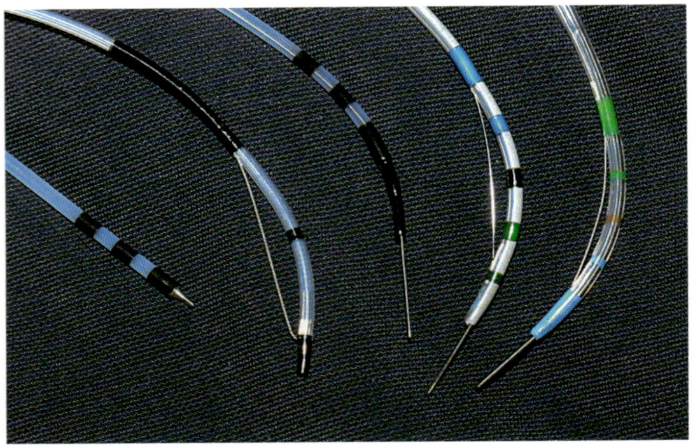

4

Fig. 3. A fluoroscopic image demonstrating a dorsal ductogram achieved using a 'long scope' position. Changes of moderately severe chronic pancreatitis are seen. **Fig. 4.** Various devices used for minor papilla cannulation. From left, Cremer metal tip cannula*, UTS Precurved Ultra Taper sphincterotome*, Glo-Tip 5-4-3 catheter* with a 0.018-inch wire, Fusion OMNI-TOME 21* with a 0.021-inch wire, and Autotome RX 44[×] with a 0.035-inch wire (*Cook Endoscopy, Inc., Winston-Salem, N.C., USA; [×]Boston Scientific, Natick, Mass., USA).

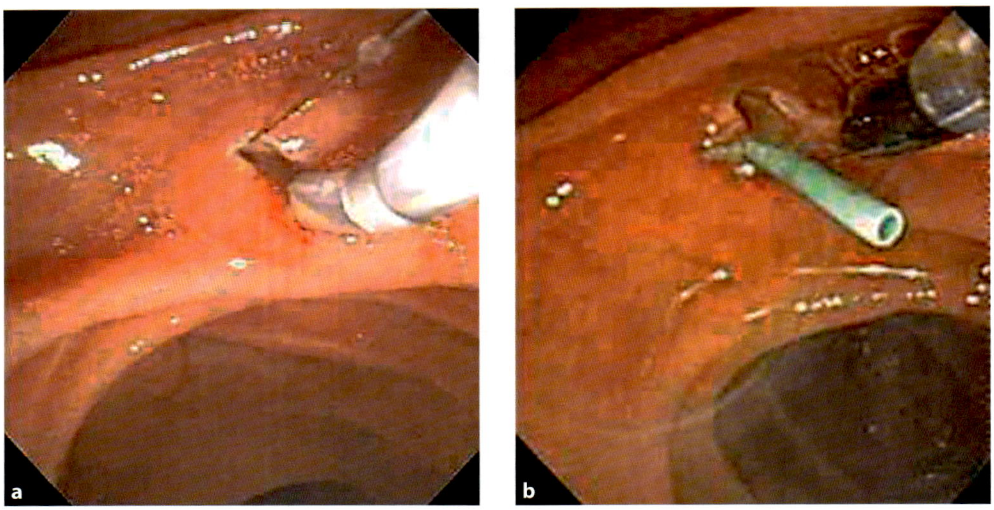

Fig. 5. **a** Endoscopic photograph of a pull-type minor papillotomy. **b** Endoscopic photograph of a needle-knife minor papillotomy over a dorsal duct stent.

have already been selected. In these instances, it is likely unnecessary to change accessories if dorsal duct access is deemed appropriate. In a recent series of 24 consecutive patients at two centers, a standard 4.4-Fr tip sphincterotome and 0.035-inch hydrophilic-tip guidewire were used to perform wire-guided cannulation of the minor papilla, with a 96% cannulation success rate [14]. Endoscopist preference for minor papillotomy technique may also influence initial device selection for achieving cannulation, as these two aspects of the ERCP are inseparably linked.

Minor Papillotomy
Several different techniques for minor papillotomy have been described. Irrespective of technique, either pure cut current or blended current (e.g. ERBE Endocut, ERBE USA, Inc., Marietta, Ga., USA) may be utilized. Whether either current type is optimal is unknown; pure cut current may theoretically induce less thermal injury and fibrosis, and thus potentially less restenosis, while blended current may potentially foster fewer bleeding complications. The length of cut is individualized, based on papillary anatomy and endoscopist judgment, but commonly electroincisions will range from 3 to 7 mm.

In a proportion of patients, a standard sphincterotome can be passed over a wire into the dorsal duct sufficiently far enough to allow PTS (fig. 5). In cases when this is not possible, a graduated dilation catheter (e.g. Soehendra 7- to 4-Fr dilation catheter, Cook Endoscopy, Inc.) may be used to first dilate the minor papillary orifice [15]. Alternatively, a 3- to 5-Fr stent can be placed over a guidewire passed deeply into the dorsal duct, and a needle-knife papillotomy may be performed over the stent (fig. 5) [16]. Another method that may be useful when PTS is not initially possible is wire-assisted access sphincterotomy (WAAS) [12]. In this technique, a needle knife is passed alongside a cannulated guidewire and used to perform minor papillotomy (fig. 6). This technique may be used either to begin a papillotomy to permit device access via the minor papilla, thus allowing subsequent papillotomy completion with a pull-sphincterotome, or to perform the entire papillotomy. A potential advantage to needle-knife papillotomy with either a stent or guidewire in situ is that (if desired) two separate incisions may be performed, 180° apart; this technique may help ensure a maximal papillotomy without increased perforation risk. Lastly, if wire access to dorsal duct cannot be attained, free-hand needle-knife sphincterotomy is an option in appropriately selected cases [17].

Minor Papilla Stenting after Papillotomy
Strong consideration should be given to leaving a stent in the dorsal duct at the conclusion of an ERP in which minor papillotomy has been performed, to mitigate the risk and severity of procedural pancreatitis. Stent composition, length, caliber, and presence or absence of internal flanges should be individualized based on case characteristics including specific ductal pathology and need for future intervention. A variety of pancreatic stents are shown in figure 7. Firmer polyethylene stents have been shown to induce ductal strictures, particularly in normal-appearing pancreatic ducts (chronic pancreatitis absent); as such, the use of softer polymer stents that are potentially less traumatic may be considered. Stents ending at a bend or genu in the pancreatic duct may also be more likely to induce fibrotic stricturing; thus, some attention should also be given to stent length, with attempts to leave the proximal end of the stent in a relatively straight section of the duct. Unless a stricture or significant ductal dilation are present, 3- to 5-Fr stents are most commonly used. Stent-induced ductal strictures have been observed as soon as 2 weeks post-placement [16]. Thus, when used for pancreatitis prophylaxis, flanged stents should be endoscopically retrieved in ≤2 weeks, and stents without an internal flange should be radiographically surveyed after 7–10 days to ensure spontaneous migration.

Alternative Access Techniques
In cases of failed access to a dilated, obstructed pancreatic duct, transgastric and transduodenal EUS-guided pancreatography have been reported, including patients with pancreas divisum. Access to the duct with either a 19- or 22-gauge needle allows different therapeutic options, including antegrade wire passage to the duodenum to facilitate a transpapillary 'rendezvous'

6
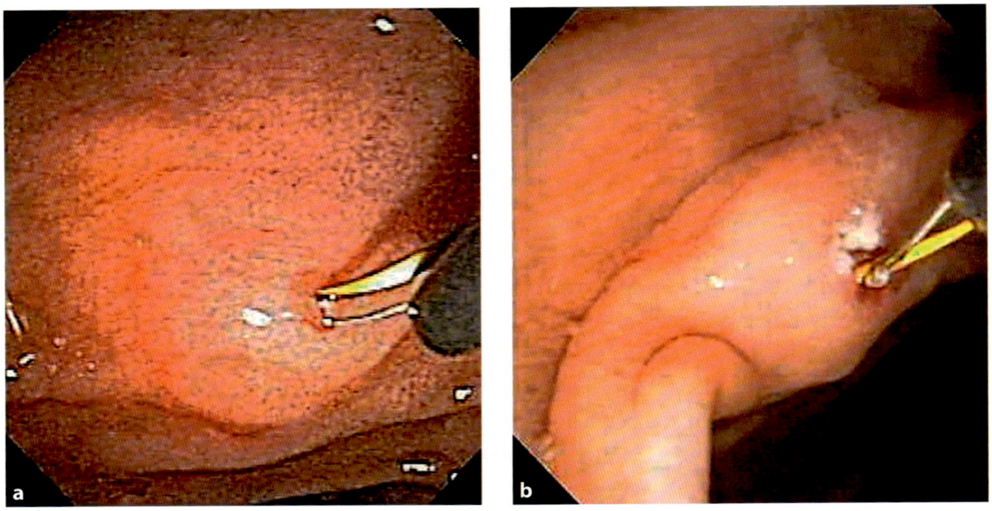
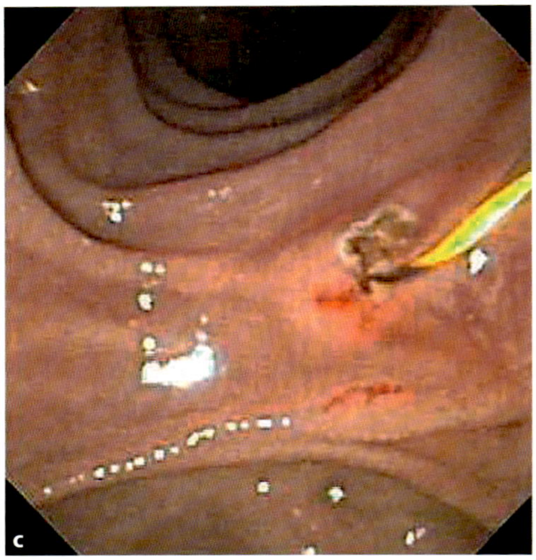

7
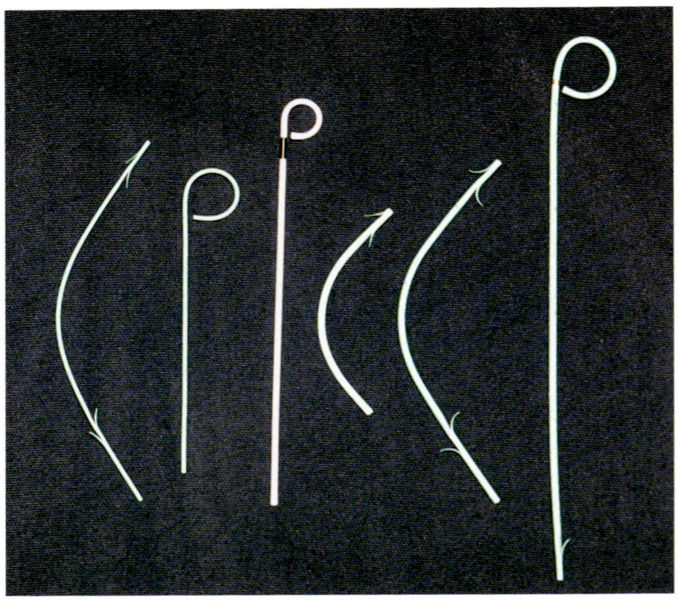

Fig. 6. Endoscopic photographs of WAAS of the minor papilla. **a** A needle knife is passed alongside a guidewire deeply cannulating the dorsal duct. **b** The needle knife is directed radially, away from the guidewire, and cutting current is applied. **c** Appearance of the minor papilla after access sphincterotomy.

Fig. 7. Several 3-, 4-, and 5-Fr pancreatic stents of different lengths, and with variable external and internal fixation designs.

procedure, or creation of a pancreaticogastrostomy or pancreaticobulbostomy for transenteric stenting and drainage [18]. Experience with these procedures is limited to small series from expert centers and severe complications have been reported; as such, careful consideration of risks, potential benefits, and available expertise should precede recommending these modalities.

Technical Outcomes

Access

In experienced centers, minor papilla access can be successfully achieved in 86–93% of cases [12, 16, 19, 20]. No data exist regarding the technical superiority of a certain technique or device for access.

Papillotomy Technique

In a retrospective series of 184 patients who underwent minor papillotomy at a large tertiary referral center, no differences were seen between the 133 patients who were treated using the needle-knife stent technique and the 51 patients who underwent PTS, with regard to adverse events, papillary restenosis, and overall need for endoscopic reintervention [21]. Similarly, in a single-center retrospective review of 64 patients undergoing minor papillotomy, the WAAS (wire-assisted) technique and PTS yielded comparable outcomes [12]. Mild post-ERCP pancreatitis and mild intraprocedural bleeding were observed more frequently in the WAAS patients, though the differences were not statistically significant, and WAAS was frequently used as a salvage technique (when PTS was not possible) in this series.

Clinical Outcomes

Clearly, the majority of patients in whom minor papilla intervention is desired are those with symptomatic pancreas divisum. In regard to these patients, however, critical evaluation of clinical outcomes of minor papilla endotherapy is hindered by the use heterogenous techniques across studies (e.g. papillotomy alone, papillotomy and stenting, dilation and stenting without papillotomy, and significant variation in durations of stenting). Furthermore, the available data regarding outcomes from minor papilla endotherapy are almost exclusively retrospective, involve small patient samples, varying definitions for pain outcomes, and have follow-up durations that are generally limited. Though this chapter is primarily focused on techniques, a brief overview of clinical outcomes with minor papilla endotherapy will be presented, while keeping these limitations in mind.

Benefit of Endotherapy

Patients with IRAP and pancreas divisum appear to be the most reasonable candidates for endotherapy. The majority of these patients will experience either an abolition or a reduction in the frequency of pancreatitis following minor papilla endotherapy [16, 20, 22–26] and the majority gain significant improvement in global pain scores during intermediate-term follow-up [16, 20, 22, 27–30] and long-term (≥2 years) follow-up [23]. A recent systematic review summarizing these data reported a pooled 'response' rate of 79% to endotherapy in patients with IRAP and pancreas divisum [2]. In the only prospective randomized trial of minor papilla endotherapy, 19 patients with pancreas divisum and IRAP were randomized to either minor papilla dilation and placement of a 5- to 7-Fr pancreatic stent (exchanged every 4 months for 1 year, then removed) or no endoscopic treatment [27]. The patients were followed for a mean of about 2.5 years, and there were significantly fewer episodes of pancreatitis, and significantly fewer emergency room visits for pain in the patients who had been randomized to endotherapy. Though the results were promising, the lack of blinding and small number of patients limits the conclusions from this trial. However, data from surgical sphincteroplasty also support a benefit in patients with divisum and IRAP [31], lending additional credence to intervention in this subset.

Patients with chronic pancreatitis and chronic pancreatic-type pain respond less robustly to minor papilla endotherapy, with significant improvements in pain scores reported for 27–69% of patients with chronic pancreatitis [16, 20, 30, 32], and the response rate for those with pancreas divisum and pain only has typically been less than 40% [16, 20, 24, 30]. In patients with chronic pancreatitis, events including parenchymal and perineural inflammation and stricturing of both main and side-branch ducts have already occurred and are difficult to ameliorate with a simple minor papilla intervention. Conversely, patients with pancreas divisum and pain alone are a diverse group, with a high prevalence of visceral hypersensitivity and chronic pain syndromes unrelated to their pancreatic anatomy, and thus poorly responsive to minor papilla endotherapy.

Some authors have described using non-invasive or less risky techniques to properly select patients with symptomatic pancreas divisum who will respond favorably to intervention on the minor papilla. Such techniques include secretin ultrasonography [31], secretin MRCP [33], and injection of botulinum toxin into the minor papilla [34]. However, most of this work has been performed in patients with IRAP, who are known to have frequent improvement (~80%) with endotherapy. Predictive tests would be more useful in selecting patients with pain only or chronic pancreatitis who would benefit from minor papilla endotherapy, given the more heterogenous and less favorable responses in these subsets.

Adverse Events

Post-ERCP pancreatitis is the most common complication of minor papilla intervention, with rates of 8–20% in series of minor papillotomies [12, 16, 20–24] and seemingly lower rates for dorsal ductography plus/minus stenting without papillotomy [11, 28]. Mild, immediate post-papillotomy bleeding prompting epinephrine injection has been reported in up to 13% [12], though more clinically significant bleeding is limited to 0–2% [16, 20, 21]. Despite the lack of landmarks guiding minor papillotomy extent, the incidence of perforation is low (0–1%) and does not appear to be more frequent than in ERCPs involving the major papilla [12, 16, 20, 21]. Restenosis of the minor papilla after initial minor papillotomy has been reported in 11–22% [12, 20, 21, 23, 24]. As previously mentioned, stent-induced changes in the dorsal duct (e.g. strictures, diffuse dilation) have been reported in significant proportions of patients with prolonged stenting, particularly those with initially normal-appearing ducts [16, 28, 35, 36]. While not all of these changes may be clinically significant and many may resolve over time following stent removal, cautious consideration is warranted with regard to timing of stent removal.

Conclusion

Endoscopic access to the minor papilla is most commonly sought in cases of symptomatic pancreas divisum. Dorsal duct access can be achieved using a variety of techniques and accessories, with technical success in about 90% cases at experienced centers. Meticulous attention to technique, and occasionally the use of adjunctive measures such as intravenous secretin or local application of methylene blue, will increase cannulation success in challenging cases. Main techniques for minor papillotomy include PTS, needle-knife over stent, and needle-knife over wire; all appear to be effective and no method has been shown to yield superior outcomes. Dorsal duct stenting may reduce the risk of post-ERCP pancreatitis, but longer durations of stenting may induce ductal strictures. Patients with IRAP are more likely to benefit from minor papilla endotherapy than those with chronic pancreatitis or pain alone. The incidence of post-ERCP pancreatitis is about three times more frequent with minor papilla cases than with unselected ERCPs, again highlighting the need for appropriate expertise in the endoscopic care of these patients.

Acknowledgment

The author thanks Dr. Rhett Jackson for his photographic assistance in the creation of figures 4 and 7.

References

1 Kamisawa T: Clinical significance of the minor duodenal papilla and accessory pancreatic duct. J Gastroenterol 2004;39:605–615.

2 Liao Z, Gao R, Wang W, et al: A systematic review on endoscopic detection rate, endotherapy, and surgery for pancreas divisum. Endoscopy 2009;41:439–444.

3 Fogel EL, Toth TG, Lehman GA, et al: Does endoscopic therapy favorably affect the outcome of patients who have recurrent acute pancreatitis and pancreas divisum? Pancreas 2007;34:21–45.

4 Dray X, Fajac I, Bienvenu T, Chryssostalis A, Sogni P, Hubert D: Association of pancreas divisum and recurrent acute pancreatitis with the IVS8-5T-12-TG allele of the *CFTR* gene and CFTR dysfunction. Pancreas 2007; 35:90–93.

5 Gelrud A, Sheth S, Banerjee S, et al: Analysis of cystic fibrosis gene product function in patients with pancreas divisum and recurrent acute pancreatitis. Am J Gastroenterol 2004;99:1557–1562.

6 Alazmi WM, Fogel EL, Schmidt S, et al: ERCP findings in idiopathic pancreatitis: patients who are cystic fibrosis gene positive and negative. Gastrointest Endosc 2006;63:234–239.

7 Song MH, Kim MH, Lee SK, et al: Endoscopic minor papilla interventions in patients without pancreas divisum. Gastrointest Endosc 2004;59:901–905.

8 Park SH, de Bellis M, McHenry L, et al: Use of methylene blue to identify the minor papilla or its orifice in patients with pancreas divisum. Gastrointest Endosc 2003;57: 358–363.

9 O'Connor KW, Lehman GA: An improved technique for accessory papilla cannulation in pancreas divisum. Gastrointest Endosc 1985;31:13–17.

10 DeWitt J, McHenry L, Fogel E, LeBlanc J, McGreevy K, Sherman S: EUS-guided methylene blue pancreatography for minor papilla localization after unsuccessful ERCP. Gastrointest Endosc 2004;59:133–136.

11 Benage D, McHenry R, Hawes RH, O'Connor KW, Lehman GA: Minor papilla cannulation and dorsal ductography in pancreas divisum. Gastrointest Endosc 1990; 36:553–557.

12 Maple JT, Keswani RN, Edmundowicz SA, Jonnalagadda S, Azar RR: Wire-assisted access sphincterotomy of the minor papilla. Gastrointest Endosc 2009;69:47–54.

13 Devereaux BM, Fein S, Purich E, et al: A new synthetic porcine secretin for facilitation of cannulation of the dorsal pancreatic duct at ERCP in patients with pancreas divisum: a multicenter, randomized, double-blind comparative study. Gastrointest Endosc 2003;57:643–647.

14 Ammar T, Maple JT, Ansstas M, Abdeen BM, Cote GA, Azar RR: Physician-controlled wire-guided cannulation of the minor papilla (abstract). Gastrointest Endosc 2009; 69:AB268.

15 Soehendra N, Kempeneers I, Nam VC, Grimm H: Endoscopic dilatation and papillotomy of the accessory papilla and internal drainage in pancreas divisum. Endoscopy 1986;18:129–132.

16 Lehman GA, Sherman S, Nisi R, Hawes RH: Pancreas divisum: results of minor papilla sphincterotomy. Gastrointest Endosc 1993;39:1–8.

17 Sahin B, Parlak E, Cicek B, Diseibeyaz S, Kuran SO: Precutting of the minor papilla for pancreatic duct cannulation in pancreas divisum patients. Endoscopy 2005; 37:779.

18 Gines A, Varadarajulu S, Napoleon B: EUS 2008 Working Group Document: evaluation of EUS-guided pancreatic-duct drainage. Gastrointest Endosc 2009;69:S43–S48.

19 Benage D, McHenry R, Hawes RH, O'Connor KW, Lehman GA: Minor papilla cannulation and dorsal ductography in pancreas divisum. Gastrointest Endosc 1990; 36:553–557.

20 Chacko LN, Chen YK, Shah RJ: Clinical outcomes and non-endoscopic interventions after minor papilla endotherapy in patients with symptomatic pancreas divisum. Gastrointest Endosc 2008;68:667–673.
21 Attwell A, Borak G, Hawes R, Cotton P, Romagnuolo J: Endoscopic pancreatic sphincterotomy for pancreas divisum by using a needle knife or standard pull-type technique: safety and reintervention rates. Gastrointest Endosc 2006;64:705–711.
22 Kwan V, Loh SM, Walsh PR, Williams SJ, Bourke MJ: Minor papilla sphincterotomy for pancreatitis due to pancreas divisum. ANZ J Surg 2008;78:257–261.
23 Heyries L, Barthet M, Delvasto C, et al: Long-term results of endoscopic management of pancreas divisum with recurrent acute pancreatitis. Gastrointest Endosc 2002;55:376–381.
24 Kozarek RA, Ball TJ, Patterson DJ, et al: Endoscopic approaches to pancreas divisum. Dig Dis Sci 1995;40: 1974–1981.
25 McCarthy J, Geenen JE, Hogan WJ: Preliminary experience with endoscopic stent placement in benign pancreatic diseases. Gastrointest Endosc 1988;34:16–18.
26 Siegel JH, Ben-Zvi JS, Pullano W, Cooperman A: Effectiveness of endoscopic drainage for pancreas divisum: endoscopic and surgical results in 31 patients. Endoscopy 1990;22:129–123.
27 Lans JI, Geenen JE, Johanson JF, et al: Endoscopic therapy in patients with pancreas divisum and acute pancreatitis: a prospective, randomized, controlled clinical trial. Gastrointest Endosc 1992;38:430–434.
28 Ertan A: Long-term results after endoscopic pancreatic stent placement without pancreatic papillotomy in acute recurrent pancreatitis due to pancreas divisum. Gastrointest Endosc 2000;52:9–14.
29 Heyries L, Barthet M, Delvasto C, et al: Long-term results of endoscopic management of pancreas divisum with recurrent acute pancreatitis. Gastrointest Endosc 2002;55:376–381.
30 Coleman SD, Eisen GM, Troughton AB, Cotton PB: Endoscopic treatment in pancreas divisum. Am J Gastroenterol 1994;89:1152–1155.
31 Warshaw AL, Simeone JF, Schapiro RH, Flavin-Warshaw B: Evaluation and treatment of the dominant dorsal duct syndrome (pancreas divisum redefined). Am J Surg 1990; 159:59–64.
32 Boerma D, Huibregtse K, Gulik TM, Rauws EA, Obertop H, Gouma DJ: Long-term outcome of endoscopic stent placement for chronic pancreatitis associated with pancreas divisum. Endoscopy 2000; 32:452–456.
33 Testoni PA, Mariani A, Curioni S, Zanello A, Masci E: MRCP-secretin test-guided management of idiopathic recurrent acute pancreatitis: long-term outcomes. Gastrointest Endosc 2008;67:1028–1034.
34 Wehrmann T, Schmitt T, Seifert S: Endoscopic botulinum toxin injection into the minor papilla for treatment of idiopathic recurrent pancreatitis in patients with pancreas divisum. Gastrointest Endosc 1999;50:545–548.
35 Kozarek RA: Pancreatic stents can induce ductal changes consistent with chronic pancreatitis. Gastrointest Endosc 1990;36:93–95.
36 Cohen SA, Rutkovsky FD, Siegel JH, Kasmin FE: Endoscopic stenting and sphincterotomy of the minor papilla in symptomatic pancreas divisum: results and complications. Diagn Ther Endosc 1995;1:131–139.

John T. Maple
Division of Digestive Diseases and Nutrition, University of Oklahoma Health Sciences Center
920 Stanton L. Young Blvd, WP 1360
Oklahoma City, OK 73117 (USA)
Tel. +1 405 271 5428, Fax +1 405 271 5803, E-Mail john-maple@ouhsc.edu

Mönkemüller K, Wilcox CM, Muñoz-Navas M (eds): Interventional and Therapeutic Gastrointestinal Endoscopy.
Front Gastrointest Res. Basel, Karger, 2010, vol 27, pp 449–458

Pancreas Divisum: Disease Association and Endoscopic Therapy

S. Ian Gan · Richard A. Kozarek

Digestive Disease Institute, Virginia Mason Medical Center, Seattle, Wash., USA

Abstract

Pancreas divisum (PD) is a relatively common congenital variant that has been associated with recurrent acute pancreatitis, chronic pancreatitis and chronic abdominal pain in a minority of affected patients. Diagnosis of PD can be achieved with magnetic resonance imaging or endoscopic ultrasound but the gold standard remains endoscopic retrograde cholangiopancreatography. Therapy of PD-associated symptoms is targeted at relief of the relative obstruction found at the minor papilla using sphincterotomy, balloon dilation sphincteroplasty or stenting. Techniques of minor duct access, therapy and outcomes are discussed.

Pancreas divisum (PD) is a congenital variant in which the ventral and dorsal ducts of the pancreas fail to fuse. It is present in approximately 10% of individuals with autopsy series demonstrating a range of 4–14% [1]. In patients undergoing endoscopic retrograde cholangiopancreatography (ERCP), the frequency tends to be lower, between 0.3 and 7.5%. Pooled data show an overall endoscopic detection rate of 2.8% with rates being significantly lower in Asia than Western countries [2]. There is some debate in the literature as to whether PD is associated with an increased risk of pancreatitis. While most patients with PD have no associated disease, it is generally accepted that a minority of patients with PD can experience complications in the form of (1) recurrent acute pancreatitis, (2) chronic pancreatitis, or (3) abdominal pain without pancreatitis. The purported mechanism of symptoms is a relative obstruction of pancreatic duct outflow at the minor papilla.

The normal embryologic development of the pancreas involves fusion of the ventral bud with the dorsal bud. The ventral bud rotates to meet the dorsal bud and normally the ventral duct and dorsal duct fuse to become the main pancreatic duct. Classically PD is a complete failure of fusion, with the residual dorsal duct draining the majority of the pancreas through the minor papilla and a small ventral duct draining the posterior inferior head through the major papilla. In incomplete PD, there is a small ductal communication between the ventral and dorsal ducts. Occasionally the entire pancreas is drained through the dorsal duct with either an absent or isolated duct of Santorini (fig. 1). Other variants include drainage of the entire gland through the minor papilla with no evidence of pancreatic duct at the major papilla (fig. 1). In all variants, the clinical manifestations are similar as the most of the gland is drained by the dorsal duct.

PD is associated with a variety of other pancreatic and biliary abnormalities. Up to 30% of patients with annular pancreas may have associated PD [3]. Associations have also been reported with partial pancreatic agenesis, and a potentially increased incidence of pancreatic carcinoma, mucinous tumors and cholangiocarcinoma [4].

Physiologic and pathologic evidence for the role of PD in pancreatitis and abdominal pain is scant. Pancreatic histology of total pancreatectomies from patients with resection of both the ventral and dorsal portions of the pancreas has confirmed chronic pancreatitis changes in the dorsal gland but not in the ventral gland [5]. Higher pressures have been documented in the dorsal duct when compared to the ventral duct in patients with PD and abdominal pain [6] correlating with the theory that the pathophysiology of clinical disease in PD patients is due to relative obstruction of pancreatic drainage. Other factors may also predispose PD patients to the development of pancreatitis. In a study of 57 patients with PD, CFTR mutations were found in 22% of PD patients with pancreatitis as compared to 0% of the control patients without pancreatitis. Ultimately, in the absence of other data, the most convincing evidence for the role of PD in disease is response to surgical and endoscopic therapy. Several studies have reported successful treatment of recurrent acute pancreatitis, chronic pancreatitis and abdominal pain with relief of relative obstruction of the minor papilla.

Diagnosis of PD

ERCP remains the gold standard for the diagnosis of PD but advances in computed tomography (CT), magnetic resonance cholangiopancreatography (MRCP) and endoscopic ultrasound (EUS) have allowed less invasive means of diagnosis (fig. 2). MRCP and CT have both been used successfully in the initial evaluation of patients with recurrent acute pancreatitis, identifying not only PD, but pancreatic duct strictures, biliary variants and congenital anomalies [7, 8]. Initial reports were promising for the use of cross-sectional imaging in the diagnosis of PD. While early studies documented a high accuracy when compared to ERCP [9, 10] particularly if secretin stimulation is used, the patients in these studies did not necessarily undergo both ERCP and MRCP, and PD may have been missed in those patients undergoing MRCP alone. A recent study suggested a relatively low overall sensitivity for the diagnosis of PD by MRCP (44%) in patients who had undergone MRCP prior to ERCP, with no increase in sensitivity using secretin stimulation [11].

EUS may play some role in the diagnosis of PD. The entire pancreatic ductal system can be visualized with both radial and linear echoendoscopes. From the second portion of the duodenum, the uncinate process, the ampulla, the distal pancreatic ducts, and bile ducts can be examined. The ventral anlage is readily visible from the duodenum in about 45–75% of patients and can be distinguished from the dorsal pancreas by its relatively hypoechoic parenchyma [12, 13]. From the bulb, the upstream pancreatic duct can be visualized and followed back to the genu and body of the pancreas. Findings suggestive of PD include: absence of a visible ventral duct, dilated or 'dominant' dorsal duct, failure to visualize the main pancreatic duct crossing the ventral anlage (fig. 3), failure to trace the main duct from ventral pancreas to the genu/body, failure to see the 'stack sign' and visualization of the Santorini duct crossing the common bile duct [14, 15]. Both linear and radial EUS have been studied with sensitivities reaching 95 and 100%, respectively [15, 16].

In addition, EUS is highly sensitive in the diagnosis of chronic pancreatitis. Both parenchymal and ductal features are visible and include hyperechoic foci and strands, lobularity, cysts,

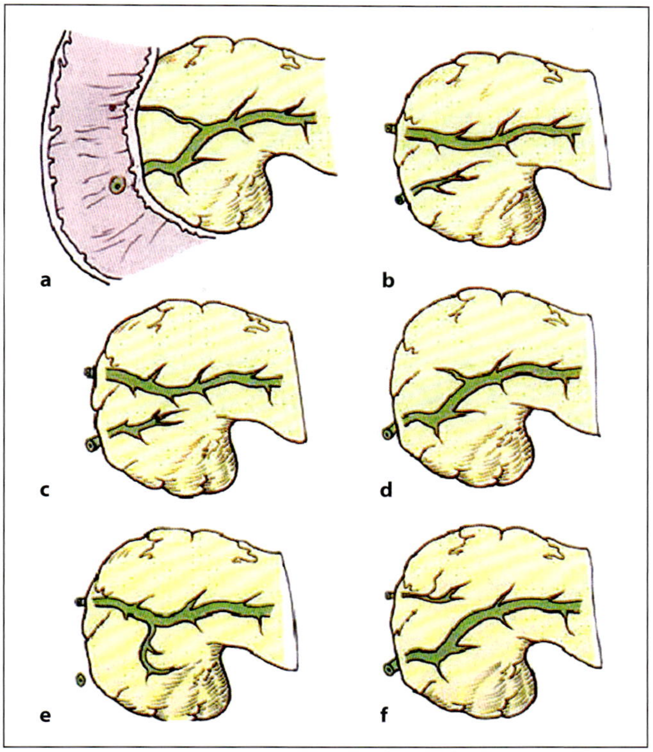

Fig. 1. Drawings illustrating pancreatic ductal variations including pancreas divisum. **a** A common variant with patent main and accessory ducts and patent major and minor papillae. **b** Typical pancreas divisum. **c** Incomplete pancreas divisum; a tiny branch connects dorsal and ventral ducts. **d** Accessory duct absent; minor papilla not patent. **e** Drainage of entire ductal system drains through minor papilla. **f** Isolated accessory duct draining through minor papilla. From Lehman, Feldman's GastroAtlas Online. Available at: URL: www.gastroatlas.com.

calcifications and ductal dilation, irregularity and hyperechoic margins. The threshold for diagnosis is unclear, but it is generally accepted that if no features are present, chronic pancreatitis is unlikely, and that if 5 or more features are present, CP is likely [17]. In patients with PD, chronic pancreatitis changes may be evident in the dorsal pancreas with no evidence of disease in the ventral pancreas. The presence of chronic pancreatitis changes, particularly if there is dorsal duct dilation which may suggest the need for therapeutic intervention and the potential for benefit.

A recent study studied the prediction of divisum on the basis of endoscopic inspection of the minor papilla [18]. Predictive factors that were included were the size of the minor papilla, the diameter of the orifice and the presence or absence of juice draining from the orifice. In 212 patients undergoing ERCP for suspected sphincter of Oddi or idiopathic pancreatitis, the positive predictive value of minor papilla appearance was 57.5% with a negative predictive value of 88.9%.

As the majority of patients with PD have no clinical disease, attempts have been made to diagnose the presence of narrowing or relative obstruction of the minor papilla. CT and MRCP may both identify dorsal duct dilation and/or features of chronic pancreatitis which may suggest relative obstruction of the minor papilla in the presence of PD. The presence of focal dilation of the distal dorsal duct before or after administration of secretin, a so-called Santorinicele, is also purported to indicate relative outflow obstruction [19] but is neither diagnostic nor predictive. A study of MRCP in PD patients failed to show proportionally more abnormal dilation after secretin administration (defined as duct diameter of >3 mm at 10 min) when compared to controls without PD. There were also no differences found between those with and without symptoms [9].

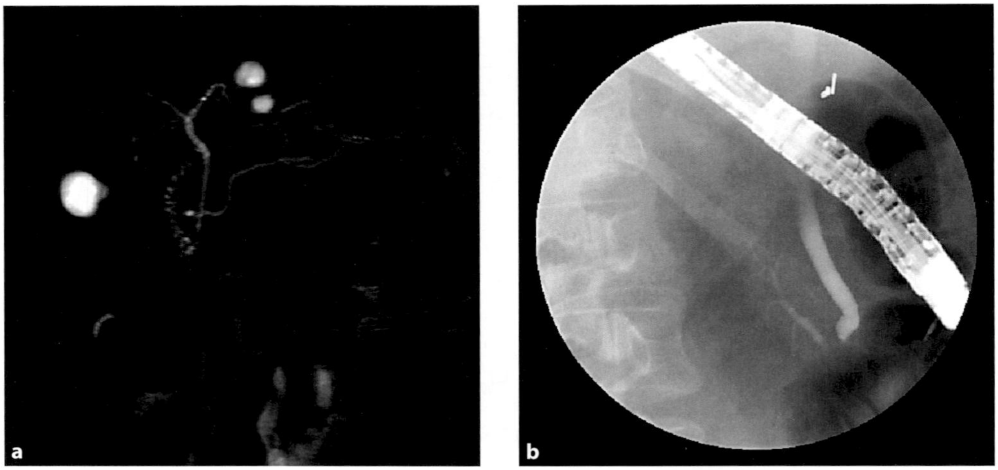

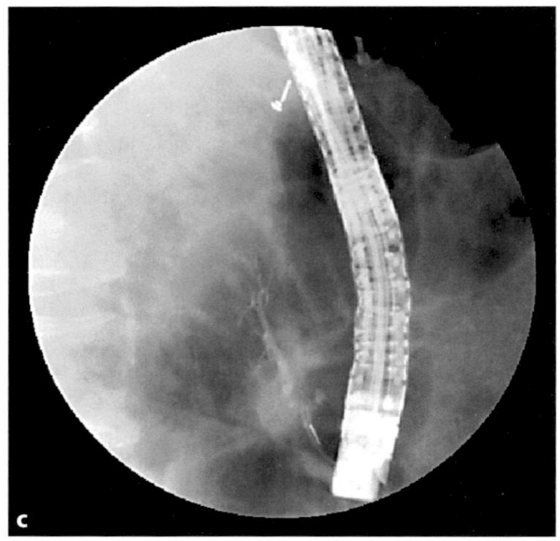

Fig. 2. **a** MRCP of patient with PD showing dominant dorsal duct of Santorini and small non-communicating ventral duct. Note presence of liver cysts adjacent to cholangiogram. **b** ERCP of same patient showing common bile duct and short ventral duct without communication with main duct. **c** ERCP showing main duct pancreatogram filling from the minor papilla.

Some groups have used transabdominal ultrasound with secretin administration to differentiate those with relative obstruction at the minor papilla [20, 21]. While transient dilation of the duct is normal after secretin administration, prolonged dilation of the PD lasting more than 15 min has been purported to be suggestive of dorsal duct outflow obstruction. Similarly, EUS may have value in the prediction of benefit from endoscopic therapy of PD patients. Catalano et al. [22] studied 22 patients with pancreatitis secondary to PD prior to treatment with stent insertion. The pancreatic duct was visualized at the level of the portal confluence before and after administration of secretin (1 IU/kg). Evidence of functional obstruction was deemed to be an increase in duct diameter of >1 mm, sustained for a 15-min period. 13 (81%) of the patients with an abnormal secretin study had reduced pain and pancreatitis whereas only 17% of the patients with a normal secretin study had benefit [22]. The definition of a positive test remains somewhat arbitrary, however, and some studies have failed to show any correlation with pancreatic symptoms [23]. Furthermore, patients with chronic pancreatitis may have scarring preventing dilation or may not generate enough pancreatic juice to facilitate ductal dilation. Larger prospective studies are necessary.

Minor papillary manometry has been used to try to determine the presence of relative obstruction but normal pressures have not been established. In the scant data available, minor papilla pressures in PD patients have been found to be comparable to the major papilla in some studies [24] and elevated in others [25]. Studies have shown a higher pressure in the dorsal duct of patients with PD, but there have been no studies to date correlating this with the presence or absence of disease states. There is anecdotal suggestion that difficulty in cannulation and a 'tight' papilla at the time of cannulation is suggestive of papillary stenosis. Ultimately, the true identification of patients with relative obstruction of the minor papilla may only be established if they respond to therapy.

Procedural Aspects

Patient Preparation

Patients should be prepared in a fashion similar to other ERCP procedures. History of potentially treatable symptoms should be obtained prior to consideration of endoscopic therapy. Patients should be nil per os for at least 6 h prior to the procedure. Informed consent should be obtained from the patient, and risks, potential benefits and alternatives such as surgery or nonspecific symptom control should be discussed. Risks of post-ERCP pancreatitis in particular should be outlined as they are generally higher with minor duct manipulation. Relevant laboratory values and results of imaging studies (US, MRCP, CT) should be reviewed prior to the procedure. Decisions on the appropriate type of sedation or anesthesia should be made on the basis of patient factors such as narcotic resistance, alcohol use, and comorbid disease and procedure factors such as the expected degree of procedural complexity and estimated procedure duration. Procedures are normally carried out with the patient in the prone position. Standard fluoroscopy, either C-arm or fixed table setup, is required for pancreatographic imaging, preferably with radiographic technical support. The authors prefer the patient to be in the prone position for ERCP.

Accessories

A duodenoscope is normally used, unless the patient has altered anatomy that precludes the use of a side-viewing scope. A therapeutic 4.2-mm channel is preferable but not necessary as large diameter (10-Fr) stents and accessories are not required for successful therapy. Cannulation instruments should include 3- or 5-Fr catheters or a 23- or 25-gauge blunt needle with contrast or thin caliber wires such as 0.04- or 0.05-cm wires with hydrophilic tips. Many endoscopists prefer to start with a conventional tapered-tip sphincterotome with a guidewire for duct cannulation. Erbe generators are preferred for needle-knife sphincterotomy over a dorsal pancreatic duct stent if using blended currents and 'endocut' settings but if pure-cut settings are used, as the authors generally do for pull-type sphincterotomy, most electrosurgical generators would suffice. If dilation is performed, initial dilation can be performed using the tapered catheter followed by serial dilation with wire-guided graduated step dilators or, in some cases, 4-mm biliary dilation balloons.

Technique

Identification of the minor papilla can prove challenging even for the most experienced endoscopist. The minor papilla is generally found 1–3 cm cephalad and anterior to the major papilla and is best approached in a long position with a duodenoscope. The minor papilla may appear as a small papule with or without an apparent orifice. In a small percentage of cases, however, the papilla cannot be readily identified endoscopically. It is important to avoid trauma to the duodenal mucosa prior to examination of the minor papilla including even gentle suction of the mucosa. Duodenal contraction can be controlled with glucagon or buscopan.

If the minor papilla cannot be identified with standard endoscopic examination, 8–16 μg of intravenous secretin can be administered intravenously. Pancreatic secretions become markedly increased often making the orifice wider and more evident. Devereaux et al. [26] found a significantly increased rate of cannulation when using secretin prior to cannulation. Furthermore, diluted methylene blue can be sprayed over the mucosa overlying the suspected region of the minor papilla to further emphasize the papilla as the clear secretions from the pancreas wash away the bluish hue of the dye [27] (fig. 4). Park et al. [27] demonstrated an 86% success rate of minor duct cannulation using this technique in patients in whom the initial examination did not reveal the minor papilla. Other groups have taken a more direct approach and injected methylene blue directly into the pancreatic duct with a needle under EUS guidance [28]. The resulting point of bluish secretions can be readily identified endoscopically.

Cannulation is often achieved using tapered 3- or 5-Fr catheters or a 23- or 25-gauge blunt needle tip, generally from the long position of the duodenoscope at which the papilla is most often visualized en face. Smaller caliber wires between 0.04 and 0.06 cm are often necessary for cannulation. Both contrast- and wire-assisted cannulation can be performed, but particular care must be taken to avoid submucosal injection or sufficient trauma that causes loss of papillary landmarks. The senior author prefers using tapered sphincterotome cannulation followed by wire access with a 0.09-cm tracer wire because of the relative tip rigidity. Care must be taken to avoid blindly perforating a side branch.

Overall cannulation rates in expert hands should be over 90% [29]. In cases where cannulation is difficult to achieve, free-hand precut sphincterotomy can be performed if the location of the minor papilla is certain. Some authors have used minor papillectomy with an electrosurgical snare to assist in difficult cannulation [30]. In cases when minor cannulation cannot be achieved using standard ERCP techniques, EUS-guided rendezvous techniques have been used by the authors and others [31]. In these procedures the pancreatic duct is accessed with a 19-gauge EUS needle and a curvilinear echoendoscope, usually at the neck of the pancreas, from the antrum of the stomach. The tail region can also be accessed through the gastric body. A pancreatogram should then be performed to outline the duct using contrast injection through the needle. A long 450-cm, 0.06-cm diameter, wire is then advanced through the needle in an anterograde fashion through the PD and into the duodenum. Once the wire is looped in the duodenum, the needle can be withdrawn, leaving the wire in place. The EUS scope can then be replaced by a duodenoscope and the wire can be retrieved through the duodenoscope with a snare or biopsy forceps. Finally a cannula or sphincterotome is backloaded along the wire and retrogradely advanced into the pancreatic duct.

During contrast injection for opacification of the pancreatic duct, caution is suggested to prevent acinarization and the risk of post-ERCP pancreatitis. This is particularly important in cases where secretin has been administered as the increased flow of pancreatic juice may prevent contrast from reaching the pancreatic tail [32].

Therapy

Two forms of therapy have been described in the literature, (1) minor papilla dilation and pancreatic duct stent placement, and (2) minor papilla dilation and sphincterotomy, or a combination of the two. Minor papilla dilation is most commonly performed using the cannulating catheter, followed by progressive dilation with tapered catheter dilation to 7–10 Fr or with small diameter balloon dilators (4 mm). Balloon dilation is associated with high rates of pancreatitis and is generally best used sparingly [32]. We generally perform sphincterotomy without long-term stenting unless a long stricture approximating the papilla is identified. Dilation is performed only if there is a stricture suspected on pancreatogram or on manometry. Similarly, stents are only left for long periods if tight or refractory strictures are encountered.

Different methods of sphincterotomy have been described. A standard pull-type sphincterotomy involves the use of a wire-guided sphincterotome directed in a 10–12 o'clock position (fig. 5). The other method requires initial insertion of a 3-, 5- or 7-Fr stent, followed by needle-knife incision of the papilla over the stent (fig. 6). Sphincterotomies should generally be approximately 5 mm in length. A recent study suggests a variation on this, cutting alongside the wire, rather than a stent [33]. Early data suggested that pure-cut currents had a lower rate of post-ERCP pancreatitis than blended 'Endocut' settings [34], but subsequent data have not substantiated this [35]. There also appears to be no difference in the rates of post-ERCP pancreatitis when comparing needle-knife sphincterotomy over stent or standard pull sphincterotomy in non-PD patients [36]. It is unknown if this is generalizable to PD patients and minor papilla sphincterotomies. The authors generally use pull-type sphincterotomies with standard pure-cut settings of 60 W/s when performing minor papilla sphincterotomies.

If long-term stenting is not performed, prophylactic stents are still recommended in all cases of minor papillary therapy to reduce the incidence of post-ERCP pancreatitis. We use 3-Fr 8-cm single pigtail stents or 5-Fr 3-cm straight stents with the internal flaps removed with a scalpel. In cases where long-term stenting is deemed helpful, we use either 5- or 7-Fr straight stents with intact internal stents. The optimal duration of stenting is unclear but due to a documented risk of stent-related ductal changes (side branch dilation, strictures, etc.) in up to 56% of patients after even short-term stenting [37], the use of long term stents is minimized.

Outcomes

There have been several studies of endoscopic therapy for PD. The studies are highly variable in size and are uniformly retrospective in nature [30, 38–41]. Studies generally suggest a decrease in chronic pain, episodes of recurrent acute pancreatitis and decreased hospital visits. In an attempt to clarify the heterogeneous results, Liao et al. [2] reported a systematic review of all publications of endoscopic and surgical therapy for PD. Fifteen studies were included and analysis demonstrated an overall 69% response to therapy. Subgroup analysis showed that acute recurrent pancreatitis patients with PD tended to respond best to endoscopic therapy with a 79% response versus 69% in chronic pancreatitis patients and 54% of chronic abdominal pain patients. Results were comparable to surgery in all 3 groups.

Initial response to therapy is often complicated by restenosis of the minor papilla and reintervention with ERCP is required in almost 30% of patients in some series [42]. Recurrent symptoms after initial response should prompt further investigation with repeat imaging and repeat ERCP if indicated. Repeat sphincterotomy and sphincteroplasty can be effective, although some patients appear to be prone to a high rate of restructuring which may be related to inadequate sphincterotomy or damage to the duct or parenchyma with thermal energy during sphincterotomy and use of ERBE (Tübingen, Germany) coagulation settings while performing sphincterotomy over a guidewire.

Complications are common with endoscopic therapy and include acute pancreatitis, stent occlusion, stent migration, stent-related stricture, post-sphincterotomy hemorrhage, pancreatic abscess and stenosis of sphincterotomy site. In one of the largest series, Lehman et al. [41] reported a sobering 13.3% rate of acute pancreatitis, 2% hemorrhage, 47% stent occlusion, 6% stent migration, and ductographic changes in 50% of patients.

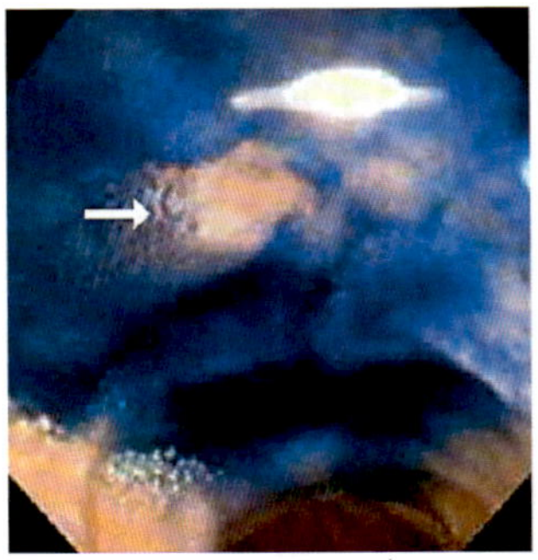

3

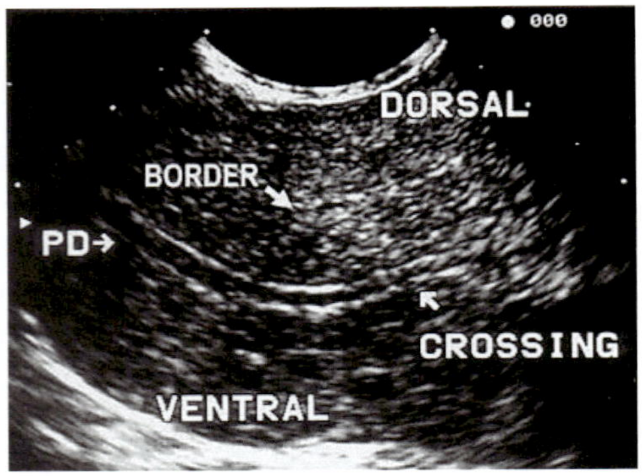

4

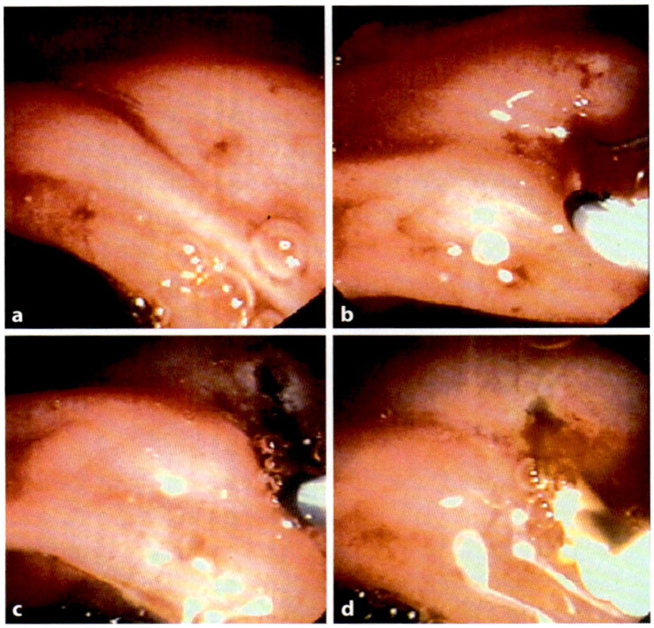

5

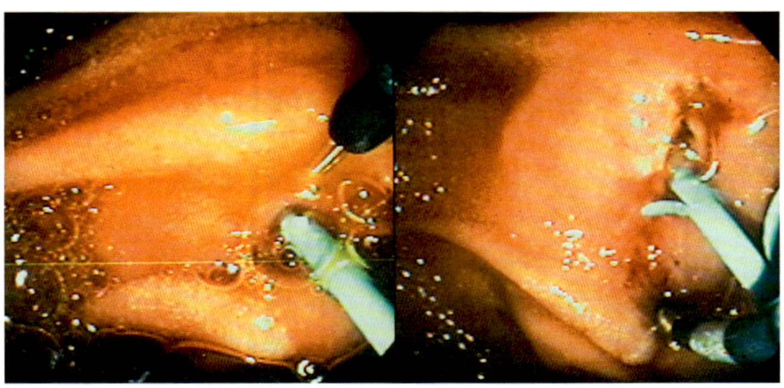

6

Fig. 3. Appearance of minor papilla (white arrow) after methylene blue spraying of the 2nd portion of duodenum and secretin infusion. Permission from Elsevier Publishing. **Fig. 4.** Linear array EUS image showing head of pancreas and the ventral anlage. The pancreatic duct (PD) can be seen coursing across the division between the dorsal and ventral pancreas (CROSSING). Permission from Thieme Publishing. **Fig. 5.** Pull-type sphincterotomy of the minor papilla. Note the passage of pancreatic duct debris (**d**). **Fig. 6.** Needle-knife sphincterotomy of the minor papilla over a pre-placed 5-Fr pancreatic duct stent.

Conclusions

PD is a common variant of ductal anatomy that is infrequently associated with clinical symptoms that include recurrent acute pancreatitis, chronic pancreatitis and chronic abdominal pain. The diagnosis of PD can be achieved on the basis of MRCP, EUS and ERCP. Relative obstruction of the minor papilla can be successfully treated by dilation and sphincterotomy or stenting. Recurrent acute pancreatitis appears to most reliably respond to endoscopic treatment, while chronic pancreatitis and chronic abdominal pain have lower response rates. Complications are relatively frequent and good outcomes require careful patient selection in high-volume centers.

References

1 Delhaye M, Engleholm L, Cremer M: pancreas divisum: congenital anatomic variant or anomaly?contribution of endoscopic retrograde dorsal pancreatography. Gastroenterology 1985;89:951–958.
2 Liao Z, Gao R, Wang W, Ye Z, Lai XW, Wang XT, Hu LH, Li ZS: A systematic review on endoscopic detection rate, endotherapy, and surgery for pancreas divisum. Endoscopy 2009;41:439–444.
3 Zyromski NJ, Sandoval JA, Pitt HA, Ladd AP, Fogel EL, Mattar WE, Sandrasegaran K, Amrhein DW, Rescorla FJ, Howard TJ, Lillemoe KD, Grosfeld JL: Annular pancreas: dramatic differences between children and adults. J Am Coll Surg 2008;206:1019–1025.
4 Nugent C, Ruffolo T, Hawes R, et al: Is pancreas divisum associated with biliary tract carcinoma? (abstract). Gastrointest Endosc 1993;39:327.
5 Cotton PB: Congenital anomaly of pancreas divisum as cause of obstructive pain and pancreatitis. Gut 1980;21:105–114.
6 Staritz M, Meyer zum Büschenfelde KH: Elevated pressure in the dorsal part of pancreas divisum: the cause of chronic pancreatitis? Pancreas 1988;3:108–110.
7 De Filippo M, Calabrese M, Quinto S, Rastelli A, Bertellini A, Martora R, Sverzellati N, Corradi D, Vitale M, Crialesi G, Sarli L, Roncoroni L, Garlaschi G, Zompatori M: Congenital anomalies and variations of the bile and pancreatic ducts: magnetic resonance cholangiopancreatography findings, epidemiology and clinical significance Radiol Med 2008;113:841–859.
8 Anderson SW, Soto JA: Pancreatic duct evaluation: accuracy of portal venous phase 64 MDCT. Abdom Imaging 2009;34:55–63.
9 Matos C, Metens T, Deviere J, Delhaye M, Le Moine O, Cremer M: Pancreas divisum: evaluation with secretin-enhanced magnetic resonance cholangiopancreatography. Gastrointest Endosc 2001;53:728–733.
10 Bret PM, Reinhold C, Taourel P, Guibaud L, Atri M, Barkun AN: Pancreas divisum: evaluation with MR cholangiopancreatography. Radiology 1996;199:99–103.
11 Carnes ML, Romagnuolo J, Cotton PB: Miss rate of pancreas divisum by magnetic resonance cholangiopancreatography in clinical practice. Pancreas 2008;37: 151–153.
12 Wiersema MJ, Hawes RH, Lehman GA, et al: Prospective evaluation of endoscopic ultrasonography and endoscopic retrograde cholangiopancreatography in patients with chronic abdominal pain of suspected pancreatic origin. Endoscopy 1993;25:555–564.
13 Savides TJ, Gress FG, Zaidi SA, Ikenberry SO, Hawes RH: Detection of embryologic ventral pancreatic parenchyma with endoscopic ultrasound. Gastrointest Endosc 1996;43:14–19.
14 Bhutani MS, Hoffman BJ, Hawes RH: Diagnosis of pancreas divisum by endoscopic ultrasonography. Endoscopy 1999;31:167–169.
15 Tessier G, Sahai A: A prospective validation of multiple EUS criteria to diagnose or to exclude pancreas divisum: EUS can accurately exclude pancreas divisum, but ERCP is still required for a definitive diagnosis(abstract AB302). Gastrointest Endosc 2005;61:5.
16 Lai R, Freeman ML, Cass OW, Mallery S: Accurate diagnosis of pancreas divisum by linear-array endoscopic ultrasonography. Endoscopy 2004;36:705–709.
17 ASGE Standards of Practice Committee, Gan SI, Rajan E, Adler DG, Baron TH, Anderson MA, Cash BD, Davila RE, Dominitz JA, Harrison ME 3rd, Ikenberry SO, Lichtenstein D, Qureshi W, Shen B, Zuckerman M, Fanelli RD, Lee KK, Van Guilder T: Role of EUS. Gastrointest Endosc 2007;66:425–434.
18 Alazmi WM, Mosler P, Watkins JL, McHenry L, Fogel EL, Sherman S, Lehman GA: Predicting pancreas divisum by inspection of the minor papilla: a prospective study. J Clin Gastroenterol 2007;41:422–426.
19 Costamagna G, Ingrosso M, Tringali A, Mutignani M, Manfredi R: Santorinicele and recurrent acute pancreatitis in pancreas divisum: diagnosis with dynamic secretin-stimulated magnetic resonance pancreatography and endoscopic treatment. Gastrointest Endosc 2000;52:262–267.

20 Warshaw AL, Simeone JF, Schapiro RH, Warshaw BF: Evaluation and treatment of the dominant dorsal duct syndrome (pancreas divisum redefined). Am J Surg 1990;159:59–66.
21 Tulassay Z, Jakab Z, Vadasz A, Kelemen E, Gupta R: Secretin provocation ultrasonography in the diagnosis of papillary obstruction in pancreas divisum. Gastroenterol J 1991;51:47–50.
22 Catalano MF, Lahoti S, Alcocer E, Geenen JE, Hogan WJ: Dynamic imaging of the pancreas using real-time endoscopic ultrasonography with secretin stimulation. Gastrointest Endosc 1998;48:580–587.
23 Lowes JR, Lees WR, Cotton PB: Pancreatic duct dilatation after secretin stimulation in patients with pancreas divisum. Pancreas 1989;4:371–374.
24 Satterfield ST, McCarthy JH, Geenen JE, Hogan WJ, Venu RP, Dodds WJ, et al: Clinical experience in 82 patients with pancreas divisum: preliminary results of manometry and endoscopic therapy. Pancreas 1988;3: 248–253.
25 Cotton PB. Pancreas divisum. Pancreas 1988;3:245–247.
26 Devereaux BM, Fein S, Purich E, Trout JR, Lehman GA, Fogel EL, Phillips S, Etemad R, Jowell P, Toskes PP, Sherman S: A new synthetic porcine secretin for facilitation of cannulation of the dorsal pancreatic duct at ERCP in patients with pancreas divisum: a multicenter, randomized, double-blind comparative study. Gastrointest Endosc 2003;57:643–647.
27 Park SH, de Bellis M, McHenry L, Fogel EL, Lazzell L, Bucksot L, Sherman S, Lehman GA: Use of methylene blue to identify the minor papilla or its orifice in patients with pancreas divisum. Gastrointest Endosc 2003;57: 358–363.
28 Dewitt J, McHenry L, Fogel E, Leblanc J, McGreevy K, Sherman S: EUS-guided methylene blue pancreatography for minor papilla localization after unsuccessful ERCP. Gastrointest Endosc 2004;59:133–136.
29 Benage D, McHenry R, Hawes RH, O'Connor KW, Lehman GA: Minor papilla cannulation and dorsal ductography in pancreas divisum. Gastrointest Endosc 1990; 36:553–557.
30 Heyries L, Barthet M, Delvasto C, Zamora C, Bernard JP, Sahel J: Long-term results of endoscopic management of pancreas divisum with recurrent acute pancreatitis. Gastrointest Endosc 2002;55:376–381.
31 Mallery S, Matlock J, Freeman ML: EUS-guided rendezvous drainage of obstructed biliary and pancreatic ducts: report of 6 cases. Gastrointest Endosc 2004;59:100–107.
32 Lehman GA, Sherman S: Pancreas divisum. Diagnosis, clinical significance, and management alternatives. Gastrointest Endosc Clin N Am 1995; 5:145.
33 Maple JT, Keswani RN, Edmundowicz SA, Jonnalagadda S, Azar RR: Wire-assisted access sphincterotomy of the minor papilla. Gastrointest Endosc 2009;69:47–54.
34 Elta GH, Barnett JL, Wille RT, Brown KA, Chey WD, Scheiman JM: Pure cut electrocautery current for sphincterotomy causes less post-procedure pancreatitis than blended current. Gastrointest Endosc 1998;47:149–153.
35 Macintosh DG, Love J, Abraham NS: Endoscopic sphincterotomy by using pure-cut electrosurgical current and the risk of post-ERCP pancreatitis: a prospective randomized trial. Gastrointest Endosc 2004;60: 551–556.
36 Lawrence C, Romagnuolo J, Cotton PB, Payne KM, Hawes RH: Post-ERCP pancreatitis rates do not differ between needle-knife and pull-type pancreatic sphincterotomy techniques: a multiendoscopist 13-year experience. Gastrointest Endosc 2009;69: 1271–1275.
37 Sherman, S, Hawes, RH, Savides, TJ, et al: Stent-induced pancreatic ductal and parenchymal changes: correlation of endoscopic ultrasound with ERCP. Gastrointest Endosc 1996;44:276.
38 Klein SD, Affronti JP: Pancreas divisum, an evidence-based review: part II, patient selection and treatment. Gastrointest Endosc 2004;60:585–589.
39 Gerke H, Byrne MF, Stiffler HL, Obando JV, Mitchell RM, Jowell PS, Branch MS, Baillie J: Outcome of endoscopic minor papillotomy in patients with symptomatic pancreas divisum. JOP 2004;5:122–131.
40 Kozarek RA, Ball TJ, Patterson DJ, et al: Endoscopic approach to pancreas divisum. Dig Dis Sci 1995;40: 1974–1981.
41 Lehman GA, Sherman S, Nisi R, et al: Pancreas divisum: results of minor sphincterotomy. Gastrointest Endosc 1993;39:1–8.
42 Attwell, A, Borak, G, Hawes, R, et al: Endoscopic pancreatic sphincterotomy for pancreas divisum by using a needle-knife or standard pull-type technique: safety and reintervention rates. Gastrointest Endosc 2006;64:705.

Richard Kozarek
Digestive Disease Institute, Virginia Mason Medical Center
C3-GAS 1100 Ninth Ave
Seattle, WA 98101 (USA)
Tel. +1 206 223 2319, Fax +1 206 223 6379, E-Mail richard.kozarek@vmmc.org

Mönkemüller K, Wilcox CM, Muñoz-Navas M (eds): Interventional and Therapeutic Gastrointestinal Endoscopy.
Front Gastrointest Res. Basel, Karger, 2010, vol 27, pp 459–476

Endoscopic Therapy for Chronic Pancreatitis

Djuna L. Cahen · Jan-Werner Poley · Marco J. Bruno

Erasmus Medical Centre, University Medical Center Rotterdam, Department of Gastroenterology and Hepatology, Rotterdam, The Netherlands

Abstract

In chronic pancreatitis, therapeutic endoscopy can be considered in three settings; drainage of the pancreatic duct, pseudocyst drainage, and treatment of biliary obstruction. In this chapter these techniques are extensively discussed with a focus on patient selection, the drainage techniques, and the optimal duration of drainage. The available evidence regarding morbidity, mortality, and long-term outcomes are summarized. Subsequently, an effort is made to establish the future role of endoscopic treatment in chronic pancreatitis.

In chronic pancreatitis, therapeutic endoscopy can be considered in different settings: drainage of the pancreatic duct to alleviate pain, pseudocyst drainage, and treatment of biliary obstruction. These techniques have become increasingly popular over the past decades, even though high-quality studies were lacking and the evidence for their efficacy was mainly based on retrospective studies. Just recently, more information from prospective studies has become available.

Pancreatic Duct Drainage

Introduction

Chronic pancreatitis is a disease characterized by an ongoing inflammatory process with severe pain as the predominant symptom. Although the origin of pain is likely to be multifactorial, pancreatic duct obstruction is considered an important etiologic factor. Therefore, ductal decompression became standard treatment for patients with painful obstructive pancreatitis [1, 2]. Obstruction of the pancreatic duct can be caused by strictures, intraductal stones, or, in the majority of cases, by a combination of both. Nowadays, improved imaging modalities (high-resolution abdominal computed tomography and 3-Tesla magnetic resonance cholangiopancreatography (MRCP)) provide sufficient information regarding the pancreatic ductal system to allow patient selection for endoscopic treatment without performing a retrograde pancreatogram. The aim of endoscopic drainage is to decompress the pancreatic duct and restore the outflow of pancreatic juice to the duodenum. It involves sphincterotomy, extracorporeal shock-wave lithotripsy (ESWL), removal of stones, and dilatation of strictures by means of temporary stent insertion.

Procedural Aspects

Pancreatic Duct Stones

Since the introduction in 1987, ESWL has become a cornerstone of endoscopic drainage in chronic pancreatitis. ESWL not only improved the results but also expanded the indications of endoscopic treatment; floating stones <5–6 mm in diameter can be extracted transpapillary with a balloon or small-caliber Dormia basket, but the majority of pancreatic stones are impacted and too large to be removed without fragmentation [3]. It is important to emphasize that ESWL of pancreatic stones is not a simple technique because it requires considerable experience and specialized equipment consisting of a forceful electromagnetic lithotripter with a fluoroscopic two-directional targeting system (the most commonly used being the Dornier Compact Delta lithotripter, Dornier Med-Tech, Wessling, Germany). Therefore, it is generally executed in expert centers. As treatment is painful and time-consuming (a single session takes about 1–2 h), it is best carried out with the patient under general anesthesia. Most ESWL sessions are immediately followed by an endoscopic procedure to clear the pancreatic duct from stones and evaluate the presence of strictures [4–7]. In the largest retrospective study, a mean of 5 sessions was necessary to achieve complete fragmentation [8]. Consecutive treatment sessions are usually carried out within a few days, during which time the patient remains admitted to the hospital. In between sessions an endoprosthesis or nasopancreatic drain can be used to prohibit pancreatic duct obstruction by stone fragments and to facilitate complete duct clearance.

ESWL is considered a low-risk procedure with a 5–10% morbidity, acute pancreatitis being the most frequent complication [8, 9]. In the past, no mortality was observed, but in a recently published prospective study, 1 patient died of a perforated duodenal ulcer in which ESWL might have played a causative role [10]. ESWL is effective in experienced hands; stone fragmentation is achieved in more than 90% of cases and complete duct clearance in 44–74% of patients [3, 5, 6, 8–18]. The best results are reported for solitary distal stones in absence of a stricture but multiple, large, and impacted stones are no contraindication because the newer lithotripters are able to pulverize these stones completely [4, 19].

Pancreatic Duct Strictures

In chronic pancreatitis, fibrotic pancreatic duct strictures require dilatation and temporary insertion of an endoprosthesis. Many questions remain regarding the technical aspects of this technique. At present, prospective studies comparing different endoscopic treatment protocols are lacking. Moreover, in retrospective reports, technical details are rarely discussed. As a consequence, evidence-based guidelines regarding the need for sphincterotomy and dilation, the choice of stents, or the duration of treatment do not exist.

Despite this lack of evidence, a selective pancreatic sphincterotomy is advocated to provide optimal access to the pancreatic duct and facilitate stone extraction. The sphincterotomy is performed towards the 1-o'clock position and can be extended safely until the first duodenal fold. It should be large enough to allow easy access of instruments and prevent post-papillotomy stenosis. Either the needle-knife technique over a stent, or a pull-sphincterotomy can be performed, with similar complication rates of 4% in retrospective studies [20, 21]. A recent prospective study reported that the needle-knife technique was safer, resulting in less post-ERCP pancreatitis [22]. In case a distal stricture is present, a short-nosed small-bore sphincterotome can also be useful. Balloon dilatation of the pancreatic sphincter, as applied by Sasahira et al. [12], seems an interesting alternative technique but needs further evaluation. One study evaluated the benefits of sphincterotomy alone in obstructive pancreatitis (pain improvement in 60% of patients), but the size, retrospective nature, and patient population prohibit drawing any definite conclusions [23]. There is no evidence to support routine biliary sphincterotomy in these patients, unless signs of biliary obstruction are present [24].

Cannulation of the pancreatic duct is usually straight forward although in patients with active inflammation identification and cannulation of the papilla can be difficult due to edema. Furthermore, in 5–10% of patients access can only be obtained via the minor papilla either due to a devised pancreas or because of an impassable stenosis of the Wirsung's duct.

Most strictures can be passed by a regular or hydrophilic 0.035-inch guidewire although sometimes the use of a thin 0.018- or 0.021-guidewire is necessary. Tight strictures, which cannot be passed by a 5- or 6-Fr guiding catheter, require dilatation, either with a 4- to 6-mm balloon or a graduated dilating catheter. Extremely tight strictures can also be dilated with a Soehendra stent retriever which is passed through the stricture over a non-metallic wire as a corkscrew.

Subsequently, stent placement can generally be performed with relative ease. For pancreatic drainage, a range of stents are available. At first, polyethylene biliary endoprostheses were used. Later, stents with multiple side holes were specifically developed for pancreatic use, to allow optimal drainage from the side branches. However, the benefit of these pancreatic stents was never studied and therefore both stent types are used in this setting. Recently, two new model stents have been introduced: these so-called S-shaped and wing-shaped stents are presumed to have a longer patency and less chance of migration, but this needs to be proven prospectively [25–27]. Stents have a wide variety in diameters from 3 to 12 Fr. Laugier and Renou [28] were the first to suggest that a larger stent circumference results in a better outcome. The current trend is to use a stent with the largest possible diameter, and to insert an increasing number of stents with each consecutive procedure to further dilate the stricture in analogy with the treatment of benign biliary strictures [29–31].

Perhaps the most interesting question regarding endoscopic dilatation of the pancreatic duct is how long a stent should be left in place. So far, the effect of stent duration on treatment outcome was never properly investigated and the two possible stent exchange protocols (either to change the stent at prescheduled intervals or to exchange 'on demand', meaning when symptoms of obstruction recur) have not been compared.

Exchanging the stent on a regular basis has the advantage of preventing recurrent symptoms due to stent obstruction [32, 33]. Furthermore, this will limit treatment duration because stricture resolution is frequently evaluated and treatment may be terminated as soon as the obstruction has resolved. Shorter treatment duration might be important in the light of two findings. First, some studies suggest that the presence of a stent leads to progression of duct damage in patients with chronic pancreatitis, but most of these changes seem reversible [34–37]. A more important reason to limit the treatment duration is the prospective observation that many patients experienced considerable pain during stent therapy, a finding that might even be aggravated if multiple stents are used [10].

The single argument in favor of a long stenting period is the belief that this will improve the efficacy of stricture dilation and reduce the chance of recurrence, although evidence to support this assumption is lacking. In published series the stent duration ranged from 5.5 to 28 months, but the reported efficacy and recurrence rate did not vary accordingly [10, 19, 28, 29, 38–45]. Only three studies have evaluated prognostic factors of outcome in pancreatic stenting, but none

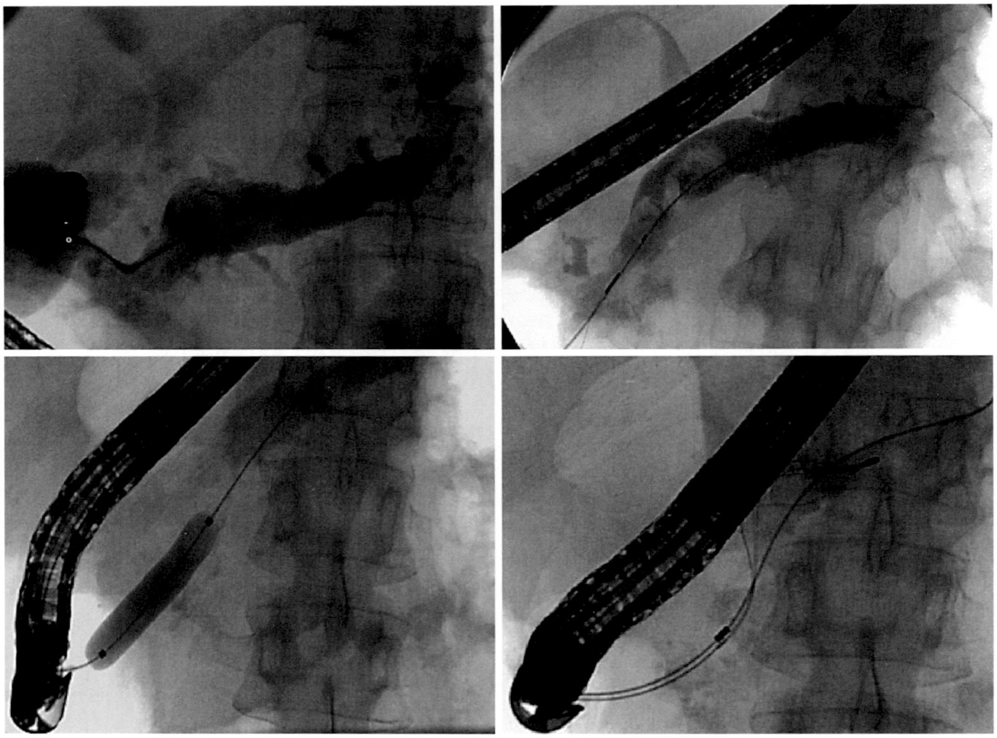

Fig. 1. a ERCP in chronic pancreatitis. Cannulation was achieved via the minor papilla because of an impassable stricture of the main pancreatic duct. **b** Minor sphincterotomy over a guidewire. **c** Balloon dilation of the stenotic part of the Santorini duct. **d** Stone removal with a small Dormia basket..

found a significant benefit of a longer treatment duration [10, 28, 38]. Furthermore, even when assuming that clinical success is achieved only after years of treatment, it is impossible to know whether pain relief was accomplished by the endoscopic intervention or if it was a consequence of the natural course of the disease [16, 46].

Outcome

There is sufficient data to conclude that endoscopic pancreatic drainage in chronic pancreatitis is technically feasible and safe. Morbidity is observed in 6–58%, but most complications are stent-related and easy to treat [10, 19, 28, 38, 39, 41–44]. However, since the introduction of endoscopic treatment, surgical techniques have evolved too, and the high complication rates of a decade ago are no longer applicable [47–49]. Therefore, the central argument in comparing endoscopic and surgical drainage has shifted from safety to efficacy. This comparison is complicated by the lack of high-quality reports on endoscopic drainage; most studies were retrospective, had a heterogeneous patient population, did not use well-defined treatment protocols, and most importantly, they failed to use uniform and validated outcome measures [19, 28, 38, 39, 42, 43].

Despite the above-mentioned limitations, some conclusions regarding the role of endoscopic drainage of the pancreatic duct in chronic pancreatitis can be drawn. Surgical drainage (by a pancreaticojejunostomy according to Partington-Rochele [50] or, in the presence of an inflammatory mass, by a Beger or Frey procedure) achieves long-term pain relief in 65–85% of patients [51–58]. After endoscopic drainage, retrospective studies report a highly variable complete pain relief of 15–84% [19, 28, 29, 38, 39, 42–44].

Only two randomized trials have been published that compare endoscopic and surgical drainage in a prospective manner and both report a clear-cut benefit of surgery [10, 41]. A possible pathophysiological explanation for this finding is offered by Reber et al. [59], who showed in an animal study that surgery is more effective in alleviating the parenchymal pressure due to the opening of the pancreatic capsule. Moreover, in both randomized trials the outcome of endoscopic treatment was disappointing and much worse than would have been expected based on the available retrospective data.

In the first study, Dite et al. [41] observed complete pain relief in 14% of patients only. However, the general opinion regarding this study is that it cannot be considered a fair comparison between the two treatment options because surgery on the one hand encompassed more than just a drainage procedure, and endoscopic drainage techniques did not meet the current standards. In the second randomized trial, which was published last year by our group in the *New England Journal of Medicine*, complete or partial pain relief was observed in 32% of patients assigned to endoscopic drainage as compared with 75% of patients who underwent surgical drainage [10]. Moreover, surgery resulted in a more rapid (within 6 weeks) and sustained pain relief during the 2 years of follow-up. For patients in the surgical group treatment consisted of a single intervention (the surgical procedure), while patients assigned to endoscopic treatment underwent a median of 5 therapeutic interventions and suffered considerable pain during this treatment period, even with a patent stent in situ. A possible limitation of this study is that the patients suffered from extensive disease and therefore, results might be different for a population with less complex pathology.

Recently a renowned center for ESWL treatment performed a third prospective randomized trial in which they compared conventional endoscopic treatment consisting of ESWL combined with endotherapy (stone clearance and stent placement in case of a pancreatic duct stricture) with ESWL alone. After 2 years, pain relapse was observed in 23 of the 55 patients that were randomized (42%) with an advantage of the ESWL alone treatment (38 vs. 45%) [14].

As prospective data suggest that the long-term success rate of endoscopic treatment is limited, the question remains if there is a role for endoscopic treatment of pancreatic duct obstructions in chronic pancreatitis. First, further development of endoscopic techniques might improve results. To date, studies that focus on the technical aspects of endoscopic treatment are rare and conflicting. On the one hand, some authors advocate a more aggressive approach: Costamagna et al. [29] have reported promising results of cumulative stenting with a success rate of 84%. Others are investigating less elaborate techniques. For instance, as mentioned above, Dumonceau et al. [14] achieved better results after ESWL treatment alone than in combination with endoscopic treatment. Future prospective studies are needed to solve these issues.

Second, a better patient selection might improve the outcome. Now that in patients with complex pathology (with multiple strictures and stones) endoscopic drainage seems to be inferior to surgery, the interest shifts to patients with less extensive disease. There is evidence that in symptomatic patients with a single obstruction or stone, the course of the disease may be favorably altered by an early intervention. Farnbacher et al. [9] found that the only parameter predictive of long-term pain relief after endoscopic pancreatic duct drainage was a short duration of disease. Also, animal studies have shown that pancreatic insufficiency develops early in the course of obstructive pancreatitis and becomes permanent within several weeks [60]. Therefore, the best way to prevent irreversible damage and pancreatic function loss may be to decompress the duct at a very early stage. Moreover, even patients without symptoms may benefit from endoscopic drainage. At present, in this third category of patients, duct decompression is postponed until symptoms of pain or recurrent flare-ups of pancreatitis develop. Future studies should evaluate if early duct decompression may prevent a course of intractable pain in such patients.

Summary

In conclusion, recent evidence suggests that surgery offers a better chance of success in patients with extensive obstructive pancreatitis and a combination of strictures and multiple stones. However, this does not write off endoscopic pancreatic duct drainage in chronic pancreatitis. It may well be that patients with less complex pathology will benefit from endoscopic treatment at an early stage of the disease, but this needs to be proven. Moreover, endoscopic therapy may still be justifiable in selected patients with extensive disease who show a favorable pain response within the first 8 weeks of stent treatment. If not, or when stricture resolution is not accomplished after a treatment period of 1–2 years, patients should be referred for surgery.

Pseudocyst Drainage

Introduction

Pseudocyst formation is a frequent complication of chronic pancreatitis with a reported incidence of 20–40% [61–63] and in contrast to acute pancreatitis, spontaneous resolution is rare [64–68]. Two mechanisms of cyst formation have been postulated. First, cysts may follow an acute exacerbation of the disease ('acute on chronic pancreatitis') when peripancreatic fluid becomes organized in a walled-off collection. The second mechanism suggests an obstruction of a side branch of the pancreatic duct that results in a saccular dilatation. Pancreatic duct disruption and obstruction often accompany pseudocysts in chronic pancreatitis and if a communication between the duct and the pseudocyst is present, cyst drainage requires addressing these duct abnormalities because otherwise they will maintain filling of the cyst [69–71].

In chronic pancreatitis, indications for pseudocyst drainage are persistent symptoms and cyst-related complications. Pancreatic pseudocysts may lead to compression of the gastrointestinal tract, the biliary system or major vessels. Furthermore, spontaneous rupturing, bleeding and secondary infection of the cyst may occur. Whether asymptomatic pseudocysts should be treated is debatable. The decision to drain is made based on the estimated chance of spontaneous resolution on the one hand, and the chance of developing complications on the other. Both figures are not exactly known for patients with chronic pancreatitis, but they are likely to be less than 10% [64–68, 72]. Available data suggests that for cysts <6 cm in diameter, the resolution rate is even higher and because complications are rare in these small cysts, a wait-and-see policy is defendable [65, 73, 74]. Moreover, also for larger asymptomatic cysts, a conservative follow-up has become more common, although a rapid increase in size is still considered an indication for drainage.

Imaging Studies
Prior to drainage, imaging studies are performed. Computed tomography has long been the key investigation in this setting. However, MRCP has evolved and provides excellent imaging of the pancreas and pancreatic region, comparable with computed tomography [75–77]. Furthermore, MRCP has additional value because it can be used to evaluate the pancreatic duct and therefore has become the first choice imaging modality when pseudocysts are suspected. Further prospective studies are necessary to assess if a MRCP can annul the need of a retrograde pancreatogram. Secretin-stimulated MRCP is able to visualize the pancreatic duct in 97% of patients but an endoscopic retrograde cholangiopancreatography is superior in depicting subtle pancreatic duct abnormalities [78]. At present, it has not been ascertained that MRCP is able to diagnose all clinically relevant duct abnormalities, in particular ductal communication with the pseudocyst [79].

Alternative drainage Modalities
Historically, surgical pseudocyst drainage was associated with significant morbidity (7–37%) and mortality (0–6%) [80–85] and therefore less invasive techniques were welcomed. However, in the future, evolvement of laparoscopic techniques might expand the role of surgical drainage again [86–88]. Percutaneous drainage is generally dismissed because it requires the presence of an external drain for an extended period of time and because it frequently leads to fistula formation [89–91]. At present, endoscopic pseudocyst drainage is the only feasible alternative to surgery and can be performed either through the gastrointestinal wall of the stomach or duodenum (transmural approach), or transpapillary if a connection of the cyst with the pancreatic duct is present.

Procedural Aspects

General Aspects
Prior to the procedure a broad-spectrum antibiotic prophylaxis should be administered to decrease the risk of infectious complications [92]. The procedure is generally carried out under conscious sedation but it can be helpful to perform the procedure under general anesthesia, especially if multiple cysts need to be drained or the procedure is combined with an ERCP.

Transpapillary Drainage
Transpapillary drainage is the most straightforward and probably the safest drainage route [39, 87, 93, 94]. It requires communication of the cyst with the pancreatic duct and is performed by inserting an endoprosthesis in the pancreatic duct over a guidewire. Whether the endoprosthesis should be advanced all the way into the cyst cavity is unknown. Placement of the stent into the cyst may optimize drainage. A possible disadvantage may be that the outflow from the pancreatic duct located upstream from the cyst is compromised.

Transpapillary drainage is indicated when duct abnormalities (strictures and/or disruptions) are present because they will maintain filling of the cyst. Therefore, imaging of the pancreatic duct system (by MRCP or ERCP) is recommended prior to drainage. Because duct strictures require prolonged dilation treatment, stent therapy is generally continued well after cyst resolution has been accomplished. The disadvantage of transpapillary drainage is that it will often not suffice if a pseudocyst is large or contains debris, because a single small-diameter stent cannot provide sufficient drainage. In that case, a combination of transpapillary and a transmural drainage is recommended [93]. In our practice we consider cysts >6 cm an indication for drainage by multiple routes.

Transmural Drainage

Transmural pseudocyst drainage is achieved by placing stents through the wall of the stomach or duodenum. Traditionally, a side-viewing endoscope was used to puncture the gastrointestinal wall at the site of most the prominent bulge. With the introduction of endosonography (EUS), cyst drainage techniques have greatly evolved. At first, a radial echoendoscope was used in a step-by-step procedure to identify the optimal drainage site [86, 95, 96]. Subsequently, a side-viewing duodenoscope was introduced to perform the drainage procedure.

Later, the single-step technique was developed using a therapeutic linear echoendoscope, with a number of potential advantages; it is likely to shorten the procedure time and does not carry the risk that the identified drainage site will be lost when the endoscopes are switched. Furthermore, real-time vision of the puncture allows better identification of the safest and shortest drainage route [97]. In addition, EUS guided drainage expanded the indications of pseudocyst drainage because it allows drainage of non-bulging cysts. Finally, it allows a better definition of the amount of debris and necrosis within the cyst.

Retrospective studies reported conflicting results of this technique and the single prospective cohort study did not find a clear difference in safety or efficacy compared to the conventional two-step approach. Only one prospective randomized trial compared the two drainage procedures and reports a 100% success rate of EUS guided drainage as compared to a 33% success rate of the conventional drainage technique, with a similar complication rate. At present, the 'EUS-guided' technique has been adopted as the preferred drainage method by most expert centers [98].

There are several techniques to perform EUS-guided drainage utilizing a range of different accessories. Application is largely based on personal preference and experience. Nevertheless, some general remarks can be made with respect to their implementation. The procedure is started by determining the optimal puncture site, either in the stomach or in the duodenum. The site is selected based on the presence of interposing blood vessels and the distance between the cyst and the gastrointestinal wall. Generally, a distance up to 1 cm is considered safe; however, drainage is possible up to a distance of 2.5 cm.

To enter the cyst, a regular sphincterotome is not recommended as it is associated with an increased risk of bleeding. Access can be gained with a 19-gauge needle, or electrocoagulation may be used to burn a hole with a specially designed cystotome. An advantage of the latter is that it is relatively easy to introduce a catheter once the inner part of the cystotome is inside the cyst. A disadvantage is that the inner part of the cystotome is floppy and that its EUS visibility is poor. Furthermore, Monkemuller observed less bleeding when puncturing was performed without electrocoagulation [99, 100]. Therefore, we prefer to use a regular 19-gauge needle.

It is important to puncture the cyst as tangentially as possible to decrease the distance that needs to be traversed. Once the needle is inside, cyst fluid is aspirated for culture, cytology and analysis of biochemical markers and 10–20 cc of contrast is injected to delineate the cyst. A stiff, long (480-cm) ERCP guidewire is then advanced into the cyst to secure access and the most difficult part of the procedure, dilation of the cyst-gastrostomy tract, begins (fig. 2). It is almost always possible to follow the wire with an 8-mm biliary dilation balloon. If the dilation balloon cannot be passed into the cyst, the outer part of the cystotome can be advanced over the guidewire into the cyst using electrocoagulation. Other options include the use of a narrow tip ERCP

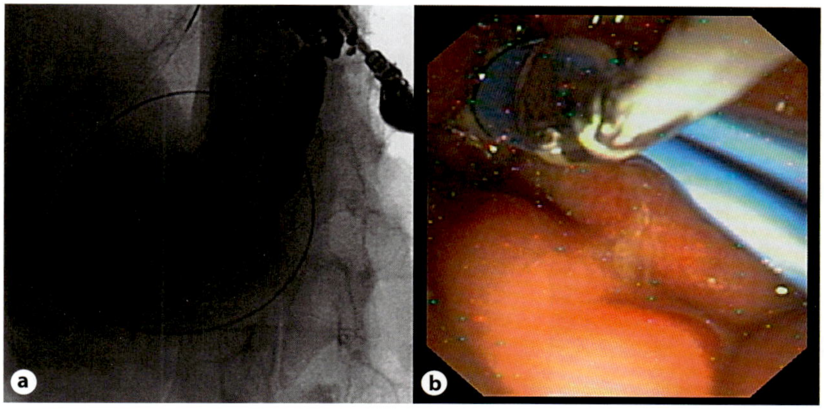

Fig. 2. Transgastric pseudocyst drainage. **a** Fluoroscopic image of the dilatation of the cystenterostomy opening with balloon. **b** Endoscopic image of the dilatation procedure after the first two pigtail stents have already been inserted.

cannula, a biliary dilation catheter, or a 6-Fr cystotome. At this stage it is important to use the ultrasound image to keep the optimal position and only convert to the endoscopic image after the dilation balloon has entered the cyst cavity.

Insertion of multiple (mostly three) endoprosthesis is recommended to prevent clogging and secondary infection of the cyst [101]. After placement of the first stent, one needs to regain access into the cyst for subsequent stent placement. This can be difficult due to a change in the position of the endoscope once the cyst is decompressed. Therefore, it is best to introduce a second guidewire before placing the first stent. If a cystotome was used to gain access, it is easy to introduce two guidewires through the outer catheter. Another option is to use an 8.5-Fr stent introduction system (Oasis®; Cook Endoscopy, Inc.) which makes it quite easy to place a second wire inside the cyst [19]. Generally, 7-Fr stents with a length of 4–6 cm suffice. Stents with a double pigtail configuration are advocated because they are safer, with less chance of migration, perforation, and bleeding due to erosion of the stent though the cyst wall [87, 96].

If there is a clinical suspicion of infection it is advisable to place a 6-Fr nasocystic catheter and start cyst irrigation with 1 liter of water or saline per 24 h with manual boluses of 100–200 ml every 4–6 h depending on cyst size and aspect. When the cyst contains debris and solid or necrotic material, an endoscopic reintervention should be performed after 1 or 2 days with further dilation of the fistulous tract up to 18 mm to allow endoscopic debridement with a forward viewing endoscope. A therapeutic gastroscope has a better suctioning capability, but is less flexible. Necrosectomy is best done with a Dormia basket or a Roth net and occasionally a grasping forceps can be useful. If stents are removed during the necrosectomy, it is important to leave at least one stent in place to reduce the chance of a blow-out of the cyst due to hyperinflation. Usually several repeat procedures are necessary until viable tissue of the wall of the cyst is clearly visible. In between these procedures cyst irrigation is maintained using a nasocystic catheter.

Before stents are endoscopically removed, cyst resolution is affirmed by an abdominal ultrasound, computed tomography or MRCP. The optimal duration of drainage is unknown, but generally the stents are left in place for at least several weeks [87, 102]. In our retrospective study, we observed superior outcome after a drainage period of at least 6 weeks, and therefore we have

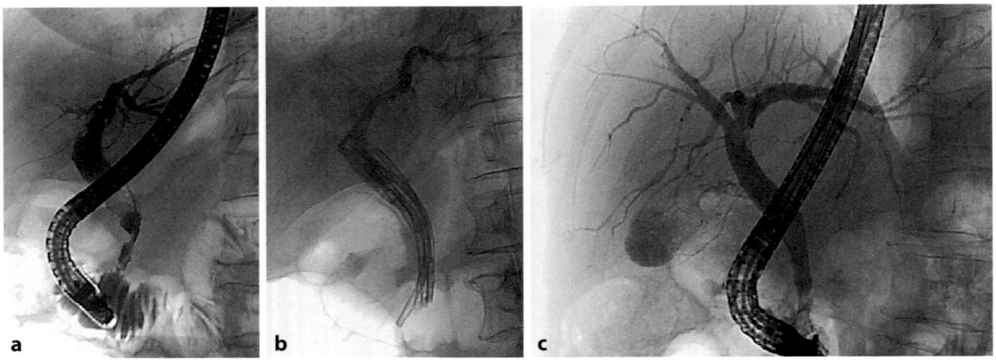

Fig. 3. **a** Stenosis of the distal common bile duct in chronic pancreatitis. **b** In 2 sessions placement of in the end 5 stents. **c** Excellent fluoroscopic result of endoscopic treatment..

adapted our drainage protocol accordingly [86]. Under specific circumstances it is probably safe to leave the stents in situ for an indefinite period, e.g. in older patients and in patients that are not able to undergo any further interventions. An interesting topic for future research is the use of covered metal stents or biodegradable stents instead of plastic stents to maintain the fistulous tract between the cyst and gastrointestinal lumen [103, 104].

Outcome

A systematic review of 25 published series regarding endoscopic pseudocyst drainage in a total of 569 patients reported an overall success rate of 81% (range 50–100%), a complication rate of 12%, a mortality rate of less than 1%, and a recurrence rate of 14% [87]. However, these studies encompassed patients suffering from both acute and chronic pancreatitis, which is relevant because the outcome seems to be more favorable for patients with chronic pancreatitis.

Beckingham was the first to observe that the success rate varied according to the nature of the underlying disease (75% in chronic pancreatitis as opposed to 25% in acute pancreatitis) [105]. Baron et al. confirmed this finding when he differentiated outcome according to acute, necrotizing and chronic pancreatitis and reported that pseudocyst drainage was the most effective and the safest for patients with chronic pancreatic with a success rate of 92% and a complication rate of 17% [95]. Retrospective studies have suggested a more favorable outcome in patients with a cyst located in the pancreatic head [106]. Furthermore, although the transgastric route is most often performed, some studies report a slight advantage of the transduodenal route [69, 87, 93, 107].

Summary

For patients with chronic pancreatitis, endoscopic pseudocyst drainage is an effective and safe therapeutic modality and should be the treatment of first choice when available. However, pseudocyst drainage is a challenging procedure and requires an experienced interventional endoscopist. Surgery and percutaneous drainage should be reserved for patients in whom endoscopic drainage has failed.

Biliary Drainage

Introduction

Approximately 10–30% of patients with chronic pancreatitis will develop a common bile duct obstruction during the course of their disease [105]. This biliary obstruction may arise from two distinct mechanisms; compression of the duct as a result of periductal swelling of the pancreas caused by acute inflammation, or fibrotic stricturing caused by ductal damage due to the chronic inflammatory process. Biliary strictures are associated with a broad spectrum of presentations, from mildly elevated liver enzymes to complete biliary obstruction. Cholangitis is a life-threatening complication and an obvious indication for drainage, but subclinical cholestasis requires drainage too, as it may lead to secondary biliary cirrhosis. Therefore, biliary drainage is indicated regardless of the presenting symptoms [108, 109]. Traditionally, a surgical bypass (i.e., choledochojejunostomy or hepatojejunostomy) was the only treatment option. Although surgery provides a definite solution, the associated morbidity and mortality lead to the investigation of alternative drainage techniques. At present, endoscopic stenting is often chosen as the initial therapy, in analogy with postoperative biliary strictures for which endoscopic treatment was reported to be successful in 43–83% of patients [108, 110–113].

Procedural Aspects

When a biliary obstruction is suspected, imaging studies (computed tomography or MRCP) are necessary to affirm the diagnosis, to rule out malignancy, and to evaluate the presence of other pancreatitis associated complications. Subsequently, an endoscopic retrograde cholangiogram is performed. A common bile duct stricture is identified as a distal narrowing of the duct with prestenotic dilatation and/or delayed runoff of the contrast agent (fig. 3). At the start of stent treatment a biliary sphincterotomy is performed to facilitate repeat access to the biliary tree and enable insertion of multiple stents later in the course of treatment. In case of a tight stricture (which cannot be passed by a regular 5- to 6-Fr ERCP catheter), dilatation is indicated, either with a balloon or graduated dilating catheter. Finally, a polyethylene Amsterdam-type stent (10-Fr) is inserted over a guiding catheter, long enough to bridge the stricture (usually 7 or 9 cm between the flaps).

Generally, after 3 months a cholangiogram is repeated. The stricture is considered sufficiently dilated when the stricture-waist and the proximal dilatation have disappeared. Furthermore, duct patency can be affirmed with a regular ERCP catheter, which should pass the stricture without resistance. In addition, observing a rapid runoff of the injected contrast agent (within 1–2 min) is proof of sufficient stricture resolution. When the stricture is resolved the stent treatment is terminated, but if the stricture persists, treatment needs to be continued. The aim of further stenting should be to maximize the dilation force. This is accomplished by inserting multiple stents in a cumulative fashion. With each procedure the stricture is first further dilated, followed by the insertion of an increasing number of endoprostheses. When stricture resolution is not accomplished within a 1-year period (after 3 stent exchange procedures), a successful outcome is highly unlikely and surgery should be considered [114].

An interesting development is the use of self-expandable metal stents as an alternative treatment. A number of small series showed metal stents to be effective in treating biliary strictures due to chronic pancreatitis, but their irremovable nature makes them unsuitable for use in this benign disease [104, 115–118]. To overcome this problem, removable metal stents were developed, equipped with a covering and extraction lasso to enable stent extraction. At present, experience with these stents is limited to several positive case reports [103, 119]. Future studies should aim at further improving this technique, because the larger stent diameter makes them an attractive alternative to dilatation with plastic stents; stent occlusion occurs less often and frequent stent exchanges are unnecessary [120]. Furthermore, treatment may be more efficient because the maximal dilatation force is effective from the very beginning of endoscopic treatment, in contrast to cumulative insertion of plastic stents, in which case the dilatation force is gradually increased with each procedure.

Outcome

Obviously, biliary stents are able to resolve cholestasis temporarily, but they are less likely to achieve long-term dilatation in patients with chronic pancreatitis. Published series reported disappointing long-term success rates of 10–38% using single stents [114, 121–124]. Despite the overall poor results of endoscopic treatment, a subset of patients might benefit from biliary drainage. Kahl et al. [124] evaluated prognostic factors of outcome in biliary stenting and showed that the presence of calcifications in the pancreatic head was a strong predictor of a more negative outcome. In the 39 patients with calcifications, long-term success was achieved in 8% only, whereas in the 22 patients without calcifications a successful long-term outcome was observed in 59%. The explanation for this finding may be found in the different mechanisms of biliary obstruction in chronic pancreatitis. Because calcifications are a sign of long-standing chronic pancreatitis, one might hypothesize that the strictures in these patients are of fibrotic nature and therefore difficult to dilate. The patients without calcifications are more likely to have developed an obstruction secondary to edema, which subsides over time and only requires temporary bridging of the stricture. For this purpose, stent placement is most appropriate. Results from our recently published series endorse this theory with the presence of concomitant acute pancreatitis resulting in a 95% chance of a successful treatment as opposed to a 24% success rate in its absence [114]. This phenomenon might also explain the unusually high 80% success rate observed by Vitale et al. [125] after balloon dilatation and stenting of biliary strictures; calcifications were present in only 4 out of the 20 patients that were studied.

An obvious way to improve outcome is a more vigorous dilatation of strictures by placing multiple stents. In the treatment of postoperative biliary strictures, this has been proven highly effective, and Draganov et al. [126] was the first to apply this method to patients with chronic pancreatitis. By inserting a cumulative number of stents with each procedure, stricture resolution was achieved in 4 of 9 patients (44%). However, in the subgroup of patients with calcifications, the results remained disappointing; stricture resolution was accomplished in 1 of 6 patients. Pozsár et al. [127] later placed the maximal number of stents that the stricture would allow (with a median of 2), which resulted in a 60% stricture resolution. Catalano et al. [31] even achieved a 100% success rate in 12 patients by inserting at least 4 stents.

Serious adverse events of biliary stenting are rare. Stent occlusion is the only complication that is frequently encountered (in most studies in approximately 35%), even when stents are exchanged on a regular basis [114, 123, 127–130]. Mostly, this complication is easily treated by stent exchange. However, in patients with pancreatitis caused by alcohol abuse, noncompliance is a considerable risk. Not showing for the arranged stent exchange can result in severe cholangitis, sepsis, and even death [127, 128].

Summary

At present, endoscopy has become the first-line approach for the treatment of postoperative biliary strictures, but strictures related to chronic pancreatitis are much more difficult to treat, especially fibrotic strictures, and patients should be informed about the limited efficacy. If, nevertheless, endoscopic therapy is chosen, an aggressive approach is preferred, with the insertion of a cumulative number of stents early in the course of treatment. When the stricture has not resolved within a 1-year period, the patient should be referred for surgery.

General Conclusions

In chronic pancreatitis, the lack of well-defined clinical trials combined with an evolving endoscopic technology has created a strong need for prospective studies to further clarify the indications, methods, and duration of endoscopic interventions. Overall, the future of endoscopic treatment in chronic pancreatitis seems to rely upon a pro-active approach; treating pancreatic duct strictures at an early stage of the disease, extensive debridement of pseudocysts, and a fierce dilatation of biliary strictures. Most importantly, surgery and endoscopic treatment should not be regarded as competing strategies but as complimentary treatments. Therefore, during the course of endoscopic treatment, patients should be carefully monitored and regularly discussed by a multidisciplinary team and when relief of symptoms and/or progression is not satisfactory, surgery must not be postponed. Moreover, when more than one complication is simultaneously diagnosed in a patient, (i.e. a pancreatic duct stricture and a common bile duct stricture) surgery might be considered at an earlier stage, because the overall chance of long-term endoscopic success decreases with each additional complication.

References

1 Karanjia ND, Widdison AL, Leung F, Alvarez C, Lutrin FJ, Reber HA: Compartment syndrome in experimental chronic obstructive pancreatitis: effect of decompressing the main pancreatic duct. Br J Surg 1994;81:259–264.
2 Ebbehoj N, Borly L, Bulow J, et al: Pancreatic tissue fluid pressure in chronic pancreatitis. Relation to pain, morphology, and function. Scand J Gastroenterol 1990;25: 1046–1051.
3 Choi KS, Kim MH: Extracorporeal shock wave lithotripsy for the treatment of pancreatic duct stones. J Hepatobiliary Pancreat Surg 2006;13:86–93.
4 Maydeo A, Soehendra N, Reddy N, Bhandari S: Endotherapy for chronic pancreatitis with intracanalar stones. Endoscopy 2007;39:653–658.
5 Tadenuma H, Ishihara T, Yamaguchi T, et al: Long-term results of extracorporeal shockwave lithotripsy and endoscopic therapy for pancreatic stones. Clin Gastroenterol Hepatol 2005;3:1128–1135.
6 Delhaye M, Vandermeeren A, Baize M, Cremer M: Extracorporeal shock-wave lithotripsy of pancreatic calculi. Gastroenterology 1992;102:610–620.

7 Deviere J, Delhaye M, Cremer M: Pancreatic duct stones management. Gastrointest Endosc Clin N Am 1998; 8:163–179.
8 Inui K, Tazuma S, Yamaguchi T, et al: Treatment of pancreatic stones with extracorporeal shock wave lithotripsy: results of a multicenter survey. Pancreas 2005;30:26–30.
9 Farnbacher MJ, Schoen C, Rabenstein T, Benninger J, Hahn EG, Schneider HT: Pancreatic duct stones in chronic pancreatitis: criteria for treatment intensity and success. Gastrointest Endosc 2002;56:501–506.
10 Cahen DL, Gouma DJ, Nio Y, et al: Endoscopic versus surgical drainage of the pancreatic duct in chronic pancreatitis. N Engl J Med 2007;356:676–684.
11 Kozarek RA, Brandabur JJ, Ball TJ, et al: Clinical outcomes in patients who undergo extracorporeal shock wave lithotripsy for chronic calcific pancreatitis. Gastrointest Endosc 2002;56:496–500.
12 Sasahira N, Tada M, Isayama H, et al: Outcomes after clearance of pancreatic stones with or without pancreatic stenting. J Gastroenterol 2007;42:63–69.
13 Adamek HE, Jakobs R, Buttmann A, Adamek MU, Schneider AR, Riemann JF: Long-term follow-up of patients with chronic pancreatitis and pancreatic stones treated with extracorporeal shock wave lithotripsy. Gut 1999;45:402–405.
14 Dumonceau JM, Costamagna G, Tringali A, et al: Treatment for painful calcified chronic pancreatitis: extracorporeal shock wave lithotripsy versus endoscopic treatment: a randomised controlled trial. Gut 2007;56: 545–552.
15 Brand B, Kahl M, Sidhu S, et al: Prospective evaluation of morphology, function, and quality of life after extracorporeal shockwave lithotripsy and endoscopic treatment of chronic calcific pancreatitis. Am J Gastroenterol 2000;95:3428–3438.
16 Delhaye M, Arvanitakis M, Verset G, Cremer M, Deviere J: Long-term clinical outcome after endoscopic pancreatic ductal drainage for patients with painful chronic pancreatitis. Clin Gastroenterol Hepatol 2004;2:1096–1106.
17 Guda NM, Partington S, Freeman ML: Extracorporeal shock wave lithotripsy in the management of chronic calcific pancreatitis: a meta-analysis. JOP 2005;6:6–12.
18 Costamagna G, Gabbrielli A, Mutignani M, et al: Extracorporeal shock wave lithotripsy of pancreatic stones in chronic pancreatitis: immediate and medium-term results. Gastrointest Endosc 1997;46: 231–236.
19 Rosch T, Daniel S, Scholz M, et al: Endoscopic treatment of chronic pancreatitis: a multicenter study of 1,000 patients with long-term follow-up. Endoscopy 2002;34: 765–771.
20 Ell C, Rabenstein T, Schneider HT, Ruppert T, Nicklas M, Bulling D: Safety and efficacy of pancreatic sphincterotomy in chronic pancreatitis. Gastrointest Endosc 1998; 48:244–249.
21 Jakobs R, Benz C, Leonhardt A, Schilling D, Pereira-Lima JC, Riemann JF: Pancreatic endoscopic sphincterotomy in patients with chronic pancreatitis: a single-center experience in 171 consecutive patients. Endoscopy 2002;34:551–554.
22 Hookey LC, RioTinto R, Delhaye M, Baize M, Le MO, Deviere J: Risk factors for pancreatitis after pancreatic sphincterotomy: a review of 572 cases. Endoscopy 2006; 38:670–676.
23 Okolo PI 3rd, Pasricha PJ, Kalloo AN: What are the long-term results of endoscopic pancreatic sphincterotomy? Gastrointest Endosc 2000;52:15–19.
24 Kim MH, Myung SJ, Kim YS, et al: Routine biliary sphincterotomy may not be indispensable for endoscopic pancreatic sphincterotomy. Endoscopy 1998;30:697–701.
25 Raju GS, Gomez G, Xiao SY, et al: Effect of a novel pancreatic stent design on short-term pancreatic injury in a canine model. Endoscopy 2006;38:260–265.
26 Eickhoff A, Weickert U, Riemann JF: Efficacy of S-type stents for the treatment of the main pancreatic duct stricture in patients with chronic pancreatitis. Scand J Gastroenterol 2007;42:537.
27 Ishihara T, Yamaguchi T, Seza K, Tadenuma H, Saisho H: Efficacy of S-type stents for the treatment of the main pancreatic duct stricture in patients with chronic pancreatitis. Scand J Gastroenterol 2006;41:744–750.
28 Laugier R, Renou C: Endoscopic ductal drainage may avoid resective surgery in painful chronic pancreatitis without large ductal dilatation. Int J Pancreatol 1998; 23:145–152.
29 Costamagna G, Bulajic M, Tringali A, et al: Multiple stenting of refractory pancreatic duct strictures in severe chronic pancreatitis: long-term results. Endoscopy 2006; 38:254–259.
30 Costamagna G, Pandolfi M, Mutignani M, Spada C, Perri V: Long-term results of endoscopic management of postoperative bile duct strictures with increasing numbers of stents. Gastrointest Endosc 2001;54:162–168.
31 Catalano MF, Linder JD, George S, Alcocer E, Geenen JE: Treatment of symptomatic distal common bile duct stenosis secondary to chronic pancreatitis: comparison of single vs. multiple simultaneous stents. Gastrointest Endosc 2004;60:945–952.
32 Testoni PA: Endoscopic stenting in benign pancreatic diseases. JOP 2007;8(suppl):141–150.
33 Ikenberry SO, Sherman S, Hawes RH, Smith M, Lehman GA: The occlusion rate of pancreatic stents. Gastrointest Endosc 1994;40:611–613.
34 Smith MT, Sherman S, Ikenberry SO, Hawes RH, Lehman GA: Alterations in pancreatic ductal morphology following polyethylene pancreatic stent therapy. Gastrointest Endosc 1996;44:268–275.
35 Morgan DE, Smith JK, Hawkins K, Wilcox CM: Endoscopic stent therapy in advanced chronic pancreatitis: relationships between ductal changes, clinical response, and stent patency. Am J Gastroenterol 2003;98: 821–826.

36 Gulliver DJ, Edmunds S, Baker ME, et al: Stent placement for benign pancreatic diseases: correlation between ERCP findings and clinical response. AJR Am J Roentgenol 1992;159:751–755.
37 Kozarek RA: Pancreatic stents can induce ductal changes consistent with chronic pancreatitis. Gastrointest Endosc 1990;36:93–95.
38 Eleftheriadis N: Long-term outcome after pancreatic stenting in severe chronic pancreatitis. Endoscopy 2005; 37:223–230.
39 Binmoeller KF, Jue P, Seifert H, Nam WC, Izbicki J, Soehendra N: Endoscopic pancreatic stent drainage in chronic pancreatitis and a dominant stricture: long-term results. Endoscopy 1995;27:638–644.
40 Renou C, Grandval P, Ville E, Laugier R: Endoscopic treatment of the main pancreatic duct: correlations among morphology, manometry, and clinical follow-up. Int J Pancreatol 2000;27:143–149.
41 Dite P, Ruzicka M, Zboril V, Novotny I: A prospective, randomized trial comparing endoscopic and surgical therapy for chronic pancreatitis. Endoscopy 2003;35:553–558.
42 Vitale GC, Cothron K, Vitale EA, et al: Role of pancreatic duct stenting in the treatment of chronic pancreatitis. Surg Endosc 2004;18:1431–1434.
43 Gabbrielli A, Pandolfi M, Mutignani M, et al: Efficacy of main pancreatic-duct endoscopic drainage in patients with chronic pancreatitis, continuous pain, and dilated duct. Gastrointest Endosc 2005;61:576–581.
44 Ponchon T, Bory RM, Hedelius F, et al: Endoscopic stenting for pain relief in chronic pancreatitis: results of a standardized protocol. Gastrointest Endosc 1995;42:452–456.
45 Weber A, Schneider J, Neu B, et al: Endoscopic stent therapy for patients with chronic pancreatitis: results from a prospective follow-up study. Pancreas 2007;34: 287–294.
46 Ammann RW, Muellhaupt B: The natural history of pain in alcoholic chronic pancreatitis. Gastroenterology 1999; 116:1132–1140.
47 Sandrasegaran K, Maglinte DD, Howard TJ, Lappas JC: Surgery for chronic pancreatitis: cross-sectional imaging of postoperative anatomy and complications. AJR Am J Roentgenol 2005;184:1118–1127.
48 O'Neil SJ, Aranha GV: Lateral pancreaticojejunostomy for chronic pancreatitis. World J Surg 2003;27:1196–1202.
49 Riediger H, Adam U, Fischer E, et al: Long-term outcome after resection for chronic pancreatitis in 224 patients. J Gastrointest Surg 2007;11:949–959.
50 Partington PF, Rochelle RE: Modified Puestow procedure for retrograde drainage of the pancreatic duct. Ann Surg 1960;152:1037–1043.
51 Izbicki JR, Bloechle C, Broering DC, Knoefel WT, Kuechler T, Broelsch CE: Extended drainage versus resection in surgery for chronic pancreatitis: a prospective randomized trial comparing the longitudinal pancreaticojejunostomy combined with local pancreatic head excision with the pylorus-preserving pancreatoduodenectomy: Ann Surg 1998;228: 771–779.
52 Strate T, Taherpour Z, Bloechle C, et al: Long-term follow-up of a randomized trial comparing the Beger and Frey procedures for patients suffering from chronic pancreatitis. Ann Surg 2005;241:591–598.
53 Frey CF, Mayer KL: Comparison of local resection of the head of the pancreas combined with longitudinal pancreaticojejunostomy (Frey procedure) and duodenum-preserving resection of the pancreatic head (Beger procedure). World J Surg 2003;27:1217–1230.
54 Rios GA, Adams DB, Yeoh KG, Tarnasky PR, Cunningham JT, Hawes RH: Outcome of lateral pancreaticojejunostomy in the management of chronic pancreatitis with nondilated pancreatic ducts. J Gastrointest Surg 1998;2:223–229.
55 Kalady MF, Broome AH, Meyers WC, Pappas TN: Immediate and long-term outcomes after lateral pancreaticojejunostomy for chronic pancreatitis. Am Surg 2001;67:478–483.
56 Schnelldorfer T, Adams DB: Outcome after lateral pancreaticojejunostomy in patients with chronic pancreatitis associated with pancreas divisum. Am Surg 2003;69:1041–1044.
57 Adams DB, Ford MC, Anderson MC: Outcome after lateral pancreaticojejunostomy for chronic pancreatitis. Ann Surg 1994;219:481–487.
58 Sielezneff I, Malouf A, Salle E, Brunet C, Thirion X, Sastre B: Long-term results of lateral pancreaticojejunostomy for chronic alcoholic pancreatitis. Eur J Surg 2000; 166:58–64.
59 Reber PU, Patel AG, Toyama MT, Ashley SW, Reber HA: Feline model of chronic obstructive pancreatitis: effects of acute pancreatic duct decompression on blood flow and interstitial pH. Scand J Gastroenterol 1999;34:439–444.
60 Lamme B, Boermeester MA, Straatsburg IH, et al: Early versus late surgical drainage for obstructive pancreatitis in an experimental model. Br J Surg 2007;94:849–854.
61 Beckingham IJ, Krige JE, Bornman PC, Terblanche J: Long-term outcome of endoscopic drainage of pancreatic pseudocysts. Am J Gastroenterol 1999; 94:71–74.
62 Baillie J: Pancreatic pseudocysts. Part I. Gastrointest Endosc 2004;59:873–879.
63 Barthet M, Bugallo M, Moreira LS, Bastid C, Sastre B, Sahel J: Management of cysts and pseudocysts complicating chronic pancreatitis. A retrospective study of 143 patients. Gastroenterol Clin Biol 1993; 17:270–276.
64 Vitas GJ, Sarr MG: Selected management of pancreatic pseudocysts: operative versus expectant management. Surgery 1992;111:123–130.

65 Gouyon B, Levy P, Ruszniewski P, et al: Predictive factors in the outcome of pseudocysts complicating alcoholic chronic pancreatitis. Gut 1997;41:821–825.

66 Beebe DS, Bubrick MP, Onstad GR, Hitchcock CR: Management of pancreatic pseudocysts. Surg Gynecol Obstet 1984;159:562–564.

67 Warshaw AL, Rattner DW: Timing of surgical drainage for pancreatic pseudocyst. Clinical and chemical criteria. Ann Surg 1985;202:720–724.

68 Bourliere M, Sarles H: Pancreatic cysts and pseudocysts associated with acute and chronic pancreatitis. Dig Dis Sci 1989;34:343–348.

69 Barthet M, Bugallo M, Moreira LS, Bastid C, Sastre B, Sahel J: Management of cysts and pseudocysts complicating chronic pancreatitis. A retrospective study of 143 patients. Gastroenterol Clin Biol 1993; 17:270–276.

70 Nealon WH, Walser E: Main pancreatic ductal anatomy can direct choice of modality for treating pancreatic pseudocysts (surgery vs. percutaneous drainage). Ann Surg 2002;235:751–758.

71 Nealon WH, Townsend CM Jr, Thompson JC: Preoperative endoscopic retrograde cholangiopancreatography in patients with pancreatic pseudocyst associated with resolving acute and chronic pancreatitis. Ann Surg 1989;209:532–538.

72 Yeo CJ, Bastidas JA, Lynch-Nyhan A, Fishman EK, Zinner MJ, Cameron JL: The natural history of pancreatic pseudocysts documented by computed tomography. Surg Gynecol Obstet 1990;170:411–417.

73 Maringhini A, Uomo G, Patti R, et al: Pseudocysts in acute nonalcoholic pancreatitis: incidence and natural history. Dig Dis Sci 1999;44:1669–1673.

74 Aranha GV, Prinz RA, Esguerra AC, Greenlee HB: The nature and course of cystic pancreatic lesions diagnosed by ultrasound. Arch Surg 1983;118:486–488.

75 Fayad LM, Kowalski T, Mitchell DG: MR cholangiopancreatography: evaluation of common pancreatic diseases. Radiol Clin North Am 2003;41:97–114.

76 Arvanitakis M, Delhaye M, De Maertelaere V, et al: Computed tomography and magnetic resonance imaging in the assessment of acute pancreatitis. Gastroenterology 2004;126:715–723.

77 Czako L: Diagnosis of early-stage chronic pancreatitis by secretin-enhanced magnetic resonance cholangiopancreatography. J Gastroenterol 2007;42 (suppl 17):113–117.

78 Hellerhoff KJ, Helmberger H 3rd, Rosch T, Settles MR, Link TM, Rummeny EJ: Dynamic MR pancreatography after secretin administration: image quality and diagnostic accuracy. AJR Am J Roentgenol 2002;179:121–129.

79 Tamura R, Ishibashi T, Takahashi S: Chronic pancreatitis: MRCP versus ERCP for quantitative caliber measurement and qualitative evaluation. Radiology 2006;238:920–928.

80 Yeo CJ, Bastidas JA, Lynch-Nyhan A, Fishman EK, Zinner MJ, Cameron JL: The natural history of pancreatic pseudocysts documented by computed tomography. Surg Gynecol Obstet 1990;170:411–417.

81 Lehman GA: Pseudocysts. Gastrointest Endosc 1999;49:S81–S84.

82 Adkisson KW, Baron TH, Morgan DE: Pancreatic fluid collections: diagnosis and endoscopic management. Semin Gastrointest Dis 1998;9:61–72.

83 Boerma D, van Gulik TM, Obertop H, Gouma DJ: Internal drainage of infected pancreatic pseudocysts: safe or sorry? Dig Surg 1999;16:501–505.

84 Rosso E, Alexakis N, Ghaneh P, et al: Pancreatic pseudocyst in chronic pancreatitis: endoscopic and surgical treatment. Dig Surg 2003;20:397–406.

85 Andrén-Sandberg A, Dervenis C: Pancreatic pseudocysts in the 21st century. Part II. Natural history. JOP 2004;5:64–70.

86 Yusuf TE, Baron TH: Endoscopic transmural drainage of pancreatic pseudocysts: results of a national and an international survey of ASGE members. Gastrointest Endosc 2006;63:223–227.

87 Cahen D, Rauws E, Fockens P, Weverling G, Huibregtse K, Bruno M: Endoscopic drainage of pancreatic pseudocysts: long-term outcome and procedural factors associated with safe and successful treatment. Endoscopy 2005; 37:977–983.

88 Cremer M, Deviere J, Engelholm L: Endoscopic management of cysts and pseudocysts in chronic pancreatitis: long-term follow-up after 7 years of experience. Gastrointest Endosc 1989;35:1–9.

89 Lohr-Happe A, Peiper M, Lankisch PG: Natural course of operated pseudocysts in chronic pancreatitis. Gut 1994;35:1479–1482.

90 Spivak H, Galloway JR, Amerson JR, et al: Management of pancreatic pseudocysts. J Am Coll Surg 1998;186:507–511.

91 Boggi U, Di Candio G, Campatelli A, Pietrabissa A, Mosca F: Nonoperative management of pancreatic pseudocysts. Problems in differential diagnosis. Int J Pancreatol 1999;25:123–133.

92 Mani V, Cartwright K, Dooley J, Swarbrick E, Fairclough P, Oakley C: Antibiotic prophylaxis in gastrointestinal endoscopy: a report by a Working Party for the British Society of Gastroenterology Endoscopy Committee. Endoscopy 1997;29:114–119.

93 Catalano MF, Geenen JE, Schmalz MJ, Johnson GK, Dean RS, Hogan WJ: Treatment of pancreatic pseudocysts with ductal communication by transpapillary pancreatic duct endoprosthesis. Gastrointest Endosc 1995; 42:214–218.

94 Barthet M, Sahel J, Bodiou-Bertei C, Bernard JP: Endoscopic transpapillary drainage of pancreatic pseudocysts. Gastrointest Endosc 1995;42:208–213.

95 Beckingham IJ, Krige JE, Bornman PC, Terblanche J: Long-term outcome of endoscopic drainage of pancreatic pseudocysts. Am J Gastroenterol 1999;94: 71–74.

96 Fockens P: EUS in drainage of pancreatic pseudocysts. Gastrointest Endosc 2002;56(suppl):S93–S97.
97 Lopes CV, Pesenti C, Bories E, Caillol F, Giovannini M: Endoscopic-ultrasound-guided endoscopic transmural drainage of pancreatic pseudocysts and abscesses. Scand J Gastroenterol 2007;42:524–529.
98 Kahaleh M, Shami VM, Conaway MR, et al: Endoscopic ultrasound drainage of pancreatic pseudocyst: a prospective comparison with conventional endoscopic drainage. Endoscopy 2006;38:355–359.
99 Antillon MR, Shah RJ, Stiegmann G, Chen YK: Single-step EUS-guided transmural drainage of simple and complicated pancreatic pseudocysts. Gastrointest Endosc 2006;63:797–803.
100 Ahlawat SK, Charabaty-Pishvaian A, Jackson PG, Haddad NG: Single-step EUS-guided pancreatic pseudocyst drainage using a large channel linear array echoendoscope and cystotome: results in 11 patients. JOP 2006; 7:616–624.
101 Giovannini M, Pesenti C, Rolland AL, Moutardier V, Delpero JR: Endoscopic ultrasound-guided drainage of pancreatic pseudocysts or pancreatic abscesses using a therapeutic echo endoscope. Endoscopy 2001;33:473–477.
102 Baillie J: Pancreatic pseudocysts. Part I. Gastrointest Endosc 2004;59:873–879.
103 Cahen DL, Rauws EA, Gouma DJ, Fockens P, Bruno MJ: Removable fully covered self-expandable metal stents in the treatment of common bile duct strictures due to chronic pancreatitis: a case series. Endoscopy 2008;40: 697–700.
104 Van Berkel AM, Cahen DL, van Westerloo DJ, Rauws EA, Huibregtse K, Bruno MJ: Self-expanding metal stents in benign biliary strictures due to chronic pancreatitis. Endoscopy 2004;36:381–384.
105 Aljarabah M, Ammori BJ: Laparoscopic and endoscopic approaches for drainage of pancreatic pseudocysts: a systematic review of published series. Surg Endosc 2007;21:1936–1944.
106 Baron TH, Harewood GC, Morgan DE, Yates MR: Outcome differences after endoscopic drainage of pancreatic necrosis, acute pancreatic pseudocysts, and chronic pancreatic pseudocysts. Gastrointest Endosc 2002;56:7–17.
107 Binmoeller KF, Seifert H, Walter A, Soehendra N: Transpapillary and transmural drainage of pancreatic pseudocysts. Gastrointest Endosc 1995;42:219–224.
108 Warshaw AL, Schapiro RH, Ferrucci JT Jr, Galdabini JJ: Persistent obstructive jaundice, cholangitis, and biliary cirrhosis due to common bile duct stenosis in chronic pancreatitis. Gastroenterology 1976;70: 562–567.
109 Afroudakis A, Kaplowitz N: Liver histopathology in chronic common bile duct stenosis due to chronic alcoholic pancreatitis. Hepatology 1981;1:65–72.
110 Stahl TJ, Allen MO, Ansel HJ, Vennes JA: Partial biliary obstruction caused by chronic pancreatitis. An appraisal of indications for surgical biliary drainage. Ann Surg 1988;207:26–32.
111 Huizinga WK, Thomson SR, Spitaels JM, Simjee AE: Chronic pancreatitis with biliary obstruction. Ann R Coll Surg Engl 1992;74:119–123.
112 Aranha GV, Prinz RA, Freeark RJ, Greenlee HB: The spectrum of biliary tract obstruction from chronic pancreatitis. Arch Surg 1984;119:595–600.
113 De Reuver PR, Rauws EA, Vermeulen M, Dijkgraaf MG, Gouma DJ, Bruno MJ: Endoscopic treatment of post-surgical bile duct injuries: long-term outcome and predictors of success. Gut 2007;56:1599–1605.
114 Cahen DL, van Berkel AM, Oskam D, et al: Long-term results of endoscopic drainage of common bile duct strictures in chronic pancreatitis. Eur J Gastroenterol Hepatol 2005;17:103–108.
115 Wadhwa RP, Kozarek RA, France RE, et al: Use of self-expandable metallic stents in benign GI diseases. Gastrointest Endosc 2003;58:207–212.
116 Yamaguchi T, Ishihara T, Seza K, et al: Long-term outcome of endoscopic metallic stenting for benign biliary stenosis associated with chronic pancreatitis. World J Gastroenterol 2006;12:426–430.
117 Deviere J, Cremer M, Baize M, Love J, Sugai B, Vandermeeren A: Management of common bile duct stricture caused by chronic pancreatitis with metal mesh self-expandable stents. Gut 1994;35:122–126.
118 Kahl S, Zimmermann S, Glasbrenner B, et al: Treatment of benign biliary strictures in chronic pancreatitis by self-expandable metal stents. Dig Dis 2002;20:199–203.
119 Kahaleh M, Tokar J, Le T, Yeaton P: Removal of self-expandable metallic wall stents. Gastrointest Endosc 2004;60:640–644.
120 Soderlund C, Linder S: Covered metal versus plastic stents for malignant common bile duct stenosis: a prospective, randomized, controlled trial. Gastrointest Endosc 2006;63:986–995.
121 Barthet M, Bernard JP, Duval JL, Affriat C, Sahel J: Biliary stenting in benign biliary stenosis complicating chronic calcifying pancreatitis. Endoscopy 1994;26:569–572.
122 Deviere J, Devaere S, Baize M, Cremer M: Endoscopic biliary drainage in chronic pancreatitis. Gastrointest Endosc 1990;36:96–100.
123 Smits ME, Rauws EA, van Gulik TM, Gouma DJ, Tytgat GN, Huibregtse K: Long-term results of endoscopic stenting and surgical drainage for biliary stricture due to chronic pancreatitis. Br J Surg 1996;83:764–768.
124 Kahl S, Zimmermann S, Genz I, et al: Risk factors for failure of endoscopic stenting of biliary strictures in chronic pancreatitis: a prospective follow-up study. Am J Gastroenterol 2003;98:2448–2453.

125 Vitale GC, Reed DN Jr, Nguyen CT, Lawhon JC, Larson GM: Endoscopic treatment of distal bile duct stricture from chronic pancreatitis. Surg Endosc 2000;14:227–231.
126 Draganov P, Hoffman B, Marsh W, Cotton P, Cunningham J: Long-term outcome in patients with benign biliary strictures treated endoscopically with multiple stents. Gastrointest Endosc 2002;55:680–686.
127 Pozsár J, Sahin P, Laszlo F, Topa L: Endoscopic treatment of sphincterotomy-associated distal common bile duct strictures by using sequential insertion of multiple plastic stents. Gastrointest Endosc 2005;62: 85–91.
128 Kiehne K, Folsch UR, Nitsche R: High complication rate of bile duct stents in patients with chronic alcoholic pancreatitis due to noncompliance. Endoscopy 2000;32:377–380.
129 Farnbacher MJ, Rabenstein T, Ell C, Hahn EG, Schneider HT: Is endoscopic drainage of common bile duct stenoses in chronic pancreatitis up-to-date? Am J Gastroenterol 2000;95:1466–1471.
130 Eickhoff A, Jakobs R, Leonhardt A, et al: Endoscopic stenting for common bile duct stenoses in chronic pancreatitis: results and impact on long-term outcome. Eur J Gastroenterol Hepatol 2001;13:1161–1167.

Djuna Cahen, MD, PhD
Erasmus Medical Centre, University Medical Center Rotterdam
Department of Gastroenterology and Hepatology
's Gravendijkwal 230, NL–3015 CE Rotterdam (The Netherlands)
Tel. +31 10 7035946, Fax +31 10 7034682, E-Mail d.cahen@erasmusmc.nl

Mönkemüller K, Wilcox CM, Muñoz-Navas M (eds): Interventional and Therapeutic Gastrointestinal Endoscopy.
Front Gastrointest Res. Basel, Karger, 2010, vol 27, pp 477–484

Endoscopic Management of Pancreatic Fluid Collections

Todd H. Baron

Division of Gastroenterology and Hepatology, Mayo Clinic, Rochester, Minn., USA

Abstract

There are a variety of pancreatic fluid collections. Purely liquefied collections include acute and chronic pancreatic pseudocysts, acute fluid collections, and pancreatic abscesses. These types of collections can be drained endoscopically using a transpapillary and/or transmural approach with placement of plastic stents. Pancreatic necrosis can be drained using a transmural approach with removal of solid material using techniques similar to those used for natural orifice transluminal endoscopic surgery.

Several types of pancreatic fluid collections (PFCs) may arise as a result of pancreatitis [1]. This chapter reviews the endoscopic management of PFCs.

Pancreatic Fluid Collections

PFCs arise as complication of acute and chronic pancreatitis or pancreatic trauma (including surgery; table 1).

It is often assumed that any PFC arising as a consequence of pancreatitis represents a pancreatic pseudocyst. However, several distinct entities fall under the general term PFCs.

Acute Fluid Collections

Acute fluid collections arise early in the course of acute pancreatitis, are usually peripancreatic in location, usually resolve without sequelae, and rarely require drainage [1, 2].

Acute Pancreatic Pseudocyst

Acute pancreatic pseudocysts arise from acute pancreatitis, require at least 4 weeks to form, and are composed of liquid (fig. 1). They usually arise from limited pancreatic necrosis that produces a pancreatic ductal leak [3]. Despite requiring at least 4 weeks to form, this time period does not mean the collection is a pancreatic pseudocyst. Patients with significant pancreatic necrosis may develop a collection that resembles a pseudocyst by CT and has been present for ≥4 weeks [see Organized pancreatic necrosis, below]. Such collections contain significant solid debris and

Table 1. Types of pancreatic fluid collections complicating acute pancreatitis

Term	Definition
Acute fluid collection	A collection of enzyme-rich pancreatic juice occurring early (within 48 h) in the course of acute pancreatitis, located in or near the pancreas, and always lacking a well-defined wall of granulation tissue or fibrous tissue
Pseudocyst	A collection of pancreatic juice enclosed by a wall of non-epithelialized granulation tissue, which arises as a consequence of acute or chronic pancreatitis, requires at least 4 weeks to form, and is devoid of significant solid debris
Pancreatic necrosis (early)	A diffuse or focal area of nonviable pancreatic parenchyma of >30% of the gland by contrast-enhanced CT, which is typically associated with peripancreatic fat necrosis
Organized or walled-off pancreatic necrosis (late)	Evolution of acute necrosis to a partially encapsulated, well-defined collection of pancreatic juice and necrotic debris
Pancreatic abscess	A circumscribed intra-abdominal collection of pus, usually in proximity to the pancreas, containing little or no pancreatic necrosis, which arises as a consequence of acute pancreatitis or pancreatic trauma.

1 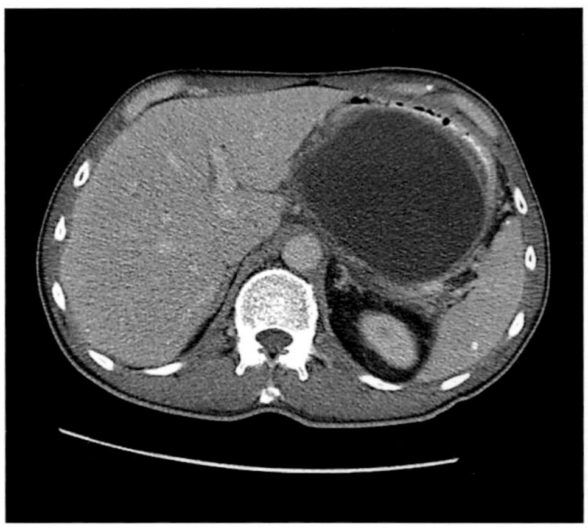

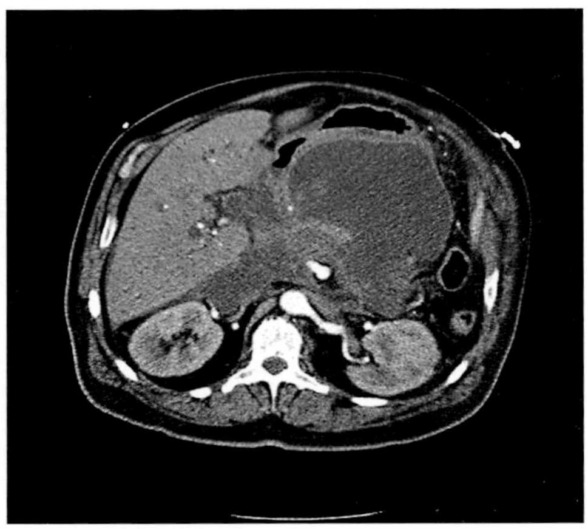 2

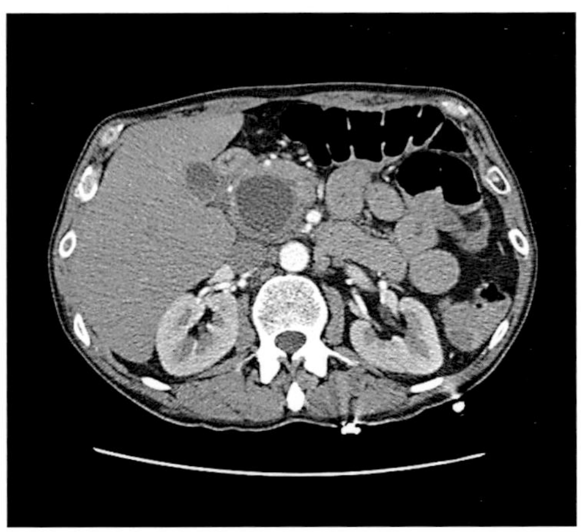 3

Fig. 1. Acute pseudocyst. CT demonstrates a homogeneous collection arising 4 weeks after clinically mild acute pancreatitis. The pseudocyst resolved with transmural drainage.

Fig. 2. Contrast CT scan demonstrating a large collection which has nearly replaced the pancreatic bed. This collection is consistent with organized pancreatic necrosis.

Fig. 3. Chronic pseudocyst. This patient had a history of chronic pancreatitis and presented with biliary obstruction from compression of the bile duct.

endoscopic treatment using pseudocyst drainage methods may result in infectious complications because solid debris are not removed [4].

Organized or Walled-Off Pancreatic Necrosis

Pancreatic necrosis is nonviable pancreatic parenchyma usually with peripancreatic fat necrosis. Contrast-enhanced CT early after onset of pancreatitis shows non-enhancing pancreatic parenchyma. Over the course of several weeks a collection may evolve and expand the initial area of necrosis that contains both liquid and solid debris (fig. 2). The resulting collection is termed organized or walled-off pancreatic necrosis (WOPN) [5]. The CT appearance may be similar and confused with an acute pseudocyst [6] and pseudocyst drainage methods may result in serious infectious complications [4, 7]. Features on CT can help distinguish WOPN from pancreatic pseudocysts [8].

Pancreatic Abscess

A pancreatic abscess is a collection of pus in close proximity to the pancreas and can include infected pancreatic pseudocysts.

Chronic Pancreatic Pseudocyst

Chronic pseudocysts result as a complication of chronic pancreatitis (fig. 3). Obstruction of the main pancreatic duct from strictures and/or stones results in upstream ductal blowout. Resultant symptoms requiring drainage are similar to that described for acute pseudocysts. In addition, pancreatic ascites and pancreaticopleural fistula can also occur [9].

Indications for Drainage of Pancreatic Fluid Collections

Indications for drainage of a pseudocyst are based upon symptoms and/or infection. Symptoms from compression of the stomach, duodenum or bile duct cause abdominal pain, gastric outlet obstruction, early satiety, weight loss, and jaundice. Progressive enlargement can be considered an indication for drainage in the absence of symptoms [10].

Pancreatic Necrosis

The indications for and the timing of endoscopic drainage of sterile organized pancreatic necrosis (OPN) are controversial. The process is not amenable to endoscopic drainage until it becomes organized, often several weeks after onset of pancreatitis. General indications for drainage of sterile OPN are refractory abdominal pain, gastric outlet obstruction or failure to thrive (ongoing systemic illness, anorexia, and weight loss) 4 or more weeks after onset of pancreatitis. Infected OPN is considered an indication for drainage.

Pancreatic Abscess

By definition, a pancreatic abscess is infected and is an indication for drainage.

Pre-Drainage Considerations

1 One must consider other collections which can be confused with pancreatic pseudocysts such as cystic pancreatic neoplasms, duplication cysts, true pancreatic cysts, and solid necrotic neoplasms [2, 11, 12]. These should be suspected when there is not a well-documented history of acute or chronic pancreatitis [13].

2 Consider underlying pancreatic adenocarcinoma in elderly patients without risk factors for pancreatitis [14].

Pre-Drainage Evaluation

1 Oral and intravenous contrast abdominal CT scan to assess the location of the collection in relation to the stomach and duodenum and to evaluate for intervening vascular structures and the presence of underlying solid debris [6].
2 Endoscopic ultrasound (EUS) can be used to assess significant solid debris that may alter the management strategy and whether the collection in question represents a true pseudocyst or a non-inflammatory cystic lesion [15]. EUS may be used to guide transmural drainage.

Endoscopic Methods of Drainage of Pancreatic Pseudocysts

Endoscopic methods to draining pseudocysts are transpapillary drainage [16, 17], transmural drainage [18], or combined transpapillary and transmural drainage [10, 19]. The approach is based upon whether the collection is adjacent to the stomach or duodenum, the presence of ductal communication, and the size of the collection.

Transpapillary Approach

If the pseudocyst communicates with the main pancreatic duct, placement of a pancreatic stent (without need for sphincterotomy) is useful for collections measuring ≤6 cm [20]. The proximal end of the stent should bridge the leak if possible (fig. 4) [21]. Transpapillary drainage avoids bleeding and perforation but pancreatic stents can cause ductal damage [22, 23].

Transmural Approach

Transmural drainage is achieved by placing one or more large-bore stents through the gastric or duodenal wall.

EUS-Guided Transmural Drainage

EUS imaging may increase the success rate and reduce complications related to transmural entry [24]. Transmural drainage can be performed entirely under EUS-guidance using Doppler-equipped therapeutic channel echo endoscopes [25].

Non-EUS-Guided Transmural Drainage

The collection is entered using needle-knife electrocautery at an endoscopically visible extrinsic compression with or without prelocalization using a needle [26]. Localization and entry can be performed using a large caliber needle without electrocautery using the Seldinger technique (fig. 5) [18]. Aspiration of fluid and/or injection of contrast confirm entry and a guidewire is passed through the needle-knife or aspiration needle and coiled within the collection (fig. 6). The tract is balloon-dilated to 8–12 mm (fig. 7) and one or more double pigtail 10-Fr stents are placed (fig. 8).

Follow-Up

A CT scan is obtained 4–6 weeks after drainage. The internal stents are endoscopically removed after documented radiographic resolution.

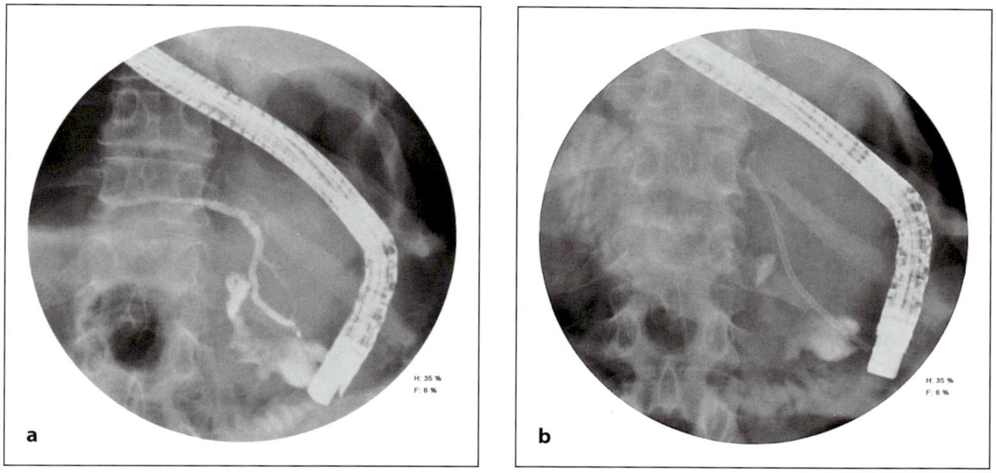

Fig. 4. Transpapillary drainage of a pancreatic pseudocyst. **a** Pancreatogram shows a leak off a side branch of the main pancreatic duct. **b** A pancreatic duct stent is in place across the leak.

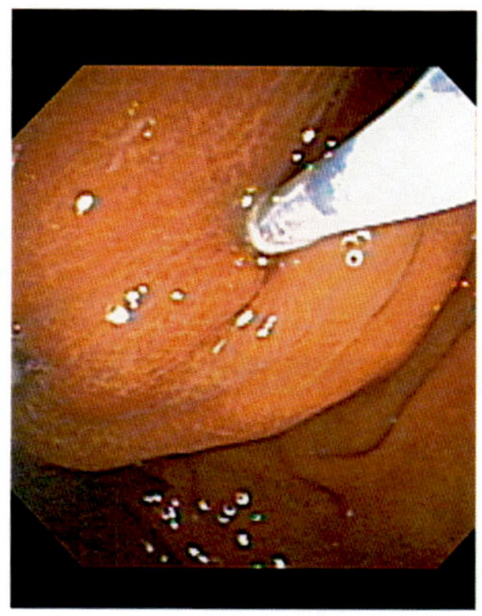

5

Fig. 5. Needle is placed through the posterior wall of the stomach at the site of extrinsic compression.

Fig. 6. **a** Endoscopic view of guidewire after withdrawal of needle. **b** Fluoroscopic image of wire coiled within the collection.

6

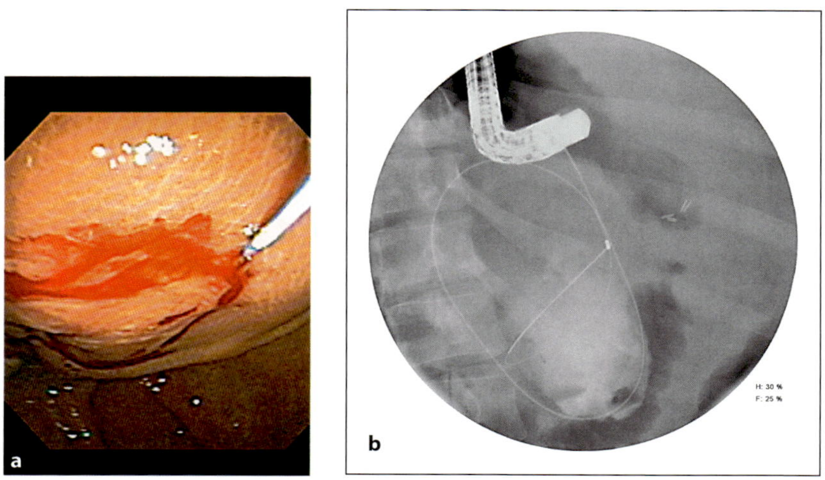

Table 2. Complications of endoscopic therapy of pancreatic fluid collections

Bleeding
Perforation
Infection
Pancreatitis
Sedation complications
Aspiration
Stent migration/occlusion
Pancreatic ductal damage

7
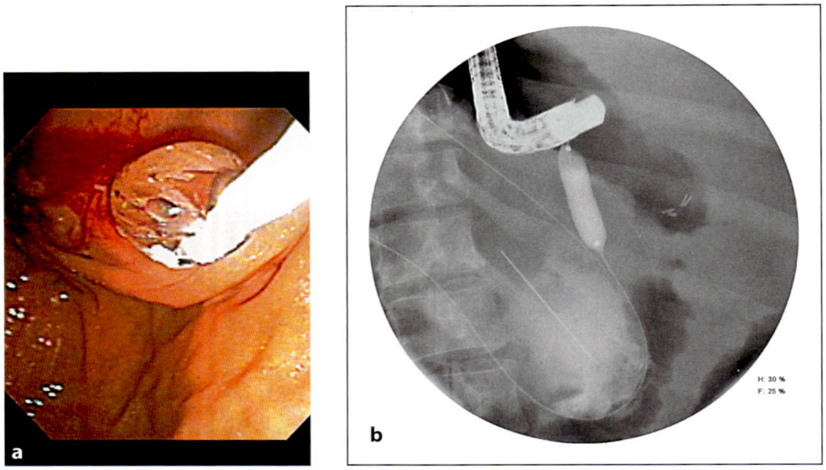

8
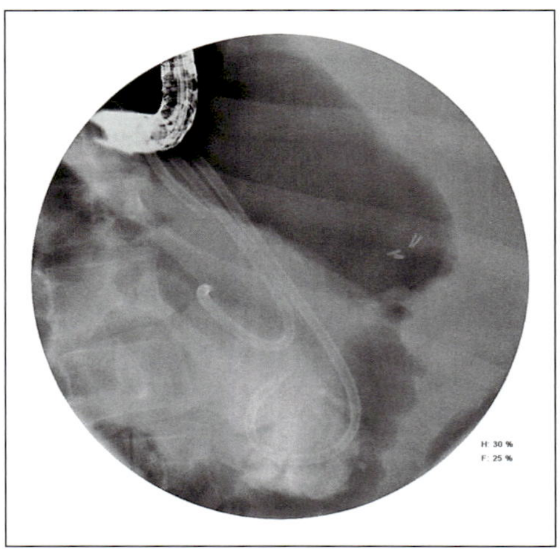

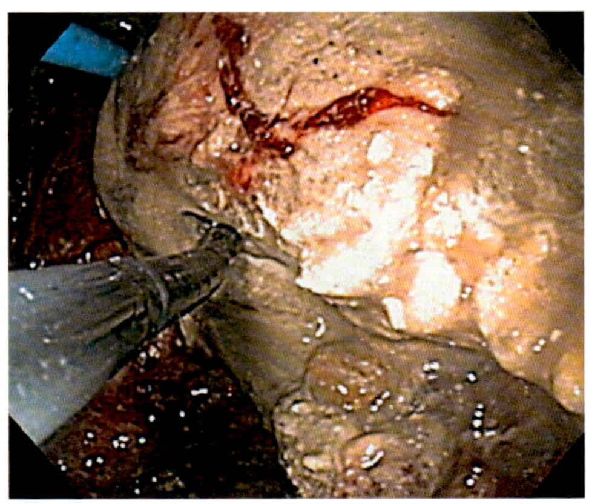
9

Fig. 7. **a** Endoscopic view of balloon dilation of transmural tract. **b** Fluoroscopic image of balloon dilation.

Fig. 8. Fluoroscopic image with two double pigtail stents placed through the wall into the collection.

Fig. 9. Endoscopic view from within necrotic pancreatic collection. Debridement is being performed with a forceps.

Endoscopic Drainage of OPN or WOPN

The transpapillary approach is not used to evacuate solid material. Transmural entry is performed and the gastric or duodenal wall is dilated to ≥15 mm on the initial endoscopy. 10-Fr stents are placed to allow re-access for subsequent debridement. A forward-viewing endoscope is passed transmurally into the necrotic cavity to allow direct endoscopic necrosectomy (fig. 9).

Complications of Endoscopic Therapy of PFCs

Life-threatening complications may arise following attempted endoscopic drainage of PFCs and are listed in table 2. Infectious complications usually occur from inadequate drainage of fluid and/or solid debris and can usually be managed by repeat endoscopy or placement of percutaneous drainage and/or irrigation catheters.

Results of Endoscopic Therapy of PFCs

Endoscopic drainage of pancreatic pseudocysts can be achieved in approximately 90% of cases with complication rates occurring in 5–10% and recurrence rates ranging from 6–18% [27, 28]. Retrospective data suggest similar success and complication rates between endoscopy and surgery for management of pseudocysts [29–31]. Pancreatic abscesses have been successfully drained endoscopically [32–34].

Organized or Walled-Off Pancreatic Necrosis

The endoscopic approach to WOPN has evolved since the initial descriptions. Successful nonsurgical resolution is achieved in approximately 80–85% of patients [35–37].

References

1 Baron TH, Morgan DE: The diagnosis and management of fluid collections associated with pancreatitis. Am J Med 1997;102:555–563.

2 Adkisson KW, Baron TH, Morgan DE: Pancreatic fluid collections: diagnosis and endoscopic management. Semin Gastrointest Dis 1998;9:61–72.

3 Kloppel G: Pathology of severe acute pancreatitis; in Bradley EL III (ed): Acute Pancreatitis: Diagnosis and Therapy. New York, Raven Press, 1994, pp 35–46.

4 Hariri M, Slivka A, Carr-Locke DL, et al: Pseudocyst drainage predisposes to infection when pancreatic necrosis is unrecognized. Am J Gastroenterol 1994;89: 1781–1784.

5 Baron TH, Morgan DE, Vickers SM, et al: Organized pancreatic necrosis: endoscopic, radiologic, and pathologic features of a distinct clinical entity. Pancreas 1999; 19:105–108.

6 Morgan DE, Baron TH, Smith JK, et al: Pancreatic fluid collections prior to intervention: evaluation with MR imaging compared with CT and US. Radiology 1997;203: 773–778.

7 Kozarek RA: Endotherapy for organized pancreatic necrosis: perspectives on skunk-poking. Gastroenterology 1996;111:820–822.

8 Takahashi N, Papachristou GI, Schmit GD, et al: CT findings of walled-off pancreatic necrosis (WOPN): differentiation from pseudocyst and prediction of outcome after endoscopic therapy. Eur Radiol 2008;18:2522–2529.

9 Pai CG, Suvarna D, Bhat G: Endoscopic treatment as first-line therapy for pancreatic ascites and pleural effusion. J Gastroenterol Hepatol 2009;24:1198–1202.

10 Libera ED, Siqueira ES, Morais M, et al: Pancreatic pseudocysts transpapillary and transmural drainage. HPB Surgery 2000;11:333–338.

11 Boggi U, Candio G, Campatelli A, et al: Nonoperative management of pancreatic pseudocysts. Problems in differential diagnosis. Int J Pancreatol 1999;25: 123–133.

12 Baron TH, Morgan DE, Vickers SM: Endoscopic transgastric drainage of a lymphocele. Gastrointest Endosc 1998;48:309–311.

13 Beckingham IJ, Krige JE, Bornman PC, et al: Endoscopic management of pancreatic pseudocysts. Br J Surg 1997; 84:1638–1645.

14 Itai Y, Moss AA, Goldberg HI: Pancreatic cysts caused by carcinoma of the pancreas: a pitfall in the diagnosis of pancreatic carcinoma. J Comput Assist Tomogr 1982;6: 772–776.
15 Brugge WR: The role of EUS in the diagnosis of cystic lesions of the pancreas. Gastrointest Endosc 2000;52:S18–S22.
16 Barthet M, Sahel J, Bodiou-Bertei C, et al: Endoscopic transpapillary drainage of pancreatic pseudocysts. Gastrointest Endosc 1995;42:208–213.
17 Catalano MF, Geenen JE, Schmalz MJ, et al: Treatment of pancreatic pseudocysts with ductal communication by transpapillary pancreatic duct endoprosthesis. Gastrointest Endosc 1995;42:214–218.
18 Monkemuller KE, Baron TH, Morgan DE: Transmural drainage of pancreatic fluid collections without electrocautery using the Seldinger technique. Gastrointest Endosc 1998;48:195–200.
19 Binmoeller KF, Seifert H, Walter A, et al: Transpapillary and transmural drainage of pancreatic psuedocysts. Gastrointest Endosc 1995;42:219–224.
20 Barthet M, Lamblin G, Gasmi M, Vitton V, Desjeux A, Grimaud JC: Clinical usefulness of a treatment algorithm for pancreatic pseudocysts. Gastrointest Endosc 2008;67:245–252.
21 Telford JJ, Farrell JJ, Saltzman JR, et al: Pancreatic stent placement for duct disruption. Gastrointest Endosc 2002;56:18–24.
22 Kozarek RA: Pancreatic stents can induce ductal changes consistent with chronic pancreatitis. Gastrointest Endosc 1990;36:93–95.
23 Smith MT, Sherman S, Ikenberry SO, et al: Alterations in pancreatic ductal morphology following polyethylene pancreatic stent therapy. Gastrointest Endosc 1996;44: 268–275.
24 Varadarajulu S, Christein JD, Tamhane A, Drelichman ER, Wilcox CM: Prospective randomized trial comparing EUS and EGD for transmural drainage of pancreatic pseudocysts (with videos). Gastrointest Endosc 2008;68: 1102–1111.
25 Seewald S, Ang TL, Kida M, Teng KY, Soehendra N; EUS 2008 Working Group: EUS 2008 Working Group document: evaluation of EUS-guided drainage of pancreatic-fluid collections (with video). Gastrointest Endosc 2009; 69(suppl):S13–S21.
26 Howell DA, Holbrook RF, Bosco JJ, et al: Endoscopic needle localization of pancreatic pseudocysts before transmural drainage. Gastrointest Endosc 1993;39: 693–698.
27 Baron TH: Endoscopic drainage of pancreatic pseudocysts. J Gastrointest Surg 2008;12:369–372.
28 Aljarabah M, Ammori BJ: Laparoscopic and endoscopic approaches for drainage of pancreatic pseudocysts: a systematic review of published series. Surg Endosc 2007; 21:1936–1944.
29 Melman L, Azar R, Beddow K, et al: Primary and overall success rates for clinical outcomes after laparoscopic, endoscopic, and open pancreatic cystgastrostomy for pancreatic pseudocysts. Surg Endosc 2009;23:267–271.
30 Johnson MD, Walsh RM, Henderson JM, et al: Surgical versus nonsurgical management of pancreatic pseudocysts. J Clin Gastroenterol 2009;43:586–590.
31 Varadarajulu S, Lopes TL, Wilcox CM, Drelichman ER, Kilgore ML, Christein JD: EUS versus surgical cyst-gastrostomy for management of pancreatic pseudocysts. Gastrointest Endosc 2008;68:649–655.
32 Vitale GC, Davis BR, Vitale M, Tran TC, Clemons R: Natural orifice translumenal endoscopic drainage for pancreatic abscesses. Surg Endosc 2009;23: 140–146.
33 Lopes CV, Pesenti C, Bories E, Caillol F, Giovannini M: Endoscopic-ultrasound-guided endoscopic transmural drainage of pancreatic pseudocysts and abscesses. Scand J Gastroenterol 2007;42:524–529.
34 Park JJ, Kim SS, Koo YS, et al: Definitive treatment of pancreatic abscess by endoscopic transmural drainage. Gastrointest Endosc 2002;55:256–262.
35 Mathew A, Biswas A, Meitz KP: Endoscopic necrosectomy as primary treatment for infected peripancreatic fluid collections (with video). Gastrointest Endosc 2008; 68:776–782.
36 Isayama H, Yamamoto K, Mizuno S, et al: NOTES and endoscopic pancreatic necrosectomy for the GI endoscopist. J Hepatobiliary Pancreat Surg 2009;16: 270–273.
37 Voermans RP, Veldkamp MC, Rauws EA, Bruno MJ, Fockens P: Endoscopic transmural debridement of symptomatic organized pancreatic necrosis (with videos). Gastrointest Endosc 2007;66:909–916.

Todd H. Baron, MD
Division of Gastroenterology and Hepatology, Mayo Clinic
200 First Street SW, Charlton 8A
Rochester, MN 55905 (USA)
Tel. +1 507 266 6931, Fax +1 507 266 3939, E-Mail baron.todd@mayo.edu

Mönkemüller K, Wilcox CM, Muñoz-Navas M (eds): Interventional and Therapeutic Gastrointestinal Endoscopy.
Front Gastrointest Res. Basel, Karger, 2010, vol 27, pp 485–500

Endoscopic Ultrasonographic Drainage of Pancreatic Fluid Collections

J.C. Subtil Iñigo · M. Muñoz-Navas

Gastroenterology Department, University of Navarra Clinic, School of Medicine, University of Navarra, Pamplona, Spain

Abstract

Fluid collections of the pancreatic area are a non-negligible complication of the pancreatitis and of the pancreatic traumas. Some of these will have clinical repercussion and will need treatment. In the last 25 years, minimally invasive treatments have slowly become the treatment of choice. Especially endoscopic ultrasonographic drainage has proven to be an effective and safe technique in these conditions. We describe the technique and comment on some critical aspects that need to be considered. The procedure may be performed in several steps or in one step, and we must choose case by case which option seems the best. We describe mainly the one-step technique because in our experience it is easier and quicker. In this chapter we wanted to set up a detailed guide that shows step by step how the technique is performed, with the hope that it may be useful for the interventional echoendoscopist.

Non-neoplastic pancreatic fluid collections may be classified as acute fluid collections, necrosis, acute pseudocysts, chronic pseudocysts or abscesses [1]. Pancreatic pseudocysts are localized collections, usually liquid, surrounded by a non-epithelial wall (granulation or connective tissue), caused by disruption or obstruction of a pancreatic duct. Other pseudocysts are related to the maturation of an acute collection, or to the liquefaction of a necrotic area, detritus and secretions, which is then encapsulated [1, 2]. A minimum of 4 weeks must pass for their wall to be considered mature. These lesions can develop as a result of acute or chronic pancreatitis, pancreatic trauma or pancreatic duct obstruction [1].

Although fluid collections are common during acute pancreatitis, they are usually too small or they disappear spontaneously, with the result that less than 10% of all cases will be clinically relevant. When pseudocysts are large they may cause symptoms such as dyspepsia, pain and abdominal fullness. Severe complications such as infection, bleeding and rupture may also occur, but in some cases, pseudocysts may be asymptomatic. In general, pseudocysts of ≤6 cm may be closely followed in time. In the past it was widely believed that pseudocysts had to be treated when they were >6 cm and persisted >6 weeks. However, spontaneous resolution may occur in a non-negligible number of patients. Today, the trend is to closely observe the pseudocysts and to treat them only when they grow, cause symptoms, or when complications occur [1–3]. Formerly, surgery was considered the gold standard but it also involved significant morbidity and mortality rates [1, 3, 4]. Thus, in the last 25 years, endoscopic and radiological drainage have slowly become the treatment of choice, and surgery is currently reserved for recurrent pseudocysts or pseudocysts associated with other (pancreatic) abnormalities that require surgical therapy [3].

Pancreatic abscesses may be classified according to their origin: postpancreatitic, postsurgical or posttraumatic. Postpancreatitic abscesses result from infection of a necrotic area, a fluid collection or a pseudocyst. This occurs spontaneously in about 10% of the cases due to bacterial translocation, usually 20–40 days after the acute episode. However, the most common cause of infection is iatrogenic due to inappropriate handling of the lesion [2]. Postsurgical and posttraumatic abscesses are often contaminated by intestinal or by external microorganisms. The treatment should always include an appropriate antibiotic therapy. However, this is insufficient and the patient might die if drainage is not performed. The approach to the abscesses is similar to pseudocysts, and currently minimally invasive treatments are also preferred [1, 3–5].

Minimally invasive treatments include percutaneous drainage under radiological guidance (transabdominal US or CT scan) or endoscopic drainage. Both drainage modalities have advantages and disadvantages. Therefore, patients with pancreatic pseudocysts or abscesses must be treated by a multidisciplinary team consisting of surgeons, radiologists, and gastroenterologists because there are specific indications for each type of procedure, and these indications are also dependent on local expertise [3, 6]. In our opinion, whenever possible, the best approach to performing drainage is the natural way – toward the intestinal lumen.

Procedural Aspects

To perform this kind of drainage, endoscopic ultrasonography (EUS) has some advantages over other techniques. Along with other authors, we believe that it should be the technique of choice [1, 3–5, 7–15]. It can characterize the lesion, thus helping to differentiate a pseudocyst, that should be drained, from other cystic lesions [3, 7]. The differential diagnosis is broad and includes benign cysts (<5%), cystic neoplasms of the pancreas (5–10%) and real non-neoplastic collections (80–90%) [2, 16]. A diagnosis of pseudocyst should be considered when previous acute or chronic pancreatitis, or etiological explanation exist. Pseudocysts are usually lesions with anechoic fluid, sometimes with an echoic level due to sedimented detritus, rarely with septa, that have a regular and echoic wall (without focal thickenings, internal projections or calcium), and with high amylase content [2, 16].

Abscesses are often morphologically similar to pseudocysts. However, their content is usually more echoic, relatively dense but fluid, with multiple hyperechoic spots in relation to detritus and microbubbles. Occasionally, if abscesses result from the infection of a necrotic area they may be more anfractuous and complex.

EUS also allows the nearest point of lesion to the wall of the digestive tract to be located. It is particularly useful in evaluating this aspect in non-protruding collections [1, 3, 14]. Furthermore, EUS imaging avoids confusion with other extrinsic potential impacts on the gastric or duodenal wall, such as the gallbladder or the caudate lobe of the liver [3]. At the same time, it measures the distance between the cavity of the cyst and the intestinal lumen. Thus, the classical approach is that the risk of leakage into the peritoneum decreases if this distance is ≤1 cm. However, this also depends on other factors such as location, degree of maturation, or presence of inflammatory adhesions between surfaces [1–4, 7]. Another consideration is the existence of true vessels or submucosal varicose veins that are not infrequently associated with this condition, and which can be interposed between the intestinal lumen and the pseudocyst. The use of color Doppler and power Doppler can help identify these structures and allow maneuvers to avoid them during puncture [1, 3, 7, 12, 14, 17]. One of the most important issues is the ability of EUS to guide the movements of the instruments in real time outside the intestinal wall.

Until a few years ago, only echoendoscopes with a small-caliber working channel were available. With this equipment, only stents with a maximum size of 7 Fr could be inserted or the endoscope had to be exchanged with a large-channel side-viewing endoscope (ERCP-type) leaving the guidewire in place [3]. With the development of large-channel echoendoscopes, 10-Fr stents can be inserted [3]. Due to the laboriousness of the classical procedure (in several steps), a one-step system has been designed [3–5, 8]. This system enables an easier and faster placement of the stent. In our opinion, this device shortens the procedure time by more than 80% and in some selected cases allows the procedure to be performed exclusively under endoscopic ultrasound control.

The availability of a previous CT scan or MRI enables a broader view of the situation to be seen [1, 3]. It allows the relationship of the collection with the intestinal wall to be characterized prior to the procedure. In some cases a CT scan can warn about the presence of abnormal vessels or a splenic artery pseudoaneurysm, but its resolution is insufficient to show varices in the gut wall [3]. Furthermore, this may be interesting to determine the attitude to take and the possible drainage method to adopt. Besides, CT scan or MRI provide a reference for subsequent follow-up. In our opinion, these imaging modalities complement the EUS image. Thus the availability of a previous CT scan or MRI is not mandatory but is advisable.

Patient Preparation

In outpatients it is advisable to keep individuals under observation in hospital for some days after the procedure. Patients with pseudocysts or pancreatic abscesses usually suffer difficulties of gastric emptying, especially if they are not on an absolute diet. Therefore, in patients who are eating, we recommend a soft midday meal without vegetables, and then an exclusively clear liquid diet. If there is a functional or organic gastric or intestinal subocclusion, it may be advisable to add prokinetic drugs and, in some cases, to leave a nasogastric aspiration tube in place. The goal is to keep the gastric and duodenal lumen clean during the procedure.

Special care must be taken with patients taking non-steroidal anti-inflammatory or anticoagulant drugs or platelet aggregation inhibitors. If drainage is necessary, it is compulsory to improve coagulation status prior to the procedure. The procedures are relatively long and must be performed under conscious sedation or under anesthesia. A mixture of midazolam and meperidine or propofol and/or remifentanil may be used depending on the patient's characteristics and local expertise. It is advisable to have pulsioximetry, electrocardiographic recording, capnography and, if necessary, the possibility of patient intubation.

Prophylactic or therapeutic antibiotic treatment should be delivered. Inpatients will already be under antibiotic treatment but this may not be the case for outpatients without infection. For patients without antibiotics, we regularly use a prophylactic intravenous broad-spectrum quinolone during the procedure in the same protocol as other punctures of cystic lesions [18]. The patient is then admitted and continues with intravenous antibiotic therapy for several days. When an abscess is drained it is better to take a culture, if possible, and to treat the infection with specific antibiotics [1, 4].

The procedure is usually performed in two possible postures. If the use of x-ray is not expected, it can be done in left lateral decubitus. When x-ray is used, it is better to perform the procedure in a supine position to obtain a good radiological projection. As patients are usually sedated or anesthetized, it is desirable to seek the maximum stability in their posture.

Accessories

The usual endoscope to perform an EUS-guided drainage of a pseudocyst or abscess is a linear ultrasonic gastrovideoscope with large diameter working channel (3.7 or 3.8 mm), forceps elevator and Doppler (usually called therapeutic echoendoscope). In some rare cases other endoscopes such as a large-channel side-viewing endoscope or different kinds of gastroscopes can be useful. There is also a novel prototype forward-viewing US endoscope (XGiF-UCT160; Olympus Medical Systems Europe, Hamburg, Germany) [14]. This prototype is a modification of a commercially available therapeutic echoendoscope (GF-UCT140; Olympus). Its main modifications are forward-viewing optics and US, plus a large working channel in alignment with the endoscope shaft. These modifications enable the endoscopist to create a cystogastrostomy/duodenostomy guided by EUS by means of a frontal incision without angle. But this device is very specific and very expensive, and it probably can be used in only a few cases. In addition, it is not commercially available. In this chapter we will refer to the conventional therapeutic linear echoendoscopes.

Although using the one-step system most drainages can be performed without radiological control, it is highly desirable to have x-ray equipment at hand. When the procedure is going to be performed using the method in several steps, it must be done with radiological control. When cutting current is going to be used, it is necessary to have an electrosurgical unit. This unit must be able to use cutting and electrocoagulation current in a blended fashion.

There are many approaches and many useful gadgets to make a perfect drainage. We will describe in detail our favorite system (one-step) and more briefly the other gadgets that are also commonly used in pancreatobiliar endoscopy.

The one-step system NWOA (Giovannini Needle Wire Oasis®, Cook Ireland Ltd, Limerick, Ireland) is available in two sizes: 8.5 and 10 Fr [4, 6, 8]. Each size is designed to place stents of 8.5 or 10 Fr respectively. The 8.5-stent is a modified Cotton-Leung® (Amsterdam) biliary stent and the 10-stent is a modified Soehendra® Tannenbaum® biliary stent. This system is only adapted to straight stents. The system consists of four basic elements telescopically positioned. The external element is a plastic positioner-pusher catheter of 8.5 or 10 Fr, according to the stent size. It has within it a plastic dilator-introducer catheter, which overhangs about 90 mm beyond the positioner-pusher catheter tip. The innermost element, within the introducer catheter, is a long guidewire with a movable core (to regulate the stiffness) and a metallic tip that allows the use of electrosurgical current in the same way as a needle knife. The stent is placed on the tip of the pusher catheter and over the introducer catheter. Stents of 5 cm length are those normally used and when they are placed on the system, they must be put with the tapered tip forward. Both sizes of stents have their advantages and disadvantages: 8.5-Fr stents are placed much more easily but they are also, in theory, more easily blocked. In later sections we will address their functioning in more detail.

To perform the procedure in several steps the required devices to puncture the collection are a normal 19-gauge endoscopic ultrasound needle and a 0.035-inch hydrophilic guidewire.

Other authors prefer a 10-Fr cystotome that is designed to electrosurgically cannulate the transgastric or transduodenal wall into a visibly bulging pancreatic fluid collection, as performed in the classical approach (without endoscopic ultrasonographic guide). A cystotome is a device manufactured by Cook consisting of a 10-Fr catheter, with another 5-Fr catheter inside it, and within this second catheter a 0.038-inch needle-knife wire [1, 19]. Smaller caliber (6- and 8.5-Fr) cystotomes (Cysto-Gastro set), manufactured by Endo-flex® GmbH (Voerde, Düsseldorf), have recently appeared on the market.

If the cystotome is not going to be used to enlarge the hole, a graduated dilation catheter or a balloon dilator has to be used [3, 4, 17]. The stents may be straight or with pigtail ends. Within the procedure in several steps, double pigtail stents are usually preferred. In order to place the stent, a normal stent introducer set is usually utilized. Some authors in selected cases have placed covered self-expanding metallic stents with different calibers with the idea of removing them later [20].

In some pseudocysts with a dense content and in abscesses it can be useful to place a nasocystic pigtail end catheter to make continuous washings [1, 3, 9, 13]. We prefer a small-caliber catheter (e.g. 5 Fr) because it is less likely for an accidental looping and strangulation to occur and, moreover, it is less troublesome for the patient. The outer end of the catheter must be connected to a gravity drip or, preferably, to a mechanical infusion volumetric pump with a normal saline solution. The mechanical pump helps avoid disruption of flow caused by obstruction of the stents due to debris or the high density of the fluid.

Technique

We start the procedure with a linear therapeutic echoendoscope because most patients have previously been studied with a CT scan, MRI and/or radial EUS. Based on these images, we often design a previous mental plan to assess the best approach: transgastric, transduodenal, or both. With the tip of the echoendoscope inside the stomach or duodenum, we explore the wall between the gut lumen and the collection, measuring its thickness and the presence of blood vessels. It is highly recommendable to perform a scan of the wall with color or power Doppler [1, 3–9, 11–13, 15, 17, 21]. We must always choose the window where the wall is thinner and without vessels between surfaces. Chronic collections with an inflammatory or infectious component would have low risk of leakage, whereas pseudocysts with little inflammation would have a higher risk. There might be other factors related to the procedure such as the use of graduate dilators or electrosurgical current. It should be borne in mind that the graduated dilation catheter exerts an axial force that could detach the surfaces. However, the diathermic effect may help to keep the surfaces together due to the melting of tissue and the inflammatory reaction [22]. Some critical aspects to consider are listed in table 1.

One-Step Technique. When we are going to use the one-step device, we usually prefer the 8.5-Fr stents because they penetrate through the stomach wall more easily [6, 8]. The stent must be preloaded on the tip of the positioner-pusher catheter and over the dilator-introducer catheter. We must be careful and place the tapered tip of the stent in a forward position to facilitate penetration. The metallic tip of the internal guidewire must protrude 1 mm beyond the tip of the dilator-introducer catheter to obtain the needle-knife effect. When this guidewire is correctly positioned, we must fix it by tightening the screw of the contact pin adapter. We must consider that in some cases, depending on the morphology of the collection, there might not be much

Table 1. Critical aspects in endoscopic ultrasonographic drainage of pancreatic fluid collections

Successful drainage
Correct diagnosis
True pancreatic fluid collection vs. cystic neoplasm
Determination optimal drainage site
Avoiding interposed vessels (Doppler)
Minor distance between collection and gut lumen
Preventing peritoneal perforation or other organ penetration
Selection of the suitable technique case by case
Ultrasonic characterization of collection content and endoscopical appearance of the liquid
Anechoic content and/or crystalline liquid: one stent
No pure anechoic fluid and/or cloudy, dark liquid or debris: multiple stents
Lumps of necrosis, microbubbles and/or purulent liquid: multiples stents + nasocystic irrigation
Assessing definitive withdrawal of stents

space between the walls. The accidental contact of the needle-knife tip with the contralateral wall of the collection might, thus, increase the risk of perforation and internal bleeding. One trick to avoid this is to place the tapered tip of the stent immediately behind the tip of the needle knife, to put the tip of positioner-pusher catheter next to the end of the stent (fig. 1), and to strongly fix the system with a surgical artery clamp placed near the catheter handle (fig. 2).

The kit has a flap positioner sleeve to lay the flap flat during the stent introduction inside the working channel of the echoendoscope. However, when 8.5-Fr stents are used, it is not necessary to utilize this gadget because the flap in the folded back position fits well through the large working channel. The contact pin adapter must be connected with the cable of the electrosurgical unit, and the patient must have the corresponding electrosurgical electrode connected, preferably on the abdominal skin but not in the x-ray field. We usually use 250 W of blended (cutting and electrocoagulation) flow current with the intention that the needle-knife incision does not slip on the intestinal surface, while the fulguration is creating a correct size hole.

When the tip of the one-step device appears in the ultrasound image, we must seek the best incision angle, as perpendicular as possible to the wall between the intestinal lumen and the collection. Therefore, we must play with the up/down angulation control and the elevator forceps control. If the incision angle is not the correct one, we could cause a false way. When the tip of the device rests on the intestinal surface in the right direction, we can step on the cutting pedal of the electrosurgical unit and push slowly but decisively the one-step system. The needle knife, the dilator-introducer catheter and the tip of the stent will penetrate into the collection. During all this time it is very important not to separate the tip of the echoendoscope from the wall because, otherwise we would lose the ultrasound image and, above all, the axial force. We can usually watch the collection content boiling on the tip of the introducer catheter and, immediately behind this tip, a change in size of the catheter that corresponds to the tip of the stent (fig. 3, 4). Moreover, in some cases it is possible to watch the stent flap inside the collection. The stent is well positioned when the internal tip and flap are inside the collection cavity.

Only at this moment can we very carefully and slowly separate the tip of the echoendoscope from the intestinal surface without losing the direction. Once this is done, we can see in the optical image the stent go through the wall and its end with the external flap out of the wall and out of the echoendoscope channel. With the positioner-pusher catheter we can control the depth of penetration (fig. 5). Then, we can release the clamp that is fixing the positioner-pusher catheter to the dilator-introducer catheter and then carefully pull out the latter until the stent is released. We can immediately see the output of collection content through the stent hole (fig. 6, 7). If we do not see the output of liquid, we should see it while aspirating with the endoscope. If despite all this the liquid does not come out, either the stent is not well placed or there is a dense or solid content.

If the liquid is clear as water (pure pancreatic secretion) and the pseudocyst has an anechoic content, one stent may be enough (fig. 6). If the liquid is dark, cloudy, hematic, or with small particles of debris, we must place more than one stent (two or more) [3]. To place another stent we must seek a new window, and perform the procedure in the same way. If the one-step device has not been deteriorated, we can use it with a new preloaded stent. If it has been deteriorated, it is necessary to use a completely new kit. In most cases with more or less fluid liquid, to place between 2 and 4 stents is usually sufficient. In these cases we should keep the patient under observation a few days and then perform the follow-up as an outpatient. In some cases, to obtain a little quantity of content of the lesion it may be desirable to take a culture and antibiogram.

When there is dense content, solid debris or pus (fig. 7), it is necessary to place a nasocystic pigtail end catheter to make continuous washings [3]. As argued above, we usually use a 5-Fr catheter. This size of nasocystic catheter has the advantage that it fits perfectly through the stents of 8.5 Fr (fig. 8). To place it we use the internal guidewire of the one-step kit or a new hydrophilic guidewire of 0.035 inch and 480 cm of length. It is necessary to place this guidewire deeply inside the collection through one of the stents. Then, we can cautiously insert the nasocystic drainage over the guidewire through the stent until its pigtail tip is placed within the collection (fig. 8, 9). Once this is done, we can withdraw the internal guidewire of the catheter and, very slowly and carefully, the echoendoscope. We must simultaneously push the nasocystic catheter at the same speed. Throughout all this step of the procedure we use only endoscopic image control.

When we have removed the echoendoscope and all the length of the catheter is out of the endoscope, we cut off the catheter surplus. Next, we must place the external end that comes out of the mouth of the patient through one of the nostrils. In order to do this, it is necessary to use the short pre-curved catheter that is available in the nasocystic catheter kit. When we have the catheter placed through the nose, it is essential to fix the nasocystic catheter in the nasal flap with adhesive plaster to prevent accidental pulling. Finally, we must connect the Luer lock adapter on the external end of the nasocystic catheter.

Using a slim gastroscope, we may check the correct position and function of the stents and the washing catheter. If the system works, when saline solution is injected under pressure through the nasocystic catheter, the collection content must exit through the unoccupied stents (fig. 9, 10). In some cases, when the patient has an abscess, we wash the collection initially with 100 ml of povidone-iodine 5%. Afterwards, we connect the nasocystic catheter to a drip with a mechanical infusion volumetric pump for washing with saline solution. We frequently use a washing flow of 20–80 ml/h, depending on the patient's clinical conditions. It is important to carefully control the balance of liquids in the patient to avoid hydric overload. The patient should be admitted and under continuous washings for at least 1 week. Then we recommend performing a new CT scan or MRI to check progression. If the clinical parameters of infection and the collection size have decreased, we must assess the removal of the washing catheter. When the lesion or clinical parameters have not changed significantly, we must carry on with the washings and reconsider the antibiotic treatment. When the lesion is bigger, we must check

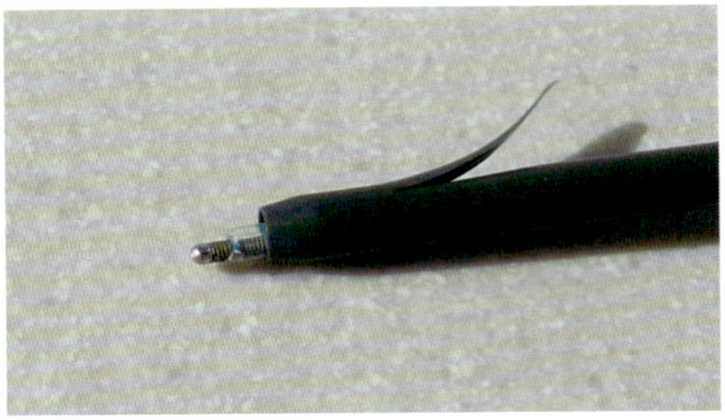

1

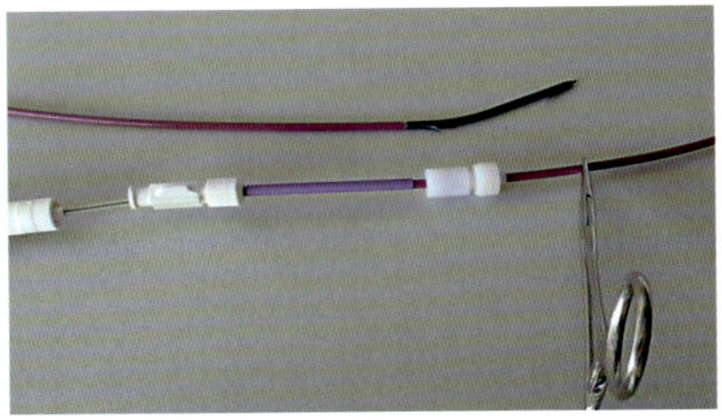

2

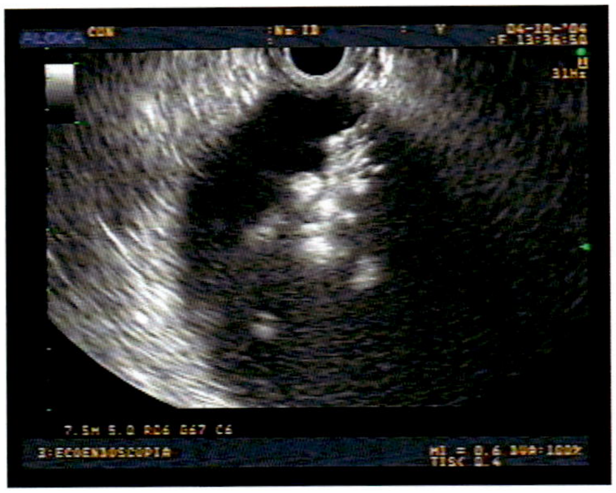

3

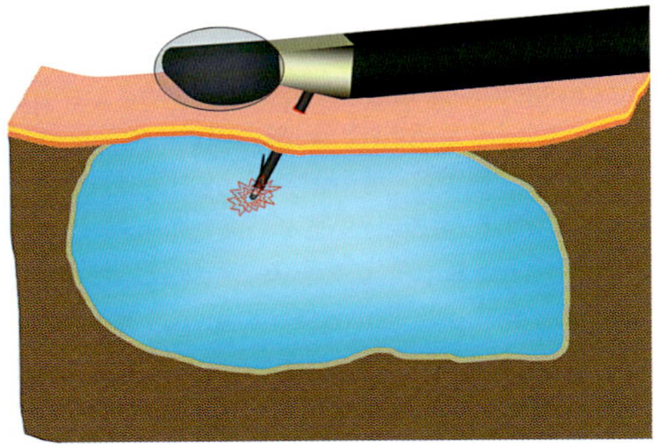

4

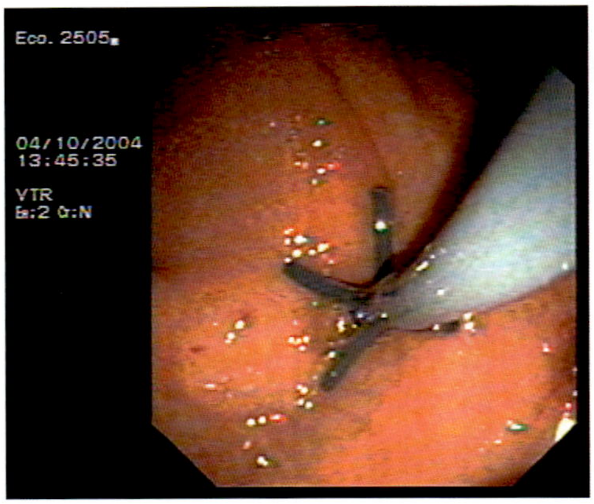

5

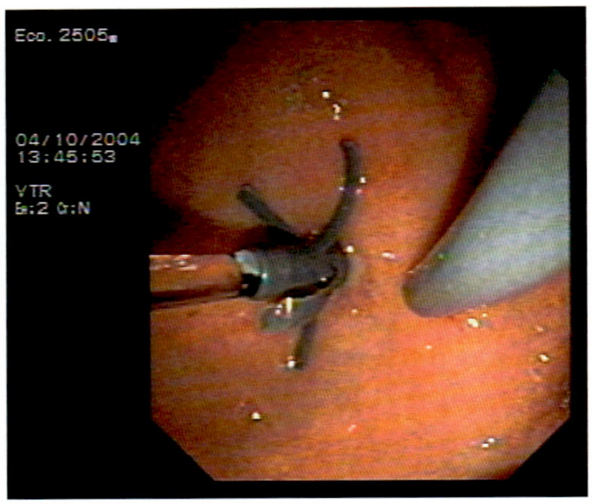

6

Fig. 1. Appropriate position of the stent, the dilator-introducer catheter and the needle-knife tip in the device. **Fig. 2.** Detail of the system with the stent and the surgical clamp positioned correctly.
Fig. 3. Ultrasonographic image showing the one-step device placing one stent. Note the content of the collection boiling. **Fig. 4.** Figure of one-step device making the hole and placing one stent at the same time.
Fig. 5. Endoscopic image showing the stent placement. We can control the deep of penetration of the stent with the positioner-pusher catheter. **Fig. 6.** Release of the prosthesis. Note the output of crystalline liquid.

the stents' permeability. This may be done by forcefully injecting 50–100 ml of saline solution through the nasocystic catheter and verifying the stents' permeability with a slim gastroscope. It is possible to perform this checking using x-ray control and radiographic liquid contrast, and if the stents are blocked we need a new endoscopic procedure to clean the system. In the event that we find ascitis, this is probably due to a leakage between the wall of the cyst and the

7

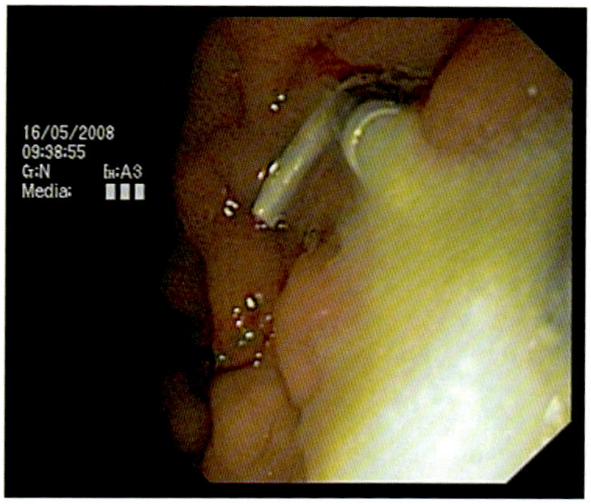

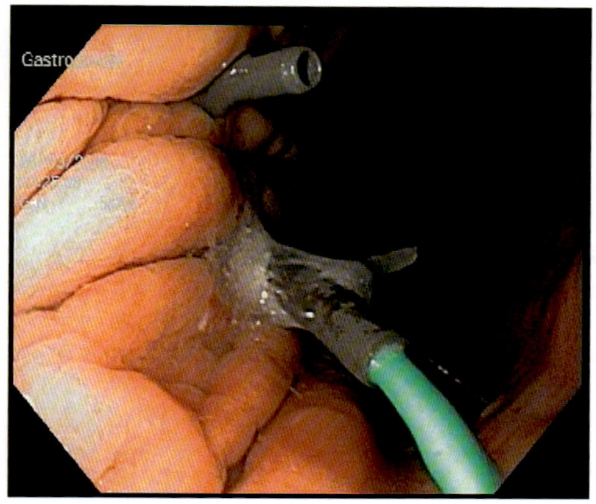

8

9

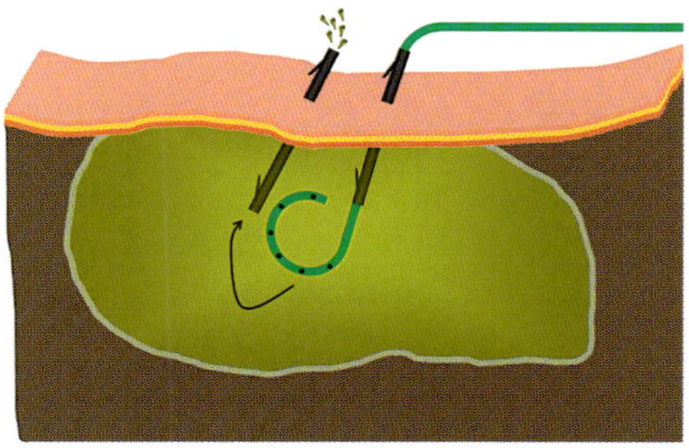

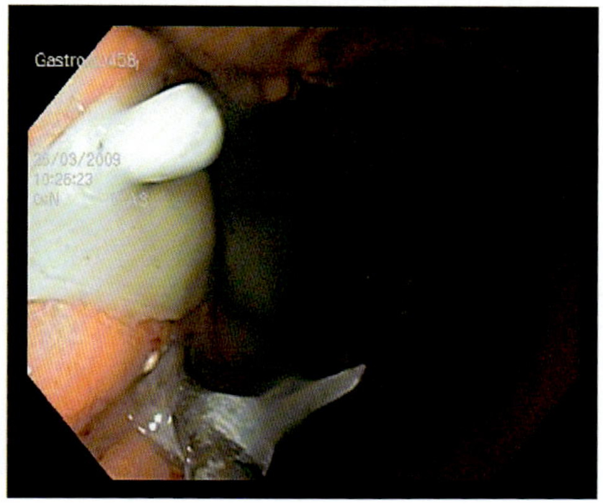

10

Fig. 7. Output of purulent material trough one stent recently placed. **Fig. 8.** Final assembly of a washing system with two stents and a nasocystic catheter. **Fig. 9.** Figure of the final assembly of a washing system to treat abscesses. **Fig. 10.** The same system as in figure 8, draining purulent content during the saline solution injection.

stomach. In this eventuality we must reduce the flow of the saline solution as little as possible and closely monitor the patient.

The nasocystic catheter should be withdrawn under endoscopic control to avoid removing the stent occupied by the catheter. In order to achieve this, we must fix the stent by holding it with a grasping forceps by the external flap, and then withdraw the entire catheter with the help of the visual control of the stent. Finally, we must check the permeability of all the stents by aspiration with the endoscope. These patients must stay admitted for 1–2 days more and then, if there are no complications, they must be discharged under oral antibiotic treatment. Some tricks are listed in table 2.

Several Steps Technique. To perform the procedure in several steps, x-ray equipment is required. When we have selected a window without vessels, we puncture the collection with a 19-gauge endoscopic ultrasound needle as in a normal diagnostic puncture. At this moment, it may be interesting to aspirate a quantity of content of the collection to decompress it and, if necessary, to perform a culture. Prior decompression of the collection may be useful in order to be able to inject radiographic contrast medium and thus reduce the risk of leakage. Next,

Table 2. Tricks (one-step technique)

- Stents of 8.5 Fr
- Place the tapered tip of the stent immediately behind the tip of the needle knife, and the positioner-pusher catheter next the end of the stent
- Fix the system strongly with a surgical artery clamp placed near the catheter handle
- Use 250 W of cutting and coagulation current blended
- Push the system slowly but decisively through the wall into the collection
- Perform the penetration time under ultrasonographic image control
- Release the stent under endoscopic image control
- If place a nasocystic catheter is needed, place a 5-Fr catheter through the last stent placed using the internal guidewire of the one-step kit
- Perform the initial washings under endoscopic image with 100 ml of povidone-iodine 5%
- Connect the nasocystic catheter with a mechanical infusion volumetric pump for washing with saline solution (20–80 ml/h)
- Nasocystic catheter should be withdrawn under endoscopic control to avoid removing the stent occupied by the catheter. Fix the stent by holding it with a grasping forceps by the external flap, and then withdraw the entire catheter with the help of the visual control of the stent

if necessary, we can inject contrast and obtain some radiological images. Then, we wash the needle lumen by injecting saline solution to lubricate its interior to facilitate the advancement of the 0.035-gauge hydrophilic guidewire. Now, we push the guidewire through the needle lumen deeply into the collection lumen. By using x-ray control we must confirm that the guidewire is coiled in the cavity to provide suitable anchorage.

Once this is done, we can use a 10-Fr cystotome to enlarge the initial hole. We prefer this device instead of using different kinds of dilators, because it is not necessary to separate the ultrasound probe from the gut wall while the hole is being enlarged. If we do not have a cystotome, a graduated dilation catheter or a balloon dilator may be used. But with this kind of device we probably lose the ultrasound probe contact and the axial force. Once we have the hole dilated and the guidewire in the cavity, we can separate the endoscope slowly and place a stent using a 10-Fr normal introducer catheter. In these cases we usually use a 10-Fr double pigtail end stent (fig. 11). If the placement of a new stent or of a nasocystic catheter is necessary, we must start again from the beginning, resulting in a more laborious technique. To avoid this, we can take advantage of the possibility that two guidewires can be simultaneously inserted into the 10-Fr cystotome or graduated dilator in a parallel position [23, 24]. Nevertheless, this procedure takes longer than the one-step method, and in our experience it is less safe, as we may lose access at any time, especially if the patient moves, because the time between the initial puncture and placement of the stents is too long.

To date, we have performed 29 procedures in 24 patients. In the first two procedures we only had available a non-therapeutic linear echoendoscope. As a result, we had to perform the procedures in two times and using the several steps technique, with a large-channel side-viewing endoscope in the second time. Once a linear therapeutic echoendoscope became available, we performed the procedures in one time. However, some of the first procedures were performed by the several steps technique using a 10-Fr cystotome and 10-Fr double pigtail end stents, because this is a well-contrasted technique commonly used in the literature. But, at the beginning, we used to employ the one-step system in a different fashion from the one previously described, and with x-ray guidance. As we gained experience, we gradually modified the procedure and usually performed it without x-ray guidance.

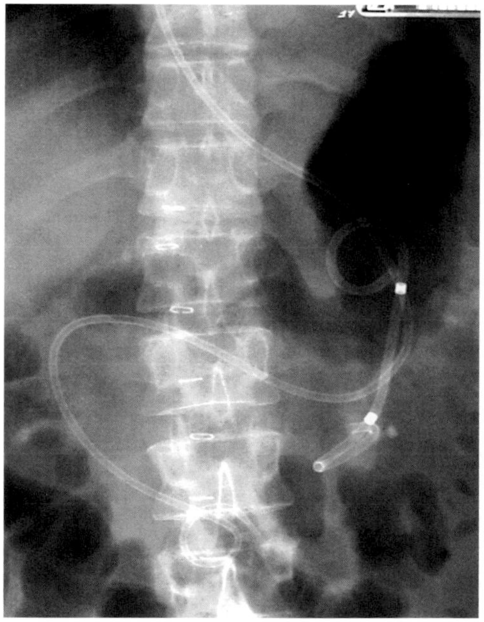

Fig. 11. Radiological image showing a double pigtail end stent and a nasocystic pigtail end catheter placed by the several steps technique.

Limitations and Complications

Limitations. There are several limitations to this technique. The presence of inaspiratable gastric content is a limitation that we have already described. This situation should be avoided because it increases the risk of bronchoaspiration and the risk of contamination of the collection content while this is being handled. The drainage, where the patient's stomach is not completely empty, should be performed only when there is a life-threatening risk (e.g. sepsis due to an abscess). Nevertheless, the airway must be protected by orotracheal intubation and the patient covered with broad-spectrum intravenous antibiotics.

Another limitation is the possibility of having a wide distance between the collection and the intestinal lumen. Classically, a distance >1 cm was considered risky [1, 3]. With the advent of EUS, this question is under review. In some articles it is considered that a distance >2 cm is risky but not an absolute contraindication, since there are other factors that also play a role to prevent perforation and leakage [1].

Endoscopic drainage is feasible only for pancreatic fluid collections located around the stomach and the duodenum. If these collections involve more distal locations, such as the paracolic regions, then these collections are not accessible through endoscopy and other adjunctive measures, such as percutaneous or surgical drainage need to be considered [15]. Postsurgical anatomic changes and impassable strictures may prevent the completion of the procedure [25]. Similarly, the presence of very large and thick varices in the ultrasound window may jeopardize the procedure. Although this eventuality is not infrequent, it is usually possible to find a low risk window [26]. This technique, as described here, is useful only in cases of collections with more or less fluid content and should not be used to treat completely solid necrosis. This topic is discussed in another chapter.

Complications. The complications of this procedure may be classified as early and late complications [3]. The most common early complications are perforation into peritoneum and leakage, bleeding, loss of a stent into the collection during its placement, and accidental puncture of other organs [3, 4, 7–9]. Perforation and leakage can usually be avoided if the procedure is correctly indicated and performed under endoscopic ultrasound guidance in real time thus allowing the selection of the best window for puncture. Factors to be considered are distance, location, degree of maturation, or presence of inflammatory adhesions between surfaces. The degree of maturation and the inflammatory adhesions between surfaces, along with the use of an electrosurgical device, are probably the most important factors to prevent perforations and/or leakages. When endoscopic ultrasonographic guidance is used the accidental puncture of other organs is a very uncommon complication [27].

There are two types of immediate bleedings: bleeding due to a laceration of wall vessels at the entry site, and the bleeding of vessels of the deep wall of the collection [3]. With echoendoscopy guidance and the use of Doppler it is possible to avoid the first type of bleedings [1, 3–9, 11–13, 15, 17, 21]. However, in these cases, the clinical implications are different depending on whether the bleeding occurs into the intestinal lumen or into the collection. If the patient bleeds on the gastric face toward the lumen, we might be able to treat it with endoscopic hemostatic techniques. If the bleeding is toward the collection, the endoscopic or echoendoscopic treatment may be more difficult, and if bleeding is uncontrollable, abundant or has hemodynamic repercussion a radiological embolization or a surgical approach might be necessary [1, 28].

In this context, we treated a patient that had a secondary vessel of the splenic artery between the gastric wall and pseudocyst wall. Prior to drainage we embolized this vessel prophylactically by using a modified cyanoacrylate (Glubran 2®) mixed with Ethiodol (Lipiodol®), guided by endoscopic ultrasound. We then placed two stents with a minimized risk. There were no complications due to this procedure and the patient progressed adequately.

The immediate bleeding of the deep wall of the collection may be the consequence of the laceration of a normal vessel caused by the accidental contact with the tip of the one-step device. A trick that we usually use to reduce this risk has been described in the previous section. Another classical origin of this complication is the rupture of a pseudoaneurysm due to the sudden decompression of the pseudocyst [1]. These eventualities will not be entirely prevented by the use of endoscopic ultrasound guidance [3]. In these cases radiological embolization or surgical treatment may be necessary. There is one report of the prophylactic embolization of a pseudoaneurysm of the splenic artery prior to the procedure which yielded good results [1].

The accidental loss of a stent into the collection during its placement is a possible complication especially when we use short straight stents. In some cases it is feasible to enlarge the hole with a 10- or 15-mm balloon dilator and to rescue the stent with a slim gastroscope. Another less aggressive trick is to create a system that fixes the stent to the catheters of the device and permits the controlled release of the stent.

Late complications may be delayed bleeding due to laceration of a deep vessel of the pseudocyst due to a decubitus of the stent, infection, progressive formation of ascites with or without associated pneumoperitoneum, and recurrence [1, 4, 9, 12]. The first complication is unusual and unpredictable. Laceration of a vessel might be facilitated by the size reduction and collapse of the cavity which causes that the internal tip of the stent, free in its interior before this eventuality, rests now on the contralateral wall to the puncture point. In this sense, some authors suggest a treatment with hydrogen pump inhibitors with the intent of reducing the potential erosion of intracystic vessels due to gastric acid [12]. However, in our opinion, the acid could play a beneficial role in reducing the number of microorganisms in the gastric lumen and contributing to the sclerosis of the wall of the collection.

Table 3. Limitations and complications

Limitations	
	Non-aspirable gastric content
	Distance between the collection and the intestinal lumen
	Collections located around the stomach and duodenum only
	Postsurgical anatomic changes and impassable strictures
	Presence of completely solid necrosis
Complications	
Early complications	
	Perforation to peritoneum and leakage
	Bleeding
	Laceration of wall vessels at the entry site
	Laceration of vessels of the deep wall of the collection
	Rupture of a pseudoaneurysm due to sudden decompression
	Accidental loss of a stent into the collection during their placement
Late complications	
	Delayed bleeding by laceration of a deep vessel of the collection due to a decubitus of the stent
	Postprocedural infection: blockage or dislodgement of the stents
	Progressive formation of ascitis with or without pneumoperitoneum: undetected or late leakage
	Recurrence: early or non-indicated withdrawal of the stent

Postprocedural infection may occur related to the blockage or dislodgement of the stents. Dysfunction of the stents in the first days after placement will induce the infection of the collection [1, 4, 8, 9, 12]. Notwithstanding, the later blockage of the stents will not cause an infection because the formation of a mature fistula around the stent tract (loose seton effect) will allow the continuous output of fluid content alongside the stents [1, 3]. The development of an infection of the collection may be prevented with an adequate number of stents and, if necessary, with the placement of a nasocystic catheter, as indicated previously (table 1) [1, 3, 9, 12]. When the infection has already occurred it must be treated as an abscess. Ascites and pneumoperitoneum are due to the existence of a leakage and its prevention has already been discussed.

When there is obstruction of the main pancreatic duct in a distal segment, or the tone of the papillary sphincter hinders the decompression of this duct, transmural drainage of the lesion might be insufficient. Theoretically, the collection may relapse in a high percentage of cases when the stent is removed. In these situations, it seems logical to place a transpapillary stent to decompress the proximal pancreatic duct. Nevertheless, authors with extensive experience are favorable to use only the transmural way. This might help to maintain a continuous flow through the stents preventing their blockage and permitting the maturation of a persistent fistula around the stent tract [1].

It is unclear when the stents must be withdrawn. Some authors propose removing the stents 3 months after their placement but, possibly, this is related to a higher recurrence rate [4]. At the beginning of our series, we usually withdrew the stents and we had one recurrence of the collection. As a result, we decided not to remove the stents at least for a long period of time. Since then, we have had no further recurrences. When performing the follow-up, some patients had spontaneously expelled some or all of the stents, and the cavity had been definitively reabsorbed and sclerosed. Because of this, in our view, the stents should not be withdrawn. In our series no patient has had problems related to permanence, late dislodgement, or intestinal migration of

Table 4. Results of some of the latest series published in the literature and our experience

Reference (first author)	Pts n	More than one collection	Total procedures	Patients who needed more than one procedure	Several steps	One step	Complications not manage-able with conservative approach	Deaths related to procedure	Immediate success of the procedure	Definitive resolution
Hookey 2006	51	24 (47%)	–	–	51 (100%)	0 (0%)	6 (11%)	0 (0%)	49 (96%)	45 (88%)
Kruger 2006	35	0 (0%)	–	9 (27%)	19 (36%)	33 (63%)	0 (0%)	0 (0%)	33 (94%)	29 (88%)
Ahlawat 2006	11	1 (1%)	12	1 (1%)	12 (100%)	0 (0%)	2 (2%)	0 (0%)	12 (100%)	9 (82%)
Lopes 2007	51	1 (2%)	62	8 (15%)	34 (55%)	28 (45%)	3 (5%)	0 (0%)	60 (96%)	48 (94%)
Varadarajulu 2008	60	6 (10%)	62	9 (15%)	62 (100%)	0 (0%)	1 (2%)	0 (0%)	57 (95%)	53 (93%)
Our experience 2009	24	1 (4%)	29	4 (17%)	5 (17%)	24 (83%)	2 (7%)	0 (0%)	28 (96%)	21 (88%)
Total	232	33 (14%)	–	–	183 (68%)	85 (32%)	14 (5%)	0 (0%)	238 (96%)	205 (88%)

stents during years of follow-up. The most important limitations and complications are outlined in table 3.

Outcomes

Results of some of the latest series published in the literature and our experience are shown in table 4 [1, 4, 8, 9, 19]. In this table we have included series with fluid collections (pseudocysts, and abscesses or necrosis more or less fluid) but no completely solid necroses. The table contains a total of 232 patients who underwent one or more drainage procedures guided by EUS. 33 patients (14%) had more than one collection. Some of these patients needed more than one drainage procedure but some publications do not specify the total number of procedures or the procedures per patient. In this table the real one-step technique has been used only in three series, in a total of 85 patients (32%). We have not found series comparing the several steps technique vs. the one-step technique specifically. 14 patients had non-resoluble complications with conservative approach. An important number of these were patients with severe pathologies. No patient died due to drainage guided by EUS. In one series that includes treatments performed with and without EUS guidance [1], 1 patient died. However, we have not included the group without EUS guidance in the table.

When assessing outcomes, it is important to distinguish between immediate success of the procedure and definitive resolution. The former refers to successfully achieving access and drainage of the fluid collection, whereas the latter pertains to complete and permanent resolution of this fluid collection [15]. This is important because, although the procedure may have been technically successful, there are other factors, some of which we have already mentioned, which can derail the final result. One of these factors is the early withdrawal of the stents solely because imaging techniques have shown the collection to have disappeared.

Conclusion

Endoscopic ultrasonographic drainage is an effective and safe technique for treatment of pancreatic fluid collections. It should be performed only by physicians expert in EUS and ERCP. There are some critical aspects of the technique that are necessary to consider: the adequate diagnosis of the collection, to determine the most appropriate puncture point (without vessels, minimum distance, avoiding other organ penetration…), and the choice of the best technique. The technique may be performed in several steps or in one step, and we must choose case by case which option we are most comfortable with. Another important issue is timing of the placement of one or more stents and a nasocystic catheter. The last important question is when we should withdraw the stents and if this is really necessary. We favor the one-step technique because in our experience it is easier and quicker. In our view, new accessories should be developed, preferably in the one-step modality, so that the procedure becomes even safer, easier and quicker.

References

1 Hookey LC, Debroux S, Delhaye M, Arvanitakis M, Le Moine O, Deviere J: Endoscopic drainage of pancreatic-fluid collections in 116 patients: a comparison of etiologies, drainage techniques, and outcomes. Gastrointest Endosc 2006;63:635–643.

2 Shami V: Benign Cysts: Pseudocysts of the Pancreas, New Orleans, Morial Convention Center, 2004.

3 Fockens P: EUS in drainage of pancreatic pseudocysts. Gastrointest Endosc 2002;56(suppl):S93–S97.

4 Lopes CV, Pesenti C, Bories E, Caillol F, Giovannini M: Endoscopic-ultrasound-guided endoscopic transmural drainage of pancreatic pseudocysts and abscesses. Scand J Gastroenterol 2007;42:524.

5 Giovannini M, Pesenti C, Rolland AL, Moutardier V, Delpero JR: Endoscopic ultrasound-guided drainage of pancreatic pseudocysts or pancreatic abscesses using a therapeutic echo endoscope. Endoscopy 2001;33:473–477.

6 Subtil JC: Manejo por ecoendoscopia de las colecciones del área pancreática en la patología inflamatoria del páncreas. EcoDigest 2006;8e(suppl 1):Art.13.

7 Mönkemüller KE, Baron TH, Morgan DE: Transmural drainage of pancreatic fluid collections without electrocautery using the Seldinger technique. Gastrointest Endosc 1998;48:195–200.

8 Kruger M, Schneider AS, Manns MP, Meier PN: Endoscopic management of pancreatic pseudocysts or abscesses after an EUS-guided one-step procedure for initial access. Gastrointest Endosc 2006;63: 409–416.

9 Varadarajulu S, Christein JD, Tamhane A, Drelichman ER, Wilcox CM: Prospective randomized trial comparing EUS and EGD for transmural drainage of pancreatic pseudocysts. Gastrointest Endosc 2008;68:1102–1111.

10 Buscail L, Faure P, Bournet B, Selves J, Escourrou J: Interventional endoscopic ultrasound in pancreatic diseases. Pancreatology 2006;6:7–16.

11 Vazquez-Sequeiros E: Drainage of peripancreatic fluid collections: is EUS really necessary? Gastrointest Endosc 2007;66:1120–1122.

12 Barthet M, Lamblin G, Gasmi M, Vitton V, Desjeux A, Grimaud JC: Clinical usefulness of a treatment algorithm for pancreatic pseudocysts. Gastrointest Endosc 2008;67:245–252.

13 Varadarajulu S, Wilcox CM, Tamhane A, Eloubeidi MA, Blakely J, Canon CL: Role of EUS in drainage of peripancreatic fluid collections not amenable for endoscopic transmural drainage. Gastrointest Endosc 2007;66:1107–1119.

14 Voermans RP, Eisendrath P, Bruno MJ, Le Moine O, Deviere J, Fockens P, et al: Initial evaluation of a novel prototype forward-viewing US endoscope in transmural drainage of pancreatic pseudocysts. Gastrointest Endosc 2007;66:1013–1017.

15 Seewald S, Ang TL, Kida M, Teng KY, Soehendra N: EUS 2008 Working Group Document: evaluation of EUS-guided drainage of pancreatic-fluid collections. Gastrointest Endosc 2009;69(suppl):S13–S21.
16 Vignesh S, Brugge WR: Endoscopic diagnosis and treatment of pancreatic cysts. J Clin Gastroenterol 2008;42: 493–506.
17 Varadarajulu S, Tamhane A, Blakely J: Graded dilation technique for EUS-guided drainage of peripancreatic fluid collections: an assessment of outcomes and complications and technical proficiency. Gastrointest Endosc 2008;68:656–666.
18 Banerjee S, Shen B, Baron TH, Nelson DB, Anderson MA, et al: ASGE Standards of Practice Committee: Antibiotic prophylaxis for GI endoscopy. Gastrointest Endosc 2008;67:791–798.
19 Ahlawat SK, Charabaty-Pishvaian A, Jackson PG, Haddad NG: Single-step EUS-guided pancreatic pseudocyst drainage using a large-channel linear array echoendoscope and cystotome: results in 11 patients. JOP 2006; 7:616–624.
20 Talreja JP, Shami VM, Ku J, Morris TD, Ellen K, Kahaleh M: Transenteric drainage of pancreatic fluid collections with fully covered self-expanding metallic stents. Gastrointest Endosc 2008;68:1199–1203.
21 Voermans RP, Veldkamp MC, Rauws EA, Bruno MJ, Fockens P: Endoscopic transmural debridement of symptomatic organized pancreatic necrosis. Gastrointest Endosc 2007;66:909–916.
22 Kwan V, Eisendrath P, Antaki F, Le Moine O, Deviere J: EUS-guided cholecystenterostomy: a new technique. Gastrointest Endosc 2007;66:582–586.
23 Jansen JM, Hanrath A, Rauws EA, Bruno MJ, Fockens P: Intracystic wire exchange facilitating insertion of multiple stents during endoscopic drainage of pancreatic pseudocysts. Gastrointest Endosc 2007;66: 157–161.
24 Ang TL, Teo EK, Fock KM: EUS-guided drainage of infected pancreatic pseudocyst: use of a 10-Fr Soehendra dilator to facilitate a double-wire technique for initial transgastric access. Gastrointest Endosc 2008;68:192–194.
25 Varadarajulu S: EUS followed by endoscopic pancreatic pseudocyst drainage or all-in-one procedure: a review of basic techniques. Gastrointest Endosc 2009;69(suppl):S–76–S181.
26 Sriram PV, Kaffes AJ, Rao GV, Reddy DN: Endoscopic ultrasound-guided drainage of pancreatic pseudocysts complicated by portal hypertension or by intervening vessels. Endoscopy 2005;37:231–235.
27 Hikichi T, Irisawa A, Takagi T, Shibukawa G, Wakatsuki T, Imamura H, et al: A case of transgastric gallbladder puncture as a complication during endoscopic ultrasound-guided drainage of a pancreatic pseudocyst. Fukushima J Med Sci 2007;53: 11–18.
28 Brandon JL, Ruden NM, Turba UC, Bozlar U, Yeaton P, Hagspiel KD: Angiographic embolization of arterial hemorrhage following endoscopic US-guided cystogastrostomy for pancreatic pseudocyst drainage. Diagn Interv Radiol 2008;14:57–60.

J.C. Subtil Iñigo, PhD
Gastroenterology Department, University of Navarra Clinic
School of Medicine, University of Navarra
ES–31008 Pamplona (Spain)
Tel. +34 948255400, Fax +34 948296500, E-Mail jcsubtil@unav.es

Mönkemüller K, Wilcox CM, Muñoz-Navas M (eds): Interventional and Therapeutic Gastrointestinal Endoscopy.
Front Gastrointest Res. Basel, Karger, 2010, vol 27, pp 501–510

Diagnostic and Therapeutic Applications of Endoscopic Ultrasound-Guided Punctures

Mohamad A. Eloubeidi[a] · Mohammad Al-Haddad[b]

[a]Division of Gastroenterology and Hepatology, Department of Medicine, University of Alabama at Birmingham, Birmingham, Ala., and [b]Division of Gastroenterology and Hepatology, Department of Medicine, Indiana University School of Medicine, and Clarian/IU Digestive Diseases Center, Indianapolis, Ind., USA

Abstract

Endoscopic ultrasound fine-needle aspiration (EUS-FNA) is a minimally invasive sampling technique that has proven to be a safe and accurate method of tissue acquisition in patients with a variety of gastrointestinal pathological conditions, including luminal and extra-gastrointestinal masses, cysts, and lymphadenopathy. In this review, we will discuss the EUS-FNA technique, and its various applications and indications in a wide variety of gastrointestinal and mediastinal indications. While interventional applications will be discussed in other chapters of this book, we will address celiac plexus block and neurolysis.

Endoscopic ultrasound (EUS) has emerged as the test of choice for accurate imaging of the gut wall and surrounding structures. Its applications have extended over the years to include fine-needle aspiration (FNA) of target lesions accessible from the gastrointestinal tract for diagnostic and therapeutic purposes [1, 2]. FNA is a minimally invasive sampling technique that has proven to be a safe and accurate method of tissue acquisition in patients with a variety of pathological conditions, including gastrointestinal and extra-gastrointestinal masses, cysts, and lymphadenopathy [3, 4].

In this review, we will discuss the EUS-FNA technique, and its various applications and indications in a wide variety of gastrointestinal and mediastinal indications. While interventional applications will be discussed in other chapters of this book, we will address celiac plexus block and neurolysis here.

FNA Technique and Devices for Tissue Sampling

EUS-FNA is performed using the linear array echoendoscope under conscious sedation and appropriate cardiovascular and respiratory monitoring. The ultrasound transducer on the distal tip of the echoendoscope permits needle advancement into the lesion under real-time guidance. A variety of needles are commercially available, ranging in size between 19 and 25 gauge. It is recommended that Doppler is used to examine the projected path of the needle to avoid puncturing intervening blood vessels, while trying to minimize the amount of normal pancreatic tissue that has to be traversed. Once the gut wall is punctured and the needle enters the target lesion, the stylet is withdrawn and suction is applied. The needle is then moved back and forth for 10 cycles or until deemed adequate by the endosonographer. The needle is then withdrawn back into the sheath and the assembly is removed. The material retrieved by aspiration is then expressed onto 2 glass slides sets; one set of slides is air-dried for immediate staining and on-site review while the other slide set is alcohol-fixed for later comprehensive pathologic examination. The presence of on-site cytopathology for rapid interpretation is recommended and has been shown to improve the diagnostic yield [5]. Our group has previously shown that there is excellent correlation between on site interpretation and final reports. We also believe that this practice decreases the work load of the practicing endosonographer [6].

When aspirating cystic lesions, complete cyst aspiration using only one biopsy is recommended to minimize the risk of infection. This risk in pancreatic cystic lesions was initially reported to be as high as 14% in early studies [3]. Therefore, it has become routine practice to administer intravenous antibiotics (such as a fluoroquinolone) prior to or immediately after EUS-FNA followed by oral antibiotics for 3–5 days to limit this risk. Recent studies have shown that this practice may limit this complication to <3% [7]. Since cytology yield is usually low when aspirating cystic lesions without a clear mass or nodule, a cytobrush device (Echobrush®, Cook Medical Inc., Winston-Salem, N.C., USA) has been developed and approved for use with a 19-gauge EUS-FNA needle. Suitable cystic pancreatic lesions (CPLs) for cytobrush use include those that are at least 2 cm in diameter and located in the neck, body or tail of the pancreas. These limitations mainly reflect the difficulty of using the relatively stiff 19-gauge needle to aspirate the pancreatic head and uncinate lesions. Once the needle is in the cyst, the stylet is withdrawn and the brush is advanced through the sheath under ultrasound guidance. The brush is moved back and forth several times to ensure adequate tangential contact with the cyst wall or any mural nodules. Patients on anticoagulation are usually excluded due to a higher risk of bleeding shown in our previously reported pilot study [8].

Other tissue sampling techniques include EUS-guided Trucut biopsy (EUS-TCB). EUS-TCB permits acquisition of a tissue fragment with a preserved histologic architecture and has been shown to be safe for tissue sampling from a variety of solid organs [9]. The Quick-Core® (Cook Medical Inc.) is a commercially available TCB device that is a 19-gauge needle equipped with a spring-loaded cutting sheath and a tissue tray [9, 10]. Initial human experience showed that EUS-TCB provides superior diagnostic accuracy for submucosal lesions, lymphoma, and autoimmune pancreatitis compared to standard EUS-FNA [11]. The same studies suggested that the use of TCB in solid lesions of the pancreas may provide a diagnosis in fewer passes.

EUS-FNA Diagnostic Applications

EUS-FNA for Cystic Pancreatic Lesions

The large number of incidental and asymptomatic CPLs noted on routine cross-sectional imaging studies challenge clinicians to identify the type of cyst, stratify the risk of malignancy and need for surgery. EUS-FNA has been shown to be an effective and safe sampling method of CPLs and thus can help guide further management [12, 13].

The ability to sample fluid for CEA, amylase and lipase, and provide cytology for interpretation, can differentiate mucinous from non-mucinous lesions of the pancreas [14]. Imaging with EUS also provides valuable information about the presence of associated masses, mural nodules which clearly suggest more advanced lesions. Yield of EUS-FNA of cystic lesions is somewhat lower than that of solid pancreatic masses due to the nature of the lesions.

The specificity of EUS-FNA cytology for the diagnosis of CPLs is excellent and exceeds 90% in most published studies [15–17]. On the other hand, the sensitivity of EUS-FNA remains widely variable and ranges between 55 and 97%, with most studies reporting a sensitivity of <50% [15–18]. Brandwein et al. [16] reported EUS-FNA sensitivity, specificity and accuracy of 50, 100 and 89%, respectively, for the diagnosis of malignancy in 26 patients with different types of CPLs. Frossard et al. [17] reported that EUS-FNA correctly identified 65 of 67 (97%) CPLs when a dedicated on-site pathologist reviewed all cytologic preparations. In a prospective, multicenter study, Brugge et al. [15] reported the results of EUS-FNA cytology and tumor markers in 112 patients who underwent surgery. This study reported a sensitivity and specificity of cytology of 35 and 83%. The sensitivity of EUS-FNA for the diagnosis of malignancy in mucinous lesions was only 22%. Possible reasons for this wide variation in the reported sensitivity of EUS-FNA cytology for the diagnosis of CPLs may include the variable use of on-site cytology interpretation and cytopathologist expertise, lesion sampling error, sporadic distribution of malignant epithelium in the cyst, presence of gastrointestinal contaminant and variability in the experience of the endosonographer. In a recent pilot study using the Echobrush® device (Cook Medical Inc.), CPLs cytobrushings (fig. 1) were shown to be superior to standard cytology specimens obtained via FNA in 7 of 10 patients [8].

Finally, the Trucut biopsies may offer a histological specimen from the wall cyst, supporting stroma or any other solid components of the cyst. Its use was initially described by Levy et al. [19] in 10 patients and was found to be diagnostic in 6 patients, partially diagnostic in 1 and non-diagnostic in the remaining 3. No complications were reported in this small study. However, until further randomized prospective trials become available, EUS-FNA remains the mainstay of sampling CPLs for cytology and obtaining fluid for tumor markers.

To further enhance the diagnostic capabilities of EUS-FNA, cyst fluid analysis is recommended. The largest prospective study to date [15] determined that a cutoff of cyst fluid CEA of 192 ng/ml provided a sensitivity of 73% and specificity of 84% for differentiating mucinous from non-mucinous CPLs. A cyst fluid CA19–9 level of 2,900 offered a sensitivity of 68% and specificity of 62% for differentiating mucinous from non-mucinous tumors. No other combination of factors including cytology, morphology and CEA levels was found to be more accurate than CEA levels alone.

Pancreatitis and bleeding are the two most common complications encountered with cystic lesions aspiration. Fortunately, and with the use of antibiotics, infections are now rare. In conclusion, we recommend evaluation of cyst fluid from EUS-FNA for CEA and cytology whenever sufficient fluid (about 1–1.5 ml) is obtained. If less fluid is obtained, cytology should always be obtained and then CEA if enough fluid remains. Other cyst fluid tumor markers such as CA19–9 appear to offer inferior diagnostic results compared to CEA alone and their use is not currently recommended.

Role of EUS-FNA in Pancreatic Masses

For the evaluation of solid pancreatic masses, EUS-FNA provides tissue diagnosis particularly in patients deemed unresectable and unsuitable for surgery. We recently reported on our cumulative data on 547 patients who underwent EUS-FNA. The operating characteristics of EUS-FNA of solid pancreatic masses was: sensitivity 95% (95% CI 93.2–95.4), specificity 92% (95% CI 86.6–95.7), positive predictive value 98% (95% CI 97–99), negative predictive value 80% (95% CI 74.9–82.7). The overall accuracy of EUS-FNA was 94.1% (95% CI 92.0–94) [20].

EUS-FNA is currently accepted throughout major centers as one of the viable options for tissue acquisition in patients with unresectable pancreatic cancer. At our and most large referral institution, EUS-FNA completely replaced percutaneous approaches for this indication. However, it is still debatable whether tissue diagnosis is needed in patients with resectable disease. We and others reported that EUS-FNA carries an acceptable rate of complications, mostly pancreatitis when sampling solid pancreatic lesions. The risk of pancreatitis varies between 0.5 and 2% [4, 21].

Pancreatic metastases account only for 2–3% of all pancreatic resections [22, 23], but early proper diagnosis may avoid unnecessary surgery and permit triage to more appropriate non-operative therapy. The most common primary malignancies that metastasize to the pancreas are lung cancer and renal cell carcinoma [24]. Other common sites of primary cancer include: lung, breast, colorectal and cutaneous melanoma. In a review of 699 cases of pancreatic metastases diagnosed by biopsy/FNA (n = 236) or autopsy (n = 463) by Mesa et al. [25], it was found that primary lung cancer (19%) was more common than renal cell carcinoma (16%).

EUS morphology alone cannot reliably distinguish primary pancreatic cancer from metastatic lesions, and EUS-FNA or EUS-TCB is recommended (fig. 2). To maximize diagnostic yield, EUS-FNA is best done with on-site, real-time cytology interpretation. The slide preparation methods are similar to those described above. It is also recommended that additional FNA passes be made for cell block examination in cases where metastatic lesions are suspected. The cell block preparation is fixed in formalin and embedded in paraffin. Hematoxylin-eosin (HE) stains and possible immunocytochemistry (ICC) on the cell block may aid in the diagnosis of the suspected metastatic lesion [25]. When EUS-FNA with or without immunocytochemistry is non-diagnostic then histology may be required to confirm a suspected diagnosis. In these patients EUS-TCB (Cook Endoscopy, Winston-Salem, N.C., USA) with a 19-gauge needle may be helpful.

While EUS can identify biliary strictures, tissue diagnosis is crucial for differentiation of malignant versus benign lesions. Few prospective studies have evaluated the role of EUS-FNA in biliary strictures. In the first study from Germany of 44 patients with strictures at the liver hilum who underwent EUS-FNA, the accuracy, sensitivity, and specificity for diagnosis of cholangiocarcinoma were 91, 89, and 100%, respectively [26]. EUS and EUS-FNA changed the preplanned surgical approach in 27 of 44 patients. In the second study from the United States by Eloubeidi et al. [27], 28 patients with previously failed tissues diagnosis underwent EUS-FNA of biliary strictures. The sensitivity, specificity, positive predictive value, negative predictive value, and accuracy of EUS-FNA were 86, 100, 100, 57 and 88%, respectively. EUS-FNA had a positive impact on patient management in 84% of patients: preventing surgery for tissue diagnosis in patients with inoperable disease or facilitating surgery in patients with unidentifiable cancer by other modalities. No major complications were reported in either study. EUS is most optimal for lesions in the mid or distal bile duct, however, lesions in the liver hilum can be sampled, albeit less successfully, especially if the lesion cannot be detected from the duodenal approach.

Since evaluating a portion of the liver is possible at the time of EUS, EUS-FNA of primary and metastatic liver lesions is possible at the time of tumor staging. Occasionally, EUS-FNA of liver lesions is the easiest way of providing tissue diagnosis particularly in patients with metastatic pancreaticobiliary malignancy and when the primary mass is not accessible. Finally, in unresectable cases of gallbladder cancer, EUS-FNA plays a vital role in providing tissue diagnosis [28]. However, sampling the gallbladder in benign-appearing lesions should be avoided since this might lead to peritonitis.

EUS-FNA in the Staging of Lung Cancer

The most common cancer-related death in the United States is from lung cancer [29]. Accurate staging is important and dictates the choice of subsequent therapy. Surgery is most appropriate for patients in whom disease is confined to the lung or hilar lymph nodes. For patients with ipsilateral mediastinal lymph node metastases, the benefit of surgery remains controversial. For patients with contralateral mediastinal lymph node metastases, surgery is generally not indicated; and chemotherapy, radiotherapy, or both are considered the standard of care [30].

Since noninvasive imaging of the chest and mediastinum, including CT scan and PET scan, have been associated with false-positive and negative results [31], invasive staging with lymph node sampling has been recommended whenever metastatic mediastinal lymph nodes are suspected [32]. EUS-FNA can be reliably and safely performed on posterior mediastinal lymph nodes (including the subcarinal lymph nodes) with higher predictive value than either the PET scan or CT scan (fig. 3) [33, 34]. Studies have demonstrated the cost-effectiveness of utilizing EUS-FNA first prior to mediastinoscopy [35]. When combined with endobronchial ultrasound, EUS-FNA was recently shown to provide a higher estimated sensitivity (93%) and negative predictive value (97%) compared with either method alone [36]. Therefore, from a practical stand point, EUS-FNA should be considered to complement the staging of lung cancer along with CT scan and PET, and preclude surgery in those with metastatic mediastinal adenopathy.

EUS-FNA of Specific Target Organs

FNA of the Adrenal Glands

EUS is able to image the left adrenal gland in almost all cases (98%) and the right adrenal gland only occasionally (30%) [37]. It has been shown that sampling the left adrenal is a very safe technique with no complications reported to date [38–40]. In a series of 31 patients with enlarged left adrenal gland, FNA was possible in all patients yielding adequate tissue for cytologic interpretation (fig. 4). Malignancy was confirmed in 13/31 patients (42%); the majority of whom had known malignancy in another site (9 in the lung, 2 in the pancreas and 1 in the bladder). In a recent report, we have demonstrated the use of EUS-FNA in 4 patients with right adrenal lesions [41]. Three of the patients had metastatic lung cancer to the right adrenal gland and 1 patient had a benign aspirate consistent with angiomyolipoma.

Therefore, examination of the left adrenal gland (and the right if accessible) is essential in all cases presenting for EUS staging of lung cancer to rule out metastatic disease, which dramatically changes the course of management.

FNA of Gastrointestinal Mesenchymal Tumors

Mesenchymal tumors of the gastrointestinal tract comprise 0.1–3% of all gastrointestinal tumors and are classified as: leiomyomas (including leiomyosarcomas) and gastrointestinal stromal

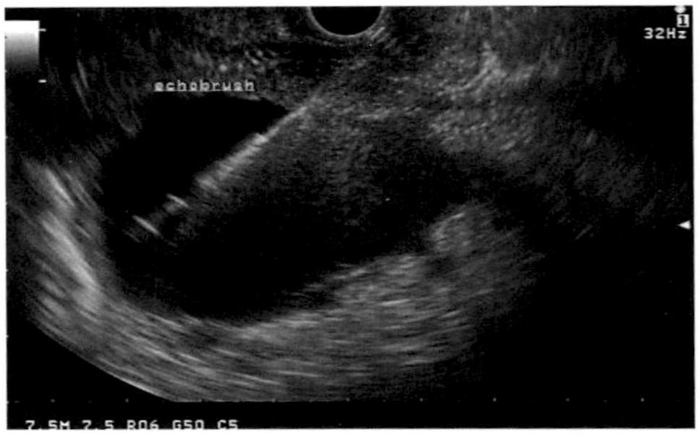

1

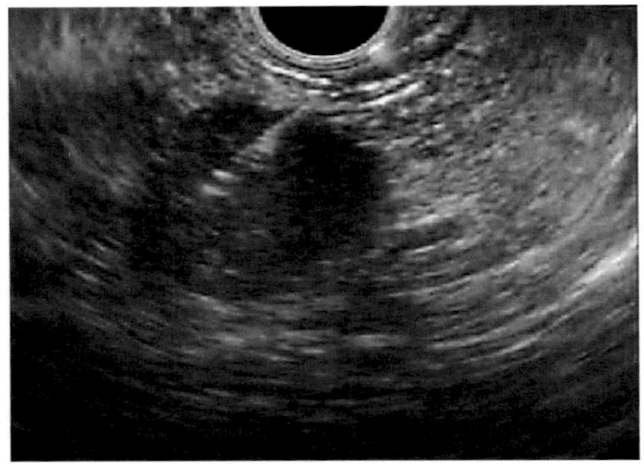

2

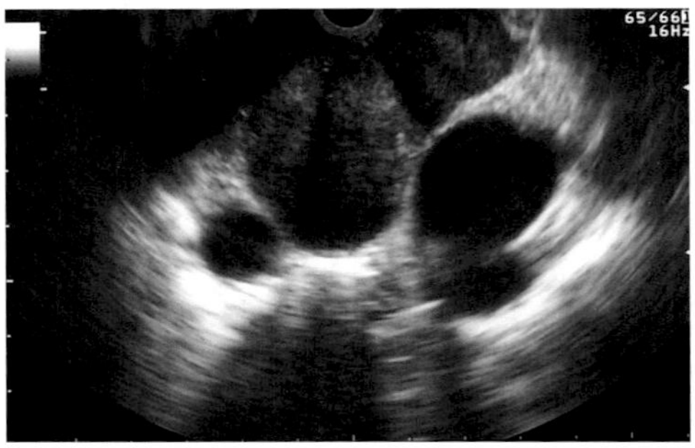

3

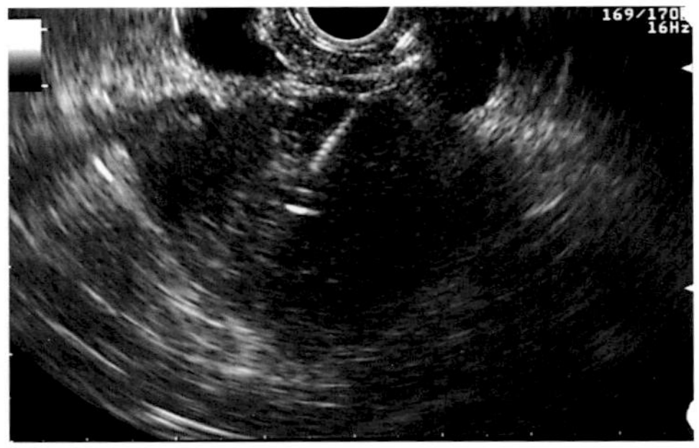

4

Fig. 1. A 3-cm unilocular pancreatic body cyst undergoing cytobrushings using the Echobrush. The communication with a side branch of the pancreatic duct (not shown) and the presence of mucinous glandular epithelium on cytobrushings were suggestive of a side branch intraductal papillary mucinous neoplasm. **Fig. 2.** A distinct hypoechoic 1.5-cm pancreatic tail lesion noted on EUS in an elderly asymptomatic patient. Fine-needle aspirate revealed metastatic renal cell carcinoma. **Fig. 3.** An enlarged subcarinal lymph node in a patient with a known lung mass referred for EUS. Fine-needle aspiration showed metastatic cells suggestive of N2 nodal staging. **Fig. 4.** A left adrenal mass in a patient with a lung mass. Cytology from fine-needle aspiration revealed metastatic squamous cell carcinoma of pulmonary origin.

tumors (GISTs). Whilst only 10–30% of GISTs are malignant, every GIST is now considered potentially malignant and therefore all GISTs may need to be resected [42, 43]. Leiomyomas are considered benign lesions and display malignant potential only in rare cases.

All mesenchymal tumors appear to originate from the 4th mucosal layer on EUS, which corresponds to muscularis propria (fig. 5). While size by EUS remains an important determining factor for the malignancy potential, there is an increasing role for FNA in determining GISTs behavior and could help direct further management. Since the typical epithelioid cytological features are seen in all of the mesenchymal tumors, immunohistochemical studies should be performed to determine their malignant potential [44, 45]. Leiomyomas have benign histology and demonstrate uptake with smooth muscle actin, desmin and less commonly CD34 (10–15%) on immunohistochemical stains. Leiomyosarcomas are histologically high-grade lesions that express smooth muscle actin and/or desmin [46]. GISTs are spindle cell or epithelioid mesenchymal neoplasms that are characterized by overexpression of the tyrosine kinase inhibitor c-kit (CD117) [47].

We recommend surgical evaluation for such submucosal lesions due to symptoms of obstruction or bleeding. For asymptomatic lesions, we recommend FNA and immunohistochemistry for confirming GISTs. Trucut biopsies could be performed to maximize tissue yield in lesions larger than 2 cm in size. GISTs that are not resected surgically should be monitored by EUS for signs of malignant progression.

FNA of the Thyroid Gland

Although more technically challenging, EUS-FNA in the superior mediastinum has been attempted. Ohshima et al. [48] described a series of 29 patients with advanced thyroid cancer who underwent EUS, esophagoscopy, and magnetic resonance imaging (MRI) to assess esophageal wall invasion. The overall accuracy of EUS (89%) was superior to that for MRI (59%) and esophagoscopy (65%). Thyroid nodules are usually sampled without US guidance by percutaneous FNA by using a 25-gauge needle. FNA provides a diagnosis in the majority of pathologies with the exception of follicular and well-differentiated adenocarcinoma, where a tissue core may be needed [49]. DeWitt et al. [50] described the first EUS-FNA of thyroid tissue in a patient presenting with a superior mediastinal mass. FNA was feasible without complications and revealed benign nodular goiter.

However, EUS-FNA in the superior mediastinum remains technically difficult due to the close proximity of the echoendoscope to the upper esophageal sphincter and difficulty maintaining a stable position. Nevertheless, this may be a suitable intervention in patients with suspected thyroid pathologies undergoing EUS-FNA for another indication. If difficulties are encountered at the time of EUS, a consideration should be to bring the patient back for repeat EUS under general anesthesia.

EUS Therapeutic Applications

EUS-Guided Celiac Plexus Block and Neurolysis

Pain resulting from chronic pancreatitis can be hard to control with conventional pharmacotherapy, which itself could have disabling side effects. A celiac plexus block (CPB) using steroid has been tried in patients with chronic pancreatitis. Gress et al. [51] described EUS-guided CPB in 90 patients with chronic pancreatitis. Significant pain relief was noted in 55% of patients for up to 8 weeks of follow-up but persisted in 10% of patients for less than 24 months. In our practice, we are increasingly offering EUS-guided celiac plexus block to patients known to have chronic pancreatitis with significant intolerance to their pain management regimens.

Technically, we identify the take off of the celiac artery from the aortic trunk, and using 19 or 22 gauge FNA needles inject 20 ml (0.25%) of bupivacaine and 6 ml (80 mg) triamcinolone (individually or premixed). This can be delivered on either one or both sides of the aorta. Injection can also be directed to the center of any visualized celiac ganglia (fig. 6).

A similar concept has been applied to manage pain from inoperable pancreatic cancer. Celiac plexus neurolysis (CPN) is a chemical splanchnicectomy of the celiac plexus, which ablates the afferent nerve fibers that transmit pain from intra-abdominal viscera. EUS-CPN performed for the palliation of pancreatic cancer pain appears to be as safe and effective as CPN performed by other routes such as CT-guided and surgical approaches. An added advantage of the EUS approach is that it can be performed during staging and biopsy of the tumor. One study of 58 such patients who underwent EUS-guided CPN showed significant decline in pain scores reported by 54% of the patients; however, the efficacy of this intervention diminished after 8–12

5
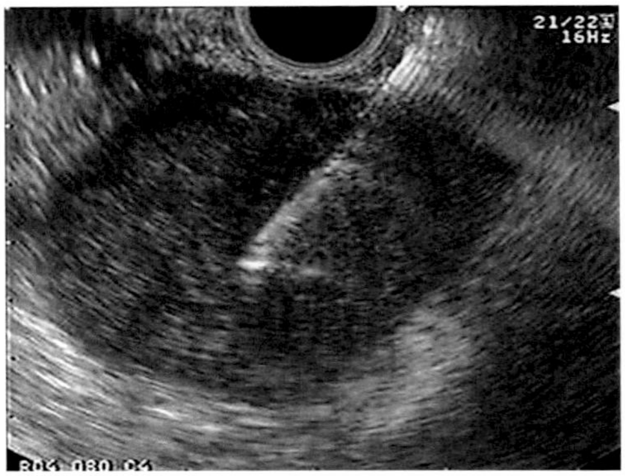
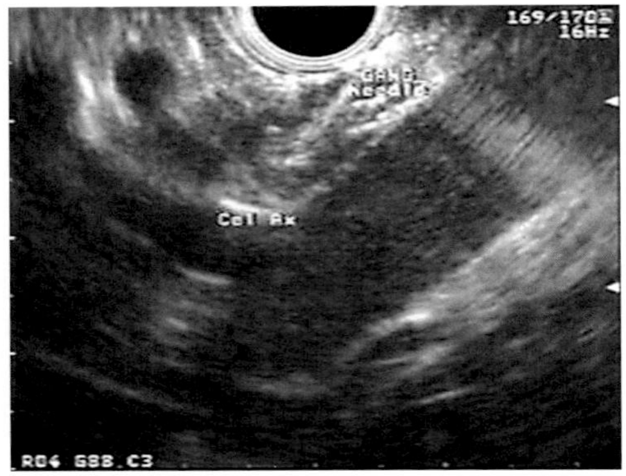
6

Fig. 5. A hypoechoic 2.5-cm lesion originating from the fourth hypoechoic layer of the gastric wall (muscularis propria). Fine-needle aspirate confirmed the diagnosis of gastrointestinal stromal tumor based on the presence of spindle cells that were positive for c-kit on immunocytochemistry. **Fig. 6.** Celiac plexus block performed using a 22-gauge EUS needle in a patient with chronic pancreatitis. A celiac ganglion was noted anterior to the celiac origin and was targeted during the block.

weeks. On multivariate analysis, the benefit of EUS-CPN was independent of morphine use, chemotherapy, and radiation [52]. The injection technique is similar to that of CPB; however, neurolysis is performed by injecting 20 ml (0.25%) bupivacaine and 10 ml (98%) alcohol into one or both sides of the celiac region, or into any visualized ganglia.

References

1 Giovannini M, Seitz JF, Monges G, Perrier H, Rabbia I: Fine-needle aspiration cytology guided by endoscopic ultrasonography: results in 141 patients. Endoscopy 1995;27:171–177.

2 Gress FG, Hawes RH, Savides TJ, Ikenberry SO, Lehman GA: Endoscopic ultrasound-guided fine-needle aspiration biopsy using linear array and radial scanning endosonography. Gastrointest Endosc 1997;45: 243–250.

3 Wiersema MJ, Vilmann P, Giovannini M, Chang KJ, Wiersema LM: Endosonography-guided fine-needle aspiration biopsy: diagnostic accuracy and complication assessment. Gastroenterology 1997;112:1087–1095.

4 Al-Haddad M, Wallace MB, Woodward TA, et al: The safety of fine-needle aspiration guided by endoscopic ultrasound: a prospective study. Endoscopy 2008;40:204–208.

5 Klapman JB, Logrono R, Dye CE, Waxman I: Clinical impact of on-site cytopathology interpretation on endoscopic ultrasound-guided fine needle aspiration. Am J Gastroenterol 2003;98:1289–1294.

6 Eloubeidi MA, Tamhane A, Jhala N, et al: Agreement between rapid onsite and final cytologic interpretations of EUS-guided FNA specimens: implications for the endosonographer and patient management. Am J Gastroenterol 2006;101:2841–2847.

7 Lee LS, Saltzman JR, Bounds BC, Poneros JM, Brugge WR, Thompson CC: EUS-guided fine needle aspiration of pancreatic cysts: a retrospective analysis of complications and their predictors. Clin Gastroenterol Hepatol 2005;3:231–236.

8 Al-Haddad M, Raimondo M, Woodward T, et al: Safety and efficacy of cytology brushings versus standard FNA in evaluating cystic lesions of the pancreas: a pilot study. Gastrointest Endosc 2007;65: 894–898.

9 Levy MJ, Jondal ML, Clain J, Wiersema MJ: Preliminary experience with an EUS-guided trucut biopsy needle compared with EUS-guided FNA. Gastrointest Endosc 2003;57:101–106.

10 Wiersema MJ, Levy MJ, Harewood GC, Vazquez-Sequeiros E, Jondal ML, Wiersema LM: Initial experience with EUS-guided trucut needle biopsies of perigastric organs. Gastrointest Endosc 2002;56: 275–278.

11 Levy MJ, Reddy RP, Wiersema MJ, et al: EUS-guided trucut biopsy in establishing autoimmune pancreatitis as the cause of obstructive jaundice. Gastrointest Endosc 2005;61:467–472.

12 Ahmad NA, Kochman ML, Lewis JD, Ginsberg GG: Can EUS alone differentiate between malignant and benign cystic lesions of the pancreas? Am J Gastroenterol 2001; 96:3295–3300.
13 Gress F, Gottlieb K, Cummings O, Sherman S, Lehman G: Endoscopic ultrasound characteristics of mucinous cystic neoplasms of the pancreas. Am J Gastroenterol 2000;95:961–965.
14 Brugge WR: The role of EUS in the diagnosis of cystic lesions of the pancreas. Gastrointest Endosc 2000;52:S18–S22.
15 Brugge WR, Lewandrowski K, Lee-Lewandrowski E, et al: Diagnosis of pancreatic cystic neoplasms: a report of the cooperative pancreatic cyst study. Gastroenterology 2004;126:1330–1336.
16 Brandwein SL, Farrell JJ, Centeno BA, Brugge WR: Detection and tumor staging of malignancy in cystic, intraductal, and solid tumors of the pancreas by EUS. Gastrointest Endosc 2001;53:722–727.
17 Frossard JL, Amouyal P, Amouyal G, et al: Performance of endosonography-guided fine needle aspiration and biopsy in the diagnosis of pancreatic cystic lesions. Am J Gastroenterol 2003;98:1516–1524.
18 Sedlack R, Affi A, Vazquez-Sequeiros E, Norton ID, Clain JE, Wiersema MJ: Utility of EUS in the evaluation of cystic pancreatic lesions. Gastrointest Endosc 2002;56:543–547.
19 Levy MJ, Smyrk TC, Reddy RP, et al: Endoscopic ultrasound-guided trucut biopsy of the cyst wall for diagnosing cystic pancreatic tumors. Clin Gastroenterol Hepatol 2005;3:974–979.
20 Eloubeidi MA, Varadarajulu S, Desai S, et al: A prospective evaluation of an algorithm incorporating routine preoperative endoscopic ultrasound-guided fine needle aspiration in suspected pancreatic cancer. J Gastrointest Surg 2007;11:813–819.
21 Eloubeidi MA, Tamhane A, Varadarajulu S, Wilcox CM: Frequency of major complications after EUS-guided FNA of solid pancreatic masses: a prospective evaluation. Gastrointest Endosc 2006;63:622–629.
22 Nakeeb A, Lillemoe KD, Cameron JL: The role of pancreaticoduodenectomy for locally recurrent or metastatic carcinoma to the periampullary region. J Am Coll Surg 1995;180:188–192.
23 Sperti C, Pasquali C, Liessi G, Pinciroli L, Decet G, Pedrazzoli S: Pancreatic resection for metastatic tumors to the pancreas. J Surg Oncol 2003;83:161–166.
24 Minni F, Casadei R, Perenze B, et al: Pancreatic metastases: observations of three cases and review of the literature. Pancreatology 2004;4:509–520.
25 Mesa H, Stelow EB, Stanley MW, Mallery S, Lai R, Bardales RH: Diagnosis of nonprimary pancreatic neoplasms by endoscopic ultrasound-guided fine-needle aspiration. Diagn Cytopathol 2004;31:313–318.
26 Fritscher-Ravens A, Broering DC, Sriram PV, et al: EUS-guided fine-needle aspiration cytodiagnosis of hilar cholangiocarcinoma: a case series. Gastrointest Endosc 2000;52:534–540.
27 Eloubeidi MA, Chen VK, Jhala NC, et al: Endoscopic ultrasound-guided fine needle aspiration biopsy of suspected cholangiocarcinoma. Clin Gastroenterol Hepatol 2004;2:209–213.
28 Varadarajulu S, Eloubeidi MA: Endoscopic ultrasound-guided fine-needle aspiration in the evaluation of gallbladder masses. Endoscopy 2005;37:751–754.
29 Jemal A, Siegel R, Ward E, et al: Cancer statistics, 2008. CA Cancer J Clin 2008;58:71–96.
30 Miller AB: Epidemiology, prevention, prognostic factors, and natural history of lung cancer. Curr Opin Oncol 1992;4:286–291.
31 Toloza EM, Harpole L, McCrory DC: Noninvasive staging of non-small cell lung cancer: a review of the current evidence. Chest 2003;123:137S–146S.
32 Silvestri GA, Tanoue LT, Margolis ML, Barker J, Detterbeck F: The noninvasive staging of non-small cell lung cancer: the guidelines. Chest 2003;123:147S–56S.
33 Eloubeidi MA, Cerfolio RJ, Chen VK, Desmond R, Syed S, Ojha B: Endoscopic ultrasound-guided fine needle aspiration of mediastinal lymph node in patients with suspected lung cancer after positron emission tomography and computed tomography scans. Ann Thorac Surg 2005;79:263–268.
34 LeBlanc JK, Espada R, Ergun G: Non-small cell lung cancer staging techniques and endoscopic ultrasound: tissue is still the issue. Chest 2003;123:1718–1725.
35 Eloubeidi MA, Tamhane A, Chen VK, Cerfolio RJ: Endoscopic ultrasound-guided fine-needle aspiration in patients with non-small cell lung cancer and prior negative mediastinoscopy. Ann Thorac Surg 2005;80:1231–1239.
36 Wallace MB, Pascual JM, Raimondo M, et al: Minimally invasive endoscopic staging of suspected lung cancer. JAMA 2008;299:540–546.
37 Dietrich CF, Wehrmann T, Hoffmann C, Herrmann G, Caspary WF, Seifert H: Detection of the adrenal glands by endoscopic or transabdominal ultrasound. Endoscopy 1997;29:859–864.
38 DeWitt J, Alsatie M, LeBlanc J, McHenry L, Sherman S: Endoscopic ultrasound-guided fine-needle aspiration of left adrenal gland masses. Endoscopy 2007;39:65–71.
39 Eloubeidi MA, Seewald S, Tamhane A, et al: EUS-guided FNA of the left adrenal gland in patients with thoracic or GI malignancies. Gastrointest Endosc 2004;59:627–633.
40 Eloubeidi MA, Varadarajulu S, Eltoum I, Jhala D, Chhieng DC, Jhala NC: Transgastric endoscopic ultrasound-guided fine-needle aspiration biopsy and flow cytometry of suspected lymphoma of the spleen. Endoscopy 2006;38:617–620.
41 Eloubeidi MA, Morgan DE, Cerfolio RJ, Eltoum IA: Transduodenal EUS-guided FNA of the right adrenal gland. Gastrointest Endosc 2008;67:522–527.

42 Miettinen M, Sarlomo-Rikala M, Lasota J: Gastrointestinal stromal tumors: recent advances in understanding of their biology. Hum Pathol 1999;30:1213–1220.
43 Miettinen M, Sarlomo-Rikala M, Sobin LH, Lasota J: Gastrointestinal stromal tumors and leiomyosarcomas in the colon: a clinicopathologic, immunohistochemical, and molecular genetic study of 44 cases. Am J Surg Pathol 2000;24:1339–1352.
44 Ando N, Goto H, Niwa Y, et al: The diagnosis of GI stromal tumors with EUS-guided fine needle aspiration with immunohistochemical analysis. Gastrointest Endosc 2002;55:37–43.
45 Ponsaing LG, Kiss K, Loft A, Jensen LI, Hansen MB: Diagnostic procedures for submucosal tumors in the gastrointestinal tract. World J Gastroenterol 2007;13:3301–3310.
46 Stelow EB, Stanley MW, Mallery S, Lai R, Linzie BM, Bardales RH: Endoscopic ultrasound-guided fine-needle aspiration findings of gastrointestinal leiomyomas and gastrointestinal stromal tumors. Am J Clin Pathol 2003;119:703–708.
47 Sircar K, Hewlett BR, Huizinga JD, Chorneyko K, Berezin I, Riddell RH: Interstitial cells of Cajal as precursors of gastrointestinal stromal tumors. Am J Surg Pathol 1999;23:377–389.
48 Ohshima A, Yamashita H, Noguchi S, et al: Usefulness of endoscopic ultrasonography (EUS) in diagnosing esophageal infiltration of thyroid cancer. J Endocrinol Invest 2001;24:564–569.
49 Suen KC: Fine-needle aspiration biopsy of the thyroid. CMAJ 2002;167:491–495.
50 Dewitt J, Youssef W, Leblanc J, et al: EUS-guided FNA of a thyroid mass. Gastrointest Endosc 2004; 59:307–310.
51 Gress F, Schmitt C, Sherman S, Ciaccia D, Ikenberry S, Lehman G: Endoscopic ultrasound-guided celiac plexus block for managing abdominal pain associated with chronic pancreatitis: a prospective single center experience. Am J Gastroenterol 2001;96:409–416.
52 Gunaratnam NT, Sarma AV, Norton ID, Wiersema MJ: A prospective study of EUS-guided celiac plexus neurolysis for pancreatic cancer pain. Gastrointest Endosc 2001;54:316–324.

Mohamad A. Eloubeidi, MD
University of Alabama at Birmingham
1530 3rd Ave. S. – ZRB 636
Birmingham, AL 35294–0007 (USA)
Tel. +1 843 934 7964, Fax +1 205 975 6381, E-Mail eloubeidi@uab.edu

Mönkemüller K, Wilcox CM, Muñoz-Navas M (eds): Interventional and Therapeutic Gastrointestinal Endoscopy.
Front Gastrointest Res. Basel, Karger, 2010, vol 27, pp 511–521

Therapeutic Endoscopic Ultrasound

Shyam Varadarajulu[a] · Jayapal Ramesh[b]

[a]University of Alabama at Birmingham School of Medicine, Birmingham, Ala., USA, and [b]University Hospital of South Manchester, Manchester, UK

Abstract

Endoscopic ultrasonography (EUS), since its development in the 1980s, has undergone a great deal of technological advancement in imaging, scopes with larger channels and accessories. This has given the endosonographer an immense reach in terms of accessing difficult areas with fewer complications. Currently, it is possible not only to obtain tissue for histological diagnosis but also to perform therapeutic procedures that hitherto would have needed surgery with its attendant morbidity. EUS has evolved over the years and EUS-guided fine-needle aspiration for histological diagnosis has become standard practice. A wide array of interventional procedures are performed under EUS guidance including celiac plexus neurolysis, drainage of pancreatic and pelvic fluid collections, drainage of obstructive biliary/pancreatic ducts, and implantation of fiducial markers/radioactive seeds into gastrointestinal tumors. Also, various experimental procedures are underway evaluating the role of EUS in radiofrequency ablation, vascular therapy, and natural orifice transluminal endoscopic surgery. In this review, we examine the various EUS-guided interventions currently undertaken and explore the potential of other emerging experimental techniques.

Endoscopic ultrasonography (EUS), since its development in the 1980s, has undergone a great deal of technological advancement in imaging, scopes with larger channels and accessories. This has given the endosonographer an immense reach in terms of accessing difficult areas with fewer complications. Currently, it is possible not only to obtain tissue for histological diagnosis but also to perform therapeutic procedures that hitherto would have needed surgery with its attendant morbidity. EUS has evolved over the years and EUS-guided fine-needle aspiration for histological diagnosis has become standard practice. A wide array of interventional procedures are performed under EUS guidance including, celiac plexus neurolysis (CPN), drainage of pancreatic and pelvic fluid collections, drainage of obstructive biliary/pancreatic ducts, and implantation of fiducial markers/radioactive seeds into gastrointestinal tumors. Also, various experimental procedures are underway evaluating the role of EUS in radiofrequency ablation (RFA), vascular therapy, and natural orifice transluminal endoscopic surgery. In this review, we examine the various EUS-guided interventions currently undertaken and explore the potential of other emerging experimental techniques.

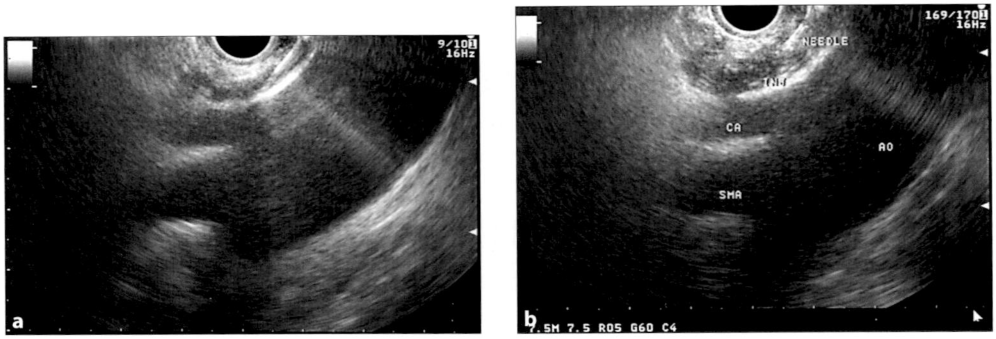

Fig. 1. **a** EUS-guided CPN being undertaken by placing the needle in the space around the celiac artery. **b** Following injection, note the soft tissue reaction at the site of neurolysis.

Celiac Plexus Neurolysis and Block

CPN is the injection of absolute alcohol to destroy the sympathetic plexus near the celiac axis while celiac plexus block (CPB) is to hinder the pain pathway by injecting triamcinolone. The former is performed in pancreatic cancer whilst the latter is undertaken in patients with chronic pancreatitis. Pain is a common symptom, with up to 90% of patients reporting pain in advanced pancreatic cancer [1]. CPN is effective in pain control in 70–90% of patients as shown in a meta-analysis [2]. However, these were radiological procedures and most adopted the posterior approach, which lead to serious complications of paraesthesia, paraplegia and pneumothorax in 1% of cases [2]. EUS has the advantage of accessing the ganglia anteriorly through the posterior stomach wall thus avoiding the spinal arteries, diaphragm and the pleura. The other notable advantages of EUS are real-time imaging, color Doppler use to avoid vasculature and the ability to visualize the ganglia for targeted block [3]. In 1996, Wiersema and Wiersema [4] evaluated 30 patients with advanced intra-abdominal malignancy and showed that following CPN, pain scores reduced significantly compared with baseline at 12 weeks, while up to 91% of patients required the same or less pain medication and 88% of patients had persistent improvement in their pain score. Similarly, in another study of 58 patients with unresectable pancreatic cancer, EUS-guided CPN lowered pain scores in 78% at 2 weeks and a sustained response was noted until 24 weeks [5].

Procedural Technique. The technique for EUS-guided CPB and neurolysis are identical with the only difference being the substances injected. Using a curvilinear-array echoendoscope, the region of the celiac plexus is visualized from the lesser curve of the stomach by following the aorta to the origin of the main celiac artery and traced, using counter-clockwise rotation (fig. 1a, b). With careful inspection it will often be possible, using slight rotational movements, to visualize directly the celiac ganglia as elongated hypoechoic structures. A 22- or 19-G EUS-FNA needle is usually used but in some countries a dedicated 20-G 'spray' needle with multiple side holes is available and allows solutions to spread over a greater area. The tip of the needle is placed slightly anterior and cephalad to the origin of the celiac artery or directly into the ganglia if these can be identified. Aspiration is first performed to ensure vascular puncture has not occurred. Bupivicaine is injected first, followed by alcohol (or triamcinolone for block).

Technical Considerations. There is considerable debate about injecting just anterior to the celiac artery take off from the aorta versus injecting on either side of the celiac artery take off. Although not proven, clinical experience suggests similar efficacy with both techniques. Also, there is increasing interest in targeting the celiac ganglion as this can be seen clearly at EUS. Levy et al. [3] have shown in 33 patients, direct celiac ganglia injections for unresectable pancreatic cancer or chronic pancreatitis can be performed safely. In their study, 94% of pancreatic cancer patients reported pain relief when alcohol was injected and 0% when steroid was injected. In chronic pancreatitis, 80% reported pain relief when alcohol was injected versus 38% receiving steroids. The role of alcohol for this indication (chronic pancreatitis) requires further evaluation.

Complications. Transient diarrhea and orthostatic hypotension have been reported in 9 and 10–15%, respectively [5]. These are usually self-limiting and respond to conservative measures such as intravenous fluid administration. Gress et al. [6] reported a complication of peripancreatic abscess in 1 of 90 patients undergoing CPB for chronic pancreatitis.

Pancreatic Fluid Collections

Pseudocysts occur in 10% of patients with acute pancreatitis and in patients with chronic pancreatitis following an acute exacerbation or due to ductal disruption [7]. Since 1989, when the first case was reported [8], endoscopy has become the modality of choice for drainage of uncomplicated pancreatic pseudocysts. Various factors need to be taken into consideration prior to endoscopic drainage of pseudocysts: clinical symptoms of patients, location of the pseudocyst, presence of luminal compression at endoscopy, single or multiple fluid collections, and communication with the main pancreatic duct.

EUS is a useful tool for the assessment and treatment of pancreatic fluid collections (PFCs) because of the close proximity of the stomach and duodenum to the pancreas [9]. EUS enables assessment of pseudocyst wall thickness, confirmation of size, delineate contents (clear fluid vs. walled-off pancreatic necrosis), check distance from the gastrointestinal lumen, evaluate for intervening vasculature, and sample cyst contents for analysis or perform transmural drainage as a single-step procedure [10–14]. Fockens et al. [16] have shown that initial EUS assessment alters management in 37% of patients. In their study of 32 patients referred for endoscopic drainage of pseudocysts, EUS did not identify a pseudocyst in 3 patients, the lesion was inconsistent with a pseudocyst in 2, transmural drainage was considered inappropriate in 7, the distance between the gastrointestinal lumen and the cyst was >1.5 cm in 4, intervening vessels were present in 2, and in 1 patient normal pancreatic parenchyma was present between the pseudocyst and the gastrointestinal lumen. Varadarajulu et al. [9] have shown that EUS alters diagnosis in 5% of cases, where cyst neoplasm was identified in cases misclassified as pseudocysts on CT imaging. At endoscopy, luminal compression is only identified in 50% of cases of PFCs [8, 17, 18]. EUS by virtue of its ability to identify PFC that does not cause luminal compression improves both the technical success rates (>90%) and safety profile (complications, <5%) of the procedure [9, 10, 13]. In a randomized trial, Varadarajulu et al. [19] showed that blind drainage with endoscopy (gastroscopy) had a higher complication rate than under EUS guidance (12 vs. 0%) and when PFCs not amenable for drainage by endoscopy underwent crossover to the EUS cohort, all patients were drained successfully. The above advantages and the safety profile accorded by EUS makes it an attractive diagnostic/therapeutic modality in the algorithm for management of PFCs (table 1).

Table 1. Studies showing success and complications of EUS-guided PFC drainage

Reference (first author)	Type of study	Patients n	Technical success	Complications
Antillon 2006 [12]	prospective	33	94%	15%
Kahaleh 2006 [15]	prospective, comparing EGD vs. EUS	99	84 vs. 91%	19 vs. 18%
Krüger 2006 [13]	prospective	35	94	0% immediate, 12% late complications
Varadarajulu 2008 [19]	randomized trial (EUS vs. EGD)	15 each arm	100 vs. 33%	0% (EUS) vs. 12% (EGD)
Varadarajulu 2008 [21]	retrospective EUS vs. surgery	20 in EUS and 10 in surgical arm	95 vs. 100%	none

EGD = Esophagogastroduodenoscopy.

Procedural Technique. EUS-guided PFC drainage is performed under conscious sedation in the fluoroscopy suite with the patient in the left lateral or prone position. The patient should receive broad-spectrum antibiotics during and after the procedure to reduce the risk of infection. The PFC is first located and the contact zone between the gastric or duodenal wall is evaluated for interposed vessels using color Doppler. After determining the optimal site for puncture, the PFC is punctured using a 19-G FNA needle and a sample of the cyst contents is aspirated and submitted for biochemical, cytological, and tumor marker analysis. If infection is suspected, a sample should be sent for Gram stain, culture and sensitivity. After passage of a 0.035-inch guidewire into the PFC, the transmural tract is sequentially dilated using a 4.5-/5-Fr ERCP cannula or a needle-knife catheter. The tract is further enlarged using a 6- or 8-mm over-the-wire biliary balloon dilator. A nasocystic drain or stent (double pigtail) is then deployed to drain the PFC. The choice between a nasocystic catheter or a stent for drainage will depend upon the density of the cyst contents. A chronic cyst with clear liquid contents can be drained with an 8.5- or 10-Fr stent alone or with two 7-Fr stents. An infected cyst mandates irrigation by nasocystic drainage catheter alongside the transmural stents.

Technical Considerations. When multiple PFCs are encountered in the same patient, the largest PFC should be drained at the index procedure. A repeat procedure is warranted for drainage of other PFCs if a patient has persistent symptoms with non-communicative fluid collection on follow-up imaging [18]. Bedside drainage of PFC can be undertaken in patients who are too unwell to be transported to the endoscopy unit. This was demonstrated in a recent study that showed successful pancreatic pseudocyst and mediastinal abscess drainage in 6 patients [17]. It is essential that a portable fluoroscopy machine is available in the intensive care unit for performing bedside EUS-guided interventions. It would also be convenient to have the ultrasound and video processors in a single endoscopy stack.

Complications. The ability to drain the pseudocyst real-time under EUS guidance minimizes the risk of complications such as perforation and hemorrhage. Intracystic hemorrhage is a rare but serious complication encountered during FNA of cyst lesions of the pancreas [20]. At EUS, the bleeding manifests as a hyperechoic area within the pseudocyst. Early identification of bleeding at EUS will enable timely intervention and thereby minimize the risk for serious adverse events.

Obstructive Bile Duct

Choledochoduodenostomy

The standard of care for patients presenting with malignant biliary obstruction is an ERCP to place a transpapillary stent to affect bile drainage. However, technical failure is encountered in up to 10% of cases due to various factors including duodenal obstruction, anatomical variations, periampullary diverticulum and tightness of the stricture. Percutaneous transhepatic biliary drainage (PTBD) or surgical drainage are other treatment alternatives. The technical success rate for PTBD placement is 90% in a dilated intrahepatic system and 70% in a non-dilated system. The procedural morbidity for PTBD is 7% and the mortality rate is 5%. Other contraindications for PTBD include ascites and coagulopathy. Although surgical drainage is a possibility, current practice does not favor that approach as most cases are drained either by endoscopic or percutaneous means and the patient cohort are usually too unwell to undergo a major surgical intervention that has a morbidity of 66% and mortality of 32% [22] Hence, the logical extension is to attempt drainage by means of EUS as the left intrahepatic system can be accessed via the stomach and the common bile duct (CBD) via the duodenal bulb. To date, 25 cases have undergone EUS-guided choledochoduodenostomy and the overall technical success rate is 92%.

Procedural Technique. After administration of intravenous antibiotics, the linear array echoendoscope is positioned in long scope position in the duodenal bulb to identify the CBD. Color Doppler is used to exclude any intervening vasculature. A 19-G needle or needle-knife catheter is used to puncture the CBD. After removal of the stylet, bile is aspirated and contrast injected under fluoroscopic guidance to image the biliary tree. A 0.035-inch hydrophilic tip guidewire is inserted into the CBD. An ERCP cannula followed by balloon dilatation may be necessary to dilate the tract to ensure easy passage of stent. With the guidewire in place, a 7- to 10-Fr plastic stent is deployed under fluoroscopic guidance. A covered metal biliary endoprosthesis may be an alternative.

Complications. The procedural complication rate is 19 with 8% being due to focal biliary peritonitis. The advantage seems to be stent patency, which has been reported to up to a mean of 211 days at long-term follow-up [23]. More studies are required with a larger cohort of patients to assess the technical feasibility and safety profile of the procedure.

Hepaticogastrostomy

There are 19 published cases examining this concept that has demonstrated a technical success rate of 90–100% and a clinical success rate of 75–100% [24–29].

Procedural Technique. The curved linear array echoendoscope is positioned along the cardia or the lesser curve of the stomach and after excluding the presence of intervening vasculature using color Doppler, a dilated peripheral radical of the left intrahepatic system is accessed using a 19- or 22-G needle. After coiling a guidewire within the intrahepatic biliary ductal system, transmural dilation and stenting is undertaken as described earlier for performing a choledochoduodenostomy.

Complications. Reported complications with this technique include bile leak, infection and stent migration. More studies with a larger cohort of patients are required before this technique can be considered as a treatment alternative to PTBD or surgery.

Obstructive Pancreatic Duct

Chronic pancreatitis is a debilitating condition causing pain, exocrine and endocrine insufficiency. The latter two complications can be treated by medical means, while pain, as a symptom, can be difficult to manage. Pancreatic endotherapy is the mainstay for management of obstructive ducts and has a high success rate in expert hands. Correction of the offending factor (stone, stricture or duct disruption) leads to an improvement in symptoms in up to 80% of cases. However, ERCP can be technically challenging in a subset of patients when there is active inflammation of the duodenum, a very tight stricture, complete disruption of the pancreatic duct or severe stenosis of the minor papilla in pancreas divisum. There is also a significant minority who develop recurrent symptoms after successful endotherapy during long-term follow-up. Surgery is an effective treatment alternative in these circumstances as it has the advantage of removing the diseased part of the gland, however it involves significant morbidity and mortality.

EUS-guided pancreatic duct drainage is an attractive treatment alternative to decompress the obstructive pancreatic ductal system. The proximity of the pancreas to the posterior stomach wall makes it easy to access the main pancreatic duct under EUS guidance. Table 2 summarizes the results of available studies in the literature.

Procedural Technique. Two approaches, similar to hepatogastrostomy, have been described. The rendezvous technique and pancreatogastrostomy. For both techniques, the curved linear array echoendoscope is positioned in the stomach or duodenal bulb depending on the least distance from the transducer to the pancreatic duct. The tip of the echoendoscope should be aligned parallel to the long axis of the dilated pancreatic duct to help ease the passage of the guidewire. After excluding the presence of intervening vasculature using color Doppler, a 19- or 22-G needle is used to puncture the main pancreatic duct. A 0.035- or 0.021-inch guidewire is inserted into the pancreatic duct and every attempt should be made to pass the wire across the papilla into the duodenum for rendezvous placement of a transpapillary stent. If this is not achievable, the guidewire should be passed retrograde to the tail of the pancreas and the transmural tract should be dilated using a 4.5-Fr cannula, needle-knife catheter or small-caliber bougie. Balloon dilatation (4–6 mm) may be necessary to dilate the tract to ensure easy passage of stent. With the guidewire in place, a transgastric 7-Fr plastic stent is deployed under fluoroscopic guidance.

Complications. Stent migration and occlusion appears to be a major problem in 20–55% of cases drained transluminally [31, 33] and stent-induced pancreatic duct strictures have been observed on follow-up [31]. The rate of procedural complications in the four series varies between 5 and 44%, and is independent of the technique adopted for drainage. Currently, the procedure should be attempted only in a research setting under a well-defined protocol.

Table 2. Studies evaluating EUS-guided pancreatic duct drainage following failed ERCP

Reference (first author)	Design	Approach	Cases n	Technical success	Complications
Tessier 2007 [30]	retrospective	transluminal	36	91.6%	hematoma (n = 1) severe pancreatitis (n = 1)
Kahaleh 2007 [31]	prospective	transluminal	13	83%	bleeding (n = 1) perforation (n = 1)
Will 2007 [32]	case series	transluminal and rendezvous	12	69%	pain (n = 4) bleeding (n = 1) perforation (n = 1) pseudocyst (n = 1)
Mallery 2004 [33]	case series	rendezvous	4	25%	fever (n = 1)

Pelvic Fluid Collections

Pelvic fluid collections can occur due to Crohn's disease, diverticlitis, appendicitis and pelvic inflammatory diseases. More commonly they occur following pelvic surgery, in particular low anterior resection for rectal carcinoma. The various approaches used conventionally to drain these collections are ultrasound-guided drainage via the transvaginal or transrectal route and CT-guided drainage via the transgluteal or transabdominal route. Alternatively, they can be managed surgically. The limitations with these approaches are the inability to access deep-seated collections, restriction on dilation of the tract to appropriate size, patient inconvenience, incomplete resolution, need for frequent reinterventions, and injury to surrounding vessels and nerves [34, 35].

Three studies have evaluated the role of EUS-guided transrectal drainage of pelvic abscesses. While Giovannini et al. [36] used transrectal stents, Varadarajulu and Drelichman [37] used a drainage catheter with intermittent irrigation. The same author later reported a hybrid approach in which both a drainage catheter and plastic stent were deployed transrectally. While the drainage catheter was flushed and aspirated intermittently and then removed after a few days when the abscess cavity reduced in size, the stents were removed after 2 weeks [38]. Technical success in these studies was recorded in 75–100% of cases and treatment success rate was 85–100%.

Procedural Technique. After administration of intravenous antibiotics and tap water enema, a curvilinear echoendoscope is passed into the rectum and the abscess cavity is identified. After using color Doppler to rule out any intervening vasculature, a 19-G needle is used to puncture the abscess cavity. Pus is aspirated in a sterile syringe and sent for Gram stain and microscopy. The abscess cavity is flushed with normal saline and aspirated multiple times so as to evacuate as much pus as possible. A 0.035-inch guidewire is coiled into the abscess cavity and the transmural tract is dilated using a 4.5-Fr ERCP cannula and a 6- or 8-mm over-the-wire biliary balloon dilator. A 10-Fr single pigtail drainage catheter is then deployed over the guide wire under fluoroscopic guidance. Additionally, 10-Fr double pigtail stents can also be placed alongside the catheter to facilitate quicker drainage. The drainage catheter should be flushed with 25-ml of normal saline and aspirated till the size of the cavity diminishes. The pigtail drainage catheter can be removed once the cavity size has reduced to at least 50% and the stents removed at a later stage by sigmoidoscopy.

Complications. No procedure-related complications were recorded in the three studies. One patient died of heart failure [37] and 25% of patients in one study [36] needed surgery because of treatment failure.

Implantation Therapy

There is a growing need for additional treatment options in cancer patients who are not surgical candidates. Due to the ability of EUS to access malignant tissue, it has the advantage of supplementing other therapeutic options that are currently available. Implantation of fiducial markers to facilitate radiotherapy and radioactive seed instillation for brachytherapy can be performed under EUS guidance.

Fiducial Implantation

Fiducials can be placed into tumors to enable more precise and targeted radiotherapy with low risk of complications. Although CT-guided placement has been attempted, EUS with its immediate access is a better option, particularly in patients with pancreatic cancer. Two studies have demonstrated a technical success rate of 84–91% [39, 40]. While EUS-guided fiducial placement is technically feasible, its direct impact on patient management is unclear.

Procedural Technique. A 19-G FNA needle is preloaded with gold fiducials and the tip of the needle is sealed with bone wax to prevent accidental dislodgement. Once the tumor is punctured under EUS guidance, the stylet is pushed to advance the fiducials slowly into the tumor. A total of 3–6 fiducials are placed within the tumor in different planes.

Complications. No immediate complications were encountered in both studies [39, 40], although 1 patient developed cholangitis after 3 weeks.

Brachytherapy

Brachytherapy is an important tool in the management of advanced pancreatic cancer and has been performed either by implanting radioactive seeds surgically or intraluminally at ERCP. As an alternative, EUS-guided brachytherapy has been performed to place radioactive iodine seeds [41] or to inject liquid-based implant into the pancreatic tumor mass [42]. Studies have demonstrated a significant improvement in pain scores in these patients. This technique needs further evaluation in multicenter trials as no survival benefit has been demonstrated and there were significant procedure-related complications [41].

Miscellaneous Applications

Botulinum Toxin Injection. EUS can identify the muscle layer in the lower esophageal sphincter as a thick hypoechoic band. This allows targeted delivery of botulinum toxin to the muscle layer of the lower esophagus in patients who are not fit for surgery or dilatation. Two studies have demonstrated technical feasibility, safety and clinical improvement in dysphagia scores [43, 44]. However, these are small studies and no randomized control trials are available to make a definitive recommendation. Another study has also reported use of botulinum toxin injections into the muscularis propria of the antrum in obese patients to induce satiation, reduce weight, and delay gastric emptying [45].

Tumor Localization. EUS is known to be very sensitive in identifying small lesions in the pancreas, particularly neuroenrodocrine tumors missed by CT imaging. As some of these lesions are difficult to identify at surgery, intraoperative ultrasound may be required in certain cases. EUS-guided tattooing of the lesion using India ink has been advocated as a technique to facilitate their intraoperative localization [46–48].

Glue Injection for Vascular Bleeding. Gastric variceal bleeding is a serious complication of portal hypertension and can be difficult to treat. Blind injections with tissue adhesives have been reported with variable success rates. One of the major complications of cyanoacrylate glue injection is spread of glue to distant areas causing vascular occlusion. EUS provides a more precise approach to target the perforating veins [49]. It has been shown in one study that periodically targeted glue injections can lead to eradication of gastric varices [50]. Others have tried to use a coil to obliterate the ectopic varices [51]. In a minority of patients with non-variceal causes, the exact site of bleeding may not be easily identifiable at endoscopy. EUS with color Doppler can identify vessels causing refractory bleeding and enables targeted therapy [52].

Experimental Applications

Portal Vein Access. Portal vein pressures are important in the management of patients with advanced liver cirrhosis. While percutaneous and transjugular approaches are current options, four animal studies have demonstrated the feasibility and safety of portal venous access by EUS [53–56]. More studies are underway evaluating this exciting treatment approach.

Radiofrequency Ablation. RFA is a well-established procedure for various malignant diseases to provide palliation. Hitherto performed under ultrasound and CT guidance, EUS-guided RFA placement was evaluated in an animal model, with specially designed umbrella-shaped probe. The probe was deployed by a 19-G needle into the liver and an impedance-based feedback system used to provide electrical energy to induce coagulative necrosis. This study demonstrated that EUS-guided RFA is technically feasible and induces coagulation necrosis of larger areas [57].

Conclusion

With further improvements in imaging and echoendoscope designs, more advanced and challenging interventions can be undertaken under EUS guidance with relative ease. Although some of the procedures are well established and performed in most centers, several others are restricted to tertiary/high volume centers and require more evidence before they are ready for primetime application. One of the challenges for the future is training of endosonographers in interventional EUS and identifying appropriate coding for procedural reimbursements.

References

1 Caraceni A, Portenoy RK: Pain management in patients with pancreatic carcinoma. Cancer 1996;78(suppl):639–653.

2 Eisenberg E, Carr DB, Chalmers TC: Neurolytic celiac plexus block for treatment of cancer pain: a meta-analysis. Anesth Analg 1995;80:290–295.

3 Levy MJ, Topazian MD, Wiersema MJ, et al: Initial evaluation of the efficacy and safety of endoscopic ultrasound-guided direct ganglia neurolysis and block. Am J Gastroenterol 2008;103:98–103.

4 Wiersema MJ, Wiersema LM: Endosonography-guided celiac plexus neurolysis. Gastrointest Endosc 1996;44: 656–662.

5 Gunaratnam NT, Sarma AV, Norton ID, et al: A prospective study of EUS-guided celiac plexus neurolysis for pancreatic cancer pain. Gastrointest Endosc 2001;54: 316–324.

6 Gress F, Schmitt C, Sherman S, et al: Endoscopic ultrasound-guided celiac plexus block for managing abdominal pain associated with chronic pancreatitis: a prospective single center experience. Am J Gastroenterol 2001;96:409–416.

7 O'Malley VP, Cannon JP, Postier RG: Pancreatic pseudocysts: cause, therapy, and results. Am J Surg 1985;150: 680–682.

8 Cremer M, Deviere J, Engelholm L: Endoscopic management of cysts and pseudocysts in chronic pancreatitis: long-term follow-up after 7 years of experience. Gastrointest Endosc 1989;35:1–9.

9 Varadarajulu S, Wilcox CM, Tamhane A, et al: Role of EUS in drainage of peripancreatic fluid collections not amenable for endoscopic transmural drainage. Gastrointest Endosc 2007;66:1107–1119.

10 Ahlawat SK, Charabaty-Pishvaian A, Jackson PG, et al: Single-step EUS-guided pancreatic pseudocyst drainage using a large channel linear array echoendoscope and cystotome: results in 11 patients. JOP 2006;7:616–624.

11 Seewald S, Thonke F, Ang TL, et al: One-step, simultaneous double-wire technique facilitates pancreatic pseudocyst and abscess drainage. Gastrointest Endosc 2006;64: 805–808.

12 Antillon MR, Shah RJ, Stiegmann G, et al: Single-step EUS-guided transmural drainage of simple and complicated pancreatic pseudocysts. Gastrointest Endosc 2006; 63:797–803.

13 Krüger M, Schneider AS, Manns MP, et al: Endoscopic management of pancreatic pseudocysts or abscesses after an EUS-guided one-step procedure for initial access. Gastrointest Endosc 2006;63: 409–416.

14 Inui K, Yoshino J, Okushima K, et al: EUS-guided one-step drainage of pancreatic pseudocysts: experience in three patients. Gastrointest Endosc 2001; 54:87–89.

15 Kahaleh M, Shami VM, Conaway MR, et al: Endoscopic ultrasound drainage of pancreatic pseudocyst: a prospective comparison with conventional endoscopic drainage. Endoscopy 2006;38:355–359.

16 Fockens P, Johnson TG, van Dullemen HM, et al: Endosonographic imaging of pancreatic pseudocysts before endoscopic transmural drainage. Gastrointest Endosc 1997;46:412–416.

17 Varadarajulu S, Eloubeidi MA, Wilcox CM. The concept of bedside EUS. Gastrointest Endosc 2008; 67:1180–1184.

18 Varadarajulu S, Tamhane A, Blakely J: Graded dilation technique for EUS-guided drainage of peripancreatic fluid collections: an assessment of outcomes and complications and technical proficiency. Gastrointest Endosc 2008;68:656–666.

19 Varadarajulu S, Christein JD, Tamhane A, et al: Prospective randomized trial comparing EUS and EGD for transmural drainage of pancreatic pseudocysts. Gastrointest Endosc 2008;68:1102–1111.

20 Varadarajulu S, Eloubeidi MA: Frequency and significance of acute intracystic hemorrhage during EUS-FNA of cystic lesions of the pancreas. Gastrointest Endosc 2004;60:631–635.

21 Varadarajulu S, Lopes TL, Wilcox CM, et al: EUS versus surgical cyst-gastrostomy for management of pancreatic pseudocysts. Gastrointest Endosc 2008;68:649–655.

22 Lai EC, Mok FP, Tan ES, et al: Endoscopic biliary drainage for severe acute cholangitis. N Engl J Med 1992;24: 1582–1586.

23 Yamao K, Bhatia V, Mizuno N, et al: EUS-guided choledochoduodenostomy for palliative biliary drainage in patients with malignant biliary obstruction: results of long-term follow-up. Endoscopy 2008;40:340–342.

24 Burmester E, Niehaus J, Leineweber T, Huetteroth T. EUS-cholangio drainage of the bile duct: report of four cases. Gastrointest Endosc 2003;57:246–251.

25 Giovannini M, Dotti M, Bories E, et al: Hepaticogastrostomy by echo-endoscopy as a palliative treatment in a patient with metastatic biliary obstruction. Endoscopy 2003;35:1076–1078.

26 Kahaleh M, Hernandez AJ, Tokar J, et al: Interventional EUS-guided cholangiography: evaluation of a technique in evolution. Gastrointest Endosc 2006;64:52–59.

27 Artifon EL, Chaves DM, Ishioka S, et al: Echoguided hepaticogastrostomy: a case report. Clinics (São Paulo) 2007;62:799–802.

28 Bories E, Pesenti C, Caillol F, et al: Transgastric endoscopic ultrasonography-guided biliary drainage: results of a pilot study. Endoscopy 2007;39:287–291.

29 Will U, Thieme A, Fueldner F, et al: Treatment of biliary obstruction in selected patients by endoscopic ultrasonography-guided transluminal biliary drainage. Endoscopy 2007;39:292–295.

30 Tessier G, Bories E, Arvanitakis M, et al: EUS-guided pancreatogastrostomy and pancreatobulbostomy for the treatment of pain in patients with pancreatic ductal dilatation inaccessible for transpapillary endoscopic therapy. Gastrointest Endosc 2007;65:233–241.
31 Kahaleh M, Hernandez AJ, Tokar J, et al: EUS-guided pancreaticogastrostomy: analysis of its efficacy to drain inaccessible pancreatic ducts. Gastrointest Endosc 2007; 65:224–230.
32 Will U, Fueldner F, Thieme AK, et al: Transgastric pancreatography and EUS-guided drainage of the pancreatic duct. J Hepatobiliary Pancreat Surg 2007; 14:377–382.
33 Mallery S, Matlock J, Freeman ML. EUS-guided rendezvous drainage of obstructed biliary and pancreatic ducts: report of six cases. Gastrointest Endosc 2004;59:100–107.
34 Onaca N, Hirshberg A, Adar R: Early reoperation for perirectal abscess. Dis Colon Rectum 2001;44: 1469–1473.
35 Harisinghani MG, Gervais DA, Maher MM, et al: Transgluteal approach for percutaneous drainage of deep pelvic abscesses: 154 cases. Radiology 2003;228: 701–705.
36 Giovannini M, Bories E, Moutardier V, et al: Drainage of deep pelvic abscesses using therapeutic echoendoscopy. Endoscopy 2003;35:511–514.
37 Varadarajulu S, Drelichman ER: EUS-guided drainage of pelvic abscess. Gastrointest Endosc 2007;66: 372–376.
38 Trevino JM, Drelichman ER, Varadarajulu S: Modified technique for EUS-guided drainage of pelvic abscesses. Gastrointest Endosc 2008;68:1215–1219.
39 Pishvaian AC, Collins B, Gagnon G, et al: EUS-guided fiducial placement for CyberKnife radiotherapy of mediastinal and abdominal malignancies. Gastrointest Endosc 2006;64:412–417.
40 Yan BM, Schellenberg D, Koong AC, Van Dam J: EUS-guided gold fiducial insertion for image-guided radiation therapy of pancreatic cancer. Gastrointest Endosc 2008;67:AB225.
41 Sun S, Xu H, Xin J, et al: Endoscopic ultrasound-guided interstitial brachytherapy of unresectable pancreatic cancer: results of a pilot trial. Endoscopy 2006;38:399–403.
42 Meenan J, Mesenas S, Mahon B, et al: Multicenter, feasibility study on the use of an EUS-delivered ^{32}P-labeled liquid-based brachytherapy implant in advanced pancreatic cancer (abstract). Gastrointest Endosc 2008;67: AB109.
43 Maiorana A, Fiorentino E, Genova EG, et al: Echo-guided injection of botulinum toxin in patients with achalasia: initial experience. Endoscopy 1999;31:S3–S4.
44 Hoffman BJ, Knapple WL, Bhutani MS, et al: Treatment of achalasia by injection of botulinum toxin under endoscopic ultrasound guidance. Gastrointest Endosc 1997; 45:77–79.
45 Topazian M, Camilleri M, De La Mora-Levy J, et al: Endoscopic ultrasound-guided gastric botulinum toxin injections in obese subjects: a pilot study. Obes Surg 2008; 18:401–407.
46 Zografos GN, Stathopoulou A, Mitropapas G, et al: Preoperative imaging and localization of small sized insulinoma with EUS-guided fine needle tattooing: a case report. Hormones (Athens) 2005;4:111–116.
47 Gress FG, Barawi M, Kim D, et al: Preoperative localization of a neuroendocrine tumor of the pancreas with EUS-guided fine needle tattooing. Gastrointest Endosc 2002;55:594–597.
48 Ashida R, Yamao K, Okubo K, et al: Indocyanine green is an ideal dye for endoscopic ultrasound-guided fine-needle tattooing of pancreatic tumors. Endoscopy 2006; 38:190–192.
49 Romero-Castro R, Pellicer-Bautista FJ, Jimenez-Saenz M, et al: EUS-guided injection of cyanoacrylate in perforating feeding veins in gastric varices: results in five cases. Gastrointest Endosc 2007;66: 402–407.
50 Lee YT, Chan FK, Ng EK, et al: EUS-guided injection of cyanoacrylate for bleeding gastric varices. Gastrointest Endosc 2000;52:168–174.
51 Levy MJ, Wong Kee Song LM, Kendrick ML, et al: EUS-guided coil embolization for refractory ectopic variceal bleeding. Gastrointest Endosc 2008;67:572–574.
52 Levy MJ, Wong Kee Song LM, Farnell MB, et al: Endoscopic ultrasound-guided angiotherapy of refractory gastrointestinal bleeding. Am J Gastroenterol 2008;103: 352–359.
53 Giday SA, Ko CW, Clarke JO, et al: EUS-guided portal vein carbon dioxide angiography: a pilot study in a porcine model. Gastrointest Endosc 2007; 66:814–819.
54 Giday SA, Clarke JO, Buscaglia JM, et al: EUS-guided portal vein catheterization: a promising novel approach for portal angiography and portal vein pressure measurements. Gastrointest Endosc 2008;67:338–342.
55 Lai L, Poneros J, Santilli J, et al: EUS-guided portal vein catheterization and pressure measurement in an animal model: a pilot study of feasibility. Gastrointest Endosc 2004;59:280–283.
56 Magno P, Ko CW, Buscaglia JM, et al: EUS-guided angiography: a novel approach to diagnostic and therapeutic interventions in the vascular system. Gastrointest Endosc 2007;66:587–591.
57 Varadarajulu S, Jhala N, Drelichman ER: Experimental study evaluating EUS-guided RFA using a prototype retractable needle electrode array. Gastrointest Endosc 2008;67:AB110.

Shyam Varadarajulu, MD
Division of Gastroenterology-Hepatology
University of Alabama at Birmingham Medical Center
410 LHRB, 1530 3rd Ave S, Birmingham, AL 35294 (USA)
Tel. +1 205 982 2874, Fax +1 205 975 6381, E-Mail svaradarajulu@yahoo.com

Mönkemüller K, Wilcox CM, Muñoz-Navas M (eds): Interventional and Therapeutic Gastrointestinal Endoscopy.
Front Gastrointest Res. Basel, Karger, 2010, vol 27, pp 522–535

Endoscopic Ultrasound-Guided Cholangiodrainage

Uwe Will[a] · Frank Meyer[b]

[a]Department of Gastroenterology, Hepatology, Nephrology and General Internal Medicine, Municipal Hospital (SRH Waldklinikum), Gera and [b]Department of General, Abdominal and Vascular Surgery, University Hospital, Magdeburg, Germany

Abstract

Endoscopic ultrasound (EUS)-guided cholangiodrainage (EUCD) following the initial steps as puncture of an extra- or intrahepatic segment of the retained biliary tree and cholangiography is a substantial and indispensable part in the spectrum of interventional EUS. Besides transluminal EUS-guided drainage of the pancreatic duct (EUPD) and endoscopic necrosectomy, it belongs to the greatest advances in interventional EUS which has been further elaborated in recent years. In addition, EUCD has been considered a reasonable therapeutic alternative over the years as a well-established percutaneous transhepatic cholangiodrainage (PTCD), since it allows permanent internal drainage of the retained bile duct or its branches to the upper gastrointestinal tract via an extra-anatomic prosthetic bypass implanted transluminally by image (EUS)-guided, real-time EUS and thus it avoids persistent disturbance of the patient's physical integrity as in PTCD. It requires extensive endoscopic expertise, experience in interventional EUS as well as interdisciplinary understanding and overview for the mostly late-stage malignant tumor disease. However, it is still an experimental clinical procedure which needs further careful evaluation of its indication, clinical courses and outcome in well-selected cases with currently exclusively malignant tumor growth.

Endoscopic retrograde cholangiography (ERC) has been established as the standard method in the treatment of biliary obstruction caused by stones or tumor lesions. Selective transpapillary cannulation and drainage of the bile duct can be achieved in almost 90–95% of clinical cases. The successful drainage depends on the expertise of the investigator, the anatomic specifics around the papilla of Vater (papilla) and the biliary tree as well as the endoscopic techniques, tools and devices which are used to cannulate the papilla and to get through stenoses [1, 2]. In case of an obstruction at or within the bile duct, transpapillary endoscopic placement of plastic stents or metal prostheses is considered the most effective therapeutic modality in a palliative approach to posthepatic jaundice [3]. In patients who formerly underwent surgical intervention (such as BII gastric resection or hepaticojejunostomy with Roux-en-Y reconstruction, kephal pancreatoduodenectomy, gastroenteroanastomosis) or who were diagnosed with tumor-induced gastric outlet syndrome or locally advanced malignant infiltration of the papilla, a primary internal endoscopic drainage is not possible in the majority of cases.

In such patients, in particular in those with incurable malignancy, percutaneous transhepatic cholangiodrainage (PTCD) is used or the biliary tree is surgically anastomosed with a Roux-en-Y jejunal loop (as the most commonly used type of biliodigestive anastomosis). Both approaches are associated with a higher morbidity and mortality when compared with ERC. In addition, a permanent external/internal drainage of the biliary tree cannot be achieved in each case using PTCD-based access [4–7]. Furthermore, a sole external drainage can cause a temporary or even permanent loss of bile and the subjective impression of an 'altered physical integrity', which is a substantial psychological problem in patients with incurable malignancy and limited life expectancy: For example, by the visible external drainage of the bile and the daily rinsing, the patient is repeatedly confronted with the incurable character and the hopelessness of the disease. This might be a remarkable problem even during the initial phase of the ongoing palliative treatment [8].

In patients with advanced and incurable malignant tumor growth as well as obstructive tumor-induced jaundice, the primary aim in the palliative therapeutic concept is a sufficient, permanent and possibly internal drainage of the biliary tree with a low complication rate and no need for a reintervention until death. Endoscopic ultrasound (EUS)-guided cholangiodrainage (EUCD) may fulfill these requirements [9–18]. Because of the anatomic adjacency of the pancreatobiliary system to the stomach and duodenum, longitudinal EUS is a suitable tool which allows puncture of the intra- and extrahepatic segments of the biliary tree and thus the subsequent placement of a transluminal cholangiography, which can be considered the basic prediction for an EUS-guided internal drainage with good prospects. Currently, three various techniques can be subdivided: (1) If the papilla can be reached but the catheter cannot be introduced into the papilla, an EUS-ERC rendezvous maneuver is preferred [11–13, 19, 20]. (2) If the papilla cannot be reached because of former surgical interventions and an obstructive jaundice due to malignant tumor growth, EUS-guided choledochoduodenostomy is preferentially chosen [13, 16, 18]. (3) In case of tumor lesions at or within the hepatic hilus, EUS-guided hepaticogastrostomy (or hepaticojejunostomy after former gastrectomy) is primarily used [11, 13, 17].

In recent years it has been shown several times, but in only small case series, that EUCD can provide a success rate of 75–100% and a low complication rate (0–18%) [9–18] (table 1). Controlled randomized studies comparing EUCD with PTCD or surgical intervention are lacking.

The present overview describes the various technical aspects of EUCD, values critically the currently available and relevant publications on the subject and compares them with own clinical experiences and also provides suggestions for an adequate approach according to the various indications.

Procedural Aspects

Approach, Material and Technique in General

The technical prediction for EUCD is a longitudinal EUS endoscope of big caliber (Aloka-Olympus GF-UCT140, Olympus, Hamburg, Germany; Pentax-Hitachi EG 3830 UT, Pentax, Hamburg, Germany). The investigation is performed under fluoroscopy control in the ERCP unit. This provides the option to carry out a rendezvous technique during the same procedure (table 2). The patients lie primarily on the left body side or on the abdomen as done for ERCP. Analgosedation is similarly administered as done for ERCP using midazolam/disoprivan/pethidine under permanent cardiopulmonary monitoring by a second physician. The biliary tree is

Table 1. Reported results of the translumenal EUCD – chronological order

Author	Cases n	Stent type	Drainage success	Complications	Clinical long-term success
Burmester 2003	4	plastic stent	75%	1 peritonitis	no data
Bories 2007	11	7 plastic stents 3 SEMS	90%	18% (1 bilioma, 1 cholangitis)	90% (2 reinterventions)
Püspök 2005	6	5 plastic stents 1 SEMS	100%	16% (1 cholecystitis)	no data
Will 2007	10	4 plastic stents 5 SEMS	90%	12.5% (1 bleeding, 1 cholangitis)	80%
Kahaleh 2006	23	11 Plastic stents 10 SEMS	91%	17% (1 bleeding, 2 pneumoperitoneum, 1 biliary leakage)	78%
Tarantino 2008	9	7 plastic stents 1 metal stent	100%	0%	100% (1 reintervention)
Yamaho 2008	5	plastic stent	100%	1 pneumoperitoneum	100%
Yasutaka 2009	5	plastic stent	80%	0%	80%
Hara 2009	10	plastic stent	100%	1 pneumoperitoneum 1 peritonitis	100%
Itoi 2008	4	plastic stent	100%	1 focal peritonitis	100%
Will DDW 2009	35	19 SEMS 6 plastic stents	80% (n = 28/35)	3 cholangitis 1 hemobilia 1 peritonitis (death) 2 stent dislocations (metal)	71% (n = 25/35)

Table 2. Technical predictions for EUCD

Longitudinal echoendoscope
(Aloka-Olympus GF-UCT140, Olympus, Hamburg, Germany;
Pentax-Hitachi EG 3830 UT, Pentax, Hamburg, Germany)
Fluoroscopy unit
Therapeutic duodenoscope
Patient monitoring (SO_2, RR, heart rate) – by a second physician
19-G needle (Wilson-Cook, Mediglobe, Olympus)
Needle-knife catheter (Olympus, Germany; Wilson-Cook, Münchengladbach, Germany)
0.035-Fr guidewire (Boston Scientific, Ratingen, Germany; Wilson-Cook, Germany)
5- to 9-Fr bougies (Olympus, Germany)
6- to 8-mm biliary dilatation balloons (Boston Scientific, Germany; Endoflex, Voerde, Germany)
8.5- to 10-Fr plastic prostheses (Amsterdam/Pigtail)
6- to 8-mm covered metal stents (Boston Scientific, Germany)

approached under focused endosonographic view by a puncture using a 19-G needle or a needle-knife catheter. The authors favor the 19-G needle since it can be faster placed into the biliary tree while the needle-knife catheter cannot be precisely visualized during the slow introduction step of the needle and the sonographic artifacts during electrocoagulation. However, the catheter is advantageous for the guidewire system since the tip of the Terumo wire cannot be sheared as possible (potential problem) in case of a sharp 19-G needle. If the biliary tree has been successfully punctured, bile is withdrawn for microbiologic investigation to initiate antibiotic treatment according to the antibiogram and results of an antibiotic resistance test if required. Independently from this, each EUCD has to be performed under peri-interventional antibiotic prophylaxis as it is well established (e.g., cefuroxime intravenously). Via the needle and catheter placed in the biliary tree, contrast media is applied to: (a) reveal the anatomy of the biliary duct and the type of biliary obstruction (proximally, distally, with flow of the contrast media into the jejunum or not), and (b) determine the next step of the approach.

In this moment, anatomy of the bile duct can be much better imaged by relocating the patient on the back. Via the 19-G needle, a 450-cm long, 0.035-inch guidewire (e.g., J wire; Boston Scientific, Ratingen, Germany) is introduced. The manipulation of the wire can be difficult through the 19-G needle, in particular, in rendezvous procedures (passage of the wire through the papilla or anastomosis) since, as already mentioned above, the tip of the Terumo wire can possibly be sheared at the sharp needle tip. If this happens, the wire cannot be moved any longer and further manipulations become impossible leading to the consequence that needle and guidewire need to be removed. To circumvent this potential problem, the bile duct should be tangentially punctured, which allows to avoid a 'zigzag' of the wire behind the needle. In case of a transgastric or transjejunal puncture of the biliary tree of the left hepatic lobe, it is recommendable to puncture in the direction to the hepatic hilus to guarantee a sufficient infeed of the wire. If the wire has to be relocated in case of an ongoing rendezvous maneuver, the puncture needle should be removed after initial infeed of the wire followed by the introduction of a 5-Fr bougie via the guidewire. By such a soft bougie, it can be attempted to overcome the malignant stenosis and to achieve the passage of the wire through the papilla. If this has been achieved, echoendoscope can be substituted by a therapeutic duodenoscope. Via the wire in situ, which is held by the duodenoscope and led out of the mouth of the papilla, conventional transpapillary drainage can be performed (fig. 1–3).

The transgastric or transduodenal position of the wire will be kept as long as the stenosis has not been passed by the prosthesis during implantation. This allows getting through very solid/dense stenoses near the hepatic hilus by countermoving the wire. Subsequently, the wire is pulled back by the duodenoscope. If the papilla can be reached but the wire cannot be passed through the papilla after former successful EUS-guided transgastric or transduodenal puncture of a(the) extra- (and/)or intrahepatic segment(s) of the biliary tree, the option of a rendezvous maneuver has to be abandoned and it can be intended to perform hepaticogastrostomy, hepaticojejunostomy or choledochoduodenostomy/choledochogastrostomy.

EUS-Guided Choledochoduodenostomy/Choledochogastrostomy

In patients with no previous surgical intervention and distal occlusion of the bile duct due to malignant tumor growth as well as extended caliber of the intra- and extrahepatic biliary tree, a primary transduodenal or transgastric antegrade drainage of the biliary tree should be attempted if the papilla cannot be reached or the wire cannot be passed through the papilla. This provides the advantage that, compared with a hepaticogastrostomy, there is an untouched anatomy of the

1 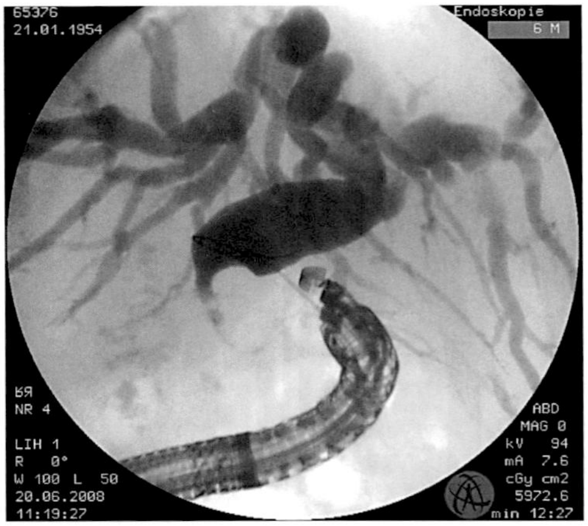

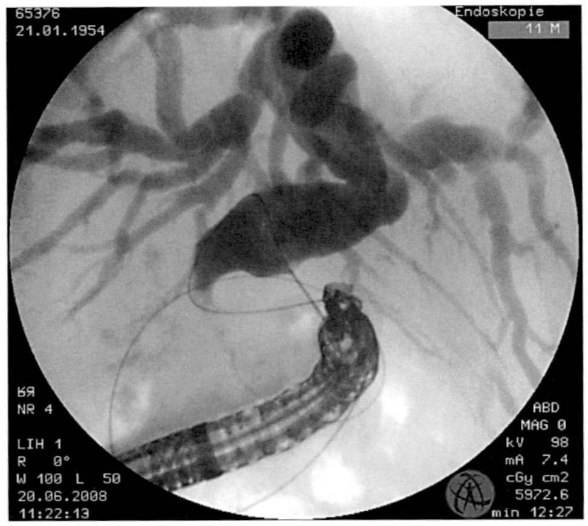 2

3 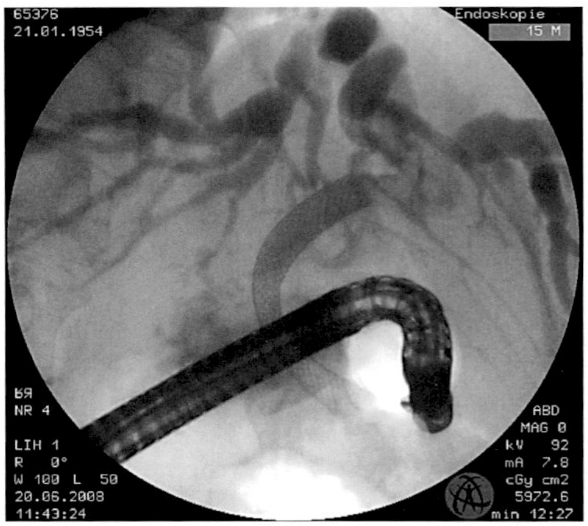

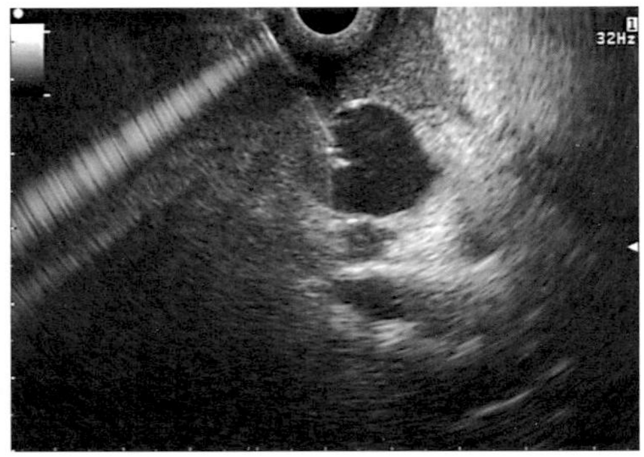 4

5 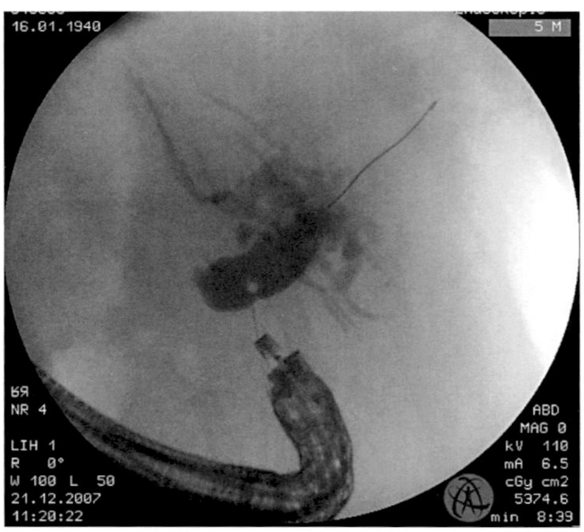

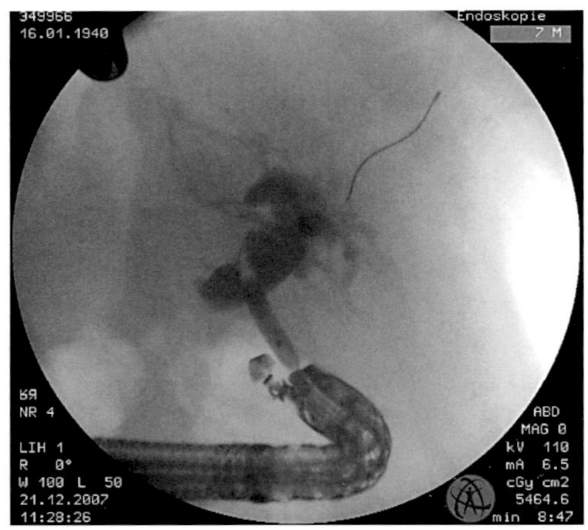 6

Fig. 1. Transduodenal EUS-guided puncture of the bile duct and subsequent cholangiography in stenosis of the papilla due to malignant tumor growth. **Fig. 2.** Infeed of the wire via the 19-G needle with passage of the wire through the papilla to prepare the rendezvous maneuver. **Fig. 3.** Substitution of the echoendoscope by a duodenoscope, holding and leading the wire out of the mouth of the papilla as well as transpapillary placement of a covered Wallstent. **Fig. 4.** EUS-guided choledochogastrostomy in a locally advanced pancreatic carcinoma: 1. Transgastric puncture of the bile duct using a 19-G needle. **Fig. 5.** EUS-guided choledochogastrostomy: 2. Placement of a guidewire within the intrahepatic segments of the biliary tree. **Fig. 6.** EUS-guided choledochogastrostomy: 3. After dilatation with 5-Fr bougies – balloon dilatation of the puncture site.

intrahepatic biliary tree as well as 'normal' physiology characterized by an antegrade flow of the bile. However, the prediction is that the common bile duct can be precisely imaged through the wall of the duodenal bulb or the antrum.

The echoendoscope is placed at the wall of the duodenal bulb or antrum at the site of the small curvature leading to a puncture direction exactly toward the hepatic hilus. It needs to be taken care of the fact that the endoscope is fixed with a stable position in situ to avoid an alteration of the subsequent interventional steps by a dislocation of the endoscope. Within the hepatoduodenal ligament, the three leading structures – portal vein, hepatic artery and common bile duct – can be easily identified also using color-coded Duplex ultrasonography for reliable differentiation of the anatomic structures. While a puncture of the middle segment of the common bile duct can be achieved transduodenally, the proximal segment of the extrahepatic bile duct can be rather accessed via a transhepatic puncture through the wall of the antrum and through the caudate lobe (fig. 4).

After successful puncture of the bilde duct using a 19-G needle, alternatively using a needle-knife catheter, the puncture distance is held by placement of a 0.035-inch guidewire (fig. 5). Via this wire, endoscopic choledochostomy is created using a sequential dilatation (initially with 5-Fr and subsequently with 7-Fr bougies) or via a wire-guided cystostome as it is used for the treatment of pseudocysts. After enlargement of the puncture site up to the width of the 5-Fr bougie, alternatively, a dilatation balloon specifically designed for the biliary tree (4 mm are adequate) can be used (fig. 6).

The width of the choledochoduodenostomy/choledochogastrostomy should be chosen according to the size of the prosthesis which is to be implanted. The authors favor a covered metal prosthesis (fig. 7). Prior to this step, preparation of the former puncture site by dilating it up to 7 Fr is sufficient. If plastic prosthesis is used, the puncture site should be predilated up to 8.5 Fr or even 9 Fr. The use of a dilatation balloon may increase the risk of provoking a pneumoperitoneum, however, implantation of the prosthesis can be thus facilitated.

Transintestinal intervention via a wire in place to achieve a sufficient drainage of the biliary tree requires simultaneous fluoroscopic and endoscopic controls of the correct wire position in situ. In particular, it has to be strictly taken care of the requirement that the wire has to be held in a straight position while introducing it and that the echoendoscope is placed near the neo-ostium. If loops of the wire form, the wire has to be straightened. Trying to correct the extraintestinal formation of such wire loops (between duodenum and bile duct) often causes dislocation of the wire leading to the consequence that the procedure has to be restarted.

If the prosthesis cannot be implanted into the bile duct after dilatation of the former puncture site using bougies or a balloon, dilatation or distension of the puncture site should be repeated. Via the wire placed in situ along the puncture site, each device of the equipment can be changed which underlines the necessity that an adequate wire position in situ is essential and should be steadily followed with great attention. The length of the prosthesis in a transgastric or transduodenal approach is recommended to be sufficient with 6–8 cm. Covered metal prostheses provide the advantage of a bigger lumen (10 mm) and of an immediate occlusion of the enteral and biliary access site but hold the risk of a peritoneal dislocation by lacking flaps. The authors try to avoid dislocation of the metal stent by a mucosal fixation of the stents using hemoclips (fig. 8).

How far the risk of a pneumoperitoneum or biliary ascites can be lowered cannot be stated currently. The transduodenal approach including the antegrade biliary fistula provides the advantage that it can also be used in patients with ascites since it is associated with a retrograde access site.

7 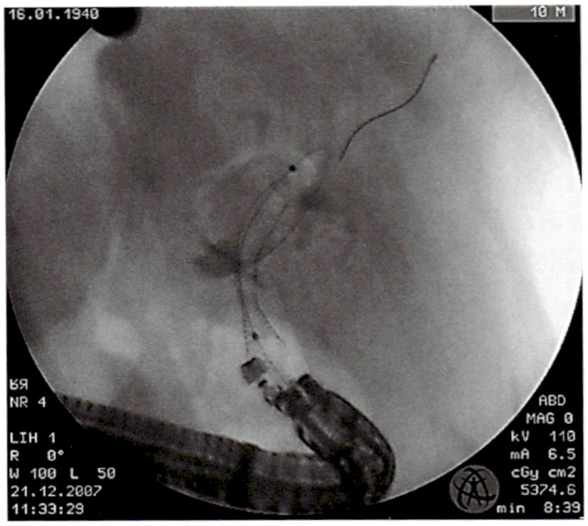

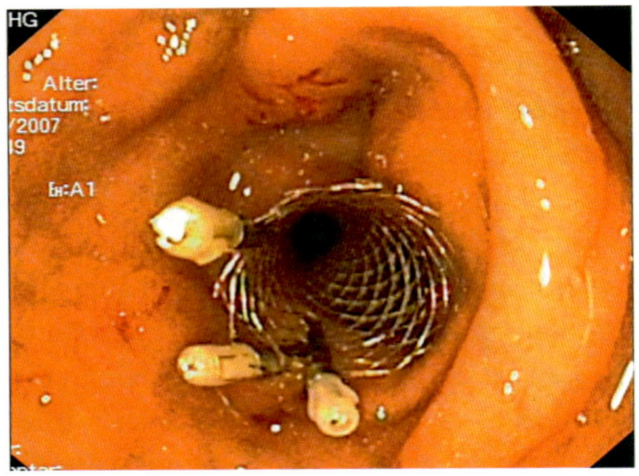 8

9 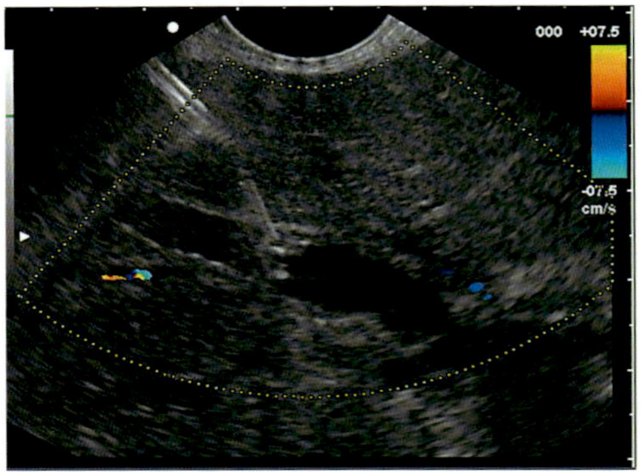

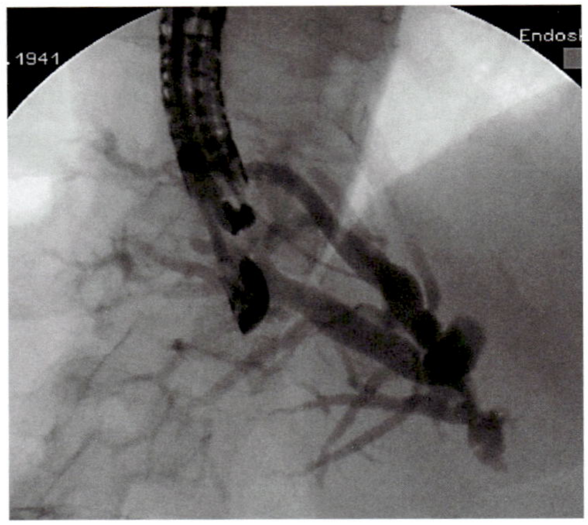 10

Fig. 7. EUS-guided choledochogastrostomy: 4. Implantation of a covered Wallstent. **Fig. 8.** EUS-guided choledochogastrostomy: 5. Fixation of the metal prosthesis at the wall of the antrum to avoid dislocation. **Fig. 9.** EUS-guided hepaticogastrostomy in recurrent tumor growth after hemihepatectomy because of gallbladder carcinoma: 1. EUS-guided transhepatic puncture of the enlarged biliary duct within the left hepatic lobe. **Fig. 10.** EUS-guided hepaticogastrostomy in recurrent tumor growth after hemihepatectomy because of gallbladder carcinoma: 2. Cholangiography with retention of bile within the biliary tree before hepaticojejunostomy.

EUS-Guided Hepaticogastrostomy/Hepaticojejunostomy

In patients with former surgical intervention(s) (such as gastrectomy, BII-gastric resection, pancreaticoduodenectomy, hepaticojejunostomy) and in case of biliary obstruction due to malignant tumor growth including an enlarged intrahepatic segment of the biliary tree or in patients with complete obstruction of the bile duct in whom an antegrade EUCD cannot be achieved, hepaticogastrostomy/hepaticojejunostomy should be aimed for. Contrarily to choledochogastrostomy/choledochoduodenostomy, the biliary tree is drained retrogradely via the transhepatic route.

While passing the aboral segment of the esophagus and the cardia, the left hepatic lobe should be translumenally identified and thus the enlarged intrahepatic ducts of the biliary tree of the third and second hepatic segment can be followed toward the hepatic hilus by a continuous right turn and infeed of the endoscope. If the anatomy of the intrahepatic biliary ducts of the left hepatic lobe has been revealed, the optimal route to approach these ducts should be selected.

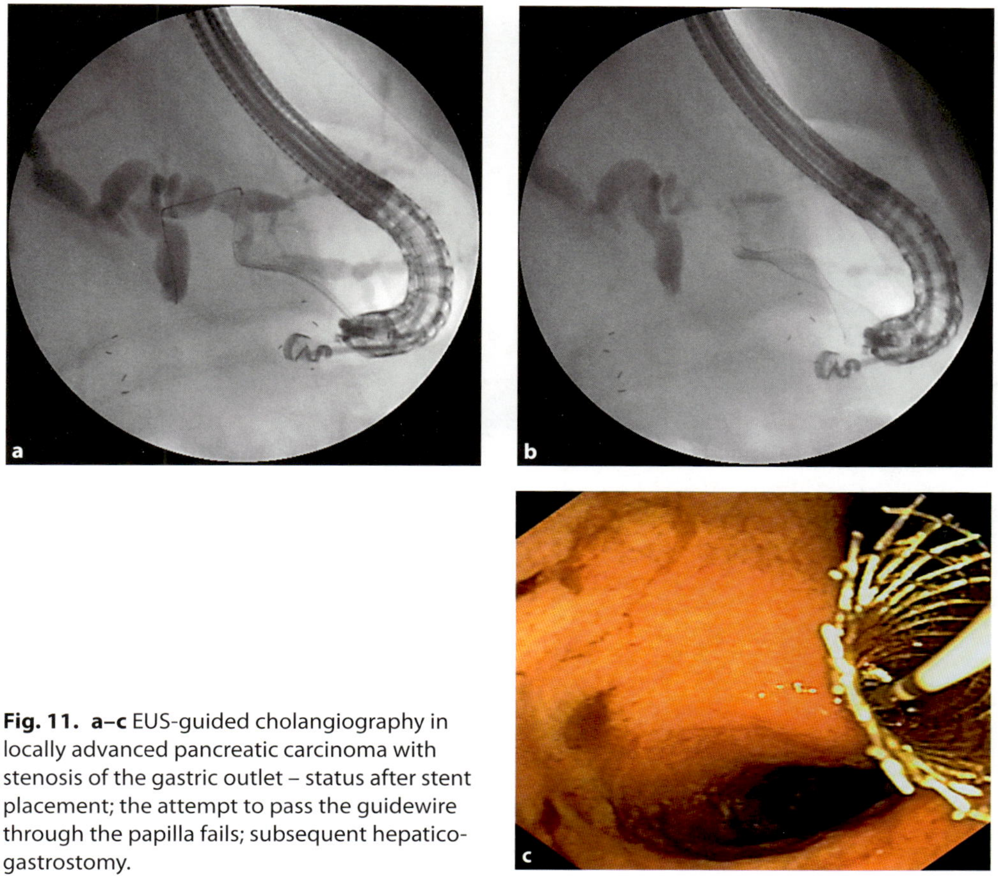

Fig. 11. a–c EUS-guided cholangiography in locally advanced pancreatic carcinoma with stenosis of the gastric outlet – status after stent placement; the attempt to pass the guidewire through the papilla fails; subsequent hepatico-gastrostomy.

Optimal conditions are: (1) stable (adherent position of the stomach/jejunum at the left hepatic lobe – be aware of possible ascites [!]); (2) stable, possibly straight position of the echoendoscope to avoid dislocation of the bougies and stents; (3) tangential puncture of a large branch of the bile duct, with no further small branches ending in this large branch in the direction to the hepatic lobe to ensure an optimal infeed of the guidewire, and (4) short distance through the liver parenchyma to limit the resistance for dilatation using bougies/balloon. If these requirements for a successful drainage are given, a puncture using a 19-G needle is performed very similar as done for duodenocholedochostomy (fig. 9). After obligatory sampling of bile for microbiological investigation, cholangiography follows (fig. 10, 11a–c).

Also under these circumstances, it appears to be reasonable to investigate the patient lying on his back to reveal and image more appropriately anatomy of the biliary tree and pathology of its obstruction, in particular, near the hepatic hilus. Simultaneously, the route to approach the bile duct or its branches should be investigated to determine the length and type of prosthesis which is needed. In case of placement of covered metal prostheses, the specific aspect that the mouths of the biliary duct branches are not 'overstented' to disfavor an appropriate drainage needs to be taken care of. If this problem cannot be satisfyingly ruled out, plastic prostheses should be preferred.

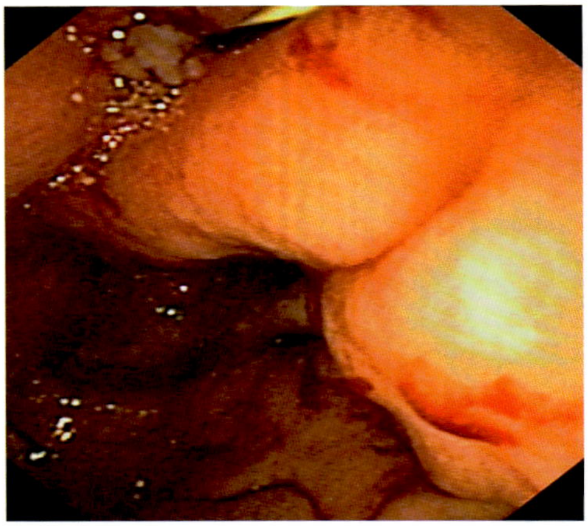

12

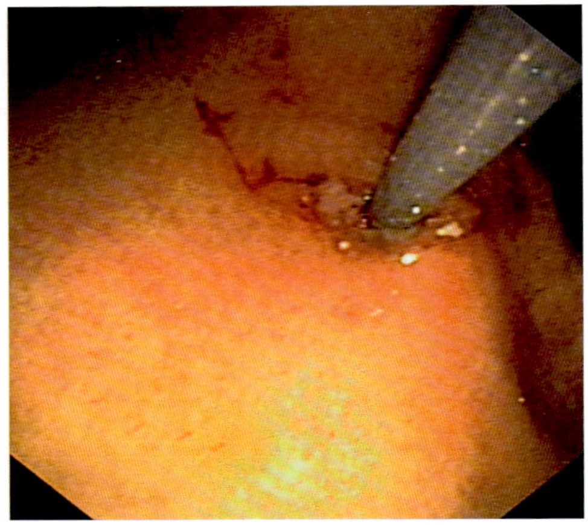

13

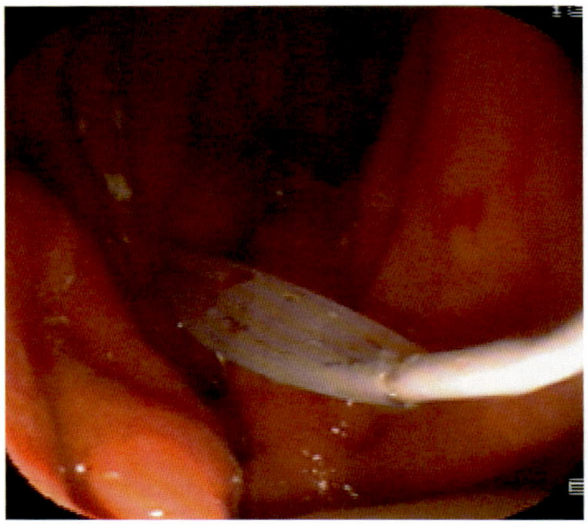

14

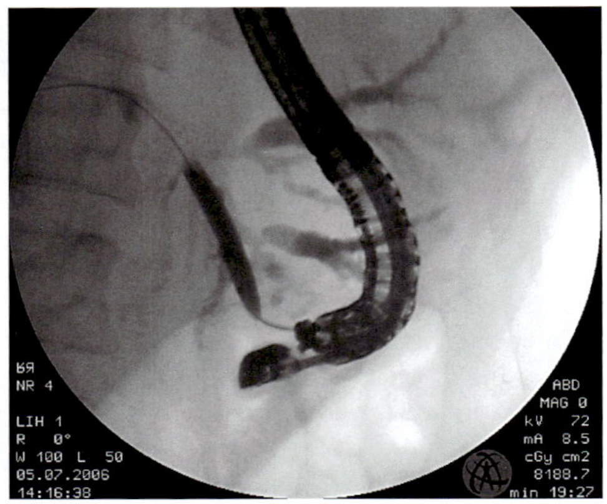

15

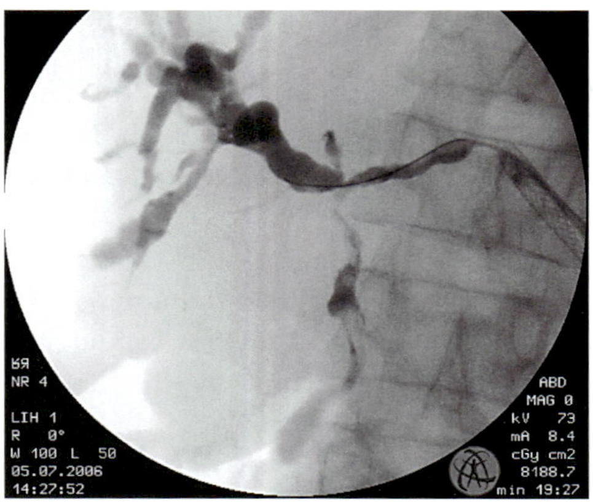

16

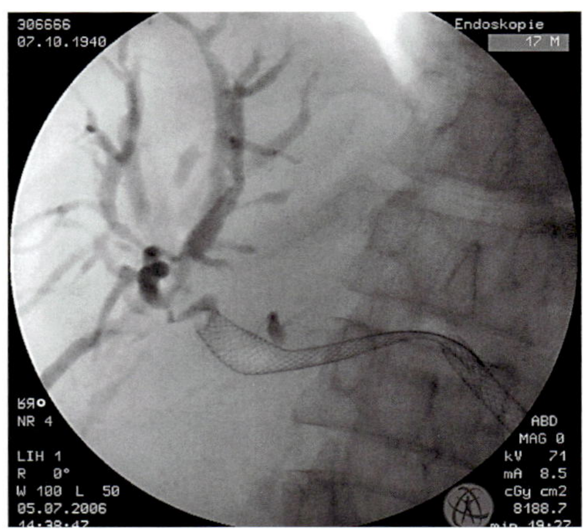

17

Fig. 12. Endoscopic view after introduction of the guidewire through a 19-G needle. **Fig. 13.** Dilatation using 5-Fr bougie via the wire in position. **Fig. 14, 15.** Endoscopic and radiological finding of a balloon dilatation to create a hepaticojejunostomy in case of locally advanced gallbladder carcinoma and status after gastric resection according to the BII procedure (cf. fig. 16, 17). **Fig. 16, 17.** Transjejunal EUS-guided placement of two covered Wallstents to drain biliary tree of the right hepatic lobe in locally advanced gallbladder carcinoma (status after former gastric resection according to the BII procedure which does not allow to reach papilla).

A 0.035-inch wire should be infeeded through the 19-G-puncture needle into the biliary tree. Wire position may not be corrected by retrograde pulling too often to avoid shearing of the tip of the Terumo wire. After substitution of the needle by a 5-Fr bougie, the wire position can be corrected with no further serious problems (fig. 12, 13).

During dilatation using bougies, formation of wire loops within the gastric lumen but, in particular, perigastrically should be avoided. Therefore, all manipulations should be controlled using fluoroscopy. During the EUS-guided puncture, the stomach is held close to the left hepatic lobe by the endoscope. After infeeding the wire, further maneuvers are endoscopically controlled but giving up the holding position and purpose of the echoendoscope leading to the generation of an empty space between liver and stomach. Primarily, there is a straight position of the wire through this space, however, during the bougie change including intermittent infeed of the wire, a wire loop can form which can be difficult to be straightened. If this is impossible, the placement of the prosthesis cannot be achieved. In case of much ascites leading to a great distance between stomach and liver, this proximal transhepatic approach should not be favored.

After sequential dilatation using bougies up to 7 Fr, placement of a covered Wallstent can be achieved. In case of plastic prostheses of 8.5 Fr in size, sometimes it is recommendable to dilate the access site up to the width provided by a 9-Fr bougie. In case of a dense liver or problems in infeeding the bougies, a dilating balloon of 4 mm in size can be helpful to enlarge the access channel (fig. 14, 15).

Peritoneal dislocation of the transgastric or transjejunal drainage can only rarely occur because of the holding flaps and the pigtail in plastic prostheses, while in metal prostheses, this might happen as has been described and observed in treated patients of the reporting department. To avoid such dislocation during the release of the prosthesis, again, the maneuver should be controlled by fluoroscopy and endoscopic view (fig. 16, 17). A delayed stent dislocation can be avoided by prophylactic placement of clips (fig. 18, 19).

EUS-Guided Transhepatic Internal Drainage with No Rendezvous

In case of a specific anatomy, in which papilla cannot be reached or in case of malignancy-induced anastomotic stenosis after former hepaticojejunostomy, it can be attempted, very similar to a PTCD with internal placement of a metal stent, to get through this stenosis using an EUS-guided internal drainage. If this can be achieved, orthograde biliary drainage can be sustained. As a possible route to the biliary duct, the transgastric approach is recommended. The initial steps are identical with those mentioned above. After getting through the central or distal stenosis of the bile duct, the length of the stenosis is measured and the transhepatic route to implant the metal prosthesis can be prepared. In contrast to hepaticogastrostomy, metal prosthesis is completely introduced into the biliary tree to get through the stenosis and it is internally released leading to a regular bile flow as usual. The transgastric access site is clipped after removal of the devices, or a second metal prosthesis can be implanted (fig. 20, 21). The advantage of the method is that the physiological bile flow can be sustained and that a peritoneal dislocation of the metal prosthesis is impossible.

In table 3, the suggested methods of EUCD are listed and were associated with the appropriate indications reflecting personal experiences and reports from the literature.

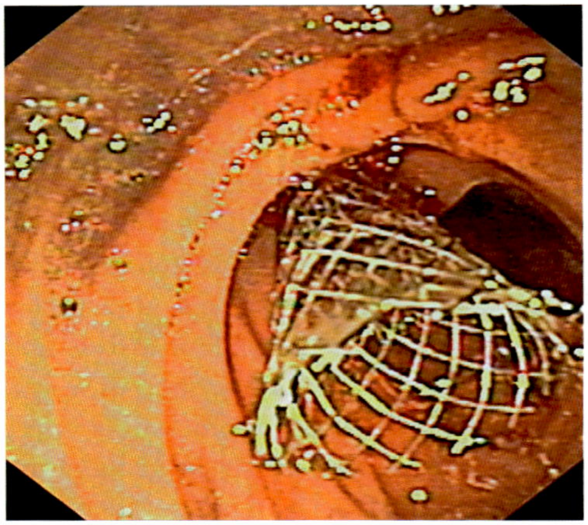

18

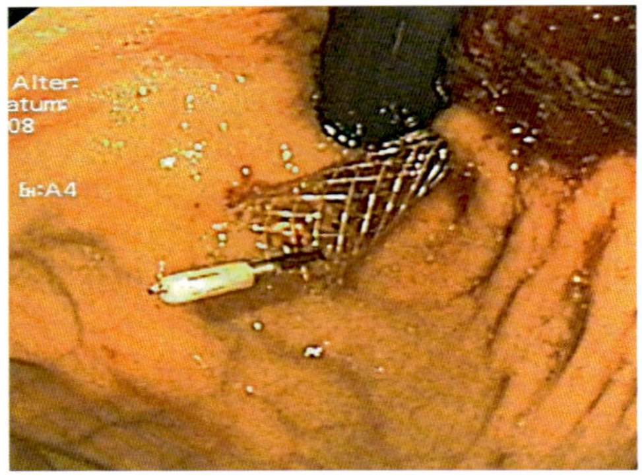

19

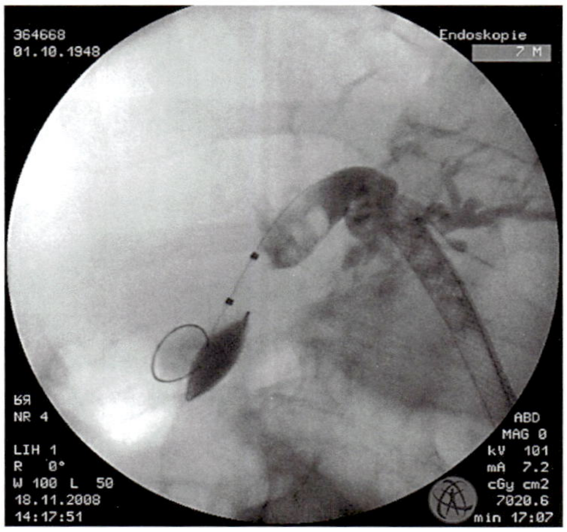

20

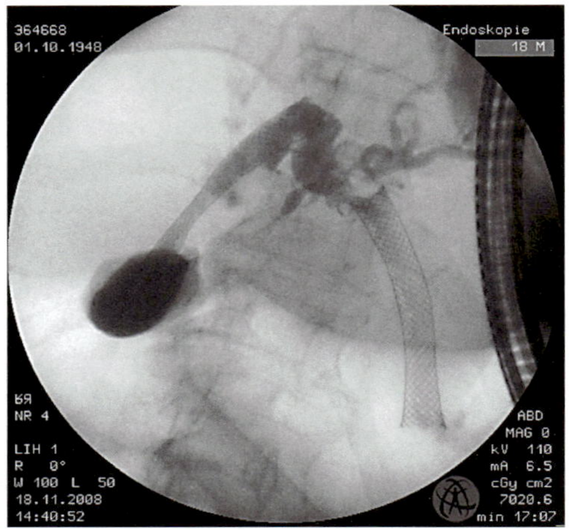

21

Fig. 18, 19. Endoscopic finding of a transjejunal hepaticojejunostomy with no clips for fixation and a transgastric hepaticojejunostomy with a clip for fixation to avoid dislocation. **Fig. 20, 21.** Status after former hemihepatectomy in case of a Klatskin's tumor showing recurrent tumor growth; EUS-guided cholangiography: tumor stenosis and cholangiolithiasis; 1. Creation of a hepaticogastrostomy; 2. Stone extraction; 3. Open up the tumor stenosis with a metal stent.

Postinterventional Care

Patients after EUCD should be equally treated as patients who have undergone ERC with drainage. Peri-interventional prophylaxis with antibiotic has already been mentioned above, however it is recommended to continue it initially as calculated therapy for 7–10 days, which needs to be optimized if necessary after bile has been microbiologically investigated.

Patients stay 'n.p.o.' through the whole day of intervention, undergo infusion and administration of analgesics if necessary. The first obligatory control of the stent patency and position should be undertaken on the first postinterventional day with percutaneous abdominal ultrasound and analysis of appropriate laboratory parameters. Using abdominal ultrasound, aerobilia should be detected as evidence for effective drainage (fig. 22, 23). The stent should be completely imaged according to its total length, in particular, the segment protruding into the intestinal

Table 3. Indications correlating to the methods of EUCD

1. Rendezvous technique with ERC – transduodenal, transgastric puncture
   Normal anatomy of the gastrointestinal tract, papilla can be reached
   After EUS-guided puncture of the biliary tree and passing the wire out of the papilla conventional ERC with transpapillary drainage
2. Choledochoduodenostomy/choledochogastrostomy
   Normal anatomy of the stomach/bulb; papilla cannot be catheterized
   Failure of rendezvous technique
   Duodenal stenosis because of malignant tumor growth
   Distal tumor stenosis of the bile duct
   Status after gastroenteroanastomosis
3. Hepaticogastrostomy/hepaticojejunostomy
   Status after gastrectomy, status after BII gastric resection
   Status after hepaticojejunostomy
   Status after pancreaticoduodenectomy
   Normal anatomy – obturated common bile duct
   Proximal tumor stenosis
4. Transhepatic EUS-guided drainage of the biliary tree
   Papilla cannot be reached
   Malignancy-induced stenosis of the bile duct or at its intrahepatic segments/branches
   Malignancy-induced stenosis at the hepaticojejunostomy.

lumen should be precisely measured. In patients with complaints, dispositioning of the stent needs to be taken into account, which can lead to the generation of a biliary peritonitis (fig. 24, 25). A postinterventional pneumoperitoneum is frequently reported but is classified to be harmless if the drainage function is satisfying.

Since all patients undergo EUCD because of a malignant incurable disease and drainage was placed under palliative intention, reinterventions are rather rare because of the long-lasting patency of metal stents. In case of stent occlusion, it can be attempted to change the stent via the neostium as it is handled in ERC or the same EUCD procedure is performed again.

Treatment Results and Outcome

EUCD is considered a novel therapeutic alternative of internal biliary drainage in patients with obstructive malignant jaundice and unsuccessful ERC or PTCD. In the literature, three technical options of EUCD have been described – rendezvous technique, hepaticogastrostomy/hepaticojejunostomy, and choledochogastrostomy/choledochobulbostomy. Until today, approximately 100 patients have been reported correcting the total number of those who underwent EUCD but were listed and described twice [9–18]. While in approximately 27 cases, successful drainage could be achieved by the rendezvous technique, the remaining cases underwent direct EUS-guided biliary drainage. Transhepatic retrograde biliary drainage via the left hepatic lobe and extrahepatic antegrade biliary drainage of the bile duct were achieved with a plastic stent in two thirds of cases whereas in the residual one third, a covered metal stent was used. While there is a success rate of almost 100% in EUS-guided cholangiography, this rate is slightly lower (mean, 91%) ranging from 75 to 100% in EUCD. However, a clinical long-term success rate has not been provided by all studies but if reported it ranges from 80 to 100% (mean, 90%). Thus, feasibility

22 23

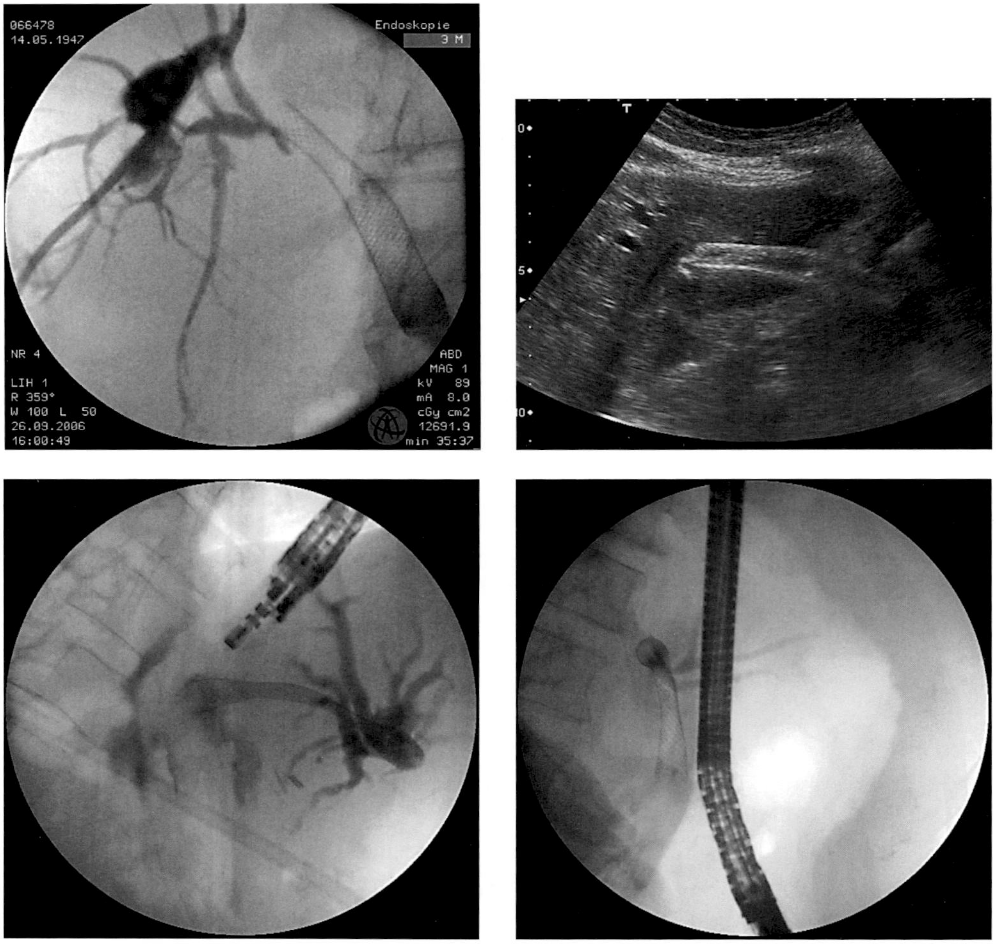

24 25

Fig. 22, 23. Hepaticogastrostomy with metal stent in situ; ultrasound control of the function (aerobilia, intraluminal length of the stents – be aware of possible dislocation). **Fig. 24, 25.** After stent release, stent dislocation occurs; endoscopic transgastric stent removal; placement of a PTCD.

of EUS-guided biliary drainage has been demonstrated, in contrast, there are only preliminary data on the clinical safety of the technique. EUCD has been performed in several high-volume endoscopy centers. Complication rates range from 0 to 25% (mean, 15.7%). The spectrum of potential complications comprises pneumoperitoneum, cholangitis, stent migration and biliary leakage with peritonitis [11, 13, 16–18].

Currently, EUCD still needs to be considered an experimental procedure which has to be performed by experienced interventional endosonographers and endoscoping clinicians in large gastroenterological centers [10, 14, 16, 17]. There is a number of open questions which finally need to be assessed: (1) Should EUCD only be used in patients with obstructive jaundice and malignancy, or can it also be used in patients with benign diseases? (2) When is EUCD reasonable in the therapeutic algorithm (primarily after unsuccessful ERC/PTCD or always before PTCD)? (3) Which type of biliary drainage is the safest if the EUS-guided rendezvous technique cannot be achieved (hepaticogastrostomy/hepaticojejunostomy; choledochogastrostomy/choledochobulbostomy)? (4) How can the access to the biliary tree be achieved (FNP with needle and atraumatic access via guidewire, bougies/balloon dilatation or more traumatically using high-frequency diathermia)? (5) Which stent can be favored (covered metal/plastic stent – straight or curved)? (6) Should a change of the stents be aimed for, and, if yes, in what time intervals?

The currently established advantage of EUCD with regard to patient comfort and morbidity in comparison to PTCD needs to be investigated in a randomized study. A general recommendation to perform EUCD in case of unsuccessful ERC can, at present, still not be given.

References

1 Fogel EL, Shermann S, Deveraux BM, et al: Therapeutic biliary endoscopy. Endoscopy 2001;33:31–38.
2 Schofl R: Diagnostic endoscopic retrograde cholangiopancreatography. Endoscopy 2001;33:147–157.
3 Carr-Locke DL: Overview of the role of the ERC in the management of diseases of the biliary tract and the pancreas. Gastrointest Endosc 2002;56(suppl):S157–S160.
4 Ferrucci JT Jr, Mueller PR, Harbin WP: Percutaneous transhepatic biliary drainage: technique, results and applications. Radiology 1980:135:1–13.
5 Smith AC, Dowsett JF, Russell RC, et al: Randomised trial of endoscopic stenting versus surgical bypass in malignant low bile duct obstruction. Lancet 1994;344: 1655–1660.
6 Winick AB, Waybill PN, Venbrux AC: Complications of percutaneous transhepatic biliary interventions. Tech Vasc Interv Radiol 2001;4:200–206.
7 Wright BE, Cass OW, Freeman ML: ERCP in patients with long-limb Roux-en-Y gastrojejunostomy and intact papilla. Gastrointest Endosc 2002;56:225–232.
8 Slovacek L, Slovackova B, Slanska I, Priester P, Petera J, Kopecky J, Vanaskowa J: Cancer and depression: a prospective study. Neoplasma 2009;56:187–193.
9 Burmester E, Niehaus J, Leineweber T, et al: EUS-cholangiodrainage of the bile duct: report of four cases. Gastrointest Endosc 2003;57:246–251.
10 Püspök A, Lomoschitz F, Dejaco C, et al: Endoscopic ultrasound guided therapy of benign and malignant biliary obstruction: a case series. Am J Gastroenterol 2005; 100:1743–1747.
11 Kahaleh M, Hernandez AJ, Tokar J, et al: Interventional EUS-guided cholangiography: evaluation of a technique in evolution. Gastrointest Endosc 2006;64:52–59.
12 Bories E, Pesenti C, Caillol F, et al: Transgastric endoscopic ultrasonography-guided biliary drainage: results of a pilot study. Endoscopy 2007;39:287–291.
13 Will U, Thieme A, Fueldner F, et al: Treatment of biliary obstruction in selected patients by endoscopic ultrasonography-guided transluminal biliary drainage. Endoscopy 2007;39:292–295
14 Yamao K, Bhatia V, Mizuno N, et al: EUS-guided choledochoduodenostomy for palliative biliary drainage in patients with malignant biliary obstruction: results of long-term follow-up. Endoscopy 2008;40:340–342.
15 Tarantino I, Barresi L, Repici A, et al: EUS-guided biliary drainage: a case series. Endoscopy 2008;40:336–339.
16 Itoi T, Itokawa F, Sofuni A, et al: Endoscopic ultrasound-guided choledochojejunostomy in patients with failed endoscopic retrograde cholangiopancreatography. World J Gastroenterol 2008;21:6078–6082.
17 Savides TJ, Shyam V, Laurent P. EUS 2008 Working Group Document: evaluation of EUS-guided hepaticogastrostomy. Gastrointest Endosc 2009;2:S3–S6.
18 Yamao K: EUS-guided choledochoduodenostomy. Gastrointest Endosc 2009;2:S194–S199.
19 Anderson RD, Mallat D: Endoscopic ultrasound-assisted transpapillary stent placement. Endoscopy 2006;38:E73.
20 Mangiavillano B, Arcidiacono PG, Carrara S, Masci E, Testoni PA: EUS-guided rendezvous technique for difficult cannulation of an intradiverticular papilla. Endoscopy 2008;40:E87–E88.

Uwe Will, MD, PhD
Department of Gastroenterology, Hepatology, Nephrology and General Internal Medicine
Municipal Hospital (SRH Waldklinikum)
DE–07548 Gera (Germany)
Tel. +49 365 828 2401, Fax +49 365 828 2402, E-Mail uwe.will@wkg.srh.de

Author Index

Subject Index